OKUDA AND NELSON'S EMERGENCY MEDICINE CERTIFYING EXAM REVIEW ILLUSTRATED

"What makes this Oral Board Exam Review stand out is how genuinely engaging it is. Each of the nearly 100 cases feels like the scenario you wish you had encountered in training – the kind that pushes your clinical reasoning, tests your composure, and then immediately rewards you with a master educator's debrief. The authors highlight the essential elements, especially the critical actions that can make or break an oral board performance, with clarity and practicality. Whether you're working through the book solo or practicing with a partner, the structure is intuitive, interactive, and actually fun – yes, fun. This is the rare review text that not only prepares you for the exam but reminds you why you love emergency medicine in the first place."

Kaushal Shah
Professor and Vice Chair of Education
Weill Cornell Medical Center, New York City

OKUDA AND NELSON'S EMERGENCY MEDICINE CERTIFYING EXAM REVIEW ILLUSTRATED

Edited by

YASUHARU OKUDA
Department of Emergency Medicine, Morsani College of Medicine

BRET P. NELSON
Department of Emergency Medicine, Icahn School of Medicine at Mount Sinai

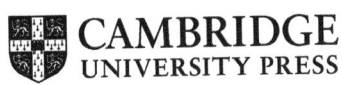
CAMBRIDGE
UNIVERSITY PRESS

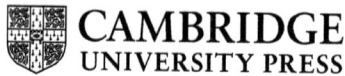

Shaftesbury Road, Cambridge CB2 8EA, United Kingdom

One Liberty Plaza, 20th Floor, New York, NY 10006, USA

477 Williamstown Road, Port Melbourne, VIC 3207, Australia

314–321, 3rd Floor, Plot 3, Splendor Forum, Jasola District Centre, New Delhi – 110025, India

Cambridge University Press is part of Cambridge University Press & Assessment,
a department of the University of Cambridge.

We share the University's mission to contribute to society through the pursuit of
education, learning and research at the highest international levels of excellence.

www.cambridge.org
Information on this title: www.cambridge.org/9781108709330

DOI: 10.1017/9781108671385

When citing this work, please include a reference to the DOI 10.1017/9781108671385

First published 2010
Second edition 2015
Third edition 2026

A catalogue record for this publication is available from the British Library

A Cataloging-in-Publication data record for this book is available from the Library of Congress

ISBN 978-1-108-70933-0 Paperback

Cambridge University Press & Assessment has no responsibility for the persistence
or accuracy of URLs for external or third-party internet websites referred to in this
publication and does not guarantee that any content on such websites is, or will
remain, accurate or appropriate.

Every effort has been made in preparing this book to provide accurate and up-to-date information that is in accord
with accepted standards and practice at the time of publication. Although case histories are drawn from actual
cases, every effort has been made to disguise the identities of the individuals involved. Nevertheless, the authors,
editors, and publishers can make no warranties that the information contained herein is totally free from error, not
least because clinical standards are constantly changing through research and regulation. The authors, editors, and
publishers therefore disclaim all liability for direct or consequential damages resulting from the use of material
contained in this book. Readers are strongly advised to pay careful attention to information provided by the
manufacturer of any drugs or equipment that they plan to use.

For EU product safety concerns, contact us at Calle de José Abascal, 56, 1°, 28003 Madrid,
Spain, or email eugpsr@cambridge.org

Contents

		page ix
List of Section Editors		page ix
List of Contributors		x
Moving from the Oral Boards to the Certifying Exam: How to Get the Most from Our Book		xvii

1	**How to Use This Book** Bret P. Nelson, MD	1
2	**EM Medical Decision-Making** Scott Weingart, MD, FCCM	15
3	**About the Oral Boards: The Approach and Practical Tips** Christina Hajicharalambous, DO, MSEd, MS and Rebecca Hellmann, DO	18
4	**About the Oral Boards: Format and Scoring** Michael Cassara, DO, MSEd	25

CASES

1	Overdose William McDowell, MD and Vinodinee Dissanayake, MD	45
2	Vomiting Infant Caroline Black, MD and Abiola Fasina, MD	50
3	Altered Mental Status Matthew Kuhns, MD and Jacob Holton, MD	54
4	Chest Trauma Wakas Ahmed, DO, Shayna Adams, MD, and Abiola Fasina, MD	60
5	Abdominal Pain and Vomiting Shefali Trivedi, MD	66
6	Weak Infant Christopher Strother, MD	70
7	Chest Pain Calloway Pichette, MD, Scott Heinrich, MD, and Alan Huang, MD	75
8	Lower Back Pain Katarzyna Gore, MD and Daniel Spearman, MD	80
9	Leg Swelling Kimbia Arno, MD, MFA, Ryan Gore, MD, and Alan Huang, MD	84
10	Weakness Alan Huang, MD and Cassandra Mackey, MD	90
11	Headache Wesley Pedicini, MD and Philip Bossart, MD	95
12	Abdominal Pain Angela Chen, MD and Joseph Chiang, MD	98
13	Ringing in the Ears Taryn Webb, MD, Michelle N. Marin, MD, and Joseph Chiang, MD	103
14	Vomiting Child Temima Waltuch, MD and Joseph Chiang, MD	108
15	Snake Bite Matthew Harris, MD and Joseph Chiang, MD	113
16	Visual Impairment Joseph Chiang, MD and Wirachin Hoonpongsimanont, MD	117
17	Syncope Maneesha Agarwal, MD and Christopher Strother, MD	121
18	Sore Throat Ian Kane, MD and Lisa Zahn, MD	126
19	Knee Pain Jennifer M. Bellis, MD, MPH and Edward R. Melnick, MD, MHS	131
20	Abdominal Pain Peter Gutierrez, MD	135
21	Abdominal Pain Yasuharu Okuda, MD	139
22	Cough Elysha Pifko, MD	145
23	Flank Pain Dhara Amin, MD	149
24	Weakness Ryan Marino, MD and Lauren Porter, DO	155
25	Facial Trauma Ryan McKenna, DO	161
26	Burn Suzanne K. Bentley, MD, MPH	166
27	Vomiting Blood Gregory Podolej, MD	172
28	Lightheadedness Kendra Amico, MD	177
29	Shortness of Breath Abraham Feshazion, MD, PharmD, MPH, and Linda Katirji, MD	182

30   Rash and Fever Nikolas Sekoulopoulos, MD, Stephanie Gaines, MD,
         and Jessica Berrios, MD   189
31   Weakness Stephanie Gaines, MD   194
32   Abdominal Pain and Vomiting Linda Katirji, MD   199
33   Chest Pain Robert M. Hughes, DO   205
34   Seizure Sylvia E. Garcia, MD   210
35   Chest Pain Sean Abraham, DO   213
36   Throat Swelling Nicole Gerber, MD   218
37   Abdominal Pain Ani Aydin, MD   221
38   Altered Mental Status Ani Aydin, MD   226
39   Rectal Pain Ani Aydin, MD   232
40   Vaginal Bleeding Ani Aydin, MD   236
41   Agitation Ani Aydin, MD   241
42   Abdominal Pain Nicholas Genes, MD, PhD   245
43   Abdominal Pain Nicholas Genes, MD, PhD   251
44   Abdominal Pain Nicholas Genes, MD, PhD   256
45   Altered Mental Status Nicholas Genes, MD, PhD   261
46   Diarrhea Nicholas Genes, MD, PhD   266
47   Seizure Shefali Trivedi, MD   270
48   Toothache Shefali Trivedi, MD   274
49   Penetrating Chest Trauma Abiola Fasina, MD, Jodi Jones MD, and
         Mandy Pascual MD   278
50   Animal Bite Shefali Trivedi, MD   283
51   Abdominal Pain Shefali Trivedi, MD   286
52   Headache Bing Shen, MD and J. Mark Rendon, MD   291
53   Pediatric Fever Alexandria Bahan Farish, MD, Jared Senvisky, MD, Nicole Rettig, MD,
         Catharine Cantrell, MD, Michelle Mendoza, MD, and Bing Shen, MD   297
54   Back Pain J. Mark Rendon, MD and Bing Shen, MD   302
55   Cardiac Arrest Bing Shen, MD and Wuya Lumeh, MD   307
56   Knee Pain Bing Shen, MD and Cassandra Mackey, MD   310
57   Rash Angela Maxwell, MD and Braden Hexom, MD   314
58   Sickle-Cell Disease Oluwakemi Badaki-Makun, MD and Braden Hexom, MD   320
59   Headache Braden Hexom, MD, Jacob M. Stritch, MD, and James P. Gillen, MD 326
60   Chest Pain Monica Sethi, MD and Braden Hexom, MD   332
61   Altered Mental Status Braden Hexom, MD, David Orban, MD, and Matthew Beattie, MD   337
62   Headache Hayley Neher, MD   343
63   Altered Mental Status Bethany Johnston, MD and Tricia Swan, MD, MEd   348
64   Shortness of Breath Michael Marchick, MD and Garrett Snipes, MD   355
65   Shortness of Breath Christopher Strother, MD   360
66   Flank Pain Haley Godwin, MD and Megan Fix, MD   365
67   Seizure Ellen Gilbertson, MD and Megan Fix, MD   370
68   Altered Mental Status Tabitha Ford, MD and Robert Stephen, MD   376
69   Vomiting Amit Patel, MD   381
70   Fever Nicholas Levin, MD and Brendan Cummins, MD   386
71   Palpitations Shawn Zhong, MD   391
72   Cough Shawn Zhong, MD   396
73   Drowning Shawn Zhong, MD   400
74   Abdominal Pain Javier Rosario, MD and Sheler Sadati, MD   406

75   Abdominal Pain David H. Cisewski, MD   412

76   Shortness of Breath Ryan McKenna, DO and Sheler Sadati, MD   418

77   Altered Mental Status Megha George, MD and Sheler Sadati, MD   423

78   Weakness Matthew Constantine, MD and Matthew Steimle, DO   429

79   Pedestrian Struck Rachel Semmons, MD and Matthew Constantine, MD   435

80   Back Pain Chanteil D. Ulatowski, MD and Nicholas G. Maldonado, MD, FACEP   443

81   Altered Mental Status Gail Knight, MD and Terri Davis MD   449

82   Abdominal Pain Christopher Strother, MD   456

83   Abdominal Pain Lisa Jacobson, MD   461

84   Respiratory Distress Lisa Jacobson, MD   465

85   Overdose Lisa Jacobson, MD   468

86   Chest Pain Lisa Jacobson, MD   473

87   Fever Edward R. Melnick, MD, MHS, Danielle Roberts, MD, and
         Marie-Carmelle Elie, MD, RDMS   477

88   Altered Mental Status Chelsea Allen, DO and David A. Caro, MD   483

89   Shortness of Breath Andrew Thomas, MD   490

90   Stab to Chest Qiaohua Zhang, MD   496

91   Abdominal Pain David Wein, MD and Edward Melnick, MD   502

92   Seizure Daniel Eraso, MD   507

93   Palpitations Edward R. Melnick, MD, MHS and Jay Khadpe, MD   511

94   Seizure Alexandra Mannix, MD   517

95   Fever Ryan McKenna, DO and Ram Parekh, MD   523

96   Abdominal Trauma Ram Parekh, MD and Carolina Pereira, MD   529

97   Hematochezia Mariam Said, MD and Ram Parekh, MD   537

98   Abdominal Pain John Kiel, DO, MPH and Anita Vashi, MD   542

99   Cough Xiao Han, MD and Anita Vashi, MD   547

100 Altered Mental Status Nicole Munz, DO and Anita Vashi, MD   552

101 Drowning Anita Vashi, MD and Ariella Nadler MD   558

102 Pallor Evelyn Chow, MD, Carrie Ng, MD, and Keegan Tupchong, MD   564

103 Diarrhea Rijo Maracheril, MD   569

104 Cough Jeanne Noble, MD   575

105 Vomiting and Altered Mental Status Nicole Munz, DO   581

106 Weakness Tomás Díaz, MD and Jacqueline Nemer, MD   587

107 Foot Pain Marianne Juarez, MD   592

108 Neck Pain Nicole Munz, DO and Evelyn Chow, MD   597

109 Abdominal Pain Jeanne Noble, MD and Evelyn Chow, MD   602

110 Shortness of Breath Jennifer Roh, MD   607

111 Arm Pain Kiyetta Alade, MD, MEd   612

112 Altered Mental Status Raashee Kedia, MD   616

113 Cardiac Arrest Benjamin H. Slovis MD and Christopher McCoy, MD   621

114 Leg Pain Mandy Pascual, MD and Jodi Jones, MD   627

115 Shortness of Breath and Swelling Bashar A. Ismail, MD   631

116 Finger Pain Alisa Wray, MD and Jeffrey R. Suchard, MD   635

117 Dizziness Robert Katzer, MD and Bharath Chakravarthy, MD, MPH   639

118 Intoxication Lars K. Beattie, MD and Henry Young, MD   642

119 Altered Mental Status Lars K. Beattie, MS, MD and Laura Scieszka, MD   648

120 Patient with Fatigue, Weight Gain, and Bruising Victor Cisneros, MD, MPH,
         Mason Shieh, MD, MBA, and Thomas Nguyen, MD   653

121 Toddler with Fever and Rash Daniel Goldstein, MD and Michael Truax Jr., MD   657

122 Arm Pain Shahram Lotfipour, MD   662

123 Headache Elisabeth Lessenich, MD, MPH   667

124 Dizziness Anne Chipman, MD, MS   671

125 Weakness Bonnie Lau, MD   677

126 Altered Mental Status Michael Cassara, DO, MSEd   682

127 Fever Julie Tokarski, MD   688

128 LVAD Emergency Giuliano De Portu, MD, FACEP and Michael Chami, MD   692

Appendix A. The Chest Pain Patient: Five Life-Threatening Causes and Critical Actions
Elaine Rabin, MD and Luke Hermann, MD   698

Appendix B. The Confused Patient: Ten Most Common Causes and Critical Actions
Denise Nassisi, MD, FACEP   702

Appendix C. The Poisoned Patient: Most Common Toxidromes and Treatments
Ruben Olmedo, MD   709

Appendix D. The Trauma Patient: The Approach and Important Principles
David Cherkas, MD, FACEP   714

Appendix E. Advanced Cardiac Life Support Review Thomas Nguyen, MD and Avir Mitra, MD   716

Appendix F. Pediatric Pearls: High-Yield Facts from Fever to Drugs Julie Tokarski, MD and
Christopher Strother, MD   726

Appendix G. Twenty Common Emergency Medicine Procedures: Indications, Contraindications,
Technique, and Complications Reuben J. Strayer, MD   732

Index   757

Section Editors

Alyssa Abo, MD
   MBA Bloom Standard
   (Cases 53, 55, 57, 58, 65, 69, 82–84, 97, 102, 111, 121)

Lars K. Beattie, MS, MD, FACEP
   University of Florida Department of Emergency Medicine, Gainesville, FL
   (Cases 59–64, 80, 81, 85, 87, 115, 118, 119, 238)

David Caro, MD
   Department of Emergency Medicine, University of Florida College of Medicine, Jacksonville, FL
   (Cases 37, 79, 88–96, 98)

Bharath Chakravarthy, MD, MPH
   Department of Emergency Medicine, University of California, Irvine, CA
   (Cases 12, 16, 21, 86, 110, 112, 113, 116, 117, 120, 122, 123)

Megan Fix, MD
   Department of Emergency Medicine, University of Utah, UT
   (Cases 11, 66–68, 70–78)

Braden Hexom, MD
   Department of Emergency Medicine, Rush University Medical Center, Chicago, IL
   (Cases 1, 3–5, 7–9, 38–42, 126)

Jennifer Li, MD
   Department of Emergency Medicine at University Hospitals, Cleveland Medical Center, at Case
   Western Reserve University School of Medicine, Cleveland, OH
   (Cases 23–33, 35)

Jacqueline Nemer, MD
   Department of Emergency Medicine, Department of Quality and Patient Safety, University of
   California San Francisco, CA
   (Cases 43, 99, 100, 103–109, 124, 125)

Jennifer E. Sanders, MD
   Departments of Emergency Medicine, Pediatrics, and Medical Education, Icahn School of
   Medicine at Mount Sinai
   (Cases 2, 6, 13–15, 17–20, 22 34, 36, 101, 127)

Dustin Williams, MD
   UT-Southwestern Medical Center, Department of Emergency Medicine, Dallas, TX
   (Cases 10, 44–52, 54, 56, 114)

Contributors

Sean Abraham, DO
Clinical Assistant Professor, Michigan State University College of Osteopathic Medicine, East Lansing, MI; Attending Physician, Ascension Genesys Hospital, Grand Blanc, MI

Shayna Adams, MD
Resident, Rush University Medical Center, Chicago, IL

Maneesha Agarwal, MD
Associate Professor, Departments of Pediatrics and Emergency Medicine, Emory University School of Medicine, Children's Healthcare of Atlanta, Atlanta, GA

Wakas Ahmed, DO
Assistant Professor, Department of Emergency Medicine, Rush University Medical Center, Chicago, IL

Kiyetta Alade, MD, MEd
Associate Professor, Director, Pediatric Point-of-Care Ultrasound, Department of Pediatrics, Baylor College of Medicine, Houston, TX

Chelsea Allen, DO
Resident Physician, Department of Emergency Medicine, University of Florida College of Medicine – Jacksonville, Jacksonville, FL

Kendra Amico, MD
Emergency Medicine Attending Physician, Orlando Health, Dr. Phillips Hospital, Orlando, FL

Dhara Amin, MD
Director of Quality Improvement and Patient Safety, Department of Emergency Medicine, Cook County Health, Chicago, IL; Assistant Professor of Emergency Medicine, Rush Medical College, Chicago, IL

Kimbia Arno, MD, MFA
Assistant Program Director, Maimonides Medical Center, New York, NY

Ani Aydin, MD
Associate Professor, Department of Emergency Medicine, Department of Surgery, Division of General Surgery, Trauma and Surgical Critical Care, Yale University School of Medicine, New Haven, CT

Oluwakemi Badaki-Makun, MD
Director of Research, Pediatric Emergency Medicine and Assistant Professor of Pediatrics, Johns Hopkins University, Baltimore, MD; Core Faculty, Center for Data Science in Emergency Medicine, Baltimore, MD; Attending Physician, The Johns Hopkins Children's Center, Baltimore, MD

Alexandria Bahan Farish, MD
Pediatric Emergency Medicine Physician, Tampa General Hospital, Tampa, FL

Matthew Beattie, MD
Lars K. Beattie, MS, MD
Associate Professor and Residency Program Director, University of Florida Department of Emergency Medicine, Gainesville, FL

Jennifer M. Bellis, MD, MPH
Clinical Instructor, Section of Emergency Medicine, Department of Pediatrics, CU School of Medicine/ Children's Hospital Colorado, Aurora, CO

Suzanne K. Bentley, MD, MPH
Chief Wellness Officer, NYC Health + Hospitals/ Elmhurst, New York, NY; Associate Professor, Emergency Medicine & Medical Education, Icahn School of Medicine at Mount Sinai, New York, NY

Jessica Berrios, MD

Caroline Black, MD
Assistant Professor of Pediatrics, Pediatric Emergency Medicine, Yale School of Medicine, New Haven CT

Philip Bossart, MD

Catharine Cantrell, MD

David A. Caro, MD
Associate Chair for Education, Emergency Medicine, University of Florida College of Medicine – Jacksonville, Jacksonville, FL

Michael Cassara, DO, MSEd
Vice President and Medical Director, Northwell Health Center for Learning and Innovation, New Hyde Park, NY; Associate Professor of Emergency Medicine and Science Education, Donald and Barbara Zucker School of Medicine, Uniondale, NY

Michael Chami, MD
Assistant Professor, Department of Emergency Medicine,UniversityofSouthFloridaCollegeofMedicine, Tampa, FL

Bharath Chakravarthy, MD, MPH
Department of Emergency Medicine, University of California, Irvine, CA

Angela Chen, MD
Assistant Professor, Icahn School of Medicine at Mount Sinai, Mount Sinai, New York, NY

Joseph Chiang, MD

Anne Chipman, MD, MS
Assistant Professor, Department of Emergency Medicine, University of Washington, Seattle, WA

Evelyn Chow, MD

David H. Cisewski, MD
Emergency Medicine Specialist, Kaiser Permanente Emergency Department, Santa Clara, CA

Victor Cisneros, MD, MPH
Director of Diversity, Equity, and Inclusion, Graduate Medical Education, Department of Emergency Medicine, Eisenhower Health, Rancho Mirage, CA

Matthew Constantine, MD

Brendan Cummins, MD
Adjunct Assistant Professor and Assistant Program Director, Department of Emergency Medicine, University of Utah, Sat Lake City, UT; Utah Emergency Physician, Intermountain Medical Center, Murray, UT

Terri Davis MD
Andalusia Health, Andalusia, AL

Giuliano De Portu, MD, FACEP
Associate Professor of Emergency Medicine, Director of Emergency Medicine Ultrasound, and Director of AEMUS Emergency Medicine Ultrasound Fellowship, University of Florida College of Medicine, Gainesville, FL

Tomás Díaz, MD
Clinical Fellow, Emergency Medicine, UCSF, San Francisco, CA

Vinodinee Dissanayake, MD
Assistant Professor, Director of Diversity, Inclusion and Racial Equity, Core Faculty, Department of Emergency Medicine, Rush University Medical Center, Chicago, IL; Advocate Role Leader, Health Equity and Social Justice Leadership Faculty, Rush Medical College, Chicago, IL

Marie-Carmelle Elie, MD, RDMS
Endowed Emergency Medicine Professor and Chair, Department of Emergency Medicine, University of Alabama Birmingham, and Heersink School of Medicine, Birmingham, AL

Daniel Eraso, MD
Assistant Professor, Department of Emergency Medicine, University of Florida College of Medicine – Jacksonville, Jacksonville, FL

Abiola Fasina, MD Medical Director and CEO
Emergency Healthcare Consultants (EHCON), Lagos, Nigeria

Abraham Feshazion, MD, PharmD, MPH
Emergency Medicine Specialist

Megan Fix, MD
Assistant Dean of Student Affairs and Professor and Vice Chair of Education, Department of Emergency Medicine, University of Utah, Salt Lake City, UT

Tabitha Ford, MD
Assistant Professor, Assistant Director, Residency Program, and Director of Didactic Education, Department of Emergency Medicine, University of Vermont Medical Center, Larner College of Medicine, Burlington, VT

Stephanie Gaines, MD
Emergency Medicine Physician, University Hospitals Cleveland Medical Center, Cleveland, OH;

Assistant Professor, Case Western Reserve University School of Medicine, Cleveland, OH

Sylvia E. Garcia, MD
Assistant Professor, Departments of Emergency Medicine and Pediatrics, Icahn School of Medicine at Mount Sinai, New York NY

Nicholas Genes, MD, PhD
Associate Professor, Ronald O. Perelman Department of Emergency Medicine, NYU Grossman School of Medicine, New York, NY

Megha George, MD
Assistant Professor, Department of Emergency Medicine, NYC Health+Hospitals, Elmhurst, and Icahn School of Medicine at Mount Sinai, New York, NY

Nicole Gerber, MD
Assistant Professor of Clinical Emergency Medicine and Pediatrics, Weill Cornell Medical College, New York, NY

Ellen Gilbertson, MD
Resident Physician, Department of Emergency Medicine, University of Utah, Salt Lake City, UT

James P. Gillen, MD
Director of Emergency Medicine Education, University of South Florida Emergency Medicine Program, Tampa, FL; Associate Professor, USF Morsani College of Medicine, Tampa General Hospital, Tampa, FL

Haley Godwin MD
Candidate, University of Utah School of Medicine, Salt Lake City, UT

Daniel Goldstein, MD
Emergency Medicine Residency, Clinical Faculty, John Peter Smith Hospital, Fort Worth, TX

Katarzyna Gore, MD
Assistant Professor of Emergency Medicine and Residency Assistant Program Director, Rush University Medical Center, Chicago, IL

Ryan Gore, MD
Assistant Professor and Director of Integrated Education, Departments of Emergency and Internal Medicine, Rush University Medical Center, Chicago, IL

Peter Gutierrez, MD FAAP FACEP
Associate Professor, Division of Emergency Medicine, Department of Pediatrics, Emory University School of Medicine, Children's Healthcare of Atlanta, Atlanta GA

Christina Hajicharalambous, DO, MSEd, MS

Xiao Han, MD
Dept of Emergency Medicine, Kaiser Permanente Walnut Creek/Antioch, Walnut Creek, CA

Matthew Harris, MD
Associate Professor of Pediatrics and Emergency Medicine, Hofstra-Zucker School of Medicine, Northwell Health, Uniondale, NY

Scott Heinrich, MD
Emergency Physician and Director of the Emergency Medicine Residency Program, Department of Emergency Medicine, Rush University Medical Center, Chicago, IL

Rebeca Hellman, DO

Luke Hermann, MD
Department of Emergency Medicine, Mount Sinai School of Medicine, New York, NY

Braden Hexom, MD
Professor, Department of Emergency Medicine, Rush University Medical Center, Chicago, IL

Jacob Holton, MD
Assistant Professor, Core Faculty, and Director of Rotating Residents, Department of Emergency Medicine, UIC College of Medicine in Peoria, Peoria, IL

Wirachin Hoonpongsimanont, MD

Alan Huang, MD

Robert M. Hughes, DO
Assistant Professor, Case Western Reserve University School of Medicine, Cleveland, OH; Medical Director, System Operations Center and Associate Medical Director, Department of Emergency Medicine, University Hospitals Cleveland Medical Center, Cleveland, OH

Bashar A. Ismail, MD
Emergency Medicine Specialist, Harris Health System, Ben Taub Hospital Texas Medical Center, Houston, TX

Lisa Jacobson, MD
Emergency Medicine Physician, Adventist Health Castle Department of Emergency Medicine, Kailua, Hawaii

Bethany Johnston, MD
Assistant Professor, Department of Emergency Medicine, University of Florida, Gainesville, FL

Jodi Jones MD
Associate Professor, Interim Division Chief, Emergency Ultrasound and Simulation, Section Chief, Clinical Ultrasound, Fellowship Director, Clinical Ultrasound, and Associate Director, EM Ultrasound Residency Education, Department of Emergency Medicine, UT Southwestern Medical Center, Dallas, TX

Marianne Juarez, MD
Associate Professor, Emergency Medicine, UCSF Medical Center, San Francisco, CA

Ian Kane, MD
Associate Professor, Pediatric Emergency Medicine, Medical University of South Carolina, Charleston, SC

Linda Katirji, MD
Assistant Professor and Associate Program Director, Department of Emergency Medicine, University of Kentucky, Lexington, KY

Robert Katzer, MD
Clinical Professor of Emergency Medicine, University of California, Irvine, Irvine, CA

Raashee Kedia, MD
Assistant Professor, Department of Emergency Medicine, UT

Jay Khadpe, MD
Assistant Professor, Department of Emergency Medicine, UT Southwestern Medical Center and Parkland Memorial Hospital, Dallas, TX

John Kiel, DO, MPH
Assistant Professor of Emergency Medicine and Assistant Professor of Orthopedics & Sports Medicine, University of Florida College of Medicine – Jacksonville, Jacksonville, FL; Field Surgeon, 256th Area Support Medical Company, Florida Army National Guard

Gail Knight, MD
Emergency Medicine Physician, Wellstar Health System, Lagrange, GA

Matthew Kuhns, MD
Assistant Professor, Department of Emergency Medicine, Rush University, Chicago, IL

Bonnie Lau, MD
Assistant Chief, Department of Emergency Medicine, Kaiser Permanente Santa Clara Medical Center, Santa Clara, CA; Clinical Assistant Professor (Affiliated), Department of Emergency Medicine, Stanford University School of Medicine, Stanford, CA

Elisabeth Lessenich, MD, MPH
Emergency Department Physician, Groupe Hospitalier Bretagne Sud Lorient, France

Nicholas Levin, MD
Chief Resident, Department of Emergency Medicine, University of Utah, Salt Lake City, UT

Shahram Loftipour, MD

Wuya Lumeh, MD

Cassandra Mackey, MD
Assistant Professor, Department of Emergency Medicine, University of Massachusetts Medical School, Worcester, MA

Nicholas G. Maldonado, MD, FACEP
Clinical Associate Professor of Emergency Medicine and Associate Program Director of the UF Emergency Medicine Residency, University of Florida College of Medicine, Gainesville, FL

Alexandra Mannix, MD
Assistant Professor and Assistant Program Director, Emergency Medicine Residency, University of Florida College of Medicine – Jacksonville, Jacksonville, FL

Rijo Maracheril, MD
Attending Physician, Nassau University Medical Center Emergency Department, New York, NY

Michael Marchick, MD
Co-Clerkship Director and Clinical Associate Professor, Department of Emergency Medicine, University of Florida College of Medicine, Gainesville, FL

Michelle N. Marin, MD
Assistant Professor of Pediatrics and Pediatric Emergency Medicine, Affiliate Faculty Florida Atlantic University Boynton Beach, FL

Ryan Marino, MD
Assistant Professor of Emergency Medicine, Department of Emergency Medicine, Division of Medical Toxicology, and Department of Psychiatry, Case Western Reserve School of Medicine, University Hospitals Cleveland Medical Center, Cleveland, OH

Angela Maxwell, MD
Assistant Professor of Emergency Medicine and Pediatrics, The George Washington University School of Medicine and Health Sciences, Washington, DC

Christopher McCoy, MD

William McDowell, MD
Emergency Medicine Attending Physician, St. Luke's Hospital, Cedar Rapids, IA

Ryan McKenna, DO
Assistant Professor, Mayo Clinic, Jacksonville, Florida

Edward R. Melnick, MD, MHS

Michelle Mendoza, MD

Avir Mitra, MD

Nicole Munz, DO
Clinical Instructor, UCSF, San Francisco, CA

Ariella Nadler MD
Assistant Professor of Clinical Emergency Medicine and Assistant Professor of Clinical Pediatrics, Advocate Health Care, Park Ridge IL

Denise Nassisi, MD, FACEP
Department of Emergency Medicine, Mount Sinai School of Medicine, New York, NY

Hayley Neher, MD
Emergency Medicine Physician, Washington Emergency Care Physicians, Tacoma, WA

Bret P. Nelson, MD
Department of Emergency Medicine, Icahn School of Medicine at Mount Sinai, New York, NY

Jacqueline Nemer, MD
Professor of Emergency Medicine, Bridges Coach at School of Medicine, Director of Advanced Procedural Skills Education, Department of Emergency Medicine, Medical Director, Clinical Documentation Integrity (CDI), Department of Quality and Patient Safety, University of California San Francisco, San Francisco, CA

Carrie Ng, MD
Assistant Professor, Division of Emergency Medicine, Department of Pediatrics, Emory University School of Medicine, Children's Healthcare of Atlanta, Atlanta, GA

Thomas Nguyen, MD
Associate Professor, Department of Emergency Medicine, Icahn School of Medicine, New York, NY

Jeanne Noble, MD
Associate Professor of Emergency Medicine, Director of Disaster Preparedness, Parnassus Emergency Department, and Residency Director of Emergency Medicine Simulation, University of California, San Francisco, CA

Yasuharu Okuda, MD
Executive Director, USF Health Center for Advanced Medical Learning and Simulation, Associate Vice President Interprofessional Education and Practice, Associate Dean Emerging Healthcare and Educational Technologies, and Vice Chair Academic Affairs, Department of Emergency Medicine, Morsani College of Medicine, University of South Florida Health, Tampa, FL

Ruben Olemdo, MD
Mount Sinai School of Medicine, New York, NY

David Orban, MD
Professor Emeritus, Division of Emergency Medicine, USF Health Morsani College of Medicine, Tampa, FL

Ram Parekh, MD
Associate Professor, Department of Emergency Medicine, Icahn School of Medicine at Mount Sinai, New York, NY

Mandy Pascual MD
Assistant Professor, Department of Emergency Medicine, UT Southwestern Medical Center, Dallas, TX

Amit Patel, MD
Assistant Professor of Emergency Medicine and Pediatrics, College of Medicine, University of Central Florida, Orlando, FL

Wesley Pedicini, MD

Carolina Pereira, MD
Emergency Medicine Physician, Emergency Medicine, Orlando Regional Healthcare, Orlando, FL

Calloway Pichette, MD
Emergency Medicine Physician, Emergency Department, Overland Park Regional Medical Center, Overland Park, KS

Elysha Pifko, MD
Pediatric Emergency Department, Nemours Children's Hospital, Wilmington, DE

Gregory Podolej, MD
Assistant Professor, University of Illinois College of Medicine at Peoria, Peoria, IL

Lauren Porter, DO
Assistant Professor of Emergency Medicine, Attending Physician of Medical Toxicology, and Clerkship Director for Medical Toxicology, University Hospitals, Case Western Reserve University, Cleveland, OH

Elaine Rabin, MD

J. Mark Rendon, MD
Associate Professor, Department of Emergency Medicine, UT Southwestern Medical Center, Dallas, TX

Nicole Rettig, MD
Assistant Professor and Residency Simulation Director, Department of Emergency Medicine, University of South Florida College of Medicine, Tampa, FL

Danielle Roberts, MD
Emergency Medicine Physician, Tactivate Medical Director

Jennifer Roh, MD

Javier Rosario, MD
Director, Emergency Ultrasound and Assistant Professor of Emergency Medicine, University of Central Florida/HCA Healthcare GME (Greater Orlando), Orlando, FL; Emergency Medicine Physician, Osceola Regional Medical Center, Kissimmee, FL

Sheler Sadati, MD

Mariam Said, MD

Laura Scieszka, MD
Emergency Medicine Physician, Department of Emergency Medicine, University of Florida, Gainesville, FL

Nikolas Sekoulopoulos, MD
Rachel Semmons, MD Associate Department Director, Tampa General Hospital, Tampa, FL; EMS Fellowship Director, University of South Florida Emergency Medicine, Tampa, FL; EMS Medical Director, Tampa Fire Rescue, Tampa, FL

Jared Senvisky, MD
Assistant Professor, Department of Anesthesiology, Case Western Reserve University, Cleveland Clinic Lerner College of Medicine, Cleveland, OH

Monica Sethi, MD
Assistant Professor, Department of Emergency Medicine, Mount Sinai Hospital, New York, NY

Bing Shen, MD
Emergency Medicine Physician, Department of Emergency Medicine, Kaiser Permanente San Leandro/Fremont, San Leandro, CA

Mason Shieh, MD, MBA

Garrett Snipes, MD
Resident, Department of Emergency Medicine, University of Florida College of Medicine, Gainesville, FL

Daniel Spearman, MD
Emergency Medicine Physician, Department of Emergency Medicine, Rush University Medical Center, Chicago, IL

Matthew Steimle, DO
Assistant Professor of Pediatrics, Division of Pediatric Emergency Medicine, University of Utah School of Medicine, Salt Lake City, Utah

Robert Stephen, MD
Associate Professor, Associate Program Director, and Student Clerkship Director, Department of Emergency Medicine, University of Utah Health Sciences Center, Salt Lake City, UT

Reuben J. Strayer, MD

Jacob M. Stritch, MD
Emergency Medicine Physician, AdventHealth Orlando, Gainesville, FL

Christopher Strother, MD
Professor, Emergency Medicine, Pediatrics, and Medical Education, Icahn School of Medicine at Mount Sinai, New York, NY

Jeffrey R. Suchard, MD

Tricia Swan, MD, MEd
Associate Professor and Program Director, Pediatric Emergency Medicine Fellowship, Department of Emergency Medicine, University of Florida, Gainesville, FL

Andrew Thomas, MD
Assistant Professor, Division of Emergency Medicine, University of South Florida Morsani College of Medicine, Tampa, FL

Julie Tokarski, MD
Assistant Professor, Departments of Emergency Medicine and Pediatrics, Icahn School of Medicine at Mount Sinai, New York, NY

Benjamin H. Slovis MD

Shefali Trivedi, MD
Assistant Professor, Icahn School of Medicine at Mount Sinai, New York, NY

Michael Truax Jr., MD
Assistant Professor, LSUHSC Baton Rouge Emergency Medicine Residency Program, Baton Rouge, LA

Keegan Tupchong, MD
Intensivist, Wellstar Pulmonary Medicine and Critical Care, Marietta, GA

Chanteil D. Ulatowski, MD
Emergency Medicine SEP, Bravera Health, Tampa, FL; Associate EMS Director of Citrus County, Inverness, FL

Anita Vashi, MD

Temima Waltuch, MD
Assistant Professor of Pediatrics,
Department of Emergency Medicine, Division of Pediatric Emergency Medicine, Hackensack Meridian Health—Hackensack University Medical Center & Joseph M Sanzari Children's Hospital, Hackensack, NJ
Department of Pediatrics, Hackensack Meridian School of Medicine, Nutley, NJ

Taryn Webb, MD
Assistant Professor, Department of Emergency Medicine, Icahn School of Medicine at Mount Sinai, New York, NY

David Wein, MD
Medical Director and Chief of Emergency Medicine Tampa General Hospital, Tampa, FL; Associate Professor, Department of Internal Medicine, Division of Emergency Medicine, USF Morsani College of Medicine, Tampa, FL; System Medical Director, Southeast Group TeamHealth

Scott Weingart, MD, FCCM
Nassau University Medical Center, East Meadow, NY

Alisa Wray, MD
Associate Residency Program Director, Department of Emergency Medicine, University of California, Irvine, Irvine, CA

Henry Young, MD
Associate Professor and Vice Chair, Department of Emergency Medicine, Ohio State University Wexner Medical Center, Columbus, OH

Lisa Zahn, MD

Qiaohua Zhang, MD
Department of Emergency Medicine, Icahn School of Medicine at Mount Sinai Hospital, New York, NY

Shawn Zhong, MD
EM Attending, Kings County Hospital, Brooklyn, NY and Staten Island University Hospital, Staten Island, NY; CCM Attending, Staten Island University Hospital, Staten Island, NY and Newark Beth Israel Medical Center, Newark, NJ

Moving from the Oral Boards to the Certifying Exam: How to Get the Most from Our Book

Nicole Rettig, MD, Bret P. Nelson, MD, and Yasuharu Okuda, MD

OPENING PERSPECTIVE: WHY THIS FOREWORD MATTERS NOW

Since 2009, Emergency Medicine residency graduates have trusted our case-based books as a practical way to prepare for high-stakes, interactive oral examinations. We have tried to distill years of residency training and study into a collection of cases because, at the end of the day, we care for patients one by one. We hope this format continues to be a helpful review and preparation for interactive examinations.

This edition is being released during a significant transition: the American Board of Emergency Medicine (ABEM) is moving from the legacy Oral Certification Examination to the in-person Certifying Exam administered at the AIME Center in Raleigh, North Carolina. ABEM describes this new Certifying Exam as the final step to becoming ABEM certified, and notes that candidates complete 10 cases during a half-day session. ABEM also explains that the exam is built around two assessment types – Clinical Care Cases and Communication & Procedure Cases – intended to reflect simulated, real-world clinical scenarios.

THE CERTIFYING EXAM AS A PROFESSIONAL MILESTONE

Regardless of format, the Certifying Exam represents a milestone: demonstrating readiness for independent practice as an emergency physician. The heart of both the prior oral boards and the new Certifying Exam is the ability to recognize typical case presentations, prioritize the most critical actions, communicate clearly, and make sound, defensible decisions under pressure.

ABEM provides preparation resources for the Certifying Exam on its website (e.g., sample case videos, case summaries, and lists of procedures and ultrasound applications). These resources can help candidates align their preparation with the competencies ABEM intends to assess – without relying on scripts or "insider" details.

The following perspectives are drawn from participation in a mock Certifying Exam administration conducted to provide structured feedback to ABEM.

WHAT TO EXPECT ON EXAM DAY: THE EXPERIENCE

If test takers are not local to the center, it is recommended to travel the day before the test. The area with the testing center and hotels is a 15- to 20-minute drive from the Raleigh–Durham International Airport, and once there, driving is not necessary. There are several hotels near the testing center, and this area is commercial and easily walkable.

Registration begins just prior to the exam session and is located at the hotel at which many candidates stay. The exact time will be provided to candidates via email when they are assigned their exam session (for the mock morning session, it was 6:45 a.m.). There is a room adjacent to the registration room where candidates can securely leave personal belongings including luggage. In the registration room, candidates check in by showing identification, then the ABEM oral board proctors explain the logistics of the day and answer questions. Candidates are instructed to turn off electronics and seal them in a provided bag that can be brought to the testing center and stored in a locker, but electronics may not be accessed until the exam session ends. Food and drink can be brought to the testing center to be stored in the locker. Next, proctors lead candidates to the testing center, which is a short, outdoor walk. Regarding the dress code, as the ABEM site states, candidates are encouraged to be comfortable, so scrubs or business casual is acceptable, but if there is a logo on the attire, it will be covered for the exam so that examiners will not be biased.

Once candidates arrive at the testing center, there is an elevator that takes groups up to the secure testing floor. There are several proctors present to direct candidates where to go for the lockers, exam rooms, bathrooms, and water. Candidates will complete 10 cases over the course of the half-day exam session: 6 of the cases test "Communication and Procedures" and are located on one side of the testing center, and 4 of the cases test "Clinical Decision-Making and Prioritization" and are located on the other side of the testing center. The candidates are split so that half complete the Communication and Procedures side and the other half completes the Clinical Decision-Making and Prioritization, followed by a break, then the candidates do the other half of the exam session. Upon arrival at the testing floor, each candidate is assigned a seat and number in a main room, and this is where candidates wait and receive more instructions on logistics before the testing starts. Each candidate is given a clipboard and an individual rotation schedule for their cases. When testing begins, proctors lead candidates to their respective rooms with chairs for candidates to sit and wait until there is an announcement to proceed.

The testing center was modern with large windows in the main gathering area, offering natural light and beautiful views of the surrounding area. Overall, the cadence of the session felt unhurried and candidates seemed to have ample time for cases and transitions. The process felt organized and standardized, and there were always proctors available to assist or take questions. For the procedure and ultrasound cases, the equipment was high quality and well functioning. The communication cases utilizing standardized patients offered an impressive and immersive element of realism.

DIFFERENCES FROM THE LEGACY ORAL BOARDS

Overall, the most significant difference between the new and legacy Certifying Exams lies in the emphases on thought process and clinical translatability. This is most notable in the "Communication and Procedures" portion of the exam as this requires proficiency in hands-on emergency medicine skills. This portion of the exam utilizes standardized patients, task trainers, and ultrasound. Some of these encounters employ cases with role-playing while others use a question-and-answer format between the examiner and the candidate to assess clinical knowledge and procedural competency. If a case does not involve role-playing, it is made explicit by the examiner.

The execution of the "Clinical Decision-Making and Prioritization" portion of the exam mirrors the classic Certifying Exam format in that the examiners ask questions to assess clinical knowledge and decision-making, but there is no hands-on component. That being said, the flow of the prioritization cases feels more immersive than the legacy exam cases. The rooms are set up with a desk on which there is a computer to display the case, and the examiner(s) and candidate are sitting face-to-face on either side of the desk. The structured interview mirrors that of the legacy Certifying Exam.

Preparation for the "Clinical Decision-Making" portion of the exam must evolve to incorporate more probing and open-ended questions to better elucidate the candidates' thought processes. The ABEM site offers examples of Certifying Exam encounters that can be used to guide preparation. If preparing for this exam alone, a candidate could practice cases and ask themselves some of these "why" questions and be able to justify decisions and actions. If studying with others, preparation could be optimized by role-playing the examiner and the candidate and making sure that the examiner prepares probing and follow-up questions to assess the candidate's clinical reasoning.

Preparation for the "Communication and Procedures" portion of the exam should focus on engagement in simulation-based education, ACGME requirements for ultrasound and procedures, and case examples and procedure lists on the ABEM site. Given the more immersive and clinically relevant features of the new Certifying Exam, preparation should similarly employ simulated, real-life scenarios, and resources should be allocated to increase simulation-based education in residency training.

THE CANDIDATE MINDSET: HOW TO SHOW UP PREPARED

As previously discussed, the new Certifying Exam focuses on thought process and reasoning, and it employs tactics to mirror the cognitive load associated with working in the clinical environment of the emergency department. In order to mentally prepare for this exam, engagement in these skills in the clinical and simulated environments is paramount. It is valuable for candidates to practice clinical decision-making aloud as this can increase one's own situational awareness and clinical reasoning, but as it related to the exam, this is evaluated by examiners to assess proficiency in communication, procedures, and medical decision-making. Thus, you must be able to verbalize what you are thinking and why. For the communication cases, maintaining empathy, a patient-centered focus, and calm under pressure can help candidates be successful. Upon review of the ABEM site examples, if there are situations in which a candidate may lack experience or proficiency, such as breaking bad news, it is necessary to develop these skills whether this is in a simulated or clinical environment. The proficiencies being evaluated in the new Certifying Exam are distinct from the knowledge tested on the qualifying exam, so preparation should be guided with this in mind.

HOW TO USE THIS BOOK IN THE CURRENT EXAM ERA

This book should be used as a resource to practice clinical reasoning, processing aloud, and communications skills. The cases in this book are intended as frameworks rather than templates, and candidates should practice these cases with the goal of applying their learning to simulated, real-world clinical scenarios rather than memorizing scripts. We encourage readers to approach their learning as developing a set of tools that can be applied to any scenario that may arise on the Certifying Exam. Readers must work through cases through the lens of strengthening the competencies established by ABEM to be successful on this new Certifying Exam.

FINAL REASSURANCE TO CANDIDATES

It is normal to feel unsettled and uncertain about taking a new exam. Keep in mind that the new Certifying Exam is more relevant to clinical practice, standardized, professionally run, and is designed to fairly assess readiness for independent practice. Per the ABEM Certifying Exam site, the intention is to "allow candidates to use the skills and methods learned in training and apply them to simulated, real-world clinical scenarios," so candidates can have confidence rooted in emergency medicine training. Thank you for all you do in taking care of patients every day and thank you for studying along with us.

DISCLOSURE STATEMENT

The perspectives shared in this foreword are based on participation in a mock Certifying Exam administration and are intentionally limited to general process, environment, and professional considerations. No ABEM exam case content, confidential assessment materials, or non-public exam information is included.

CHAPTER 1

How to Use This Book

Bret P. Nelson, MD

The amount of information that must be transferred from books, patients, journals, mentors, and so on into the brain of an aspiring emergency physician is overwhelming. Many physicians create study plans, purchase books, fall behind schedule, and readjust timelines in an endless process akin to yo-yo dieting. Whatever the means we use to study while not actively caring for patients, inevitably we learn as our forebears did – one patient at a time.

Thus, this book was crafted as a case-based approach to the art and science of emergency medicine. Although the format stresses an approach useful in preparation for the emergency medicine certifying exam, the cases serve as a review (or introduction) to the practice of emergency medicine. These pages contain heuristics on the general approach to patient management, pearls on the care of children, tips on performing common bedside procedures, and a litany of cases.

CERTIFYING EXAM PREPARATION

Working with a Partner

As described in Chapter 3, during the certifying exam you will be taken through a series of cases by an American Board of Emergency Medicine examiner. To mimic this process as closely as possible, you should review the cases in this book with a partner. Pairing with another emergency physician is ideal, as they will be familiar with the format of the exam and the medical decision-making in the cases, and they will have more fun throwing curveballs at you to make the cases more interesting (or difficult)! If you cannot find a colleague with a medical background to take you through the cases, a friend, family member, or significant other will do. The "examiner instructions" for each case are written to help a nonphysician approach the case. It is quite likely that your family and friends already know a lot of the jargon in this book. Like most physicians, you have probably regaled them with enough stomach-turning stories over the dinner table to make them experts. If you are fortunate enough to have a partner (examiner), read through the introductory section and appendices and become familiar with the format for the exam, but do not look at the images or cases. The examiner will take you (the candidate, to use ABEM's term) through the cases. You should read through each case on your own after working through it with your examiner, and look up any areas you had difficulty with. Standard emergency medicine texts are included for each case: *Tintinalli's Emergency Medicine: A Comprehensive Study Guide*, 9th edition by Tintinalli et al., 2020; *Rosen's Emergency Medicine: Concepts and Clinical Practice*, 10th edition by Walls et al., 2023. Please ask your partner to read the next section (Examiner Instructions) and the sample case before you tackle the cases in the rest of the book.

Examiner Instructions

Thank you for helping your friend, family member, or colleague (the candidate) to review for the certifying exam. This is the final step in their quest to become a board-certified emergency physician.

It is probably not the first (and certainly not the last) time you will ask yourself, "What have I gotten myself into?" when dealing with them. Your efforts will greatly exceed whatever reward you have been offered, especially if you were convinced by dinner in any restaurant they can afford on a resident's salary. If you are a physician, nurse, emergency medical technician (EMT), or other medical provider, the case-based format should be familiar to you. Your goal is to provide the candidate with bits of information about the case and to take the case in different directions based on their actions (or inaction). If you have no medical background, don't be intimidated! You already understand enough about medical care to appreciate the daily struggles the candidate faces in taking care of patients. Keep in mind that none of the actors on today's "doctor shows" ever attended medical school – yet they can sound convincing, and you can appreciate the medical plot points, with a little coaching.

Each case focuses on a patient presenting with some acute manifestation of illness. Some will have subtle signs such as headache or nausea, and others will be quite obviously sick (vomiting blood, major motor vehicle accident, etc.). Many patients will have straightforward problems such as broken bones, while others will have diagnoses that are difficult to pin down (poisonings, drug reactions, or more rare illnesses). Start by reading the examiner instructions for each case; these will give you an overall picture of what the medical problem and major critical actions are. Within the description there will often be additional points on how to deal with situations that will arise in the course of the case – playing the part of a consultant, when to reveal certain key information, how to deal with common medical errors, and so on. Next, read the case from beginning to end to see the flow, starting with the chief complaint (reason for evaluation), then initial impressions (What do I see when I walk into the room?), then basic historical information about the patient and the physical examination, followed by ordering tests, giving medications, interpreting the test results, calling upon consultants, and establishing patient disposition (admitting to the hospital, going to the operating room, discharging them, etc.).

The cases are meant to be fun (in a nerdy sort of way). At first, you'll probably present the cases pretty "straight." You can state the patient's complaint and examination as written in the text, speak about consultants in the third person ("the cardiologist says they will see the patient in the morning"), and "stick to the script." As you become more comfortable with the certifying exam format, feel free to get into the character a bit more. Patients, consultants, nurses, and other "characters" in certifying exam cases are typically portrayed in the first person by examiners. Instead of saying, "the patient reports they are in pain," try, "Doctor, my arm still hurts" or "Why isn't my son getting anything for pain? Who's in charge here?" You probably know someone who thought karaoke was stupid but then would not give up the microphone after trying it. Taking a friend through these cases can be similarly entertaining, even without the aid of alcohol.

When you become fairly comfortable with the format (this is easier for medical professionals), you can deviate a bit from the cases to make them more interesting and challenging. Examples of how to do this are given in some cases with a "curveball" described. Some of these curveballs will involve reluctant consultants, patients who aren't forthcoming with the truth, or other factors that can make proper diagnosis and treatment difficult. Many of these types of curveballs can appear on the real certifying exam, because the candidate is being tested partially on their ability to work effectively in the emergency medicine practice system. Some are so important that they should be expected in every case, even when not explicitly stated in the instructions. For example, if the candidate orders a medication before checking the patient's allergies, that patient should exhibit an allergic reaction to the medication. This is good practice for the exam (where points can be deducted for such mistakes), but more important in real life, where "points" are people.

Working Alone

Don't worry if you couldn't convince anyone to nurse you through all of the cases. You can still use this book effectively to engage in "active learning," which is much more effective for adult learners than flipping through pages and passively reading the text. You'll have to use a bit of discipline in approaching the cases and force yourself to think about your management for each case.

After reading the sample case, take each case one by one. Read through the chief complaint and think about what you would do with that patient immediately. Usually, the next question to ask is, "What do I see when I look at the patient?" After the text reveals the answer, stop and think of your next action. For example, if you see an ashen, unresponsive patient, you will want to move immediately toward resuscitation. For a well-appearing patient in no distress, you will likely start with a primary survey, history, and physical examination.

Try to think ahead as much as possible, focusing on what specific historical or physical examination items you are especially interested in. You will get more out of asking yourself, "Does this patient have a carotid bruit?" than simply thinking, "Now I'll examine the patient." Remember that the real examiners will not just give away the entire examination; they will often ask for what specific actions you would like to perform. There are no tricks in this book, and there should not be any on the certifying exam either. When a test or physical examination is described as "normal," move on with the case as if it is.

By the end of each case, you will see a checklist of critical actions. These types of actions are the basis for scoring on the real certifying exam. The examiner instructions are near the end. These will often provide insights into the case, confirming or revealing the diagnosis, and often elucidating why certain actions were or were not mandated, why that computed tomography (CT) scan was never available, or why the consultant gave you such a hard time. While the case is fresh in your mind, refer to the appropriate chapters in *Rosen's* or *Tintinalli's* to ensure you are comfortable with the material.

EMERGENCY MEDICINE STUDY GUIDE

Sometimes it's more interesting and engaging to go through cases rather than to read textbook chapters. An individual case can be reviewed in a very short time, making it ideal for reading on public transportation or when you have only a few minutes. Ideally, use the "active" reading method described in the board review section. You can also give the cases a straight read-through, though it's not as effective as engaging your limbic system a bit by challenging yourself to think, "What should I do next?"

The cases should then be used as a springboard for further reading or discussion. Primary textbook references are given, but these should be supplemented by a search for more current literature (using PubMed, UptoDate, or other online research tool). Ask colleagues or mentors about similar cases they've encountered and how they managed them. The management decisions in this book are meant to represent "textbook" answers, but real-world management often differs significantly. By anchoring your supplemental reading in cases, you will have a greater retention of the management pearls and other facts discussed.

SAMPLE CASE

The following sample case is presented twice. First, the case is written in the standard format used throughout the book. Next, a sample dialogue describes the case as it would be presented by an examiner to a candidate. By looking back and forth between the case and the dialogue, you should get some sense of how the book can be used and how the certifying exam is administered.

CASE A: Back Pain

A. Chief complaint
a. 55-year-old male with backache

B. Vital signs
a. Blood pressure (BP): 165/90, heart rate (HR): 90, respiratory rate (RR): 16, temperature (T): 36.8°C orally, oxygen saturation (Sat): 98% on room air (RA)

C. What does the patient look like?
a. Patient lying on stretcher, appears stated age; appears in mild distress as he attempts to find a position of comfort

D. Primary survey
a. Airway: speaking in full sentences
b. Breathing: no respiratory distress, no cyanosis
c. Circulation: warm and moist skin, normal pulses, and capillary refill

E. History
a. History of present illness (HPI): the patient is a 55-year-old male with no significant past medical history who presents with a backache for several hours. He reports walking to work when he noted a sharp, burning pain in his mid to lower back, worse on the left than the right side. The pain began rather abruptly and was severe. He felt that it radiated up to his posterior chest and down to his leg when it was most pronounced. It has since improved a bit. There is no position that makes the pain better or worse, and the patient is unable to localize the pain to an exact point on his back. He denies any difficulty urinating, blood in the urine, or trauma.
b. Past medical history (PMHx): none
c. Past surgical history (PSHx): none
d. Allergies: none
e. Medications: none
f. Social: lives with wife; drinks alcohol socially, smokes one-half pack of cigarettes per day, denies the use of other drugs. Works as a manager at a box company.
g. Family history (FHx): no significant family history
h. Primary medical doctor (PMD): Dr. Underhill

F. Action
a. Monitor: BP: 165/95 HR: 95 RR: 18 Sat: 100% on 2L NC

G. Secondary survey
a. General: mild pain, discomfort
b. Head: normocephalic, atraumatic
c. Eyes: normal
d. Ears: normal
e. Nose: normal
f. Neck: supple, nontender, normal range of motion, no carotid bruit
g. Pharynx: normal dentition, no lesions, no swelling
h. Chest: nontender, no lesions
i. Lungs: normal air movement, clear breath sounds bilaterally

j. Heart: normal rate, rhythm regular; no murmurs, rubs, or gallops
k. Abdomen: normal bowel sounds, soft, nontender or distended
l. Rectal (if performed): normal tone, brown stool, occult blood negative
m. Urogenital (if performed): normal examination
n. Extremities: full range of motion; no deformity; normal femoral, radial, and dorsalis pedis pulses
o. Back: nontender, no costovertebral angle tenderness, no muscle spasm, no signs of trauma
p. Neurologic: alert and oriented; cranial nerves intact; normal strength, sensation, gait
q. Skin: warm to touch. No rash noted
r. Lymphatic: no lymphadenopathy

H. Studies

a. CBC, BMP, coagulation studies, blood type and crossmatch
b. Lactate, UA
c. EKG (electrocardiogram, also known as ECG)

I. Nurse

a. EKG (Figure 1.1)

J. Action

a. Imaging
     i. Chest x-ray (CXR)
b. Medications
     i. Morphine IV
c. Reassess
     i. Pain improved with morphine

K. Results

Table 1.1 Results table

Test	Result	Test	Result
Complete blood count (CBC):		**Liver function panel:**	
White blood cells (WBC)	$11.1 \times 10^3/\mu L$	Aspartate aminotransferase (AST)	31 U/L
Hematocrit (Hct)	40.3%	Alanine aminotransferase (ALT)	29 U/L
Platelets (Plt)	$438 \times 10^3/\mu L$	Alkaline phosphatase (Alk phos)	52 U/L
		Total bilirubin (T bili)	0.9 mg/dL
		Direct bilirubin (D bili)	0.1 mg/dL
Basic metabolic panel (BMP):			
Sodium (Na)	134 mEq/L	Amylase	42 U/L
Potassium (K)	3.9 mEq/L	Lipase	19 U/L
Chloride (Cl)	101 mEq/L	Albumin	4.1 g/dL
Bicarbonate (CO_2)	29 mEq/L		

Table 1.1 (cont.)

Test	Result	Test	Result
Blood urea nitrogen (BUN)	20 mEq/dL	**Urinalysis (UA):**	
Creatinine (Cr)	1.2 mg/dL	Specific gravity (SG)	1.019
Glucose (Gluc)	113 mg/dL	pH	6
		Protein (Prot)	Neg
Coagulation panel:		Glucose (Gluc)	Neg
Prothrombin time (PT)	11.9 sec	Ketones	Neg
Partial thromboplastin time (PTT)	24.0 sec	Bilirubin (Bili)	Neg
International normalized ratio (INR)	1.1	Blood	Neg
		Leukocyte esterase (LE)	Neg
		Nitrite	Neg
		Color	Yellow

a. Lactate: 1.5
b. CXR (Figure 1.2)

L. Reassess
a. Patient describes worsening of pain, now with nausea and some chest discomfort as well

M. Action
a. Imaging
b. Computed tomography (CT) scan of chest and abdomen (must describe differential diagnosis to radiologist protocoling study)

N. Nurse
a. CT scan (Figure 1.3) demonstrates dissection of the descending thoracic aorta extending to the abdominal aorta and the left iliac artery. There is no involvement of the aortic arch.

O. Action
a. Establish two large-bore IV lines
b. Consultation
   i. Vascular surgery
   ii. Intensive care unit
   iii. Notify primary care doctor
c. Meds
   i. Esmolol, labetalol, or other β-antagonist IV
   ii. Morphine IV
   iii. Sodium nitroprusside IV

P. Reassess
a. (β-antagonists given) Monitor: BP: 110/55 HR: 55 RR: 18 Sat: 100% on 2L NC; pain improved
b. (β-antagonists not given) Monitor: BP: 170/100 HR: 100 RR: 18 Sat: 100% on 2L NC; pain continues

Q. Diagnosis
a. Type B aortic dissection

R. Critical actions
a. EKG
b. CXR
c. Analgesia
d. Thorough neurologic and vascular examinations
e. CT scan to assess for dissection
f. Verbalize differential diagnosis (dissection, aneurysm, renal colic) with consultant (radiologist, ICU staff, etc.)
g. Blood pressure control
h. ICU consultation and admission

S. Examiner instructions
a. This is a case of aortic dissection. The aorta is the largest artery in the body and carries blood from the heart to the chest and abdomen. Its wall is composed of several layers that can tear, causing blood to dissect in between the layers. High blood pressure, smoking, and chronic medical conditions can increase the risk of this disorder. The patient's back pain and shortness of breath were due to tearing of the layers of the aorta, and therefore will not be improved with moving to a different position. The aorta should be suspected because of the severity and radiation of pain, and taking into account the patient's risk factors (smoking) and abnormal vital signs (high blood pressure). If the patient is not placed on a cardiac monitor, they should complain of feeling "woozy." The patient's pain will continue to worsen in the ED until he is treated with a β-antagonist (such as labetalol, esmolol, or propranolol) and a pain medication such as morphine. If the patient does not undergo imaging or is discharged, he should lose consciousness. A CT scan should be readily available if requested, but ultrasound and MRI will "take a few hours."

T. Pearls
a. Dissections are often classified according to their anatomic involvement: Type A involves the ascending aorta; type B does not.
b. Up to 12% of patients with aortic dissection have a normal CXR; the test should not be used to exclude the diagnosis.
c. Magnetic resonance imaging (MRI) has the best sensitivity and specificity for the diagnosis of aortic dissection; however, this test is often not feasible as it requires a stable patient and more time than other modalities, such as transesophageal echo (TEE) or CT scan. Among these options, CT scan is most commonly employed as the test of choice in the ED.
d. When considering aortic dissection in a patient with chest pain or difficulty breathing, other diagnoses in the differential include myocardial ischemia, congestive heart failure, pericarditis, and pulmonary embolus (PE). The diagnosis should also be considered for atypical back pain where renal colic or musculoskeletal causes are being considered, especially in patients with risk factors, such as advanced age, smoking, or hypertension.
e. Goals of emergency department therapy for dissection include blood pressure reduction and decreasing shear forces acting on the dissection site. Thus, β-blockers such as esmolol, metoprolol, and propranolol are considered first-line agents. Vasodilators such as sodium nitroprusside may be administered after these agents are used. Analgesia is important for patient comfort; it reduces sympathomimetic drive contributing to blood pressure and shear forces.

f.   Surgical management reduces in-hospital mortality for type A dissections and is the standard
of care. Initial treatment of type B acute aortic dissections is generally medical (blood pressure
control and observation). Patients with persistent pain, uncontrolled hypertension, occlusion
of a major arterial trunk, aortic leak or rupture, or development of a localized aneurysm may
require surgical intervention.

U. Figure legends

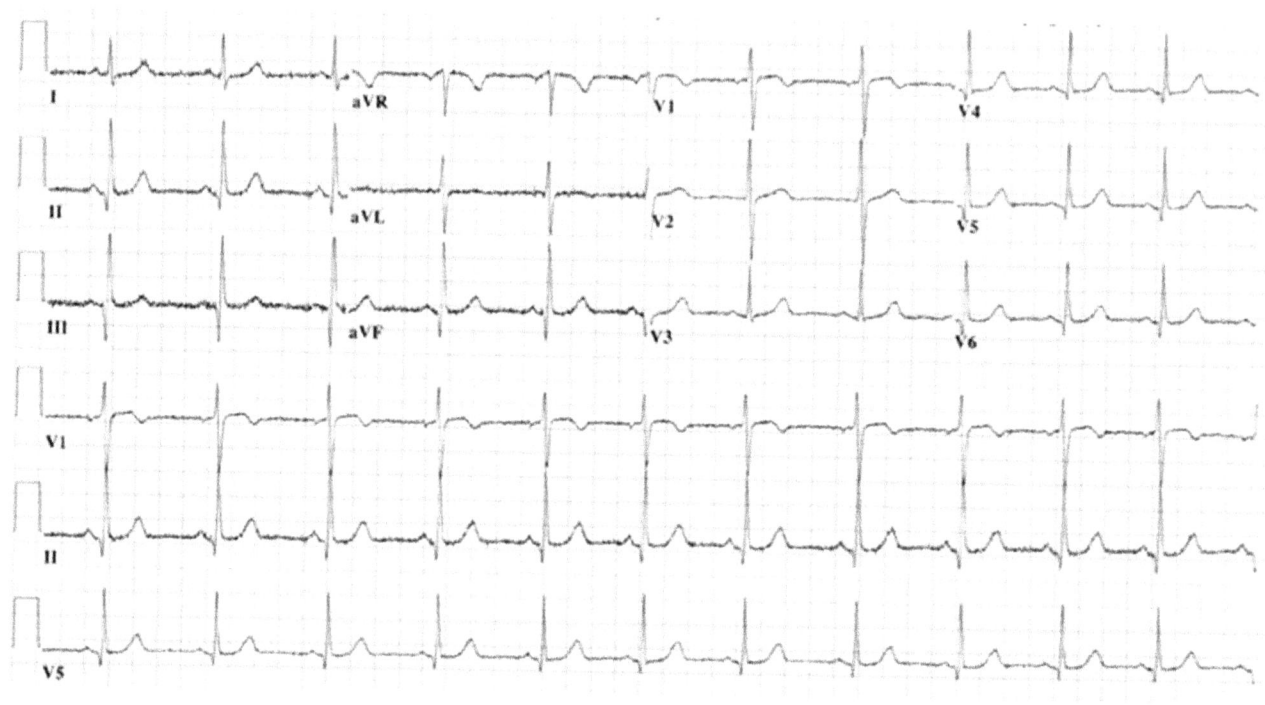

Figure 1.1 EKG.

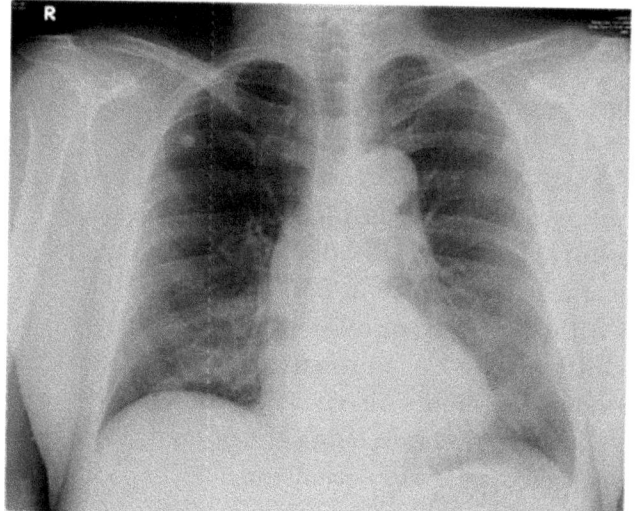

Figure 1.2 Chest x-ray.

A

B

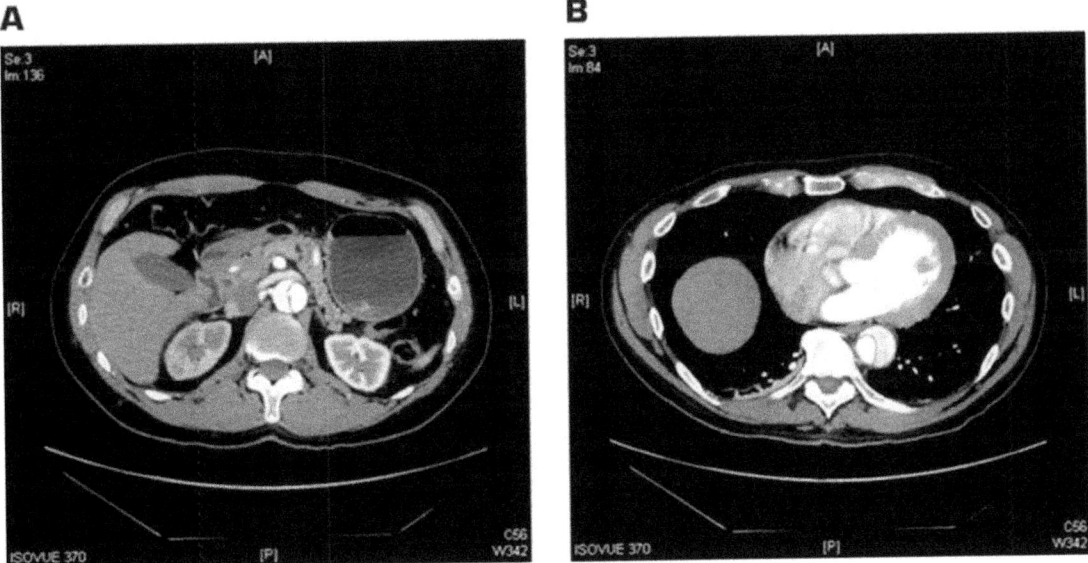

Figure 1.3 CT scan.

V. References
a. *Tintinalli's*: Chapter 59. Aortic Dissection and Related Aortic Syndromes
b. *Rosen's*: Chapter 71. Aortic Dissection

SAMPLE CASE SCRIPT

Here is one example of how the sample case could play out between an examiner and a candidate. Each case will run a very different course, depending on the examiner and the choices the candidate makes. This example is intended to highlight a few common circumstances that will come up during the cases. This is *not* an example of a "perfectly run" case.

EXAMINER:
You are working an overnight shift at General Hospital, and the next patient is a 55-year-old man with back pain. *(If you are making up the case, you get to name the hospital! Most cases should take place in an emergency department associated with a large hospital, but you can alter the scenarios as you like. During the certifying exam, "ABEM General" is the default location.)*

CANDIDATE:
What do I see when I walk into the room?

EXAMINER:
(From What does the patient look like?) The patient is lying on a stretcher, appears stated age; he is in mild distress as he attempts to find a position of comfort.

CANDIDATE:
May I have the vital signs?

EXAMINER:
(From Vital signs) Blood pressure: 165/90, heart rate: 90, respiratory rate: 16, temperature: 36.8°C orally, oxygen saturation: 98% on room air.

CANDIDATE:

I'd like to perform a primary survey. Is the patient able to speak?

EXAMINER:

(From the Primary survey) Yes, he is speaking in full sentences.

CANDIDATE:

How is his breathing? What does his skin look like?

EXAMINER:

(From the Primary survey) He is in no respiratory distress; there is no cyanosis. His skin is warm and moist, and he has normal capillary refill.

CANDIDATE:

The patient seems stable enough to obtain a further history. Sir, what brings you to the emergency department today?

EXAMINER:

(From the HPI section) Well, Doc, my back's been hurting me for a few hours now. I got this sharp pain in my lower back while I was walking to work. It came out of nowhere. It seemed to go down my left leg and up to my chest. *(If you are just starting out, you can just read the HPI as written. Once you become comfortable with the cases, it will be more interesting and true to the certifying exam format to act out the case a bit and speak as the patient in the first person.)*

CANDIDATE:

Is there a particular position that makes the pain worse or better?

EXAMINER:

No, and I can't seem to get into a comfortable position now, either. I've never had anything like this before.

CANDIDATE:

Were you exerting yourself at all? Have you been working out recently, or have you had any injury to the area?

EXAMINER:

No, nothing I can think of.

CANDIDATE:

Are you having any chest pain, trouble breathing, or palpitations?

EXAMINER:

The back pain seemed to go toward the chest as well. No trouble breathing or palpitations. *(If a symptom isn't mentioned in the case, feel free to say it is negative.)*

CANDIDATE:

I'd like to put this patient on a cardiac monitor, place an intravenous line, and start him on oxygen. We should hold some blood tubes for laboratory testing as well.

EXAMINER:

All right. The nurse has established a cardiac monitor, IV access, and placed the patient on oxygen. *(If you are comfortable with the way cases typically run, you can ask the candidate what type of IV and how much oxygen. If all these words are like a foreign language for you, just play the cases straight. Also, note how the candidate has the nurse place a line and draw labs early in the case. Since it is not yet clear which labs will need to be sent, the candidate just requests the nurse "hold" the blood for now. The cases in the rest of the book list lab tests early on, but that doesn't mean the candidate needs to order them before examining the patient or obtaining a history. They are listed early so the examiner has a rough idea of what might be requested or relevant. The examiner can have the nurse ask, "What labs would you like?" as the IV is placed, and the candidate should practice the reply, "Let's hold the samples for now until I have a bit more information.")*

CANDIDATE:

I'd like to examine the patient. How is the head and neck examination?

EXAMINER:

(Read the Secondary survey section, but do not give it away yet because the candidate was too vague.) What are you looking for?

CANDIDATE:

I'd like to examine the head for signs of injury. I'll check the pupils for reactivity, examine the retina for vascular abnormalities, check carotid pulses in the neck, listen for carotid bruits, ensure that the neck is supple and nontender …

EXAMINER:

(Now satisfied that the candidate knows how to examine the head and neck region.) The head and neck examination is normal. The neck is nontender, and there are no bruits. *(Some specific findings are listed, both normal and abnormal, to help the candidate in the case. In this case, it will be useful to note the lack of carotid bruits. The retina examination can be described as normal, because the entire eye examination was normal according to the case.)*

CANDIDATE:

Now I'll look at the chest and abdomen for signs of injury or other visible abnormalities. I'll listen to the lungs and heart as well.

EXAMINER:

The chest, heart, and lung examination is normal. *(Let's skip ahead a bit – the remainder of the physical examination in this case was unremarkable. Just remember to have the candidate specify what they are examining before giving them the examination results from the case.)*

CANDIDATE:

Sir, are you a smoker? Do you have any other medical problems? Are you allergic to any medications?

EXAMINER:

(From the History section) Yes, I smoke approximately three to four packs per week. I don't have any other medical problems or allergies. *(Note the candidate seems to be skipping around a bit. That's fine – you have all the answers in front of you and the examiner instructions tell you where the case should go. The candidate, however, may have an easier time if they follow a more algorithmic method of assessing the patient, as described in Chapter 3. This will significantly reduce the candidate's chances of missing something, and it should reduce anxiety on test day.)*

CANDIDATE:

I'd like to order some tests. May I have an EKG, chest x-ray, and labs including a CBC, chemistry panel, coagulation panel, UA, and type and hold?

EXAMINER:

(Check the Studies section and Examiner instructions.) No problem; the tests have been sent, and the patient will have an EKG and chest x-ray. Is there anything else you'd like?

CANDIDATE:

No, that's all for now.

EXAMINER:

(Following Examiner instructions) The nurse informs you that the patient is still having quite a bit of pain.

CANDIDATE:

Thank you. I'd like to order 6 mg of morphine intravenously.

EXAMINER:

The patient's pain is improved after receiving the morphine. *(If you are familiar with drug dosing, ask the candidate to be more specific with drug dosages and routes. Dosages are generally not mentioned in this book for simplicity.)*

EXAMINER:

Results of the tests are back. *(Also show candidate the laboratory results as printed in the case. Since the table can't be split up, show all the laboratory results in the table even if they weren't all requested. However, do not show images [EKG, CXR, etc.] for tests that were not ordered. Note there is no reading for the CXR and EKG in the case – the candidate is expected to interpret these images on his or her own. The interpretations are discussed at the end of each case. For other types of tests that the candidate is not expected to interpret on their own [such as an MRI], results will be communicated to the candidate by the examiner.)*

CANDIDATE:

Sir, how is your pain now?

EXAMINER:

(Following case, Reassess section) It was better for a while, but now it's back as bad as ever. I'm starting to feel a little chest pain and nausea.

CANDIDATE:

Let's repeat the vital signs.

EXAMINER:

(There are some repeat vital signs listed – since the patient hasn't received a β-antagonist, we'll use the vitals in the "no β-antagonists" section of Reassess.) Blood pressure: 170/ 100, heart rate: 100, respiratory rate: 18, oxygen saturation: 100% on 2L NC.

CANDIDATE:

All right. I'd like to consult cardiology.

EXAMINER:

(This consultation was not described in the instructions! When this happens, the consultant will offer no useful information to the candidate, and the candidate will have to continue with the case as they would manage the case on their own. If the candidate is having trouble with some aspect of the case, the consultant can be used to give them a hint. For the purposes of the exam, consultants generally serve to perform some specific action that an emergency physician

cannot, such as performing an operation, admitting a patient, or performing a specialized study. When asked to give their opinion on a case or provide a diagnosis, they will not be helpful.) We have Dr. Harmon from cardiology on the phone. (In character) This is Dr. Harmon, what's going on?

CANDIDATE:
I have a patient here with back pain radiating to the chest *(describes the case)*. I need a consult.

EXAMINER:
I'm not sure what you need me to do. What do you think is going on with the patient?

CANDIDATE:
Well, it could be a heart attack, renal colic, an aortic aneurysm, or dissection, or some trauma we've missed. But I think he might be sick.

EXAMINER:
Why don't you figure it out a bit more and call me if you need me. *(Hangs up.)*

CANDIDATE:
I'd like to order a CT scan of the abdomen.

EXAMINER:
All right. The radiologist wants to know what you're looking for so they can protocol the study appropriately.

CANDIDATE:
Renal colic, an aortic aneurysm, or dissection; less likely to be some occult trauma.

EXAMINER:
The patient gets the CT scan. *(Show the candidate Figure 1.3.)*

CANDIDATE:
This looks like an aortic dissection. Do we have an official reading on this?

EXAMINER:
Yes. It is read as a dissection of the descending thoracic aorta extending to the abdominal aorta and left iliac artery. There is no involvement of the aortic arch. *(Candidates would not normally be expected to interpret this type of study. Thus, the results are given in the text of the case. These images are included in this book for their educational value.)*

CANDIDATE:
I'd like to move the patient to the critical care area of the ED. Place a second large-bore intravenous line, please. I'd like to start an esmolol drip.

EXAMINER:
Done. Would you like anything else?

CANDIDATE:
I'd like to repeat the vital signs and contact vascular surgery.

EXAMINER:
(Now we can use the vitals in the "β-antagonists" section of Reassess.) Blood pressure: 110/55, heart rate: 55, respiratory rate: 18, oxygen saturation: 100% on 2L NC. Vascular surgery *(Dr. Mcdia)* is on the phone for you.

CANDIDATE:

Dr. Media, this is Dr. Candidate in the ED. We have a type B aortic dissection in the ED who arrived with back pain radiating to his chest and leg. He was initially hypertensive but we've started him on an esmolol drip and his vital signs and symptoms have improved.

EXAMINER:

Thank you; can you admit him to the ICU and we'll see him there? *(The candidate has a similar discussion with the ICU staff and the patient's primary care physician, and the patient is admitted.)*

At this point, the candidate should read through the case themselves, focusing on the critical actions, examiner instructions, and pearls. References should be examined to solidify understanding of the disease processes from the case. Each case will contain a reference from *Rosen's* and *Tintinalli's*. The formal references are detailed below.

REFERENCES

Walls RM, Hockberger R, Gausche-Hill M, Erickson TB, Wilcox SR. eds. (2023). *Rosen's Emergency Medicine: Concepts and Clinical Practice.* 10th ed. Elsevier.

Tintinalli JE, Ma O, Yealy DM, Meckler GD, Stapczynski J, Cline DM, Thomas SH. eds. (2020). *Tintinalli's Emergency Medicine: A Comprehensive Study Guide*, 9th ed. McGraw-Hill Education.

CHAPTER 2

EM Medical Decision-Making

Scott Weingart, MD, FCCM

This chapter discusses the cognitive processes of emergency medicine (EM). It is applicable to our approach in the department and to the more artificial environment of the board exam. Decision-making in EM is quite different than most of the other fields in medicine. The novice may assume that we make most of our decisions using conscious contemplation, perhaps because this is the path the novice is forced to take. The reality is that if we had to think about every diagnosis and treatment during the course of a shift, we would be crushed under the cognitive load. Imagine for a moment how effortlessly you walk or speak; would these be as easy if you were consciously guiding each muscle contraction?

ILLNESS SCRIPTS

Thinking is the last resort; it is slow and – counterintuitively – predisposes us to error. Most of our decisions are made by pattern matching. Using only a few lines from the patient's history, a brief physical examination, some basic tests such as glucose level, and most importantly a gestalt impression of how the patient looks, we can usually narrow the differential to one or perhaps a couple of possibilities. The process takes only seconds. We match the patient's presentation to an accumulation of all of the similar presentations we have seen or read about throughout our careers; this accumulation is referred to as an illness script. It is only when we do not have an illness script to match with the patient in front of us that we are forced to resort to other decision-making techniques.

All of the cases on the oral board exam should be approached by pattern matching. These patients should not be anomalies; they will be bread and butter presentations. If you cannot match the case, you are probably missing something, but do not give up hope. In this situation and in real life, we can fall back on three strategies: heuristics, analytic thinking, and shotgunning.

HEURISTICS

Heuristics are mental shortcuts; they are a pathway to rapid action without formal analysis. We use many heuristics in the practice of EM. Some of them can predispose us to error – for example, all reproducible chest pain is benign. However, there are many heuristics that are indispensable and lead to good outcomes on both the exam and for our patients. Some examples of useful EM heuristics are as follows.

Sick/Not Sick Paradigm

The immediate dichotomization between sick/not sick is the most important heuristic in EM. Sometimes, we'll have no idea what is going on with a patient, but we have an intuition that they are unwell. That patient is going to be admitted and we are going to fix every vital-sign abnormality and address any positive diagnostic tests. If the patient looks well, but has a vague complaint, we may send them home with close follow-up even if we do not have a final diagnosis. Unfortunately, this heuristic can fail if the patient looks pristine but has a life-threatening illness. For instance, an acute acetaminophen overdose can cause this heuristic to fail.

Age Heuristic

Another valuable heuristic relates to the elderly. Very few presentations should lead to the discharge of a patient older than 75 years old; similarly, a patient under 40 years old needs to be pretty sick to get admitted. *If they're old we hold, if they're young they're sprung* will often lead to an appropriate decision.

The ABCs Heuristic

Fundamental to EM is falling back on the ABCs for our initial approach to any sick patient. Over the years, I have added to this alphabetical heuristic. Box 2.1 lists an approach to a sick patient for the boards or in the resuscitation room.

Box 2.1

Airway
Breathing
Circulation
Disability-pupillary reaction, GCS (Glasgow coma scale), and ability to move all four extremities
Exposure/environment – see every inch of skin and then keep the patient warm
Finger stick (can also mean finger-do rectal if appropriate)
Girls and women get a pregnancy test
Hang antibiotics (early antibiotics for all of your sepsis patients and preprocedural antibiotics in your trauma patients)
Inject tetanus when appropriate (you may forget it later on)

ANALYTIC THINKING

Careful use of deductive reasoning is the proper approach when the previous strategies have not yielded answers. Thinking is hard; we should reserve it for when it serves us best. As we gain experience, we need to think about fewer cases; most of our answers will come to us through subconscious pattern matching and the use of proven heuristics. If, during the oral boards, you are forced to resort to analytic thinking, you are in a difficult situation. Thinking under enormous stress is difficult, but not insurmountable. It is acceptable to take a second, close your eyes, and reorganize your perceptions. By the same token, in the hectic, chaotic environment of the emergency department, finding a quiet corner for a moment can often improve our analytic processing.

SHOTGUNNING

This is a cognitively bereft heuristic, but every so often you are left with little else. Shotgunning involves sending every laboratory test and radiographic study that is vaguely applicable and hoping something comes back that reveals an answer. This is very low-level cognitive reasoning. If you are resorting to shotgunning during your exam, it is doubtful that a passing score will be the result. Using this technique in the department will lead to wasted money and unnecessary testing.

Cognitive Checkpoint

Before completing our care of any patient, we need to stop and consciously ask ourselves if we are missing anything. This is perhaps the most important error-prevention strategy we can use in our field. During the board exam, it is just as important. Take a moment and review your performance; you may pick up errors that you initially missed. For example, after taking a history and completing a primary and secondary survey, it may be helpful to review the facts of the case thus far before ordering tests. This will give you an opportunity to fill in any gaps, allow yourself to see a pattern that you may have missed, and will better crystallize your thought processes for the examiner.

In conclusion, our approach to decisions in EM bears similarities to the fields of anesthesiology and critical care, but is different than the other fields in medicine. We arrive at thousands of decision nodes in the course of a shift. If we had to think about every one of them, we could not function at a high level. Most of our decisions are made by unconscious processes that can predispose us to error if our knowledge base is poor, our experience lacking, or our vision clouded by emotion or stress. However, when we are prepared and clear-minded, a shift can feel cognitively effortless; I hope your board exam experience is the same.

CHAPTER 3

About the Oral Boards: The Approach and Practical Tips

Christina Hajicharalambous, DO, MSEd, MS and Rebecca Hellmann, DO

Emergency medicine (EM) is rich in what is known as narrative medicine. Stories are the foundation of our practice. Patients tell us their stories. We edit them and add in our own details (test results, radiography, etc.). We often retell these stories: if we are students to attending physicians during clinical rotations; if we are attendings or residents to colleagues and consultants when we seek input into a complex case; and even back to patients when we have solved the case, or at least written the next chapter.

It is wholly appropriate that the American Board of Emergency Medicine (ABEM) and the American Osteopathic Board of Emergency Medicine (AOBEM) incorporate an oral examination into their certification process. As a process, the oral examination involves elements of an Observed Structured Clinical Encounter (OSCE) and simulation, though it does not incorporate high-fidelity simulation (yet). As with an OSCE, the process must be organized and thorough because it is observed and scored. Like a simulated patient, it evolves in a version of "real time" in which decisions and commitment to certain pathways must be made. You must interact with the examiner as if you are speaking to a real patient, a real family member, a real consultant, or other real staff.

The oral board examination "stories" unfold over a virtual platform. Prior to your examination date, you will do a technology check with an ABEM team to ensure your equipment and setup is compatible with the exam requirements. After the tech check is complete, you will receive a link that will go live on the day of the exam. On examination day, you will log on and be placed in a virtual waiting room. Examiners will come into your virtual room for each testing session, with a small break between sessions.

An oral exam case differs from a conventional story in that you are very much a part of how the story unfolds, but you must always remember that it is already written. The authors have created a story for you with a beginning, a middle, and an ending. The beginning will appear as a written prompt on your screen: patient name, gender, mode of arrival, chief complaint, and triage vitals. The middle of the story is a series of critical actions that you must take along the way. Many of these are similar from case to case: undress the patient; check a rapid blood glucose; ask EMS to stay to give further history. Others will be quite case-specific – for example, checking salicylate levels in an elderly patient with altered mental status. The ideal ending may be known, but it is flexible. Success on the test doesn't always mean that the patient walks away unharmed. Perhaps the patient is meant to die no matter what, and the goal of the case is to marshal the resources of your department (social worker, private family room) to deliver the news to the family and discuss organ donation.

The process is one of asking for more details, descriptions, and taking actions. After reading the initial prompt, often the best way to start is "I approach the patient; what do I see?" Though things may change rapidly as they do in real life, you should get a first impression of what intervention is needed. For example, ABCs for a patient in full arrest; lines and monitoring if the patient is critical; time for a further history if the patient is awake and talking to you. As you move through the case, as with any good story, you must constantly ask, "And then? What happened next?" If you order tests, ask for the results. If you made an intervention, be sure to go back and reassess the patient and their vital signs afterward.

The examiner holds onto the details of the story until you ask for them. There are a series of results – some necessary, some unnecessary – that the examiner will show you on your screen when asked. If you do not ask *specifically* for a blood urea nitrogen (BUN) or creatinine, do not expect to be given one. If you do not *specifically* say, "Please put the patient on a cardiac monitor with a continuous oxygenation saturation," it will not happen. You will need to ask, "What is the oxygen saturation?" to learn the result. If you place a hypoxic patient on oxygen, reassess their saturation. If you fail to do so, you may miss methemoglobinemia or a patient who will require intubation. Remember, you must explicitly ask for whatever piece of information you need. One strategy is to cognitively offload the task of following up to your examiner. By saying, "Nurse, please send the following labs and let me know when the results have returned," you place the onus of reporting results to you on the examiner – but keep in mind that they are not obligated to follow this request.

Over the course of 5 hours, each participant goes through seven scenarios: five single case encounters, two structured interview cases. The single case encounters are typically around 15 minutes; listen for subtle clues where the examiner is hinting at speeding up or slowing down the case. Though direct pathophysiology questions were dropped in 2002, the examiners still test knowledge base by asking for electrocardiogram (ECG) or radiography interpretations, doses for critical medications, or even the information that you provide to a consultant or a family member in a scenario. The best strategy for this is to think through the interpretation of any labs, imagining aloud as you are working through the scenario.

Your examiners are master storytellers. They are leaders in the field of EM. They have been well trained in the cases they are giving and will probably only work with two or three cases over the days that the test is administered. They know the details of their stories inside out. Some will try more than others to act out the script: You might be expected to interact with them as if they were the pregnant teenager in their case. Others might just stick to narrating the case for you. Though the resources of the hospital are available to you, examiners will not let you use consultants for answers to questions or look up information in a textbook if the question is within the scope of knowledge expected as an EM physician (e.g., common drugs, fracture patterns, ECG interpretation); your examiner may tell you that the consultant is not available if they expect you to know this information.

The key to preparation is practice. The medical knowledge content is similar to that of the written exam, which you will have already passed as a prerequisite to sit for the oral exam. There is a slight focus on cardiovascular topics, toxicology, and trauma; if these have been your weak areas in the past, they definitely require review. It is best to sit down with this book and practice as many scenarios as possible, aloud, with a friend. If you are able to practice with someone in a virtual setting, it is helpful to get used to the feeling of the technology and interacting through the computer screen. The back-and-forth exchange is different from your typical conversations about patients at work, though the content will be similar.

The oral certifying examination can be nerve-wracking. Remember, though, that you have been doing this through residency and every working day since finishing your residency – only in a different format. Instead of getting the story from a patient, you are getting it from your examiner. Your confidence will grow with repetition as you practice cases in this book. At the most basic level the examiner holds a story about a patient. Your challenge is to get the details of that story from the examiner in a smooth and rational manner. The rest of this chapter contains practical tips for the day, as well as one approach to the oral board encounter.

PRACTICAL TIPS

- Ensure you have a computer that can easily run the software required for the exam.
- Set yourself up in a quiet area with a reliable Wi-Fi connection to avoid technological or interpersonal interruptions.
- Sleep and eat well. Nothing too heavy to eat the night before; make sure you eat and go to sleep at a reasonable time. You want to keep your mind sharp for the next day. Eat breakfast the following morning but don't eat something that may make you uncomfortable during the exam. If you think you might get hungry, have a small snack and a glass of water on your desk or surrounding area – you are able to eat or drink as needed during your breaks.
- Dress professionally but comfortably. Dress as you would for a job interview.
- Smile and be polite. Once you are placed in your breakout room for your encounter with the examiner, introduce yourself and greet them with a smile. Though these exams are standardized, it never hurts to be pleasant to the examiner. We are all human, including the examiners. Never argue with the examiner, no matter what.
- Play the game. Don't think, "This is so artificial" or "I'd get it if it were a real patient." The examination is what it is: an exam to test your skills. Be compassionate when you are talking to the family or a patient. Suspend any disbelief about the artificial environment and try to pretend you are in the clinical environment.
- Have something that will help you keep track of time – you will not be allowed to wear a watch or have a phone, so having a clock in view is helpful.
- Have a pen/pencil and a few back-ups just in case. You will be provided an exam packet to print out, including seven sheets of paper with a human body on it, standardized for the oral exam. Use them. This will be detailed in the next section.
- You will have a 2-minute warning prior to the examiner entering the virtual space. Take this time to reset your work space, take deep breaths, and prepare yourself. Once the examiner enters the room, you will confirm your identity, the examiner will read a standard introduction, and the exam will begin.
- The examiner will let you know when you have finished the encounter. They will ask you to tear up your notes in front of them. Do not read into what they say or do not say when the case is over. They are not supposed to give you any hints on how you did during or after and they are coached to not change facial expression during the exam. Just because you do not hear "great job" or see a smile on their face does not mean you did not do well. Just clear your mind and go to the next case.

THE APPROACH

There are many ways to approach the oral boards cases. It is likely that you have done some mock oral boards exams during your residency and have learned a format that works for you. If it works, stick with it. As described in Chapter 2, EM physicians' brains work in ways that differ from many specialties. Because we work in a chaotic environment with multiple patients and typically high volumes, we rely on pattern matching and heuristics. The experienced EM physician knows when a patient is sick because of their "look," abnormal vital signs, or concerning trends in their appearance upon reassessment.

Unfortunately, the oral boards are an artificial environment and we lose the edge that we have come to rely on – our senses. The smell of melena, recognition of cyanotic lips, the use of accessory muscles to breathe, and subtle hints of delirium in an older patient must be revealed through asking questions instead of automatically presenting themselves to the candidate. As a result, the candidate theoretically starts at a slight disadvantage in the encounter compared to the true clinical environment. Fortunately, there is one aspect of the oral boards that we can use to our advantage: The examiner cannot lie and they are not there to trick you. This means if you ask them about breath sounds on the left side of the chest, they have to say "yes" or "no." We do not have to second guess ourselves and wait for the chest x-ray (CXR) to place a chest tube in a penetrating trauma.

To overcome the situational disadvantage of the artificial physician–patient encounter, we have to maximize our data collection in an efficient way. The following approach may seem overly detailed and time-consuming, but if done correctly, with practice it will likely save you time in the long run. This is so you do not have to go back to ask, "What was the rectal exam again?" or say, "Whoops, that patient had a penicillin allergy?"

You will be permitted seven standardized pieces of scratch paper with a human body drawn on each, along with pens/pencils. Take the initial time upfront to set yourself up for success. Use your paper and outline key portions of the encounter you will want to remember. Divide the rest of the paper into four quadrants, labeled as illustrated in Figure 3.1. Do this just *before* starting the case. This should take you less than 1 minute.

History (HPI) box: The top-left box will be where you record information relevant to the patient's chief complaint, as well as history and review of systems (ROS).

Exam box: The bottom-left box is the vitals and physical examination box. Memorize and write down all of the abbreviations before beginning so that you will not forget to ask about certain aspects of the examination. You might not end up asking for all of them (like a rectal examination in a patient with an ankle sprain). But some things may not be obvious unless you ask about it. For example, you may encounter a patient with left-sided sharp chest pain for 3 days, which is constant and not made worse with breathing. Unless you ask about the skin examination, you may miss the vesicular lesions along a dermatomal distribution seen in zoster. Be vague initially; if a portion of the examination is normal, the examiner will just say "normal" and you can move on. If it is especially relevant to the case or there are abnormalities to be discovered, they may ask you, "What are you looking for?" Then you would need to be more detailed by asking questions, such as, "Are there equal breath sounds, crackles, wheezes, rubs, crepitus, etc.?"

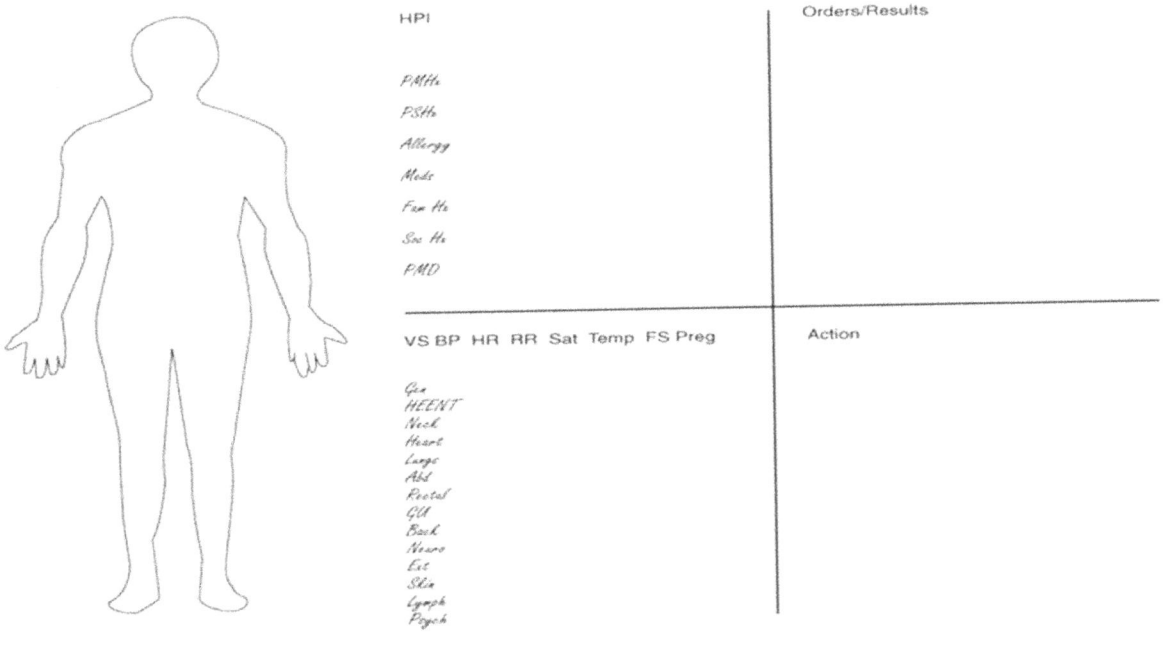

Figure 3.1 Sample oral boards note sheet with suggested labels.

Orders and results: The top-right box is where you order tests and put the results. If you ask for a test such as a complete blood count (CBC) or basic metabolic panel (BMP), be sure to ask for the results later; they are not obligated to give them to you automatically. One technique is to say, "Nurse, can I have a CBC, BMP, PT/PTT, and type and cross and can you give the results to me as soon as they are available." Keep in mind, this is not always a fool proof method and make sure to circle back on everything you have ordered. The other way to keep track is to write it down in the box. Once you have the result, you can write it down or put a check next to it.

Action: The bottom-right box is your action box. Here you'll record what you've done: whether antibiotics or tetanus was administered, consults you've requested, and disposition (such as the OR or ICU). While using this book, if you find you always forget to do a critical task or action, write this task here too (e.g., given antibiotics or making a patient NPO). It may not be relevant to the case on exam day, but you will not forget to do it if you write it down.

The picture on the left of the paper can be used to help visualize the patient.

Now you're ready to start the case – it begins when you tell the examiner, "I'm ready." The examiner will show you the prompt, as described earlier.

Name: Frank Jordan
Chief complaint: Abdominal pain
Age: 50
Mode of arrival: Private vehicle
Temp: 36.8
HR: 87 bpm
BP: 157/82
Resp: 18
SpO2: 98% on RA

At this point you need to assess whether the patient is sick or not sick and perform the ABCDEs, intervening when necessary.

The first question should always be either "What does the patient look like?" or "What do I see, hear, and smell as I walk into the room?" Either will give you a gestalt of how sick the patient is. If the patient is critical, you will need to act immediately to stabilize them.

The next step is to consider vital signs. Vitals are extremely important and will tell you a lot about the status of the patient. Continue throughout the case to frequently repeat vital signs *especially* after an intervention, such as medication administration or procedure.

The third step is the *primary survey* – ABCDEs. This is also done when you want to ask the nurse to start an intravenous line (IV), O_2, and monitor if appropriate. Specifically, place two large-bore (16- to 18-gauge) angiocatheters in the antecubital fossa, start oxygen either by nasal cannula or nonrebreather mask, and place the patient on a monitor. Not all patients may warrant these steps (the patient with an ankle sprain, for example), but most sick patients will need these as a minimum. If the patient has an abnormal A, B, C, D, or E, you may need to intervene before moving on.

- The patient with GCS < 8 in a trauma or respiratory distress may need to be intubated.
- With altered mental status, check a blood sugar and intervene if suspicion for a specific underlying cause.
- Place a chest tube or needle decompression in a tension pneumothorax.
- Start blood or fluid boluses in a hypotensive patient.
- Apply pressure to large wounds that are bleeding.

This is also when you may ask for stat items like EKG or CXR if the patient has severe chest pain or respiratory distress.

Now the history. EMS offers valuable information, but if you wait too long they will leave the ED. Ask them to stick around early in the case, so you do not lose them if you need to stabilize the patient first. They can give you valuable information about the mechanism of injury, pills at the bedside, or the condition of the patient's home, as well as what treatments were given in the field.

Use the history box to record the history of present illness (HPI) and other history. Do not forget important things such as drug, alcohol, smoking history, do not resuscitate (DNR) status, and allergies. Use all resources available, such as the patient, nursing home papers, family or friends, and primary medical doctor. *Do not order medication for a patient until you have checked their allergies.*

Once you have some idea of the history and have stabilized the patient, you can move on to the *secondary survey.* Refer to the physical examination box. As discussed earlier, ask general questions such as "What is the lung exam like?" If the examiner wants to know what you're thinking, they will ask, "What are you looking for?" Otherwise, they will say "Normal."

Continue to repeat vital signs throughout the case, especially after an intervention (such as oxygen or drug administration). It can be helpful to ask for the reevaluation. For example, say "Nurse, please put the patient on 3L nasal cannula and let me know of any changes, up or down, of the oxygen saturation immediately." Also, ask the patient how they are doing after each intervention (e.g., ask "How is the pain?" after giving morphine).

Orders and results box: Once you have an idea of what's going on with the patient, you will usually order laboratory tests, radiology studies, and so on. You may have already sent basic laboratory work, but you can add relevant data here. Avoid trying to shotgun lots of tests, as the examiner can deduct points if you are wasting resources. Mark down what you ordered because you may forget, and the nurse does not have to voluntarily offer you the information once the results are available. Ask the nurse to give you the results when available.

Action box: Treat pain, give antibiotics for infections early, order tetanus for wounds, get appropriate consultants, and manage all the issues relevant to the chief complaint. You may be asked to describe how you would perform a procedure, so be prepared (refer to Appendix G). Also, don't forget social workers or child protective services in abuse cases, calling primary care doctors to discuss the patient, talking to family and the patient to update them on their status, explain all procedures, and appropriate disposition.

Upon completion of the case, the examiner will tell you that the time is up. They will ask you to tear up your notes, then they will exit the breakout room. You will have a short break between cases, but your camera and microphone must remain on at all times. After the case, clear your mind from it and move on to mentally prepare for the next case.

THE STRUCTURED INTERVIEW

Every day during a patient encounter, we take in hundreds of small clues that inform our decision-making and diagnostic algorithms. Most of the time, this analysis is done in our heads, quickly and almost instinctively. But what we choose to focus on and how we choose to incorporate it into the management of our patient can ultimately determine diagnosis and outcome. The structured interview is designed so that the ABEM examiner can understand your thought process and how you sift through all of the information presented to you about a given patient presentation. It is to evaluate your critical thinking skills, ensuring that your thought process – and not just algorithmic thinking – is correct. Throughout the structured interview, the interviewer will give you different pieces of information and ask how you are using or assessing that information. It is as if they are giving you individual pieces of a puzzle and asking you how you are putting it together and why you are making the choices you are.

The Approach

The structured interview will begin similarly to the cases: The examiner will enter your virtual space, tell you they are evaluating you via structured interview, and give you a prompt just as they did with the cases. They will go through a series of questions, starting with the history, then physical, diagnostics studies, then interventions to assess your approach to different chief complaints. They may ask you to clarify an answer you give, asking why you chose to order a test or what you were looking for during a part of your physical exam. Some sample structured interview questions are:

1. Knowing this chief complaint, what other information would you want to elicit from this patient?
2. What specifically are you looking for when you are examining the abdomen?
3. How will a urinalysis change your management for this patient?
4. What specifically are you looking for on a CT scan?
5. What would need to change in this patient's condition for you to change your disposition?

The interview progresses very similarly, if not exactly the same, as the sample interview that ABEM has on their website (www.abem.org/public/become-certified/oral-exam/types-of-cases-and-samples). Watching that video will fully prepare you for the style and order of the structured interview.

Just as with the sample cases, when the interview is finished, the examiner will tell you that the time is up. They will ask you to tear up your notes, then they will exit the breakout room. Once they leave, take a deep breath and start readying yourself for the next case or interview.

ABEM AND AOBEM DIFFERENCES

There are not many differences between the ABEM and AOBEM oral examinations. The key distinctions are discussed here. If not mentioned specifically, assume the exam is identical to what has already been described in this chapter.

AOBEM does not have a structured interview case. The exam consists of eight single cases that are tested two cases at a time for a total of 30 minutes for the two cases.

Given the ever-changing circumstance with regards to the format of either exam, it is always best to visit each of the following websites for the most up to date information.

- ABEM exam: www.abem.org/public/become-certified/oral-exam
- AOBEM exam: https://certification.osteopathic.org/emergency-medicine/certification-process-overview/specialty-certification-process/oral-exams

In 2026, ABEM plans to launch an in-person certifying exam to replace the oral certification exam. All candidates will be required to complete this examination in person at a testing center in Raleigh, North Carolina.

CHAPTER 4

About the Oral Boards: Format and Scoring

Michael Cassara, DO, MSEd

INTRODUCTION AND BRIEF HISTORY

For over 40 years, major emergency medicine (EM) certification boards worldwide[1] have used objective structured oral examinations ("oral examinations") as summative assessments of physician candidates seeking initial board certification. In the United States, these examinations are key components of board certification pathways sponsored by the American Board of Emergency Medicine (ABEM) and American Board of Osteopathic Emergency Medicine (AOBEM). Both organizations use oral examinations as complementary assessment methods to computer-based tests containing single best answer multiple choice questions (MCQs). The oral examinations of both organizations have similar features, resulting from their common grounding in the theory and science of simulation-based education. Candidates are immersed in hypothetical scenarios where they must verbalize the management of simulated patients presenting for emergency care. Candidates are expected to apply and demonstrate the cognition, skills, and affective characteristics expected of independently practicing emergency physicians, including the clinical reasoning, decision-making, and diagnostic interpretations they make while engaged in these simulated scenarios. Examiners portray simulated nonplayer characters and provide descriptions of environments and situational contexts, including responses to candidates' actions. In most oral examinations, the decisions made by candidates influence the turns and twists cases take and, ultimately, the outcomes of patients being managed. Candidates' actions reveal their underlying thought processes and knowledge and are used as surrogate measures informing judgments supporting or refuting their claim for board certification.

Surprisingly, the structure and content for the oral examinations for both certification boards remained largely unchanged until only very recently. Most oral examinations implemented prior to 2017 are best described as low-technology ("pencil and paper" or "tabletop") simulations. The pre-2017 ABEM Oral Certification Examination (OCE) included five simulated patient encounters (SPEs) and two simulated situation encounters (SSEs). Simulated patient encounters ("single case scenarios") were assessments of candidates' abilities to describe the simulated diagnostic and therapeutic management of individual patients. Simulated situation encounters ("triple case scenarios") differed in that the assessment focus was candidates' abilities to verbalize the contemporaneous management of and task-switching among three simulated patients. AOBEM's Emergency Medicine Oral Exam during this same period consisted of three testing stations during which candidates

---

[1] For brevity, the scope of this chapter is focused on OCE formats used by the two major EM certifying boards (ABEM, AOBEM) in the United States. EM certifying boards in other countries that also rely on OCE incorporate similar principles of sound assessment and rigor while incorporating formats, styles, and standards specific to their learners, patients, norms, customs, cultures, and society. These other OCEs are not discussed in this chapter. Any consequence or offense generated by the author's editorial decision to omit these from discussion is unintended.

managed two simulated patients simultaneously. A fourth station was used to assess candidates' interpretations of diagnostic tests and other visual stimuli (e.g., 12-lead electrocardiogram traces).

In 2017, ABEM began pilot testing the transformation of its single patient encounter low-technology simulations into technology-enhanced computer-based simulations (coining the phrase "eOral[2] patient case" for this examination case format). ABEM quickly integrated this novel format of case delivery within a few cycles of pilot testing. Almost simultaneously, AOBEM began modifying its oral examination processes. In 2020, however, both ABEM and AOBEM were compelled to make significant adaptations to the testing experience in response to the global COVID pandemic. A concise summary of these changes includes the following:

- Both ABEM and AOBEM migrated to entirely synchronous, online learning environments,[3] enabling examiners and examinees to interact and communicate without the need for travel or direct physical interaction. ABEM renamed the oral examination as the Virtual Oral Exam (VOE); AOBEM continues to use the Emergency Medicine Oral Exam.
- ABEM suspended use of the eOral Patient Case with its move to the VOE format. ABEM examiners who previously delivered cases under the eOral format reverted to administering cases using modifications to the methods used previously for the SPE. This new virtual SPE is rebranded as the *single-patient case.*
- ABEM retired the SSE format, implementing the *structured interview* as its replacement. The structured interview is an entirely new testing format that will be covered more extensively later in the chapter.
- AOBEM integrated the content from an independent fourth station ("special diagnosis identification cases") – dedicated to the assessment of candidates' abilities to interpret conventional radiographs, electrocardiograms, and a variety of other visual stimuli – into its simulated case scenarios. Previously, these were projected on a large screen in a conference room. To accommodate this change, AOBEM has expanded the number of stations (four instead of three) and cases (eight instead of six) it delivers to candidates as part of its Emergency Medicine Oral Exam. In contrast to ABEM's decision to retire the SSE, AOBEM continues to deliver two simulated patients within each station of its oral examination.
- AOBEM retired the Clinical Exam for all candidates who have applied for initial primary board certification in EM after 2013.
- ABEM made slight modifications to the content areas from the Model of Clinical Practice of EM emphasized on the VOE (thoracic-respiratory disorders replaced toxicologic emergencies).
- As of January 2023, ABEM recodified the skills and abilities assessed, by percentage of overall performance, during the VOE; these include: communication (10–15%); data gathering (10–15%); synthesis (20–30%); management (15–25%); disposition (15–25%); and judgment/other (10–15%).

Oral examinations as summative assessments remain controversial. Critics of summative oral examinations describe them as intimidating and disorienting assessments that impose significant real and potential costs (e.g., direct financial burdens and opportunity costs) upon candidates and key stakeholders without sufficient validity evidence supporting their use. Proponents of summative oral examinations assert that this format assesses competencies necessary for the independent practice of EM that remain unobservable and, therefore, unassessed through completion of the single best answer MCQ examinations alone. Proponents also assert that summative oral examinations

---

[2] "eOral" is the short form for the term "enhanced Oral" as described by Kowalenko et al. (2017).

[3] At the time of publication, ABEM is using Zoom (Zoom Video Communications, Inc., San Jose, CA); AOBEM is using MonitorEDU (MonitorEDU, Spring Hill, TN).

align well with the enhanced emphasis on competency-based outcomes prevalent in undergraduate and graduate medical education. Regardless, oral examinations and the adaptations described are poised to remain as significant components of the EM board certification process in the United States until other methods emerge.

The aim of this chapter is to reassure and prepare the prospective candidate about to engage in this segment of their board certification pathway by providing them with the most current information about the oral examination format and scoring to promote optimal performance. Candidates preparing for these simulation-based examinations benefit immensely from understanding the structure, content, procedures, technical characteristics, and scoring rubrics defining the "game." Whenever possible, similarities and differences between the ABEM and AOBEM examinations will be presented. As the intended audience for this textbook includes all physician candidates preparing for ABEM and AOBEM board certification examinations, this chapter has been intentionally framed with these examinations exclusively in mind. Finally, readers should acknowledge that any attempt to provide immediately current information in the format of a textbook carries the inherent risk of rapidly becoming obsolete. Nevertheless, the editors and I suspect the insights and discussions that follow will benefit current and future cohorts of board certification examination candidates until more significant process changes are made.

NEW CERTIFYING EXAM

ABEM has announced plans to retire the current virtual OCE in 2025. In its place, ABEM will initiate the in-person Certifying Exam for 2026. While many similarities between the OCE and the Certifying Exam exist, the new format will allow better assessment of procedural skills, ultrasound skills, communications, prioritization, task-switching, and other key skills for emergency physicians. The Certifying Exam will take place in person at the AIME Center, a professional assessment center in Raleigh, North Carolina.

STRUCTURE AND PROCESS OF THE ABEM VOE

The ABEM VOE is the second part of a two-step certification pathway that is offered biannually in the spring and fall of each calendar year. Candidates who successfully complete the ABEM Qualifying Examination are eligible to sit for the ABEM VOE. ABEM assigns candidates to a precise day and session; this assignment is made by email far in advance of the VOE testing period. Each ABEM examination day is subdivided into two 3-hour and 50-minute sessions ("morning" and "afternoon"). Invitations provide examinees with check-in and exam start times and links to external webpages where candidates register and create login passwords. These web pages provide the links candidates use to connect to their individualized Zoom meetings with examiners.

The VOE testing sessions start with a 25-minute check-in period (beginning 45 minutes prior to the first case), during which identification credentials are confirmed and video "sweeps" of testing environments are performed. Following the check-in period, candidates experience seven 15-minute time blocks during which five single-patient cases and two structured interviews are administered. All ABEM VOE formats (single-patient cases and structured interviews) are timed; candidates must complete all critical actions and case-related tasks within 15 minutes. A brief break (10–20 minutes) is provided between the fourth and fifth testing period. Finally, one simulation is used for "field-testing" a new scenario or for research purposes and does not contribute to one's overall summative assessment.

The summative judgment is based on each candidate's overall performance across all scored oral examination formats. Therefore, each candidate must effectively manage up to seven simulated encounters (five single-patient cases and two structured interviews) over the entire testing period. A comprehensive description of the content, process, policies, procedures, implementation, and scoring of the ABEM VOE, along with a comprehensive video demonstration of both the single-patient case and structured interview oral examination formats, is available on the ABEM website.

ABEM STRUCTURED INTERVIEW

As the structured interview represents a distinctly novel departure from oral examination formats previously employed by ABEM, candidates would benefit from a more comprehensive discussion and analysis before moving onward. The structured interview is intended as a guided discussion between examiners and candidates, where patients with "everyday" ED conditions, illnesses, and injuries presented in unfolding case vignettes are discussed. Each structured interview event centers on one patient. During the interview, examiners use scripted questions to prompt candidates to "think aloud" and verbally describe and justify how they would proceed along the diagnostic and therapeutic management pathways related to the patient presented. Scripted interview questions are organized and aligned with one of eight physician tasks: *history, physical, differential diagnosis, diagnostic studies, treatment and other actions* (pharmacologic and nonpharmacologic interventions), *final diagnosis, disposition,* and *transition of care.* For each domain, examiners ask candidates initial questions, usually beginning with the interrogative "what." For a subset of domains, examiners will follow initial questions with secondary questions beginning with the interrogative "why." An example of the flow and order of the domains covered during the structured interview, and the questions asked at each interval, is provided in Table 4.1.

Key features of the structured interview are summarized below:

- Structured interviews are interviews, not dialogs or role-plays. Examiners are in control of the questions that are asked. Candidates are expected to answer questions, not ask them. Unlike the single-patient case format, there is not a back-and-forth exchange of information, nor is there any role-play component.
- In almost every domain of the structured interview, the first question asks "what" candidates would or should do (the phrasing of this question is domain-specific).
- In almost every domain of the structured interview, the most likely second question is a follow-up question asking candidates to justify their answers.
- Once a domain has been addressed (e.g., examiner and candidate have discussed a domain, and all interview questions asked by the examiner have been answered by the candidate), consider it closed for future exploration. Candidates are unable to return to previously asked questions and revise responses later in the interview. Candidates are therefore advised to be thoughtful and comprehensive in their responses, especially early in the structured interview.

The key features associated with scoring the structured interview are covered later in the chapter.

STRUCTURE AND PROCESS OF THE AOBEM EM ORAL EXAM

Much like the ABEM VOE, the AOBEM EM Oral Exam is a component of a two-step certification pathway. It is offered once in the fall of each calendar year, with each examination day subdivided into morning and afternoon testing sessions. Registration for the examination opens approximately six months prior to the testing period; specific information, including the assignment of the precise session–day pairing, is made in advance of the testing day. In contrast to the ABEM process, examiners administer two simulation case scenarios per station during the AOBEM EM Oral Exam. Unlike the ABEM VOE, candidates move through four testing stations. Therefore, each candidate

Table 4.1 Representative questions, by domain, and proposed answer framework for ABEM structured interview (SI)

Domain	Question is asked …	Initial SI question	Author recommended framework for candidate answers to first SI question	Secondary (follow-up) SI question	Author recommended framework for candidate answers to second SI question
History	Following launch of the structured interview, after the initial case vignette, including vital signs, is presented (Stimulus #1)	"What additional historical information would you want to ask the patient?"	Verbalize exploration of the following • CC and HPI using a known framework (e.g., OPQRST) • Past histories# • SDOH • Medications and allergies • ROS	"You asked about X. Why X?"	• Provide one or more reasonable justifications when asked "why." • Be sure to answer the specific question that is being asked. • Consider incorporating evidence-based practice when possible in answers (e.g., knowledge of likelihood ratios to justify questions asked in the history, examination maneuvers performed during the physical, or other actions like diagnostic and therapeutic interventions ordered during the case).
Physical	Following history, after additional historical information is presented verbally	"What specific physical examination findings would you be looking for?"	Verbalize a problem-focused physical examination • Include repeat vital signs. • Consider missing monitoring adjuncts. • Incorporate key physical examination maneuvers, where applicable.	"You examined X during the physical exam. How did that help you?"	

Table 4.1 (cont.)

Domain	Question is asked ...	Initial SI question	Author recommended framework for candidate answers to first SI question	Secondary (follow-up) SI question	Author recommended framework for candidate answers to second SI question
Differential diagnosis	Following physical, after additional information from the physical assessment is presented verbally	"What are the top three items on your differential diagnosis based on the most likely conditions?"	Consider multiple systems if feasible • For a patient with RLQ abdominal pain: appendicitis, obstructing ureteral stone, ovarian torsion. Provide three specific, likely conditions • For a patient presenting with fever and shock: do not state "sepsis, sepsis, sepsis."	n/a	
Diagnostic studies	Following the candidate's listing of three differential diagnoses	"What, if any, diagnostic studies would you order?"	Consider • serology • XR, US, CT, MRI • diagnostic procedures	"Why did you order X? What you would be looking for on X?"	
Treatment and other actions	Following presentation of Stimulus #2	"What treatment, if any, would you order?"	Consider • pharmacologic interventions (especially pain management) • nonpharmacologic interventions • Reassessments • Consultations • Discussions with key stakeholders	"You ordered X. Why X?"	

Final Diagnosis	Following the candidate's description of treatment and other actions to be taken	"Based on everything you know, what is your final diagnosis?"	Provide one diagnosis (the best, most likely diagnosis)	n/a
Disposition	Following the candidate's determination of final diagnosis	"What should be the disposition of this patient?"	Provide the best disposition • Unless clearly obvious, admission is generally favored over discharge.	"Why would you [admit/discharge] this patient?"
Transition of care	Following the candidate's disposition decision	"How would you hand off this patient?" or, alternatively, "How would you discharge this patient?"	Describe essential information to include to stakeholders at handoff or discharge • Consider mention of known frameworks (e.g., IPASS). • Mention reassessments (e.g., current vitals, repeat measurements of pain), diagnostic and therapeutic interventions and responses, and critical results	n/a

CC, chief concerns; HPI, history of present illness; OPQRST, onset, provocation/palliation of symptoms, quality, region/radiation, associated signs/symptoms, severity, timing; SDOH, social determinants of health (e.g., employment, living environment, social supports, health insurance, etc.); ROS, review of systems. # Past histories include past medical history, past surgical history, past obstetrical/gynecological history, past psychiatric history, social history (tobacco, ethanol, recreational and illicit drugs), and family history.

must effectively manage eight simulated patients (four pairs of simulated case scenarios) over the course of the entire testing period. All AOBEM simulation-based assessments are timed. Candidates must complete all critical actions and case-related tasks within the designated time limits. Candidates are given a maximum of 30 minutes in which to manage two simulated patients simultaneously at each of the four testing stations. The summative assessment for each candidate is based on one's performance across all four stations. Comprehensive description of the content, process, policies, procedures, implementation, and scoring of the AOBEM EM Oral Exam may be found on the AOBEM website.

EXAMINATION CONTENT

Content for the ABEM OCE is derived from the 2022 Model of the Clinical Practice of Emergency Medicine (Beeson et al., 2023; "the Model"). The Model defines the scope of EM as a medical specialty. Twenty content domains are highly matrixed across three acuity frames (critical, urgent, and nonemergent presentation states) and 20 physician tasks. Unlike the ABEM Qualifying Examination, the percentage breakdown of the content upon which the ABEM VOE is based is not explicitly described. ABEM may select content from any content area within the Model for the VOE, although the conditions, presentations, and diseases within the domains of cardiovascular, traumatic, thoracic-respiratory disorders, and systemic infectious disorders are emphasized. Half of all simulated case scenarios on the VOE will portray conditions with emergent ("critical") acuity time frames. Testing sessions will generally include at least one pediatric and geriatric patient.

Previously, all content for AOBEM oral examinations was derived from the AOBEM Table of Specificity for Certification Examinations, which was adapted from the Core Content in Emergency Medicine. Recent review of publicly available published descriptions of the content for the AOBEM oral examinations does not provide specific content delineations or breakdown other than 20 content areas (as described for the written examination/computer-based testing section of AOBEM's *Candidate Handbook*) and 11 physician tasks (as noted on the AOBEM website). For all practical exam preparation purposes, the content described in the Model appears analogous, applicable, and suitable for AOBEM candidates seeking a comprehensive resource on which to base their examination preparation.

PERFORMANCE RATING AND EXAMINATION SCORING FOR THE ABEM SINGLE-PATIENT CASE FORMAT

Candidate performance on the ABEM single-patient case is assessed across eight domains ("performance criteria") using an interval scale from 1 (worst) to 8 (best). The eight performance criteria are: data acquisition, problem-solving, patient management, resource utilization, health care provided (outcome), interpersonal relations and communication skills, comprehension of pathophysiology, and clinical competence (overall). ABEM provides detailed explanations of the expected performance standards for each criterion, which have been summarized below:

- Data acquisition (DA): This rating is based on the candidate's demonstration of a plan to collect data critical for correctly diagnosing and managing the patient. The candidate's approach should be orderly, efficient, and timely. The candidate should easily integrate the data obtained into the overall management plan to provide quality patient care.
- Problem-solving (PS): This rating is based on the candidate's ability to appropriately organize data collection so that differentiation and selection among reasonable alternative diagnoses is possible while contemporaneously stabilizing/managing the patient and anticipating complications.

- Patient management (PM): This rating is based on the candidate's treatment decisions, including appropriately sequenced management actions. The candidate's management decisions (including the sequence of diagnostic and therapeutic interventions) are judged in contrast to the data acquisition and problem-solving activities. The candidate directs the proper interventions at the right times, makes appropriate referrals, and manages multiple patients simultaneously.
- Resource utilization (RU): This rating is based on the candidate's logical, organized, judicious, parsimonious, and efficient use of resources (e.g., laboratory, diagnostic tests, nurses, consultants) in the context of the simulation.
- Health care provided (HCP): This rating is derived from the simulated patient's actual outcome as based on the candidate's overall performance. The candidate provides timely and appropriate medical care, stabilizes the patient in alignment using current evidence-supported practices and guidelines, and maximally improves the patient's condition.
- Interpersonal relations and communication skills (IRCS): This rating is based on the candidate's ability to communicate clinical information (e.g., possible and likely diagnoses, management, test results, procedures, options) clearly with patients, family, staff, and consultants, while simultaneously demonstrating respect, empathy, concern, and an appreciation of the patient's culture, preferences, and health literacy.
- Comprehension of pathophysiology (CP): This rating is based on the candidate's understanding of the underlying pathophysiology of the conditions being treated and of the scientific rationale and evidence base for treatments and procedures. The candidate is able to interpret diagnostic tests, implement procedures and perform other aspects for care while avoiding reliance on "rote" recognition of cause, "knee-jerk" routines, or algorithms without mindful consideration of intended and unintended effects resulting from these actions.
- Clinical competence (CC): This rating represents the examiner's overall assessment of the candidate's cognitive and procedural skills throughout the simulation.

Along with these eight performance criteria, ABEM explicitly defines "critical actions" for each simulated case scenario. Critical actions are "predetermined behaviors" that are judged essential for the completion of tasks or successful outcomes. They are usually constructed as imperative sentences (e.g., "order chest x-ray," "treat pneumothorax," or "explain procedure to patient"). Examiners use critical actions as guides to provide more objective and differentiated rating among different levels of performance. They are integral to the scoring of each single-patient case. A typical single-patient case has 3–5 clearly defined critical actions.

A key feature of critical actions is that they are linked to one (and only one) of the aforementioned eight performance criteria. Possible critical action–performance criteria links, using the previous examples, could include the following: "order chest x-ray" linked with "data acquisition"; "treat pneumothorax" linked with "patient management"; and "explain procedure to patient" linked with "interpersonal relations and communication skills." A review of the ABEM website explicitly demonstrates this linkage. When a candidate performs a critical action, examiners typically rate the candidate's performance at 5 or greater on the rating scale of the performance criteria with which the critical action is aligned. When a candidate fails to perform a critical action, examiners typically rate the candidate's performance at 4 or lower on the rating scale of the performance criteria with which the critical action is aligned. Two or more critical actions may be linked to the same performance domain.

As described above, each of the eight domains of performance are rated for each case using an eight-point interval scale. ABEM divides the scale into quartiles of performance using the following category headings: very acceptable (7, 8); acceptable (5, 6); unacceptable (3, 4); and very unacceptable (1, 2). ABEM defines these categories using the following anchors:

Very acceptable (7, 8)

- Candidate performs *all* critical actions related to the domain criteria being rated and avoids committing dangerous actions.
- Examiner without significant objections or criticisms.
- Candidate demonstrates efficient, confident, correct data acquisition skills and provides a correct diagnosis.
- Candidate uses current, evidence-supported, generally accepted principles and guidelines to guide diagnostic and management decisions.
- Candidate demonstrates a sophisticated and sound understanding of the pathophysiology inherent in the case.
- Candidate anticipates and addresses psychological, social, and economic needs of patients and their families.

Acceptable (5, 6)

- Candidate performs *all* critical actions related to the domain (performance criteria) being rated while avoiding the commission of dangerous actions. Exceptions are possible at the discretion of the examiner if correctly documented (these exceptions were previously known as "critical action equivalents" or "4/5 exceptions," but they are no longer described in publicly available material from ABEM).
- Candidate demonstrates minor inefficiencies, error, or incomplete data acquisition and patient management, but performance remains within the range of generally accepted guidelines and practice standards; patient received "adequate care" while avoiding "significant unnecessary pain or life-threatening procedures or medications."
- Candidate may have exposed the patient to significant, unnecessary prolonged time or expense as a consequence of diagnostic or therapeutic management decisions.
- Candidate ultimately successfully diagnoses and correctly manages the case, but with some difficulty.
- Candidate performs an "adequate" history and physical examination.
- Candidate demonstrates a sufficient underlying "working knowledge" of pathophysiology and of safe medical practice.
- Candidate demonstrates a reasonable concern about the patient's psychological, social, and economic issues.

Unacceptable (3, 4)

- Candidate misses *one or more* critical actions related to the domain (performance criteria) being rated.
- Candidate commits inappropriate or dangerous actions.
- Candidate demonstrates significant gaps in data acquisition and management.
- Candidate provides care that is incomplete, disorganized, and inefficient, but may recognize their own limitations, and may demonstrate a concern for the patient's welfare by recruiting help from consultants and using other resources to overcome deficiencies.
- Candidate demonstrates a partial, inadequate, or incomplete knowledge of pathophysiology, procedures, and generally accepted evidence-based management principles.
- Candidate does not anticipate complications or problems.
- Candidate demonstrates a lack of concern for the patient's psychological, social, and economic issues.

Very unacceptable (1, 2)

- Candidate *misses two or more* critical actions.
- Candidate commits inappropriate or dangerous actions.
- Candidate demonstrates gross negligence or mismanagement without recognizing their own deficiencies and inadequacies.
- Candidate demonstrates rudimentary history acquisition and patient stabilization/management skills along with a deficient fund of knowledge.
- Candidate does not obtain appropriate consultation when indicated.
- Candidate discharges the patient when hospitalization and emergent specialized care is necessary.

Each category described above provides the examiner with two possible ratings (a high and low point within each quartile of level of performance) with which to score the candidate's performance. For example, an examiner assessing a candidate who functions at the "very acceptable" level for the performance criteria of data acquisition may apply (at his or her discretion) a rating of either 7 or 8. ABEM does not explicitly describe how examiners discriminate candidate performance between these two points on the scale within each category (quartile of level of performance). ABEM provides extensive rater training, however, to sharpen and optimize examiners' assessment skills and ensure adequate intra- and interrater reliability across all candidates. ABEM includes case-specific "scoring guidelines" and "play of case guidelines" aligned with each critical action to assist raters with these nuanced, high-stakes judgments of performance.

To summarize, ABEM is explicitly seeking to assess candidates' abilities to verbalize patient management, including their abilities to synthesize case-related information, select and prioritize diagnostics and therapeutic interventions, and make sound disposition decisions.

PERFORMANCE RATING AND EXAMINATION SCORING FOR THE ABEM STRUCTURED INTERVIEW FORMAT

ABEM examiners assess candidates' performances on the ABEM structured interview using a unique rating instrument (the structured interview scoresheet). Close inspection of the sample structured interview scoresheet provided by ABEM on its website provides valuable insights, of which ABEM examination candidates should be aware. Each structured interview scoresheet lists 25 scenario-specific critical actions. A critical action is aligned with only one structured interview domain. The distribution of critical actions across domains, however, varies and is dependent on the specific scenario upon which the structured interview is based. The majority of these critical actions are linked to key elements that ABEM expects candidates to include as components of their formulated answers to the examiners' initial scripted interview questions (the "what" questions). A minority of critical actions relate to the quality and comprehensiveness of the rationales (justifications) candidates offer to the secondary, follow-up "why" questions. Examiners rate candidates' attainment of all critical actions during the structured interview using a binary scale: "No" (not verbalized) or "Yes" (verbalized). Similar to the other oral examination formats, ABEM uses standard setting specific for each structured interview scenario to establish the minimum number of critical actions candidates must attain to successfully pass the structured interview scenario.

ABEM APPROACH TO STANDARD SETTING

ABEM examiners assess candidates' performances on the single-patient cases and structured interview scenarios using criterion-referenced standards. There is no "curve." Pass/fail decisions are made in alignment with these standards. If all of the criteria set forth by ABEM are met, the candidate passes the examination.

Examiners use scoresheets to record their ratings of candidates' performances and calculate a case score. The ratings on these scoresheets inform pass/fail decisions; these have been replaced with a newer, simpler approach given the changes in test format: the mean of the scores from the five single-patient cases (the mean of the ratings for each of the eight performance domains for each case scenario) and the scores from the two structured interview scenarios is calculated, and then compared to a "cut score" (passing score) derived from ABEM's standard-setting process. The "cut score" represents ABEM's minimum performance expectations for demonstrating expertise in EM. ABEM has not made public the exact method it uses to establish a cut score for its summative pass/fail decisions (although the Angoff method, a well-established, defensible method, is likely).

EXAMPLE: SIMULATED ABEM VOE SINGLE-PATIENT CASE

The examiner presents the candidate with Mr. Red, a 63-year-old man with 1 hour of substernal chest pain resulting from ST-segment elevation myocardial infarction (STEMI). Initial vital signs are: pulse, 84/minute; respirations, 14/minute; blood pressure, 160/80 mmHg; temperature, 37°C (98.6°F); and oxygen saturation, 99% ($FiO_2 = 0.21$). The patient has a past medical history of hypertension, type 2 diabetes mellitus, and hypercholesterolemia. He has no medication allergies. His medications include metformin, sildenafil (taken within the past three hours), and amlodipine. The candidate is presented with the initial case information, and then should move forward with the primary survey, initial diagnostic and stabilizing management interventions, history and data acquisition, and the secondary survey. ECG, if requested by the candidate, reveals an obvious anterior wall STEMI. Chest x-ray, if requested, reveals clear lung fields and a normal mediastinum. During the case play, the patient's condition will suddenly deteriorate; he develops ventricular fibrillation and sudden cardiac arrest. The examiner and candidate role-play 4 minutes of the resuscitation, including CPR, procedures (endotracheal intubation, defibrillation), medication administration (epinephrine), and post-resuscitation management (ongoing arrhythmia management, discussion with consultants and the patient's family, admission to ICU). For the examples below, the critical actions (and performance criteria to which they are linked) for this sample case are:

1. Order ECG (data acquisition)
2. Obtain chest x-ray (problem-solving)
3. Administer aspirin (patient management)
4. Perform defibrillation (patient management)
5. Consult cardiologist (resource utilization)

Scoring example 1

The candidate performs all critical actions and demonstrates "very acceptable" performance. The candidate performs a problem-focused history and primary survey as initial stabilization measures are implemented. The candidate demonstrates the integration of all data obtained in the formulation of the initial management plan. The candidate anticipates alternative diagnoses (e.g., aortic dissection) and obtains an ECG and chest x-ray. The candidate recognizes anterior wall STEMI and orders aspirin. The candidate appropriately avoids nitroglycerin (dangerous action). The candidate anticipates complications and applies defibrillator pads to the patient before the cardiac arrest happens. The candidate demonstrates knowledge of and applies evidence-based guidelines when sudden cardiac arrest occurs (initiates immediate CPR, defibrillation and sequences medications and interventions appropriately). The candidate succinctly and accurately describes how to perform endotracheal intubation and defibrillation when asked. The candidate requests consultation with a cardiologist, effectively explains the situation to the consultant and family members, and admits the patient to the ICU until cardiac catheterization can be arranged. The patient survives the event.

The examiner provides the ratings for the eight performance criteria (using the scoring rubric and eight-point integer scale) shown in Figure 4.1. Note that the overall individualized score for the simulated patient case scenario would equal 7.63 (the calculated mean of all performance criteria ratings). ABEM applies the calculated means of all scored simulation case scenarios to the cut score derived from their standard-setting process to inform on their pass/fail decisions.

Critical actions
Order ECG (data acquisition)
Obtain chest x-ray (problem solving)
Administer aspirin (patient management)
Perform defibrillation (patient management)
Consult cardiologist (resource utilization)

Ratings (1-8)	
DA	8
PS	7
PM	8
RU	7
HCP	8
ICRS	8
CP	7
CC	8
Mean	**7.63**

Figure 4.1 Visualization of the scoring for single-patient case example 1.

Scoring example 2

The candidate performs a problem-focused history and primary survey but is inefficient and disorganized with implementing initial stabilization measures. The candidate does not anticipate alternative diagnoses (e.g., aortic dissection, pneumothorax), only ordering an ECG (does not obtain a chest x-ray). The candidate recognizes anterior wall STEMI and orders aspirin. The candidate avoids nitroglycerin (dangerous action). The candidate does not anticipate sudden cardiac arrest as a potential complication, however, and does not apply defibrillator pads to patient before the sudden cardiac arrest. The candidate requests immediate defibrillation when sudden cardiac arrest occurs but cannot fluently describe the procedure. The candidate requests consultation with a cardiologist but provides only a rudimentary explanation of the situation to the consultant and does not engage family members. The candidate admits the patient to the ICU. The patient survives the event.

The examiner provides the ratings for the eight performance criteria (using the scoring rubric and eight-point ordinal scale) shown in Figure 4.2. Note that the overall individualized score for the simulated patient case scenario would equal 4.88 (the calculated mean of all performance criteria ratings). The effect of missing one critical action on the performance domain rating is clear.

Critical actions
Order ECG (data acquisition)
~~Obtain chest x-ray (problem solving)~~
Administer aspirin (patient management)
Perform defibrillation (patient management)
Consult cardiologist (resource utilization)

Ratings (1-8)	
DA	5
PS	4
PM	5
RU	5
HCP	5
ICRS	5
CP	5
CC	5

Figure 4.2 Visualization of the scoring for single-patient case example 2.

This candidate, however, could still pass the VOE, depending on the standard-setting process, the unique cut score for this specific case, and the overall cut score for the entire exam.

PERFORMANCE RATING AND EXAMINATION SCORING FOR THE AOBEM EM ORAL EXAM

Equivalent to the ABEM process, examiners for the AOBEM EM Oral Exam rate candidates' performances using criterion-referenced standards. Pass/fail decisions are made in alignment with these standards. If all of the criteria set forth by AOBEM are met, the candidate passes the examination. There is no "curve." Standards for the AOBEM EM Oral Exam are likely set using similar if not identical procedures to those used by ABEM for its single-patient cases. On its website, AOBEM explicitly states it uses the Angoff standard-setting method to establish cut scores for pass/fail decisions. AOBEM has published specific criteria for failure, which are:

- final examination scores below minimum thresholds set by AOBEM;
- failure of a minimum of two of the eight clinical cases, regardless of the final examination score;
- failure of a minimum of three of the six clinical cases regardless of final examination score;
- omission of significant magnitude;[4]
- commission of an error of significant magnitude; and
- violation of the American Osteopathic Association's Code of Conduct and Code of Ethics

These concepts are summarized in Table 4.2.

Table 4.2 Comparison of the ABEM and AOBEM examination formats

	ABEM Virtual Oral Exam	AOBEM EM Oral Exam
Testing cycle	Biannually (spring, fall)	Annually (fall)
Stations	7	4
Single-patient case format	4–6[b]	0
Allotted time per	15 minutes	n/a
Multiple case scenarios	0	4
Allotted time per multiple case scenario	n/a	30 minutes
Number of patients per multiple case scenario	n/a	2
Structured interview format	1–3[b]	n/a
Allotted time	15 minutes	n/a
Diagnostic test and other visual stimuli[a] interpretation	Embedded within case simulations No separate assessment of proficiency	Embedded within case simulations No separate assessment of proficiency

---

[4] AOBEM defines "significant magnitude" as "resulting either in the mortality of a patient or high probability of causation of morbidity or mortality regardless of the final examination score."

Table 4.2 (cont.)

	ABEM Virtual Oral Exam	AOBEM EM Oral Exam
Content basis	Model of Clinical Practice of EM 20 content domains, 20 physician tasks (structured interview incorporates 8) KSA and Standards	20 content domains, 11 physician tasks[c] AOA Code of Ethics AOA Rules and Guidelines on Physician' Professional Conduct
Scoring and pass/fail decision	Criterion-referenced Critical actions Standard setting (no method specified)	Criterion-referenced Critical actions Standard setting (Angoff method specified)

[a] Diagnostic tests include, but are not limited to, static and dynamic audiovisual stimuli, including electrocardiographs (12-lead and continuous ECG traces), conventional radiographs, computed tomography images, magnetic resonance images, ultrasounds, and results of serologic and other body fluid tests. The use of dynamic stimuli and audiovisual files within an ABEM Oral Examination has only been described by ABEM within the eOral format (suspended with the transition to the VOE in 2020).

[b] The ABEM website presents slightly conflicting information: www.abem.org/public/become-certified/oral-exam/types-of-cases-and-samples indicates five single-patient cases and two structured interviews, but www.abem.org/public/become-certified/oral-exam/exam-content implies more variability

[c] Presumed to be derived from or analogous to the 2022 Model of Clinical Practice of EM, but not explicitly stated.

ADDITIONAL THOUGHTS

- Frederick et al. (2011) demonstrated a predictive correlation between candidate scores on the ABEM In-Training Examination (taken as the PGY-3) and the ABEM OCE.
- Bianchi et al. (2003) demonstrated a high level of agreement (interrater reliability) among raters scoring candidate performance using the critical actions and eight performance criteria within an ABEM OCE testing session.
- Lunz and Bashook (2008) demonstrated that the candidate communication ability (cited by some as a source for construct-irrelevant variance) does not influence candidate outcomes on OCEs in orthopedic surgery administered by trained examiners.
- Kowalenko et al. (2017) gathered validity evidence to support the use of the scores and ratings generated from the eOral format and establish its equivalence with the traditional SPE case delivery.

CONCLUSIONS

To optimize performance in the role-play formats (ABEM single-patient cases and AOBEM EM Oral Exam), candidates should:

- demonstrate an organized approach to the emergent assessment and management of one or more critically ill or injured adult or pediatric patients;
- describe the appropriate sequence and methods for acquiring data, solving problems, and stabilizing patients;
- anticipate and perform the expected critical actions;
- maximize ratings by fully understanding the criteria on which summative assessments are based;

- avoid dangerous actions (commissions and omissions);
- practice using this textbook; and
- consider taking an OCE review course.

Strategies and recommendations specific for the novel structured interview format for candidates include:

- Do not assume strategies effective for the single-patient case format apply to the structured interview format.
- Thinking aloud, and comprehensively answering the question asked when it is asked, is important during the structured interview (remember, once a candidate completes a section of the structured interview, the candidate cannot move backward to rectify omissions; additional thoughts about the history will not be solicited or accepted once the question has been answered and the examiner moves the interview forward).
- Consider allocating more time to answering questions asked at the beginning of the structured interview, especially those aligned with the history and physical domains (learners who allocate as much as one-third of the total test time – approximately 3–5 minutes – to addressing prompts in the history and physical domains are still generally able to effectively complete the structured interview within the 15-minute limit, as later portions of the test move more quickly).

BIBLIOGRAPHY

American Board of Emergency Medicine (2023a). Detailed performance criteria: oral exam. www.abem.org/public/become-certified/oral-exam/results-scoring. Accessed November 27, 2023.

American Board of Emergency Medicine (2023b). KSA and standards. www.abem.org/public/resources/emergency-medicine-milestones-ksas. Accessed November 27, 2023.

American Board of Emergency Medicine (2023c). Oral exam. www.abem.org/public/become-certified/oral-exam. Accessed November 27, 2023.

American Board of Emergency Medicine (2023d). Sample single case score sheet. www.abem.org/public/docs/default-source/default-document-library/sample-single-case-notesheet.pdf. Accessed November 27, 2023.

American Board of Emergency Medicine (2023e). Sample standard interview score sheet. www.abem.org/public/docs/default-source/default-document-library/score-sheet-and-rating-scales-example.pdf?sfvrsn=6a20c8f4_12. Accessed November 27, 2023.

American Osteopathic Association (2022a). Code of ethics. https://osteopathic.org/about/leadership/aoa-governance-documents/code-of-ethics/. Accessed November 27, 2023.

American Osteopathic Association (2022b). AOA rules and guidelines on physicians' professional conduct. https://osteopathic.org/about/leadership/aoa-governance-documents/aoa-rules-and-guidelines-on-physicians-professional-conduct/. Accessed November 27, 2023.

American Osteopathic Board of Emergency Medicine (2022). Oral exam. https://certification.osteopathic.org/emergency-medicine/certification-process-overview/specialty-certification-process/oral-exams/. Accessed July 1, 2022.

Beeson MS, Bhat R, Broder JS, et al. (2023). The 2022 Model of the Clinical Practice of Emergency Medicine. *Journal of Emergency Medicine*, 64(6), 659–695.

Bianchi L, Gallagher EJ, Korte R, Ham HP (2003). Interexaminer Agreement on the American Board of Emergency Medicine Oral Certification Examination. *Annals of Emergency Medicine*, 41(6), 859–864.

Frederick RC, Hafner JW, Schaefer TJ, Aldag JC (2011). Outcome Measures for Emergency Medicine Residency Graduates: Do Measures of Academic and Clinical Performance during Residency Training Correlate with American Board of Emergency Medicine Test Performance? *Academic Emergency Medicine*, 18, S59–S64.

Kowalenko T, Heller BN, Strauss RW, et al. (2017). Initial Validity Analysis of the American Board of Emergency Medicine Enhanced Oral Examination. *Academic Emergency Medicine*, 24(1), 125–129.

Lunz ME, Bashook PG (2008). Relationship Between Candidate Communication Ability and Oral Certification Examination Scores. *Medical Education*, 42, 1227–1233.

Schwartz JT & Babineau MR (2021). Quarantine the oral boards. www.acepnow.com/article/quarantine-the-oral-boards/ Accessed June 30, 2022.

Sherbino J, Bandiera G, Frank J (2008). Assessing Competence in Emergency Medicine Trainees: an Overview of Effective Methodologies. *Canadian Journal of Emergency Medicine*, 10(4), 365–371.

Tekian A, Yudkowsky R, Downing S, Yudkowsky R (2009). Oral Examinations. In R Yudkowsky, YS Park, SM Downing, eds., *Assessment in Health Professions Education*. New York: Taylor and Francis, 269–285.

CASES

Overdose

William McDowell, MD and Vinodinee Dissanayake, MD

A. Chief complaint
a. 19-year-old female presents via EMS for abdominal pain and vomiting after taking "a bottle of pills"

B. Vital signs
a. BP: 90/55, HR: 105, RR: 24, T: 37.0°C, Sat: 99% on room air

C. What does the patient look like?
a. Appears stated age, actively vomiting, in moderate discomfort

D. Primary survey
a. Airway: Speaking in full sentences, protecting airway despite vomiting
b. Breathing: No respiratory distress, mild tachypnea
c. Circulation: Skin dry and cool, normal capillary refill

E. Action
a. Two large-bore IV lines
b. POC glucose: 105 mg/dL
c. 1 L crystalloid bolus
d. EKG
e. Antiemetics: ondansetron or metoclopramide
f. Monitor: BP: 90/55, HR 110, RR: 24, T: 37.0°C, Sat: 100% on 2 L NC
g. Labs
   i. CBC, BMP, LFT, lipase, PT/INR, PTT, type and cross, ethanol level, serum acetaminophen level, serum salicylate level, VBG/ABG, lactate
   ii. UA, urine pregnancy test, urine toxicology screen

F. History
a. HPI: 19-year-old female with PMH of heavy menstrual periods and anemia took "a bottle of pills" 3 hours prior to arrival because she was a victim of online bullying and she "wanted to die." She denies drinking alcohol or taking any other substances. Approximately 1 hour after the ingestion, she developed nausea with three episodes of vomiting. The last episode of vomiting had "some blood in it." She has moderately crampy epigastric pain. She denies diarrhea, fevers, chills, shortness of breath, chest pain, recent antibiotics or travel, vaginal discharge, or urinary symptoms. EMS was called and brought patient to the ED. EMS found an empty bottle labeled ferrous sulfate, 325 mg tablets. The label reveals that it had contained 60 pills with a fill date of yesterday (must ask).

G. Nurse
a. EKG (Figure 1.1)
b. Monitor:
    i. If fluids given:
        1. BP: 100/65, HR 100, RR: 24, T: 37.0°C, Sat: 100% on 2 L oxygen by nasal cannula
    ii. If no fluids given:
        1. BP: 85/50, HR 125, RR: 24, T: 37.0°C, Sat: 100% on 2 L oxygen by nasal cannula
c. Urine pregnancy test negative

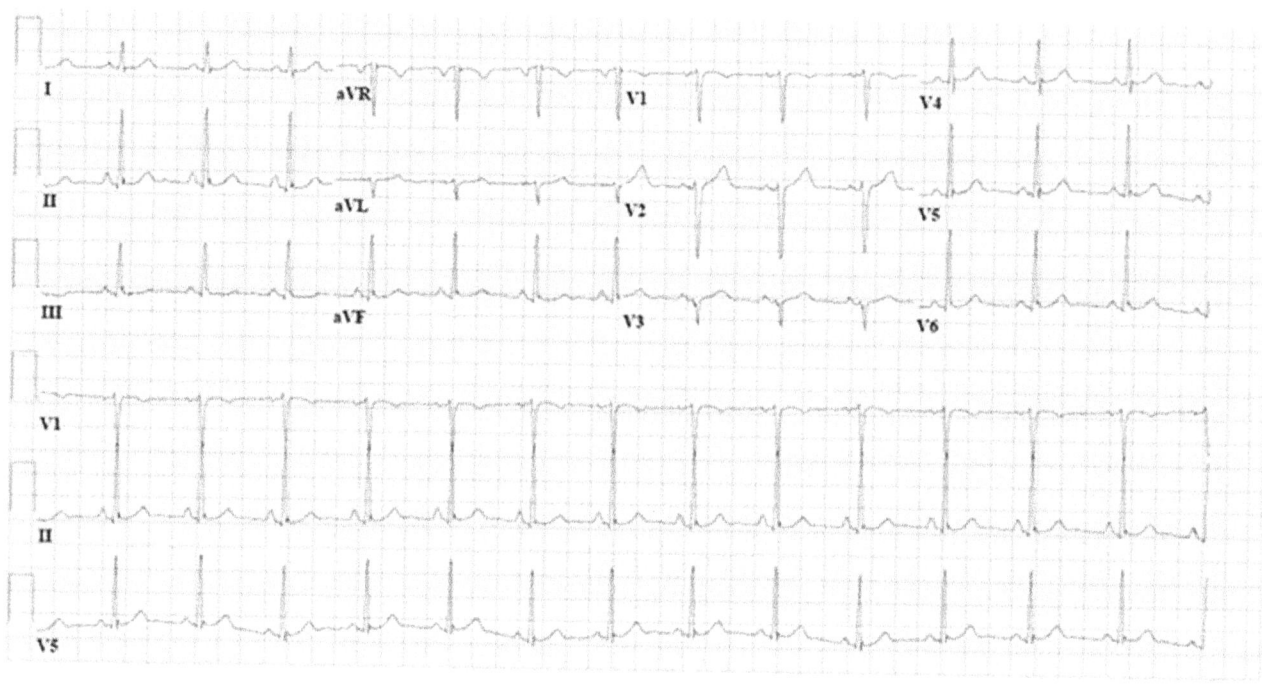

Figure 1.1

H. Secondary survey
a. General: alert and oriented ×3, has had two episodes of vomiting since she has been in the ED, appears uncomfortable. Weight: 60 kg
b. HEENT: Dry mucous membranes
c. Neck: Normal
d. Chest: Normal, nontender
e. Heart: Mild tachycardia, regular rhythm, no murmurs
f. Lungs: Clear to auscultation bilaterally
g. Abdomen: Mild epigastric tenderness, nondistended, no masses or organomegaly, negative Murphy's sign, no rebound/guarding/rigidity
h. Rectal: dark-colored stool, guaiac negative, normal tone
i. Extremities: Normal
j. Back: Normal
k. Neuro: No focal deficits
l. Skin: Cool and dry

I. Action
a. Reassess
    i. BP mildly improved now 110/70, HR 95
    ii. Nausea moderately improved but not resolved, no longer vomiting if given antiemetic

b. Second liter fluid bolus
c. Imaging
   i. Abdominal x-ray/KUB
d. Calculate dose of elemental iron: 325 mg/pill × 60 pills × 20% (elemental iron composition of ferrous sulfate) = 3900 mg (65 mg/kg)
e. Placement of NG tube
f. Medications
   i. Reassess need for repeat antiemetics
   ii. Whole-bowel irrigation
   iii. Deferoxamine
g. Additional labs
   i. Add serum iron levels to be obtained at 4 hours from ingestion

J. Results

Table 1.1 Results table

Test	Result	Test	Result
Complete blood count:		**Liver function panel:**	
WBC	$9.1 \times 10^3/\mu L$	AST	28 U/L
Hgb	10%	ALT	30 U/L
Plt	$300 \times 10^3/\mu L$	Alk phos	62 U/L
		T bili	1.1 mg/dL
Basic metabolic panel:		Albumin	4.2 g/dL
Na	140 mEq/L	Lipase	42 U/L
K	4 mEq/L		
Cl	105 mEq/L	**Urinalysis:**	
CO_2	20 mEq/L	SG	1.020
BUN	15 mEq/dL	pH	6.1
Cr	1 mg/dL	Prot	Neg
Glucose	110 mg/dL	Gluc	Neg
		Ketones	Neg
		Bili	Neg
Coagulation panel:		Blood	Neg
PTT	30 sec	LE	Neg
PT	12 sec	Nitrite	Neg
INR	1.0	Color	Yellow

a. Serum iron concentration: 550 mcg/dL

K. Nurse
a. BP: 120/80, HR: 90, RR: 20, Sat: 100% on 2 L oxygen by nasal cannula
b. Patient's abdominal pain has improved, vomiting has resolved

L. Action

a. Admit to ICU

b. Consult toxicology or poison control
  i. Consultant agrees with plan
  ii. If candidate has not ordered acetaminophen level, salicylate level, urine toxicology screen, alcohol level, or serum iron level, consultant recommends obtaining these labs
  iii. If candidate has not ordered both whole-bowel irrigation and deferoxamine, consultant will recommend that therapy

c. Consult psychiatry regarding the patient's suicide attempt.
  i. Psychiatry will evaluate patient, recommends 1:1 direct observation

M. Diagnosis

a. Iron overdose, moderate to severe toxicity

N. Critical actions

a. Large-bore IV access and minimum 1 L fluid bolus

b. EKG

c. Calculate elemental iron dose

d. Obtain 4 hour serum iron level

e. Start deferoxamine, consider whole-bowel irrigation

f. Consult toxicology or poison control

O. Examiner instructions

a. This is a case of intentional iron overdose presenting a few hours following ingestion. Effects of iron overdose can range from GI irritation with vomiting and diarrhea to hepatic failure, coagulopathy, coma, and death. This patient has classic symptoms of the first stage of iron overdose with abdominal pain, vomiting, hematemesis, and diarrhea. The patient took a dose of iron associated with moderate to severe toxicity. Important early actions in the case include large-bore IV access with fluid resuscitation for hypotension, EKG to evaluate for tricyclic antidepressant overdose, and urine pregnancy test. Obtaining a serum iron level is critical to guide treatment. This patient requires whole-bowel irrigation, deferoxamine, toxicology consult, and ICU admission.

P. Pearls

a. The clinical manifestations of iron overdose are classically split into five stages:
  i. Stage 1, local GI toxicity (1–6 hours): abdominal pain, vomiting, and diarrhea. Patients either recover from this stage or progress to systemic toxicity.
    1. If no GI symptoms within 6 hours of ingestion, significant toxicity is unlikely.
  ii. Stage 2, latent stage (6–24 hours): GI symptoms resolve, systemic toxicity may begin to develop. May have worsening metabolic acidosis and hypoperfusion.
  iii. Stage 3, systemic toxicity (12–24 hours): GI symptoms may return, coagulopathy, worsening acidosis, and renal failure may develop.
  iv. Stage 4, hepatic stage (2–5 days): elevation of AST/ALT, fulminant hepatic failure, worsening coagulopathy.
  v. Stage 5, delayed sequelae (4–6 weeks): rare, pyloric scarring and bowel obstruction.

b. Pathophysiology
  i. Iron generates free radicals which causes both GI irritation by direct damage to the mucosal surface and systemic toxicity by inhibiting oxidative phosphorylation in the mitochondria.
  ii. Systemic toxicity results in an anion gap metabolic acidosis resulting from lactic acidosis.

   c. Toxicity of ingestion is determined by dose of elemental iron. Doses of less than 20 mg/kg elemental iron are generally nontoxic, 20–60 mg/kg has the potential for systemic toxicity, and 60 mg/kg and greater is associated with moderate to severe toxicity.

      i. Elemental iron dose is calculated by tablet dose × proportion of elemental iron in preparation × number of tablets ingested.

      ii. Elemental iron composition of common formulations:

         1. Ferrous fumarate: 33%

         2. Ferrous sulfate: 20%

         3. Ferrous gluconate 12%

      iii. Ferrous sulfate 325 mg tablet formulation is the most commonly prescribed iron preparation. Moderate toxicity would be expected after ingestion of 20–35 tablets.

   d. Serum iron levels can help predict toxicity, but iron overdose remains primarily a clinical diagnosis.

      i. Serum iron concentrations of 300–500 mcg/dL are associated with mild toxicity, 500–1000 mcg/dL with moderate toxicity, and greater than 1000 mcg/dL with severe toxicity.

   e. Iron tablets are radiopaque. Visualization on x-ray promotes the need for GI decontamination to decrease absorption. Large iron loads or bezoars may require endoscopy for removal. False-negative x-rays are associated with chewable and liquid forms of iron.

   f. Activated charcoal should not be given, as it does not adsorb iron.

   g. Whole-bowel irrigation should be considered for GI decontamination in significant ingestion (such as ingestions of more than 60 mg/kg) or those with systemic toxicity. Adult dosing is 2 L/hr of polyethylene glycol by NG tube until rectal effluent is clear and there is no radiographic evidence of retained iron.

   h. Deferoxamine is a chelating agent that binds iron and forms renally excreted complexes.

      i. Indications: serum iron concentrations greater than 500 mcg/dL, severe systemic toxicity including metabolic acidosis, hypotension/shock, lethargy, persistent vomiting.

      ii. Dose: 5 mg/kg/hr IV to total max daily dose of 6 g. Can titrate rate up to 15 mg/kg/hr slowly if no hypotension occurs.

      iii. Duration: end of therapy defined by clinical improvement, if patient has severe toxicity after 24 hours, may continue deferoxamine at lower dose.

      iv. Iron–deferoxamine complex causes a rusty brown urine color, "vin rose." In theory, when this color change resolves there is no longer significant toxicity.

   i. Hemodialysis (HD) is not indicated for iron overdose as it does not remove iron, but patients on deferoxamine may require HD if in renal failure to excrete the iron–deferoxamine chelation complex.

   j. Disposition: Patients requiring deferoxamine should be admitted to the ICU.

Q. Figure legends

   a. Figure 1.1 (EKG) Normal sinus rhythm, normal EKG.

R. References

   a. *Tintinalli's Emergency Medicine: A Comprehensive Study Guide* (9th ed.): Chapter 198, Iron.

   b. *Rosen's Emergency Medicine: Concepts and Clinical Practice* (10th ed.): Chapter 146, Iron and Heavy Metals.

Vomiting Infant

Caroline Black, MD and Abiola Fasina, MD

A. Chief complaint
a. 3-week-old baby brought in with vomiting and poor feeding

B. Vital signs
a. HR: 170 BP: 50/palp, RR: 60, T: 37.2°C, Wt: 2.8 kg

C. What does the patient look like?
a. Small pale baby that is sucking air hungrily. The baby has sunken eyes and is lethargic.

D. Primary survey
a. Airway: weak cry
b. Breathing: tachypneic, no cyanosis
c. Circulation: pale skin with decreased elasticity, slow capillary refill, and weak pulses

E. Action
a. Establish IV access
b. Labs
    i. BMP, CBC, ABG, and liver function tests
    ii. Bedside serum glucose (result: 85 mg/dL)
    iii. Serum lactate
    iv. Blood and urine cultures if sepsis suspected
    v. Lumbar puncture for CSF studies if meningitis suspected
c. 20 mL/kg saline bolus × 2, Followed by D5 ½ NS infusion at 1.5–2 times maintenance
d. Nothing by mouth (NPO)

F. History
a. HPI: This is a 3-week-old male infant brought in by his mother with vomiting and poor feeding. The mother states that three days ago the baby started to spit up formula after several of his feedings. Symptoms have progressively worsened; he now vomits food forcibly after every feeding. The mother reports that the vomit appears clear with only occasional streaks of blood. She states the baby always appears hungry but is unable to keep food down. He has become progressively more lethargic and weaker. She reports having to change a diminishing number of wet diapers over the past few days. The mother occasionally sees the baby's "stomach churning," and the baby is starting to turn "yellow." She denies fever, fatigue with feeds, or night sweats. There are no sick contacts at home. She reports that the infant had an uncomplicated prenatal course and was born by normal spontaneous vaginal delivery. The baby has received all age-appropriate vaccinations.
b. PMHx: none, birth wt: 3 kg

c. PSHx: none
d. Allergies: none
e. Meds: none
f. FHx: only child
g. PMD: Dr. Roberts

G. Nurse
a. NS bolus
b. Vital signs: HR: 160, BP: 60/p, RR: 60, T: 37°C
c. Patient now NPO

H. Secondary survey
a. General: small pale lethargic baby with a weak cry, sucking air avidly
b. HEENT: depressed fontanelles, sunken eyes, and dry mucous membranes
c. Neck: normal
d. Chest: normal
e. Heart: tachycardic, regular rhythm, no murmurs, rubs, or gallops
f. Abdomen: Firm, peristaltic waves noted passing from the left to the right across the upper abdomen
g. Rectal: normal, no stool in the vault
h. GU: normal
i. Back: normal
j. Extremities: decreased tone, moving all four extremities weakly
k. Neuro: normal male infant brought in by his mother
l. Skin: poor skin turgor; jaundice over torso

I. Action
a. Abdominal x-ray
b. Abdominal US
c. Meds/IV fluids: continue IV hydration with D5 ½ NS at 1.5–2 times maintenance rate
d. Reassess
   i. Patient appears more comfortable following rehydration.
e. Surgical consult

J. Nurse
a. Vital signs: HR: 160, BP: 70/30, RR: 50, afebrile (after two 20 mL/kg boluses)

K. Results

Table 2.1 Results table

Test	Result	Test	Result
Complete blood count:		Alk phos	40 U/L
WBC	$4.8 \times 10^3/\mu L$	T bili	1.5 mg/dL
Hgb	13 g/dL	D bili	0.1 mg/dL
Hct	38%	Lipase	250 U/L
Plt	$165 \times 10^3/\mu L$	Albumin	3.6 g/dL

Table 2.1 (cont.)

Test	Result	Test	Result
Basic metabolic panel:		**Urinalysis:**	
Na	140 mEq/L	SG	1.030
K	2.9 mEq/L	pH	6
Cl	90 mEq/L	Prot	Neg
CO_2	30 mEq/L	Gluc	Neg
BUN	11 mEq/dL	Ketones	Neg
Cr	0.8 mg/dL	Bili	Neg
Gluc	90 mg/dL	Blood	Neg
		LE	Neg
Coagulation panel:		Nitrite	Neg
PT	12.5 sec	Color	Yellow
PTT	26 sec		
INR	1.0	**Arterial blood gas:**	
		pH	7.55
Liver function panel:		pO_2	85 mmHg
AST	20 U/L	pCO_2	40 mmHg
ALT	25 U/L	HCO_3	30 mmol/L

a. US (Figure 2.1) thickness: 4 mm, length 14 mm

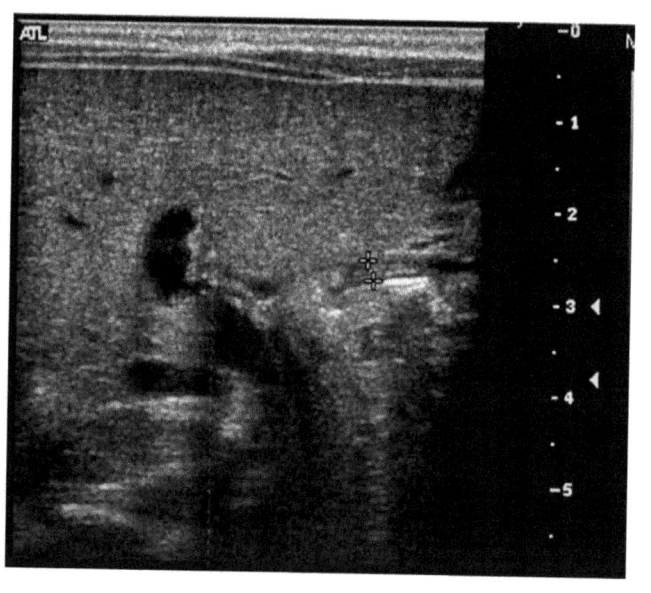

Figure 2.1

L. Action

a. Admit to pediatrics and continue to monitor electrolytes, fluid input and output, daily weights
b. Continue maintenance fluids, including potassium supplementation
c. Pyloromyotomy in OR, not emergent in this case

M. Diagnosis

a. Congenital hypertrophic pyloric stenosis

N. Critical actions

a. IV/IO access and adequate rehydration
b. Abdominal examination
c. Nasogastric tube, NPO
d. Abdominal US

O. Examiner instructions

a. This is a case of congenital hypertrophic pyloric stenosis. In this illness, muscles at the stomach outlet become overgrown (hypertrophied) and obstruct normal food transit from the stomach to the small intestine. Digestion and absorption are consequently impaired. Initial vital signs demonstrate tachycardia and hypotension resulting from hypovolemia (hypovolemic shock; normal neonatal vital signs include: HR between 120 and 160; systolic BP greater than 70; RR less than 60). These will correct only with fluid administration. If no fluids are given, have the nurse remind the doctor of the vital signs. Labs early in the course of the disease are generally normal; once significant vomiting and dehydration occurs, hypochloremic hypokalemic metabolic alkalosis is commonly seen. Ultrasound is the preferred diagnostic study and demonstrates a hypertrophied pylorus (pyloric muscle thickness > 4 mm; pyloric diameter > 14 mm is significant). To make this particular case more challenging, state that care providers cannot obtain venous access upon arrival. In this case, the neonate is ill enough to warrant intraosseous (IO) needle placement if IV access is not rapidly established.

P. Pearls

a. Abdominal US is the preferred diagnostic study.
b. Physical exam is important:
    i. Peristaltic waves may be seen after a feeding.
    ii. Palpation of an "olive" is pathognomonic. When this is present, no further diagnostics are necessary.
c. Fluid resuscitation and nasogastric decompression in sick infants.
    i. Hypochloremic hypokalemic metabolic alkalosis is pathognomonic of electrolyte derangement.
    ii. Potassium chloride added to fluids once urine output observed.
d. Typically presents in the second to sixth week of life and is usually in first-born males.

Q. Figure legends

i. Figure 2.1 Ultrasound image of the right upper quadrant in the longitudinal plane showing an elongated pylorus (>14 mm) with thickened pyloric muscle (>4 mm).

R. References

a. *Tintinalli's Emergency Medicine: A Comprehensive Study Guide* (9th ed.): Chapter 131, Vomiting, Diarrhea, and Dehydration in Infants and Children.
b. *Rosen's Emergency Medicine: Concepts and Clinical Practice* (10th ed.): Chapter 166, Pediatric Gastrointestinal Disorders.

Altered Mental Status

Matthew Kuhns, MD and Jacob Holton, MD

A. Chief complaint
a. 60-year-old male arrives by car with a headache

B. Vital signs
a. BP: 145/60, HR: 85, RR: 14, T: 37°C, Sat: 100%

C. What does the patient look like?
a. The patient appears his stated age. Sitting in a chair holding his head, appears uncomfortable.

D. Primary survey
a. Airway: speaking in full sentences
b. Breathing: no respiratory distress
c. Circulation: warm and dry skin, normal pulses, and capillary refill

E. Action
a. Peripheral IV line
b. Monitor (unchanged if no bolus) if a bolus is given: BP: 149/69, HR: 55, RR: 18, Sat: 100% on room air
c. Finger stick glucose (result = 395 mg/dL)

F. History
a. HPI: A 60-year-old male with a history of hypertension and recurrent lower-extremity DVT is brought in by his wife for a headache. The patient states he was at home preparing dinner when he developed a sudden-onset headache. He notes a severe diffuse headache that is the worst of his life. The patient's headache is associated with photophobia and nausea, with one episode of non-bloody non-bilious emesis. He denies any chest pain, shortness of breath, abdominal pain, or diarrhea. He has been in his normal state of health without any recent fevers, neck stiffness, numbness, weakness, or balance problems. He denies any previous history of similar headaches.
b. PMHx: hypertension, DVT (chronic)
c. PSHx: none
d. Allergies: none
e. Meds: warfarin, lisinopril, HCTZ
f. Social: no history of smoking, drinking, or drugs; patient lives with his wife
g. FHx: noncontributory
h. PMD: Dr. Smith

G. Secondary survey

a. General: uncomfortable but nontoxic appearing male
b. HEENT: normocephalic, atraumatic, 3 mm pupils reactive to light, moist mucus membranes
c. Neck: no midline tenderness, normal ROM, no lymphadenopathy
d. Chest: clear bilaterally, no crackles or rales
e. Heart: regular rate and rhythm, no murmur, gallops, or rubs
f. Abdomen: soft, nontender, no guarding or rebound, normal bowel sounds
g. Rectal: normal tone, hemoccult negative, brown stool
h. GU: normal external genitalia
i. Back: no abrasions, hematomas, or ecchymoses
j. Neuro: normal motor strength, sensation intact, no tremor, no ataxia, cranial nerves intact. Glasgow coma scale: eye = 4, verbal = 5, motor = 6
k. Extremities: no peripheral edema noted; normal radial and dorsalis pedis pulses bilaterally
l. Skin: dry, warm, no rashes
m. Lymph: normal

I. Action

a. Labs:
   i. CBC, BMP, PT/PTT/INR, type and crossmatch
b. Meds: IV antiemetic such as metoclopramide, hold NSAIDs or aspirin if intracranial hemorrhage is being considered
c. CT head

J. Nurse

a. BP: 145/80, HR: 60, RR: 14, Sat: 100%
b. Reassess:
   i. Patient pain mildly improved

K. Results

Table 3.1 Results table

Test	Result	Test	Result
Complete blood count:		T bili	1.2 mg/dL
WBC	$10.9 \times 10^3/\mu L$	D bili	0.2 mg/dL
Hct	33%	Amylase	204 U/L
Plt	$261 \times 10^3/\mu L$	Lipase	223 U/L
		Albumin	3.2 g/dL
Basic metabolic panel:			
Na	134 mEq/L	**Urinalysis:**	
K	3.9 mEq/L	SG	1.028
Cl	102 mEq/L	pH	6.5
CO_2	24 mEq/L	Prot	Neg
BUN	16 mEq/dL	Gluc	+

Table 3.1 (cont.)

Test	Result		Test	Result
Cr	0.8 mg/dL		Ketones	Neg
Gluc	405 mg/dL		Bili	Neg
			Blood	Neg
Coagulation panel:			LE	Neg
PT	30 sec		Nitrite	Neg
PTT	26 sec		Color	Yellow
INR	2.9			
			Arterial blood gas:	
Liver function panel			pH	7.4
AST	25 U/L		pO_2	85 mmHg
ALT	33 U/L		pCO_2	40 mmHg
Alk phos	44 U/L		HCO_3	25 mmol/L

a. Head CT (Figure 3.1)

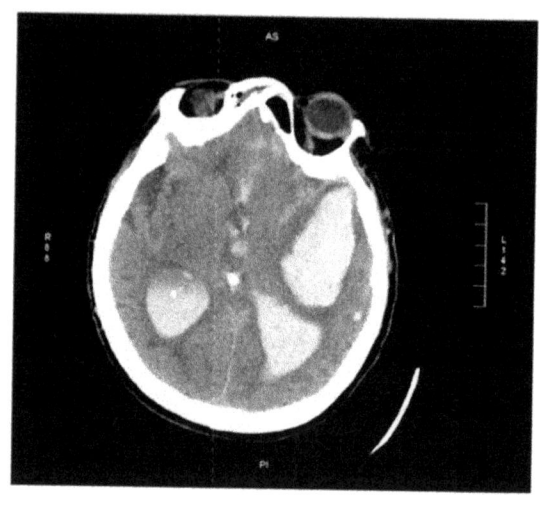

Figure 3.1

L. Action
a. Neurosurgical consult and neurosurgical intensive care unit (ICU) admission
b. Two large-bore peripheral IV lines (if not already placed)
c. Central line and arterial line placement (optional for ED evaluation)
d. Prothrombin complex concentrate (PCC) or vitamin K and fresh frozen plasma if PCC unavailable to reverse anticoagulation

M. Nursing
a. Vitals: BP: 199/104, HR: 45, RR: 16, T: 37.2°C, Sat: 100%
b. Reassess: patient has become somnolent and difficult to arouse. Respirations are sonorous with gurgling.

N. Action

a. Endotracheal intubation
    i. Bag valve mask with good technique (oral airway, good mask seal, jaw thrust, etc.) or nasal cannula and nonrebreather at flush rate to optimally preoxygenate.
    ii. Rapid sequence intubation using medications to protect against possible increased intracranial pressure:
        a. Consider premedication with fentanyl to blunt sympathetic response to laryngoscopy. Lidocaine pretreatment not recommended.
        b. Induction with etomidate or ketamine
        c. Paralysis with rocuronium or succinylcholine
        d. Post-intubation CXR and VBG/ABG, Foley catheter, sedation

b. Consider slight hyperventilation only if $PaCO_2$ 30–35 mmHg can be maintained and monitored; otherwise do not attempt this as over- or undershooting this range is harmful.

c. Elevated head of the bed 30 degrees

d. Mannitol (1 g/kg IV bolus) or hypertonic saline (250 mL IV bolus 3% NaCl)

e. EKG

O. Results

a. CXR (Figure 3.2)

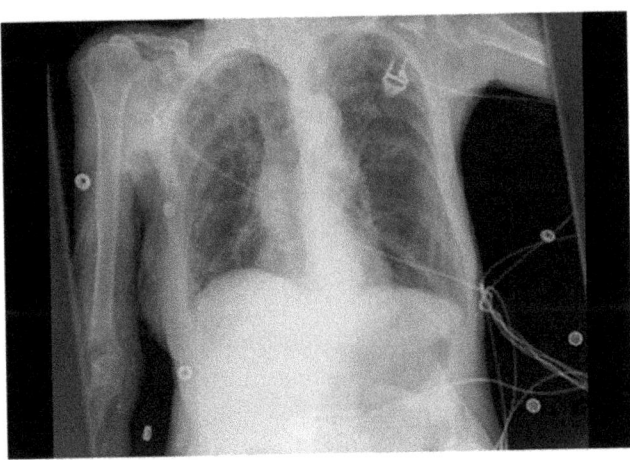

Figure 3.2

b. EKG (Figure 3.3)

P. Diagnosis

a. Nontraumatic intracranial hemorrhage (ICH)

Q. Critical actions

a. Head CT for new-onset coma
b. Large-bore IV access
c. Laboratory evaluation (coagulation factors)
d. Manage airway
e. Address increased ICP with mannitol or hypertonic saline
f. Reversal of anticoagulation (with one or more of the following: PCC, FFP, vitamin K)
g. Neurosurgical consultation
h. ICU admission

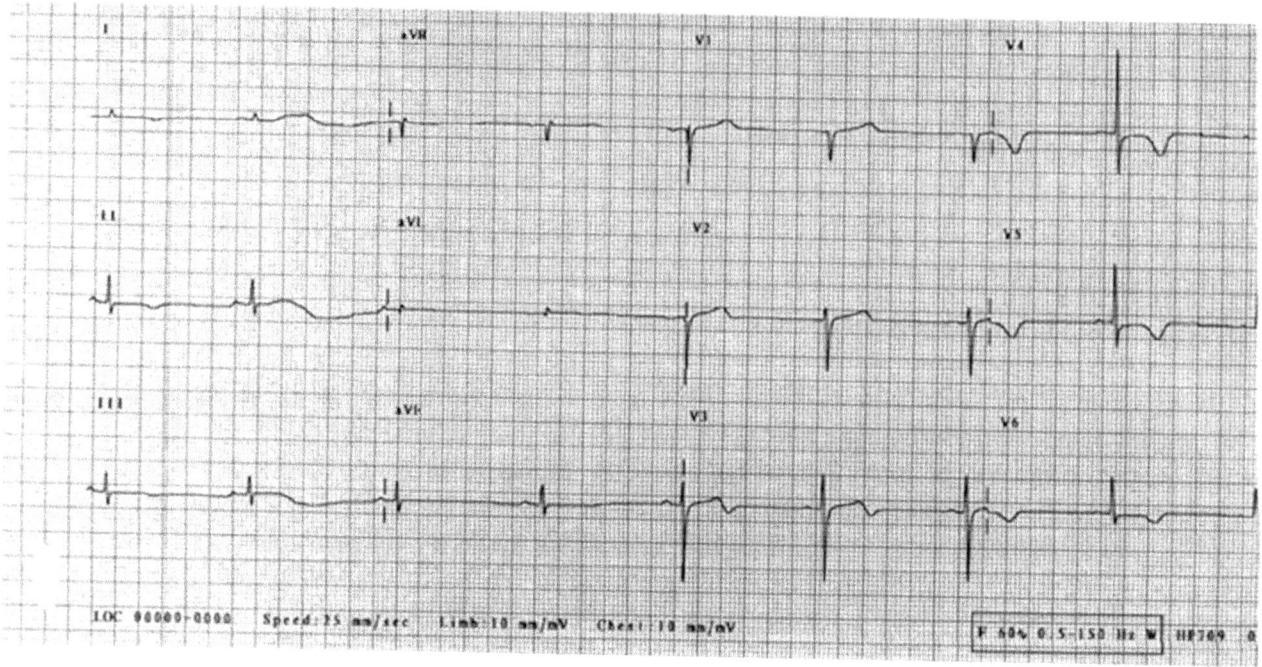

Figure 3.3

R. Examiner instructions

a. This is a case of nontraumatic intracranial hemorrhage (ICH) in a patient on anticoagulation for recurrent DVT. Anticoagulation is a risk factor for life-threatening bleeding complications, including intracranial bleeding. Intracranial hemorrhage should be suspected in patients with sudden onset or "thunderclap" headaches and can often be associated with nausea and vomiting. Early actions should include obtaining coagulation studies as well as a stat CT head to confirm the diagnosis.

b. Reversal of anticoagulation is a priority in the treatment of this patient. The patient's anticoagulated status will place him at high risk for continued bleeding and clinical decompensation. Prothrombin complex concentrates (PCCs) are the fastest method of reversing the patient's anticoagulation and require less volume. However, if PCCs are not available, vitamin K and FFP should be used.

c. The patient clinically decompensates through the course of this case with the development of altered mental status and abnormal vital signs. These changes are representative of increasing intracranial hypertension secondary to continued intracranial bleeding. Important next steps to address this change should include intubation to secure the patient's airway, mannitol or 3% saline to decrease cerebral edema, elevating the head of the bed, and consideration of hyperventilation to a $PaCO_2$ to 30–35 mmHg. It is important not to hyperventilate prophylactically, but only in impending herniation and only for brief periods. Hyperventilation can lead to cerebral ischemia. The measures are only temporizing, until definitive surgical management can be obtained.

S. Pearls

a. Intracranial hemorrhage should be suspected in patients with sudden-onset severe headaches. The most important diagnostic step is to obtain a stat CT head.

b. Prothrombin complex concentrates are faster than the more traditional FFP and vitamin K in reversal of anticoagulation in life-threatening bleeds.

   c. The Cushing reflex is a sign of increased intracranial hypertension and consists of hypertension associated with bradycardia.

   d. Temporizing measures including mannitol, hypertonic saline, and (rarely) hyperventilation should be employed pending more definitive surgical management.

T. Figure legends

   a. Figure 3.1 (Head CT) Subarachnoid, intraparenchymal, and intraventricular hemorrhage.

   b. Figure 3.2 (CXR) ET tube in place; osteoporosis/degenerative joint disease.

   c. Figure 3.3 (EKG) Sinus bradycardia with broad T-wave inversions throughout.

U. References

   a. *Tintinalli's Emergency Medicine: A Comprehensive Study Guide* (9th ed.): Chapter 166, Spontaneous Subarachnoid and Intracerebral Hemorrhage. Chapter 168, Altered Mental Status and Coma.

   b. *Rosen's Emergency Medicine: Concepts and Clinical Practice* (10th ed.): Chapter 12, Depressed Consciousness and Coma.

Chest Trauma

Wakas Ahmed, DO, Shayna Adams, MD, and Abiola Fasina, MD

A. Chief complaint

a. 34-year-old male stabbed in the chest

B. Vital signs

a. BP: 88/42, HR: 110, RR: 28, T: 37.9°C, Sat: 92% on nonrebreather mask

C. What does the patient look like?

a. Young disheveled male, appears intoxicated. Patient is gasping and complaining of difficulty breathing and right-sided chest pain. Patient appears slightly somnolent but is following commands and answering questions.

D. Primary survey

a. Airway: speaking in short sentences and gasping for air

b. Breathing: moderate respiratory distress with decreased breath sounds on the right. Hyper-resonant to percussion. Tracheal deviation to the left (candidate must ask)

c. Circulation: patient has slightly cool extremities but capillary refill is normal, distended neck veins

E. Action

a. Supplemental oxygen

b. Bedside ultrasound to evaluate for pneumothorax, hemothorax, and cardiac tamponade (Figure 4.1)

    i. Remainder of E-FAST exam is normal (if performed)

c. Two large-bore peripheral IV lines

d. Needle decompression or finger thoracostomy, hiss of air audible after insertion

e. Pain medication

f. Tube thoracostomy (pigtail catheter or chest tube)

g. Labs

    i. CBC, BMP, PT/PTT, ABG, serum toxicology screen, blood type and crossmatch

h. Monitor: BP: 130/80, HR: 96, RR: 18, Sat: 98% on nonrebreather mask (after thoracostomy)

i. EKG (Figure 4.2)

j. Prepare for emergent intubation (if needed)

F. History

a. HPI: A 34-year-old male with no significant past medical or surgical history reports being stabbed in the right chest by a broken bottle. Patient admits to drinking several beers but

Case 4: Chest Trauma

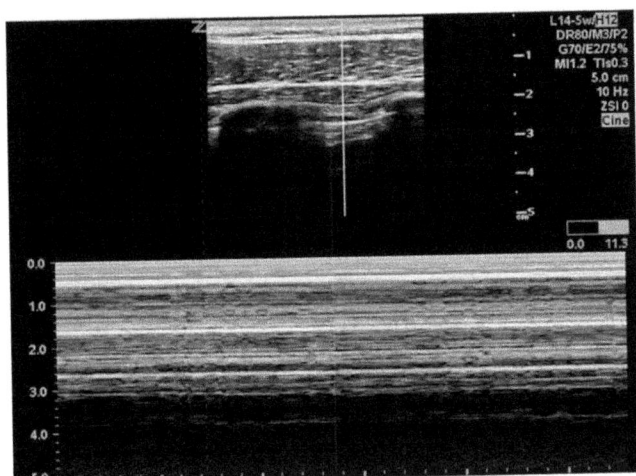

Figure 4.1

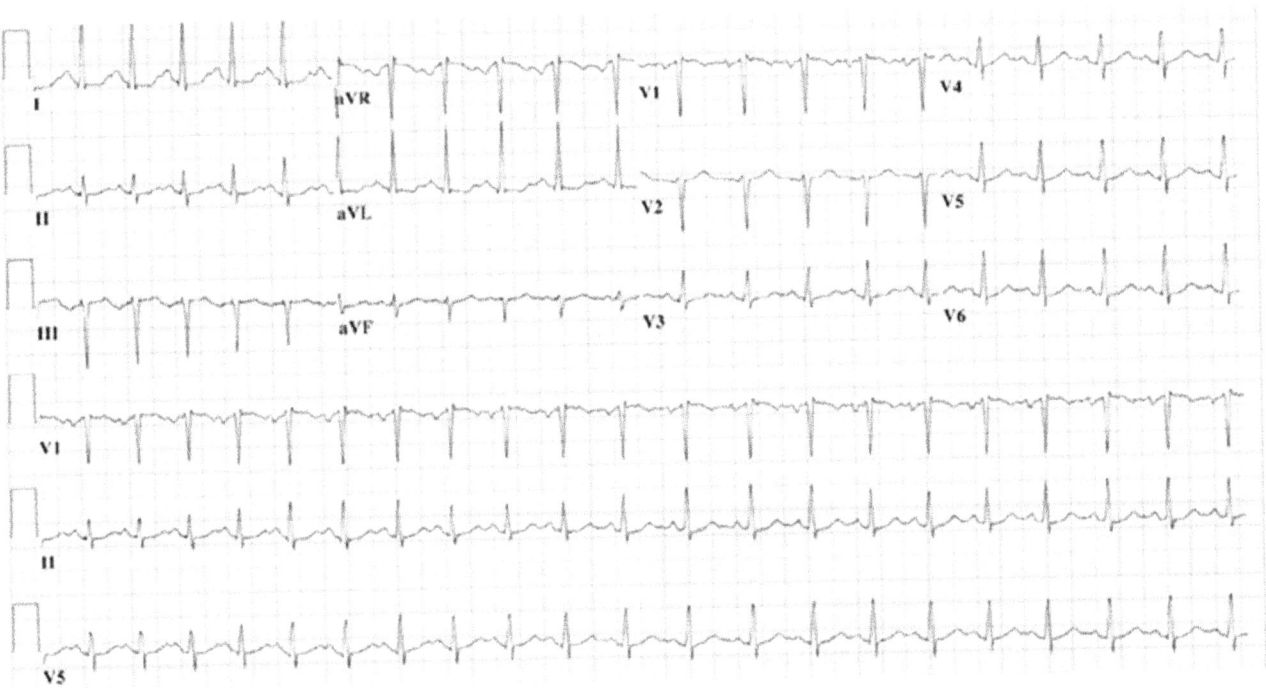

Figure 4.2

denies additional drug use. There was no loss of consciousness. Patient denies any head or neck trauma.

b. PMHx: none
c. PSHx: none
d. Allergies: penicillin
e. Meds: none
f. Social: works in construction, lives with three friends; denies tobacco and illicit drug use, but admits to recent alcohol use ("a few beers")
g. FHx: noncontributory

G. Nurse

a. Monitor and pulse oximetry
b. Repeat vital signs after needle/tube thoracostomy
   i. BP: 130/80, HR: 96, RR: 18, Sat: 98% on nonrebreather mask

H. Secondary survey

a. General: young, disheveled male, somnolent, arousable, oriented, appears intoxicated
b. HEENT: normal except injected conjunctiva, no injury or bruising noted, pupils equal, reactive
c. Neck: trachea is now midline; neck veins appear normal, no stridor noted
d. Chest: chest tube or pigtail catheter in right chest; breath sounds are still slightly diminished on the right; no crackles or rales, symmetric excursion; deep 6 cm laceration present along the right anterior chest wall, near fourth to fifth rib space. No visible foreign body, no active bleeding
e. Heart: normal; no murmurs or rub
f. Abdomen: soft, nondistended; no peritoneal signs; bowel sounds normal
g. Rectal: normal, fecal occult blood (guaiac test) negative
h. GU: normal
i. Extremities: moving all four extremities well, normal pulses bilaterally, slightly pale, good tone and 5/5 strength
j. Back: normal
k. Neuro: patient is following commands easily, normal on examination
l. Skin: as stated earlier
m. Lymph: normal

I. Action

a. Tube thoracostomy (pigtail catheter or chest tube) if not placed earlier (describe procedure)
b. Portable upright CXR to confirm placement and assess for other cardiopulmonary dysfunction (Figure 4.3)
c. Right-sided anterior chest wall laceration dressed
d. Surgical consult

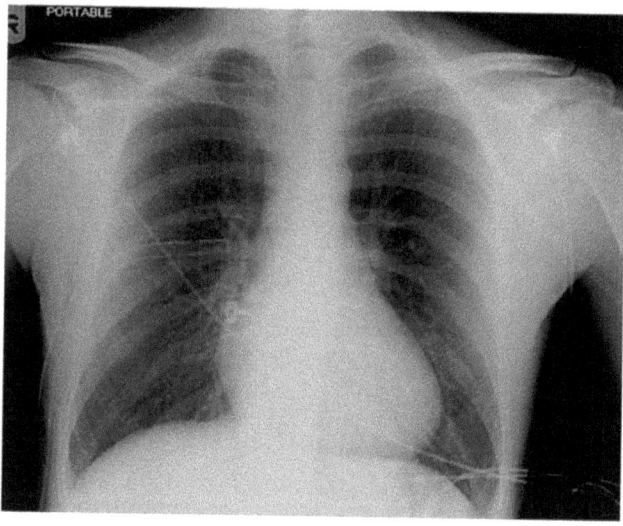

Figure 4.3

J. Nurse

a. Vital signs stable after tube thoracostomy and 1 L crystalloid bolus
    i. BP: 130/80, HR: 96, RR: 18, Sat: 98% on 2 L oxygen by nasal cannula
b. Patient complaining of some chest pain

K. Results

Table 4.1 Results table

Test	Result	Test	Result
Blood Type	AB+	**Liver function panel:**	
		AST	44 U/L
		ALT	34 U/L
Complete blood count:		Alk phos	55 U/L
WBC	$14.2 \times 10^3/\mu L$	T bili	0.8 mg/dL
Hct	39%	D bili	0.1 mg/dL
Plt	$300 \times 10^3/\mu L$	Amylase	200 U/L
		Lipase	23 U/L
		Albumin	3.9 g/dL
Basic metabolic panel:			
Na	140 mEq/L		
K	3.8 mEq/L	**Urinalysis:**	
Cl	107 mEq/L	SG	1.028
CO_2	27 mEq/L	pH	6
BUN	21 mEq/L	Prot	Neg
Cr	0.9 mg/dL	Gluc	Neg
Gluc	110 mg/dL	Ketones	Neg
		Bili	Neg
Coagulation panel:		Blood	Neg
PT	12.3 sec	LE	Neg
PTT	31 sec	Nitrite	Neg
INR	1.0	Color	Yellow
Ethanol	190 mg/dL		
Acetaminophen	Neg	**Arterial blood gas:**	
Salicylates	Neg	pH	7.4
		pO_2	90 mmHg
		pCO_2	40 mmHg
		HCO_3	27 mmol/L

L. Action
a. Meds
    i. Morphine IV
    ii. Antibiotics
    iii. Tetanus toxoid IM

  b. Reassess
      i. Patient is more comfortable, breathing easier, and saturating well; awaiting surgical consult
          to assess and repair chest laceration, admitted to SICU

M. Diagnosis
  a. Tension pneumothorax

N. Critical actions
  a. Needle thoracostomy or finger thoracostomy
  b. Tube thoracostomy
  c. CXR
  d. Pain management
  e. Diligent search for other traumatic injuries
  f. Surgical consult

O. Examiner instructions
  a. This is a case of tension pneumothorax resulting from penetrating trauma. Air has become
      trapped outside the lung within this patient's chest, impairing the normal mechanics of
      respiration and causing obstructive shock. Preload decreases with increased intrathoracic
      pressure, as venous return to the heart by the inferior and superior vena cava is diminished.
      It is a diagnosis that the candidate should make during the primary survey before ordering
      radiologic or laboratory tests based solely on the physical examination findings. Classic
      signs and symptoms include: labored breathing, hypotension, distended neck veins, tracheal
      deviation to the unaffected (contralateral) side, diminished or absent breath sounds, and
      ipsilateral hyperresonance. The most important early action is to perform immediate needle
      decompression to convert the tension pneumothorax to a simple pneumothorax. It is also
      reasonable to perform a chest thoracostomy (incision through the chest wall and pleura;
      the first steps of a tube thoracostomy), which will release the tension even before definitive
      tube placement. The patient's vital signs will deteriorate (oxygen saturation and blood
      pressure will drop, heart rate will rise, and the patient will lose consciousness) until needle
      or tube thoracostomy is performed. The patient should be kept on supplemental oxygen and
      monitored while a thoracostomy tube is placed. Ideally, only after these critical steps should a
      chest radiograph be ordered and obtained. Other important early actions include continuous
      cardiac monitoring and oximetry, diagnostic testing (serum, ultrasound, etc.) as part of a
      diligent search for other traumatic injuries, and early surgical consultation.

P. Pearls
  a. Tension pneumothorax should be diagnosed clinically; no CXR needed initially.
  b. Immediate needle thoracostomy followed by tube thoracostomy are critical actions.
  c. Tracheal deviation is a rare and very late finding in tension pneumothorax. Although this
      finding is often used as a pathognomonic sign for tension pneumothorax, its absence certainly
      does not exclude the diagnosis.

Q. Figure legends
  a. Figure 4.1 (Ultrasound) barcode (aka stratosphere) sign demonstrating lack of pleural sliding
      concerning for pneumothorax.
  b. Figure 4.2 (EKG) sinus tachycardia.
  c. Figure 4.3 (CXR) right sided chest tube and resolved pneumothorax.

R. References

a. *Tintinalli's Emergency Medicine: A Comprehensive Study Guide* (9th ed.): Chapter 254, Trauma in Adults. Chapter 261, Pulmonary Trauma

b. *Rosen's Emergency Medicine: Concepts and Clinical Practice* (10th ed.): Chapter 37. Thoracic Trauma.

Abdominal Pain and Vomiting

Shefali Trivedi, MD

A. Chief complaint
a. 45-year-old female suffering from abdominal pain

B. Vital signs
a. BP: 145/85, HR: 93, RR: 16, T: 38.6°C, Sat: 99% on RA

C. What does the patient look like?
a. Patient appears stated age, overweight, lying in stretcher holding abdomen, uncomfortable due to pain, in mild distress.

D. Primary survey
a. Airway: patent, speaking in full sentences
b. Breathing: no apparent respiratory distress, no cyanosis
c. Circulation: warm, dry skin, normal capillary refill

E. History
a. HPI: A 45-year-old female with a past medical history of hypertension, hypercholesterolemia, and gallstones presents with worsening abdominal pain for 1 day. She states that her pain is constant, sharp, and worst in the right upper quadrant, occasionally radiating to the right shoulder. She has had several similar episodes over the past 2 years that have either resolved spontaneously or with pain medications after about 1–2 hours. All episodes have begun after eating a "heavy" meal, as did this episode. She complains of a subjective fever and chills for 1 day and nausea and three episodes of nonbilious, nonbloody vomiting. She denies diarrhea, constipation, chest pain, shortness of breath, sick contacts, recent travel history, unusual food intake, trauma, or urinary symptoms.
b. PMHx: hypertension, hypercholesterolemia
c. PSHx: none
d. Allergies: no known drug allergies
e. Meds: none
f. Social: lives with her husband and two children, denies smoking, alcohol, or drug use; sexually active with her husband only
g. FHx: mother with hypertension, father with hypercholesterolemia and hypertension
h. PMD: none

F. Secondary survey
a. General: alert and oriented, overweight, mild distress due to pain
b. HEENT: normal
c. Neck: normal
d. Chest: normal
e. Heart: normal
f. Abdomen: normal bowel sounds, soft, severe tenderness in the right upper quadrant with voluntary guarding, positive Murphy's sign, nontender at McBurney's point, no pulsatile masses, no hepatosplenomegaly, no hernia, no rebound or guarding
g. Rectal: brown stool, fecal occult blood (guaiac test) negative, normal rectal tone
h. GU: normal
i. Extremities: normal
j. Back: normal, no costovertebral angle tenderness
k. Neuro: normal
l. Skin: normal
m. Lymph: normal

G. Action
a. One or two large-bore peripheral IV lines
b. Labs
    i. CBC, BMP, liver function panel, PT/PTT, blood type and hold, urinalysis, blood culture, urine culture, qualitative or quantitative hCG (urine or serum)
c. 1 L crystalloid bolus
d. Monitor: BP: 139/83, HR: 96, RR: 16, Sat: 100% on oxygen 2 LPM by nasal cannula
e. Imaging
    i. CXR
    ii. Right upper quadrant ultrasound
    iii. EKG
f. Meds
    i. Third-generation cephalosporin (cefotaxime or ceftriaxone) IV *plus* metronidazole IV *or* single broad-spectrum IV antibiotic (piperacillin-tazobactam)
    ii. Morphine sulfate IV or ketorolac IV
    iii. Odansetron IV or sublingual
    iv. Acetaminophen PO
    v. IV fluids
g. Reassess
    i. Patient's pain has improved somewhat, but still complains of right-sided upper quadrant abdominal pain

H. Nurse
a. BP: 142/76, HR: 86, RR: 16, Sat: 100% on oxygen 2 LPM by nasal cannula

I. Results

Table 5.1 Results table

Test	Result	Test	Result
Complete blood count:		**Liver function panel:**	
WBC	$15.6 \times 10^3/\mu L$	AST	22 U/L
Hct	41.70%	ALT	20 U/L
Plt	$350 \times 10^3/\mu L$	Alk phos	325 U/L
		T bili	5.0 mg/dL
Basic metabolic panel:		D bili	3.5 mg/dL
Na	142 mEq/L	Amylase	56 U/L
K	4.2 mEq/L	Lipase	24 U/L
Cl	105 mEq/L	Albumin	4.0 g/dL
CO2	24 mEq/L		
BUN	15 mEq/dL	**Urinalysis:**	
Cr	0.9 mg/dL	SG	1.015
Gluc	110 mg/dL	pH	6
		Prot	Neg
Coagulation panel:		Gluc	Neg
PT	13.2 sec	Ketones	Neg
PTT	27 sec	Bili	Pos
INR	0.9	Blood	Neg
		LE	Neg
		Nitrite	Neg
		Color	Yellow

a. Urine pregnancy test: negative
b. EKG: normal sinus rhythm
c. CXR: clear lungs, no acute pulmonary process
d. Right upper quadrant US: gallstones, pericholecystic fluid, gallbladder wall thickening, and sonographic Murphy's sign. Normal common bile duct

J. Action
a. Surgery consult
   i. Admit for IV antibiotics and possible OR for cholecystectomy
b. Discussion with patient regarding need for admission and possible cholecystectomy

K. Diagnosis
a. Cholecystitis

Case 5: Abdominal Pain and Vomiting

L. Critical actions

a. Large-bore IV access
b. Right upper quadrant US
c. Pain management
d. Surgery consultation
e. Antibiotics

M. Examiner instructions

a. This is a case of acute cholecystitis. Symptoms are often worse after eating fatty meals. The patient continues to complain of fever until acetaminophen or other antipyretic is administered and will continue to complain of pain until an analgesic is given. It is important that the candidate administers antibiotics early and describes their concern for cholecystitis adequately to the surgical consultant (fever, Murphy's sign, elevated white blood cell count, vomiting, etc.).

N. Pearls

a. Fever and tachycardia are often absent in cholecystitis.
b. Ultrasound is the preferred imaging modality in acute care settings. Positive ultrasound findings could include gallstones, a thickened gallbladder wall, sonographic Murphy's sign, and pericholecystic fluid. The presence of gallstones and a positive sonographic Murphy's sign have a positive predictive value greater than 90%.
c. The differential diagnosis includes ascending cholangitis, choledocholithiasis, hepatitis, biliary colic, hepatic abscess, Fitz–Hugh–Curtis syndrome (fibrinous perihepatitis as a consequence of pelvic inflammatory disease), pyelonephritis, right lower lobe pneumonia/pleurisy, pleural effusion, pancreatitis, peptic ulcer disease (of the duodenum with perforation), and appendicitis.
d. Consider atypical myocardial infarction, particularly in elderly or diabetic patients presenting with similar symptoms.
e. In pregnant patients and young women, elicit a sexual history and consider performing a pelvic examination to exclude Fitz–Hugh–Curtis syndrome (as described above).
f. Patients with diabetes have an increased risk for bacterial invasion into the gallbladder wall and emphysematous cholecystitis.
g. Acalculous cholecystitis can occur in up to 5–10% of cholecystitis cases.
h. Patients with acalculous and emphysematous cholecystitis are at increased risk for a more rapid course, gangrene, and perforation, and require emergent cholecystectomy.

O. References

a. *Tintinalli's Emergency Medicine: A Comprehensive Study Guide* (9th ed.): Chapter 42, Pancreatitis and Cholecystitis.
b. *Rosen's Emergency Medicine: Concepts and Clinical Practice* (10th ed.): Chapter 76, Liver and Biliary Tract Disorders.

Weak Infant

Christopher Strother, MD

A. Chief complaint
a. 4-week-old female with fever, lethargy, and weakness, worsening over the past 2 days

B. Vital signs
a. HR: 205, BP: 50/20, RR: 58, T: 39.2°C, Sat: 94% on RA, Wt: 5 kg

C. What does the patient look like?
a. Patient appears stated age, lethargic, tachypneic, febrile, and flushed.

D. Primary survey
a. Airway: patent, weak cry
b. Breathing: tachypnea, no cyanosis, lungs clear
c. Circulation: warm flushed skin, capillary refill three seconds, tachycardia

E. Action
a. Oxygen supplementation (nasal cannula or nonrebreather mask)
b. Largest possible peripheral IV × 2, likely in the antecubital fossa; interosseous (IO) line if any difficulty with peripheral line
c. Labs
   i. Bedside serum glucose = 30 mg/dL
   ii. Lactate (blood gas), CBC, BMP, LFT, PT/PTT, blood culture, UA, urine culture
   iii. Lumbar puncture and spinal fluid studies deferred until patient stabilized
d. 20 mL/kg bolus NS
e. Monitor: HR: 200, BP: 50/25, RR: 58, Sat: 100% on O_2
f. Dextrose bolus 0.5 g/kg (dosing: 10% dextrose = 5 mL/kg; 25% dextrose = 2 mL/kg)

F. History
a. HPI: A 4-week-old female, born full term by normal spontaneous vaginal delivery without complications, doing well until past two days. Initially she was noted by the parents to have fussiness, sleepiness, and poor feeding. These symptoms and signs were followed by "really high" tactile fever and lethargy today. Fever, lethargy, poor feeding, and irritability were noticed today and are present on initial examination. There is no history of vomiting, diarrhea, cough, travel, or recent exposure to other sick contacts.
b. PMHx: full term, no complications
c. PSHx: none

d. Allergies: none
e. Social: lives with parents, two older siblings
f. FHx: not relevant
g. PMD: Dr. Chris

G. Nurse
a. NS bolus 20 mL/kg (100 mL)
  i. HR: 190, BP: 60/40, RR: 50, Sat: 100% on O_2
b. If no fluids, then
  i. HR: 205, BP: 50/25, RR: 55, Sat: 100% on O_2

H. Secondary survey
a. General: lethargic, very weak cry and motions, tachypnea, febrile
b. HEENT: anterior fontanelle open soft and sunken
c. Neck: normal
d. Chest: normal
e. Heart: mild vibratory systolic murmur, tachycardia
f. Abdomen: normal
g. Rectal: normal
h. GU: normal
i. Extremities: normal
j. Back: normal
k. Neuro: normal
l. Skin: warm, flushed, capillary refill 3 seconds
m. Lymph: normal

I. Action
a. Recheck blood glucose: now 120 mg/dL
b. Prepare for early endotracheal intubation for airway protection in sepsis/lethargy
  i. Ventilator settings: volume 5–10 mL/kg, rate 30, O_2 100%
c. Meds
  i. Cefotaxime IV or cefepime IV
  ii. Ampicillin IV
  iii. Multiple fluid boluses 60 mL/kg up to 100 mL/kg total
  iv. Acetaminophen rectally
d. Reassess
  i. Patient with mild improvement in fever after 15 minutes so decreased warmth and flush, some decrease in HR and tachypnea, but only after multiple fluid boluses (as stated above)
e. Imaging
  i. CXR (Figure 6.1)

J. Nurse
a. HR: 170, BP: 65/45 (after NS boluses), RR: 50, Sat: 100% on O_2 (or vent)
b. Patient: mild global improvement

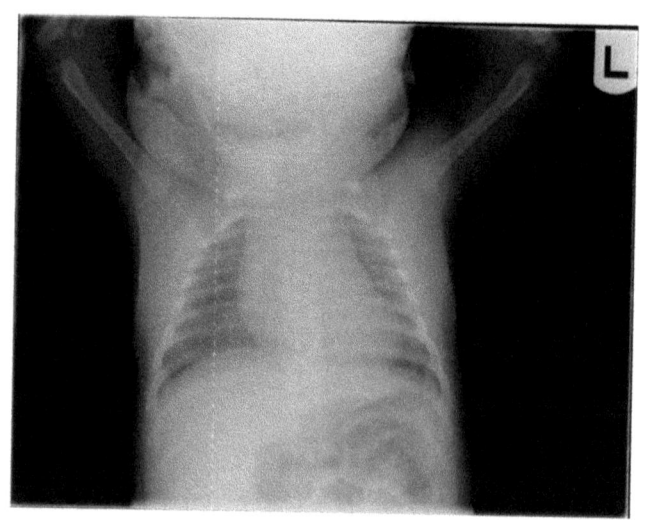

Figure 6.1

K. Results

Table 6.1 Results table

Test	Result	Test	Result
Complete blood count:		T bili	3.1 mg/dL
WBC	$22.1 \times 10^3/\mu L$	D bili	0.8 mg/dL
Hct	45.50%	Amylase	40 U/L
Plt	$425 \times 10^3/\mu L$	Lipase	20 U/L
		Albumin	3.5 g/dL
Basic metabolic panel:			
Na	140 mEq/L	**Urinalysis:**	
K	3.8 mEq/L	SG	1.030
Cl	110 mEq/L	pH	7
CO_2	13 mEq/L	Prot	Neg
BUN	3 mEq/dL	Gluc	Neg
Cr	0.6 mg/dL	Ketones	Neg
Gluc	35 mg/dL	Bili	Neg
		Blood	Neg
Coagulation panel:		LE	Neg
PT	11.4 sec	Nitrite	Neg
PTT	29 sec	Color	Yellow
INR	1.0		
		Arterial blood gas:	
Liver function panel:		pH	7.1
AST	90 U/L	pO_2	160 mmHg
ALT	75 U/L	pCO_2	35 mmHg
Alk phos	200 U/L	HCO_3	12 mmol/L

Case 6: Weak Infant

a. Lactate: 4.6 mmol/L
b. LDH: 610 U/L

L. Action
a. Pediatric intensive care unit (PICU) consult
b. Discussion with family and PMD on need for ICU admission and monitoring for likely septic shock
c. Meds
   i. Continued fluid support, antibiotics, antipyretics

M. Diagnosis
a. Sepsis

N. Critical actions
a. IV or IO access
b. Administer dextrose
c. Multiple fluid boluses
d. Early antibiotics
e. ICU consult

O. Examiner instructions
a. This is a case of an infant in septic shock from bacteremia. Early and generous fluid support is essential to maintain blood pressure and cardiac output. Antibiotics should be given early. If the infant is very lethargic, intubation should be performed to protect the airway and to decrease the metabolic demands (work) of breathing. In a stable infant, a full work-up is required, including a lumbar puncture to obtain cerebrospinal fluid for culture and analysis. In an unstable infant, blood and urinalysis are usually obtained quickly, but lumbar puncture may not be; this procedure may be deferred, as it may delay emergent stabilizing interventions and could unnecessarily physiologically stress the critically ill neonate. This patient will need to be expeditiously moved to an intensive care setting as continuous hemodynamic monitoring and frequent serial reassessments will be needed.

P. Pearls
a. Septic shock is a form of distributive shock. Other forms of shock (e.g., hypovolemic shock) may be superimposed. The recommended initial management for septic shock is the rapid administration of crystalloid fluids (a minimum volume of 20 mL/kg up to 100 mL/kg may be required; 60 mL/kg rapidly is the goal if in shock). Vasopressor support should be considered for patients with septic shock and hypotension refractory to 60 mL/kg of fluid administration.
b. Broad-spectrum antibiotics should be given early in the management of an infant who may be septic.
c. Sepsis should be considered high on the differential diagnosis of any newborn presenting *in extremis*; empiric treatment should be initiated before diagnostic testing confirms the diagnosis.
d. Sick infants frequently become hypoglycemic; always check glucose in an ill-appearing child and give dextrose when needed. After dextrose, recheck to ensure adequate treatment.

Q. Figure legends
a. Figure 6.1 Normal chest x-ray.

R. References

a. *Tintinalli's Emergency Medicine: A Comprehensive Study Guide* (9th ed.): Chapter 119, Fever and Serious Bacterial Illness in Infants and Children.

b. *Rosen's Emergency Medicine: Concepts and Clinical Practice* (10th ed.): Chapter 161, Pediatric Fever.

Chest Pain

Calloway Pichette, MD, Scott Heinrich, MD, and Alan Huang, MD

A. Chief complaint
a.   19-year-old male complaining of chest pain

B. Vital signs
a.   BP: 100/60, HR: 104, RR: 28, T: 37.8°C, Sat: 99% RA
b.   Glucose 96 mg/dL (must ask)

C. What does the patient look like?
a.   He is alert but appears uncomfortable, anxious, and diaphoretic.

D. Primary survey
a.   Airway: speaking normally
b.   Breathing: tachypneic, but in no respiratory distress
c.   Circulation: skin diaphoretic, pulses are full in the peripheral extremities

E. Action
a.   Oxygen via nasal cannula
b.   Two large-bore peripheral IV lines
c.   Monitor: BP: 100/60, HR: 104, RR: 28, T: 37.8°C, Sat: 99% RA
d.   1 L fluid bolus
e.   EKG
f.   CXR
g.   Draw labs here and hold tubes

F. History
a.   HPI: a 19-year-old male college student with a history of asthma presents with sudden onset of burning chest pain while at rest this morning. The pain is rated a 10 out of 10, diffuse, and radiates to the shoulders and back. His chest pain is worse with swallowing (must ask for exacerbating symptoms). He denies emesis this morning, but had multiple episodes of nonbloody, nonbilious vomiting through the night. He binge-drank alcohol last night at a college party prior to the emesis starting (must ask about alcohol use). He denies having any shortness of breath. He denies tobacco, cocaine, or other illicit drug use. He denies any personal history of blood clots and any family history of cardiac disease. He reports no history of swelling in his legs.
b.   PMHx: asthma
c.   PSHx: none
d.   Allergies: none

e. Meds: albuterol inhaler PRN
f. Social: no tobacco or illicit drug use; occasional alcohol "binges"
g. FHx: noncontributory

G. Nurse
a. EKG (Figure 7.1)
b. If fluids given: BP: 115/65, HR: 100, RR: 22, T: 37.8°C, Sat: 99% RA
c. If no fluids given: BP: 90/56, HR: 125, RR: 24, T: 37.8°C, Sat: 99% RA, and patient appears
    more ill

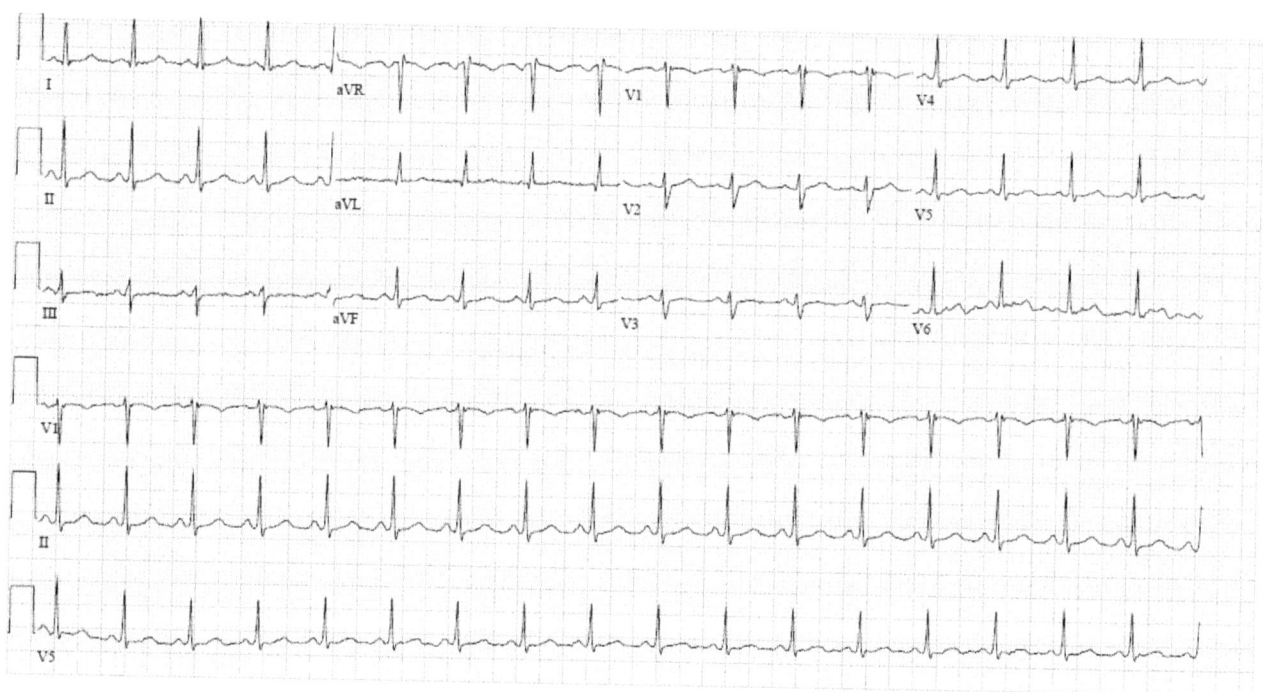

Figure 7.1

H. Secondary survey
a. General: alert, oriented, diaphoretic, remains uncomfortable
b. Head: normal
c. Eyes: normal
d. Neck: full range of motion, no jugular vein distension, crepitus bilaterally (provide only if
    asked)
e. Chest: nontender
f. Lungs: clear bilaterally
g. Heart: tachycardic, rhythm regular. If examinee asks: crunching, rasping sound, synchronous
    with the heartbeat is heard over the precordium on auscultation.
h. Abdomen: normal bowel sounds, soft, nondistended, moderate epigastric tenderness, no
    rebound or guarding
i. Skin: warm, diaphoretic; if fluids not given, cool, clammy skin

CASE 7: Chest Pain

I. Action

a. Review portable CXR (Figure 7.2)
b. Labs
    i. CBC, CMP, cardiac enzymes (optional), lipase, coagulation studies, blood type and hold
c. Meds
    i. Morphine IV
    ii. Antibiotics: imipenem-cilastatin (500–1000 mg IV Q6– Q8H) IV or vancomycin (15 mg/kg) and piperacillin-tazobactam (3.375 g)
    iii. H2 blocker IV
d. Gastroenterology (GI), cardiothoracic surgery, or otolaryngology (ENT) consult
e. Arrange CT neck/chest with contrast (Figure 7.3)

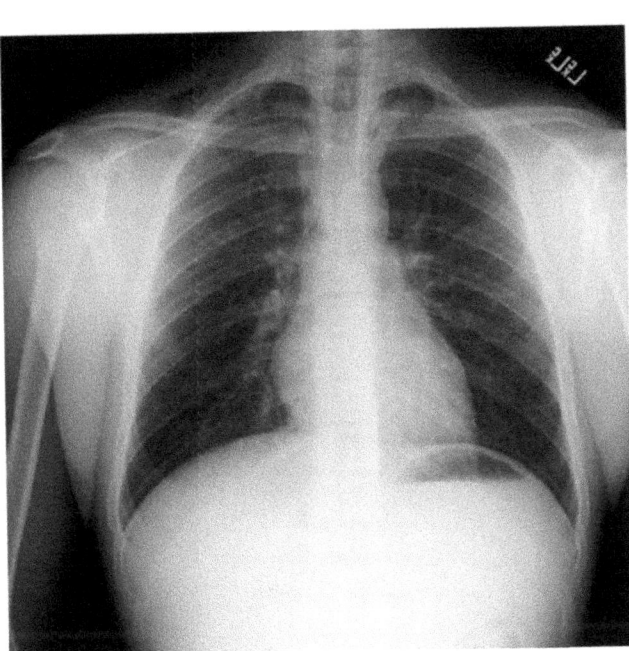

Figure 7.2

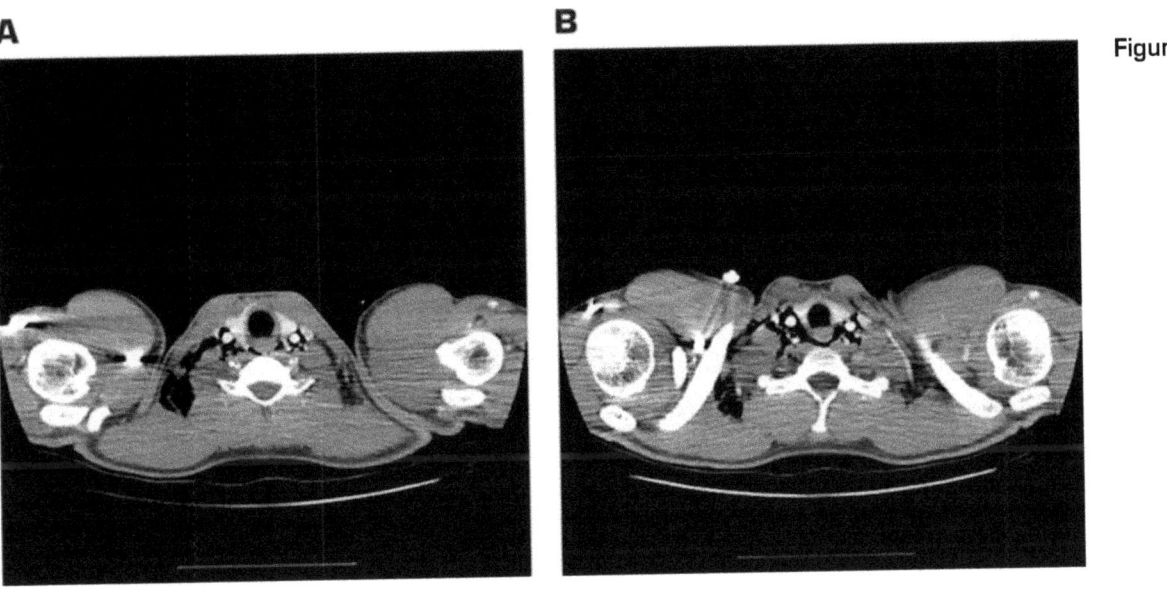

Figure 7.3

J. Results:

Table 7.1 Results table

Test	Result	Test	Result
Complete blood count:		T bili	0.5 mg/dL
WBC	$15.8 \times 10^3/\mu L$	D bili	0.1 mg/dL
Hgb	11.5 g/dL	Albumin	3.8 g/dL
Hct	35.20%	Lipase	200 U/L
Plt	$258 \times 10^3/\mu L$	Calcium	9.6 mg/dL
Complete metabolic panel:		**Urinalysis:**	
Na	135 mEq/L	SG	1.018
K	4.5 mEq/L	pH	7
Cl	102 mEq/L	Prot	Neg
CO_2	20 mEq/L	Gluc	Neg
BUN	15 mEq/L	Ketones	Neg
Cr	0.8 mg/dL	Bili	Neg
Glucose	85 mg/dL	Blood	Neg
		LE	Neg
Coagulation panel:		Nitrite	Neg
PT	14.1 sec	Color	Yellow
PTT	28.4 sec		
INR	1.0	**Arterial blood gas:**	
		pH	7.37
Liver function panel:		pO_2	80 mmHg
AST	33 U/L	pCO_2	44 mmHg
ALT	38 U/L	HCO_3	20 mmol/L
Alk phos	45 U/L		

a. If ordered: cardiac enzymes, D-dimer, alcohol: negative
b. Lactate: 2.5 mmol/L

K. Diagnosis
a. Boerhaave's syndrome

L. Critical actions
a. Consider esophageal tear in differential of chest pain in this patient
b. CXR to evaluate lungs and mediastinum
c. Emergent GI, ENT, and/or CT surgery consultations (for endoscopy and operative intervention)

d. Resuscitation with fluids
e. Broad-spectrum antibiotics to treat mediastinitis
f. Admit to intensive care setting or operating room

M. Examiner instructions

a. This is a case of Boerhaave's syndrome (tear of the esophagus) due to episodes of vomiting. Keys include recognition of this etiology as an extremely deadly cause of chest pain, especially in the setting of vomiting and very uncomfortable-appearing patient. Aggressive fluid resuscitation should begin early, or the patient's vital signs will deteriorate (heart rate will rise, blood pressure will fall, skin will become more clammy and mental status will deteriorate).
b. Curveball: consultants should be reluctant to see a "vomiting college student with recent binge drinking." They will only become interested when the candidate describes concern for esophageal rupture given crepitus on physical examination and x-ray findings. At examiner discretion, CT scanning could be made unavailable while the candidate evaluates the case using other means (e.g., CXR, physical exam findings, consultation with GI, etc.).

N. Pearls

a. A large proportion of esophageal tears are iatrogenic. However, spontaneous esophageal ruptures (10–15% of ruptures), or Boerhaave's syndrome, is associated with acts that increase intraluminal pressures, including vomiting (75%), coughing, straining, seizures.
b. Most common location of distal esophageal tear is left posterolateral.
c. Mackler's triad (subcutaneous emphysema, chest pain, and vomiting) is the classic presentation of spontaneous esophageal perforation, but occurs in less than 50% of patients.
d. Hamman's crunch is a raspy, crunching sound with each heartbeat, thought to be caused by the heart sliding against air-filled tissues in the mediastinum.
e. It can be associated with pleural effusion on CXR. Findings on CXR may not be visible in the first few hours of the presentation.
f. Severity of systemic toxicity dictates conservative versus operative management.
g. Mortality of full-thickness ruptures is very high.
h. If unsure of diagnosis, you can evaluate with chest CT or esophagram (use water-soluble contrast).

O. Figure legends

a. Figure 7.1 (EKG) Sinus tachycardia, no acute ischemic changes.
b. Figure 7.2 (CXR) Subcutaneous emphysema right shoulder and suspected pneumomediastinum.
c. Figure 7.3 (a) (Chest CT) Right pneumothorax. (b) (Chest CT) Subcutaneous emphysema neck.

P. References

a. *Tintinalli's Emergency Medicine: A Comprehensive Study Guide* (9th ed.): Chapter 77, Esophageal Emergencies.
b. *Rosen's Emergency Medicine: Concepts and Clinical Practice* (10th ed.): Chapter 75, Esophagus, Stomach, and Duodenum.

Lower Back Pain

Katarzyna Gore, MD and Daniel Spearman, MD

A. Chief complaint
a. Lower back pain

B. Vital signs
a. BP: 132/88, HR: 108, RR: 16, T: 38.3°C, Sat: 100% on RA

C. What does the patient look like?
a. Patient is uncomfortable-appearing due to pain, but is in no acute distress.

D. Primary survey
a. Airway: speaking in full sentences
b. Breathing: breath sounds clear and equal bilaterally
c. Circulation: skin is well perfused with strong pulses

E. History
a. HPI: Patient is a 42-year-old male presenting with lower back pain. Symptoms started one week ago. The back pain is dull and nonradiating. Patient reports taking ibuprofen without relief. He cannot pinpoint any inciting event that led to his back pain. He reports feeling generally weak but no focal weakness. Denies incontinence or sensory loss. He does not report altered mental status, fever, neck stiffness, photophobia, lower back trauma, nausea, vomiting, abdominal pain, cough, or shortness of breath.
b. PMHx: none
c. PSHx: none
d. Meds: ibuprofen
e. Allergies: none
f. Social history: current IV heroin user
g. FHx: noncontributory

F. Secondary survey
a. General: nontoxic appearing; in no acute distress
b. HEENT: normal
c. Chest: normal
d. Heart: tachycardic, normal rhythm; no murmurs or extra heart sounds
e. Abdomen: soft, nontender, nondistended, normoactive
f. Back: lumbar tenderness diffusely
g. Neuro: cranial nerves II–XII intact. Reflexes 2/5 bilaterally. Diminished rectal tone. Strength 5/5. Sensation intact
h. Skin: 3 cm in diameter abscess with surrounding erythema on the skin at the right inner thigh.

CASE 8: Lower Back Pain

G. Actions
a. Place peripheral IV(s)
b. Labs:
   i. CBC, BMP, ESR, type and screen, PT, INR, UA, blood cultures, urine cultures, wound cultures
d. 1 L crystalloid
e. Monitor
f. Medications
   i. PO acetaminophen
   ii. IV morphine
g. MRI spinal survey

H. Results

Table 8.1 Results table

Test	Result	Test	Result
Complete blood count:		D bili	0.2 mg/dL
WBC	$12 \times 10^3/\mu L$	Amylase	31 U/L
Hct	36.90%	Lipase	32 U/L
Plt	$320 \times 10^3/\mu L$	Albumin	4.1 g/dL
Basic metabolic panel:		**Urinalysis:**	
Na	140 mEq/L	SG	1.020
K	4.6 mEq/L	pH	6
Cl	98 mEq/L	Prot	Neg
CO_2	27 mEq/L	Glucose	Neg
BUN	9 mEq/dL	Ketones	Neg
Cr	0.9 mg/dL	Bili	Neg
Glucose	123 mg/dL	Blood	Neg
		LE	Neg
Coagulation panel:		Nitrites	Neg
PT	12.4 sec	Color	Yellow
PTT	31 sec		
INR	1.0	**Arterial blood gas:**	
		pH	7.39
		pO_2	85 mmHg
Liver function panel:		pCO_2	42 mmHg
AST	37 U/L	HCO_3	26 mmol/L
ALT	41 U/L		
Alk phos	54 U/L		
T bili	1.2 mg/dL	ESR	87 mm/hr

a. MRI (Figures 8.1 and 8.2)

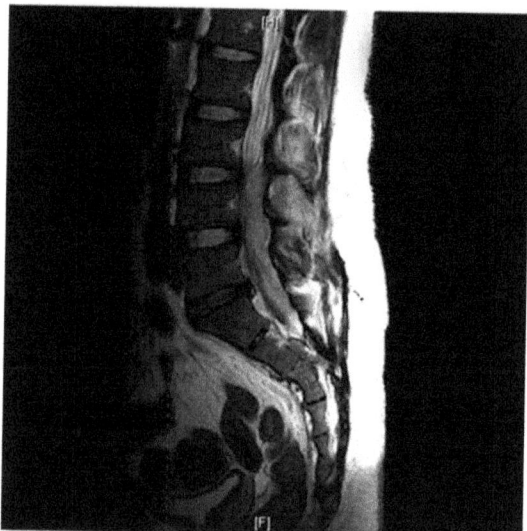

Figure 8.1

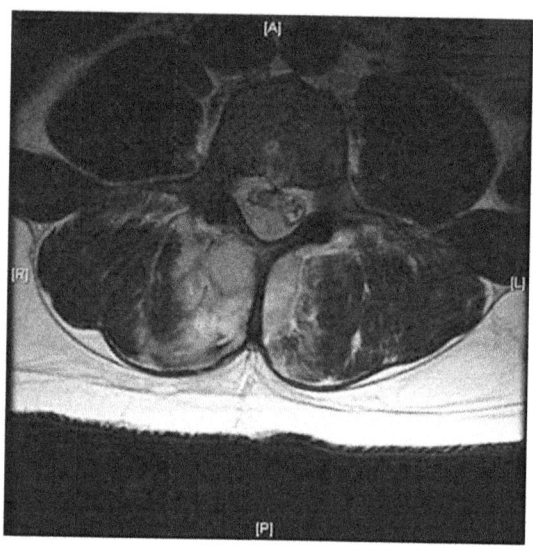

Figure 8.2

I. Actions
a. Consult neurosurgery
b. Start broad-spectrum IV antibiotics
c. Perform incision and drainage of skin abscess

J. Diagnosis
a. Epidural abscess

K. Critical actions
a. Obtain social history (IV drug use)
b. Complete skin exam (any lesions, track marks, abscesses)
c. Complete neuro exam (any neurologic deficits)
d. MRI of lumbar spine
e. Neurosurgery consultation
f. IV broad-spectrum antibiotics
g. Incision and drainage of abscess

CASE 8: Lower Back Pain

L. Examiner instructions
a. This is a case of spinal epidural abscess. The examiner should portray the radiologist, nurse, and neurosurgeon. The neurosurgeon should be reluctant to examine the patient as back pain is a common ED complaint. In communication with the neurosurgeon, the candidate should mention back pain, fever, elevated ESR with a source, and a focal neuro deficit. The candidate should insist that the patient be evaluated emergently despite push back from the neurosurgeon.

M. Pearls
a. *Staph aureus* is the most commonly involved bacteria and is responsible for 70% of cases.
b. Risk factors include IV drug use, diabetes, prior spinal surgeries or procedures, and immunocompromised states.
c. Classic triad of back pain, fever, and neurologic deficit is seen only in 8–37% on initial presentation.
d. Leukocytosis is not sensitive or specific enough for the diagnosis.
e. ESR is elevated in 94% of cases.
f. MRI imaging is the gold standard imaging with a sensitivity and specificity greater than 90%.
g. Treatment includes broad-spectrum IV antibiotics and possible surgical decompression.

N. Figure legends
a. Figure 8.1 (MRI 1) Epidural abscess near spinous process of L4.
b. Figure 8.2 (MRI 2) Epidural abscess near spinous process of L4.

O. References
a. *Tintinalli's Emergency Medicine: A Comprehensive Study Guide* (9th ed.): Chapter 174, Central Nervous System and Spinal Infections.
b. *Rosen's Emergency Medicine: Concepts and Clinical Practice* (10th ed.): Chapter 92, Spinal Cord Disorders.

Leg Swelling

Kimbia Arno, MD, MFA, Ryan Gore, MD, and Alan Huang, MD

A. Chief complaint
a. 77-year-old male with leg swelling

B. Vital signs
a. BP: 139/103, HR: 109, RR: 18, T: 38.0°C, Sat: 98% on RA

C. What does the patient look like?
a. Patient is lethargic and oriented to person and place but not time.

D. Primary survey
a. Airway: speaking normally, in full sentences
b. Breathing: no respiratory distress
c. Circulation: moist skin, thready pulses

E. Action
a. Peripheral IV line
b. Labs
    i. CBC, BMP, LFT, coagulation studies, cardiac enzymes, CRP type and screen, urinalysis, blood cultures
c. Monitor as listed above
d. EKG
e. CXR
f. Finger stick glucose: 185 mg/dL

F. Nurse
a. If no finger stick is obtained, the patient becomes completely unresponsive.
b. EKG (Figure 9.1)
c. CXR (Figure 9.2)

G. History
a. HPI: A 77-year-old male nursing home resident brought in for progressive left leg swelling over the past 24 hours. He rapidly developed leg blisters and skin weeping.
b. PMHx: heart failure with reduced ejection fraction, hypertension, diabetes, venous stasis disease
c. PSHx: gastric bypass three years ago
d. Allergies: none
e. Meds: furosemide, isosorbide nitrate, omeprazole, carvedilol, aspirin, gabapentin

Case 9: Leg Swelling

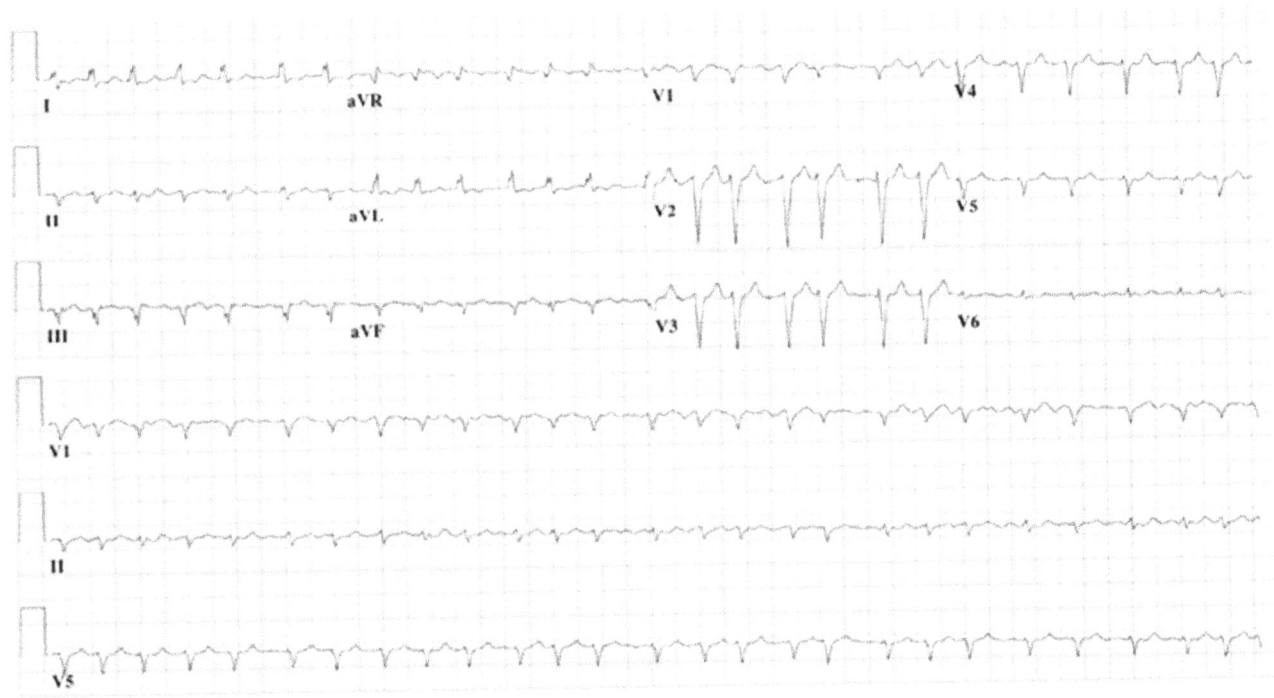

Figure 9.1

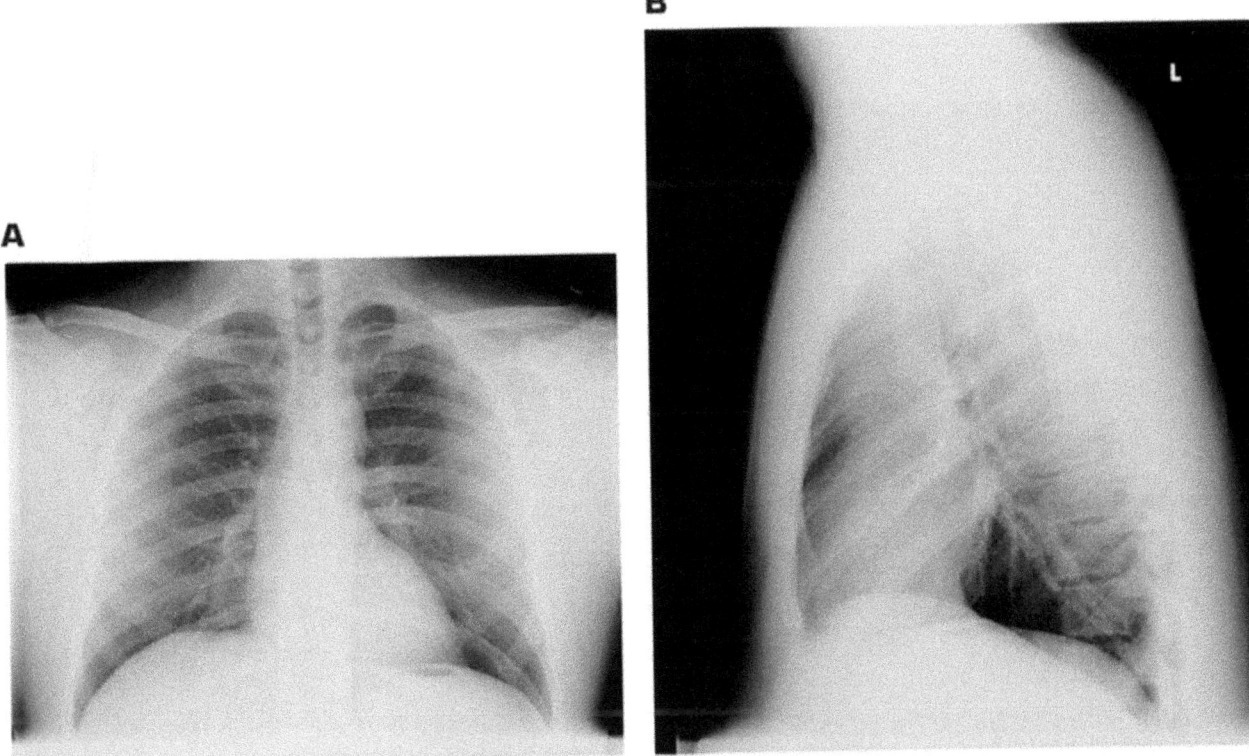

Figure 9.2

f. Social: former tobacco use (quit 10 years ago), former IV drug use (quit 15 years ago), social alcohol use

g. FHx: noncontributory

H. Secondary survey

a. General: remains lethargic
b. Head: normal
c. Eyes: normal
d. Neck: normal
e. Chest: nontender, bilateral basilar rales
f. Heart: tachycardic, no murmurs, rubs, or gallops
g. Abdomen: normal
h. Skin:
    i. Left leg: 2+ pitting edema to the knee, multiple hemorrhagic bullae, faint distal pulses
    ii. Right leg: chronic venous stasis changes with no ulcers, warmth, or erythema
i. Recheck vital signs:
    i. BP: 100/65
    ii. HR: 150
    iii. RR: 25
    iv. SpO_2: 97% on 2 L nasal cannula

I. Action

a. IV antibiotics: imipenem/meropenem + vancomycin + clindamycin + ciprofloxacin
b. 1 L crystalloid bolus
c. Stat general surgery consult
d. X-ray of left lower extremity (Figure 9.3)

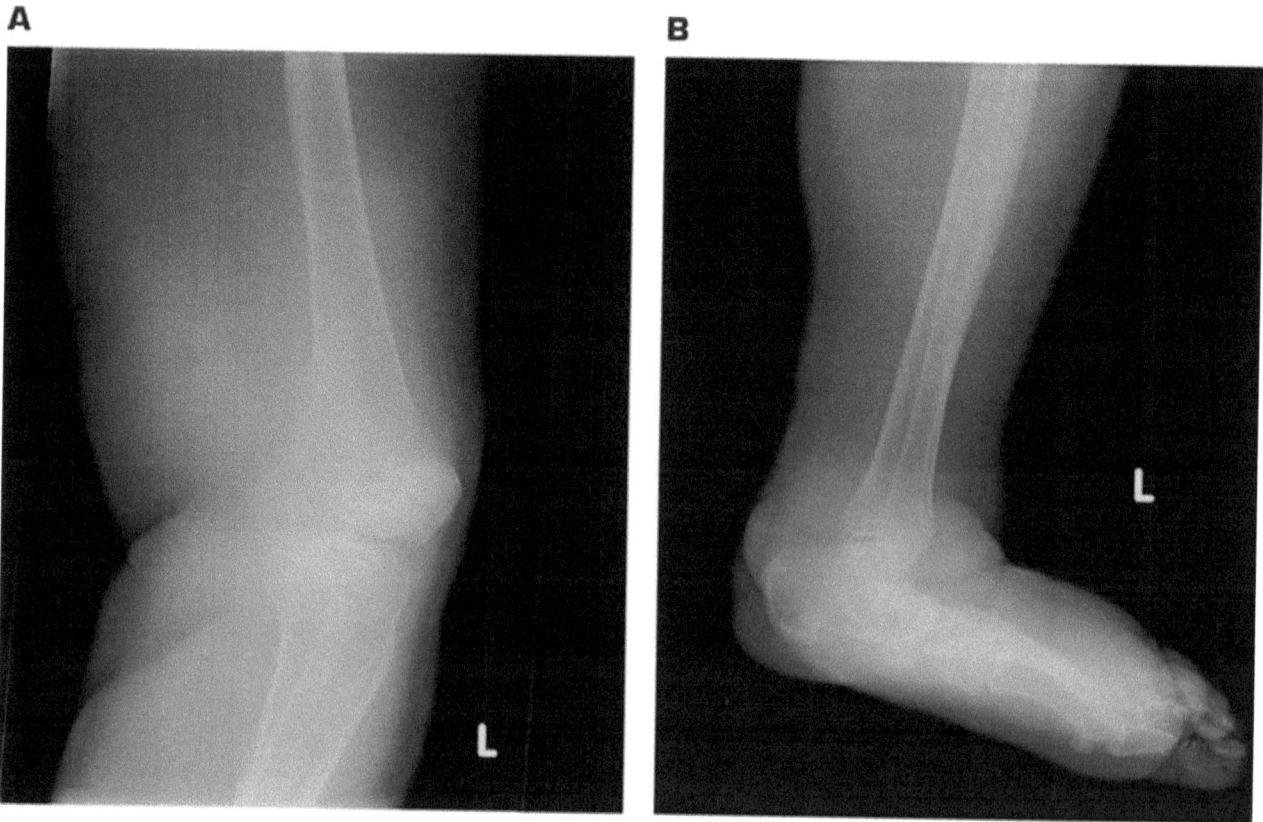

A   **B**

Figure 9.3

J. Results

Table 9.1 Results table

Test	Result	Test	Result
Complete blood count:		**Liver function panel:**	
WBC	$27.9 \times 10^3/\mu L$	D bili	0.2 mg/dL
Hct	36%	Amylase	246 U/L
Hgb	10.7 g/dL	Lipase	155 U/L
Plt	$229 \times 10^3/\mu L$	Albumin	3.9 g/dL
		AST	40 U/L
Basic metabolic panel:		ALT	44 U/L
Na	132 mEq/L	Alk phos	100 U/L
K	4.5 mEq/L	T bili	0.1 mg/dL
Cl	5.4 mEq/L		
CO_2	17 mEq/L	**Urinalysis:**	
BUN	95 mEq/dL	SG	1.030
Cr	4.8 mg/dL	pH	5
Glu	183 mg/dL	Prot	Neg
		Gluc	Neg
		Ketones	80
Coagulation studies:		Bili	Neg
PT	15 sec	Blood	Neg
PTT	34.9 sec	LE	Neg
INR	1.1	Color	Yellow

a. Cardiac enzymes negative
b. C-reactive protein 18

K. Nurse
a. Surgery consult returns call
   i. Requests CT of leg; recommends fluids, continued antibiotics, will follow as an inpatient, admit to medicine

L. Action
a. Candidate should decline request for CT.
b. Candidate should insist on need for immediate operative intervention.

M. Diagnosis
a. Necrotizing fasciitis

N. Critical actions

a. Early recognition of condition based on appearance, rapidity of symptom development, amount of pain, and possible development of sepsis
b. Aggressive fluid resuscitation
c. IV antibiotics
d. Immediate surgical consult
e. Do not delay operative intervention (definitive treatment is surgical debridement)

O. Examiner instructions

a. This is a case of necrotizing fasciitis. Necrotizing fasciitis is a rapidly progressive bacterial infection of the deep tissues of the body. It is associated with extremely high morbidity and mortality. Surgical consultants will delay evaluating the patient and patient's condition will worsen (mental status will deteriorate, blood pressure will fall, and heart rate will rise) unless the candidate articulates the reasons for concern about necrotizing fasciitis.

P. Pearls

a. Necrotizing fasciitis is usually a polymicrobial infection of aerobes and anaerobes.
b. Clindamycin has been shown to decrease toxin production in animal models and is typically given in combination with other bactericidal antibiotics.
c. Mortality is high.
d. Diabetes is a risk factor for spontaneous disease (even without pre-existing manipulation or trauma)
e. The course can often be indolent, though this case was not.
f. Be cautious about using absence of gas on imaging as a diagnostic rule out; this is a clinical diagnosis and imaging should not delay surgical consultation.
g. Surgical debridement is definitive management.
h. Avoid vasopressors if at all possible as they will only decrease blood flow to the dying limb/body part.
i. Lower extremity is the most common site, followed by upper extremities.
j. Consider hyperbaric oxygen therapy.
k. Consider calculating a laboratory risk indicator for necrotizing fasciitis (LRINEC) score (Table 9.1)

Table 9.2 LRINEC score

Test	Value	Score
CRP (mg/dL)	<15	0
	≥15	4
WBC (per mm³)	<15	0
	15–25	1
	≥25	2
Hemoglobin (g/dL)	>13.5	0
	11–13.5	1
	<11	2

Table 9.2 (cont.)

Test	Value	Score
Sodium (mEq/L)	≥135	0
	<135	2
Creatinine (mg/dL)	≤1.6	0
	>1.6	2
Glucose (mg/dL)	≤180	0
	>180	1
Total score	Score <6	Low risk
	Score 6–7	Intermediate risk
	Score ≥ 8	High risk

Q. Figure legends
a. Figure 9.1 (ECG) Tachycardia, atrial fibrillation, low voltage.
b. Figure 9.2 (CXR) Normal chest x-ray.
c. Figure 9.3 (Left lower extremity x-ray) Normal lower extremity x-ray.

R. References
a. *Tintinalli's Emergency Medicine: A Comprehensive Study Guide* (9th ed.): Chapter 147, Soft Tissue Infections.
b. *Rosen's Emergency Medicine: Concepts and Clinical Practice* (10th ed.): Chapter 126, Skin and Soft Tissue Infections.

Weakness

Alan Huang, MD and Cassandra Mackey, MD

A. Chief complaint
a. 77-year-old male complaining of chest pain, shortness of breath, and weakness

B. Vital signs
a. BP: 137/64, HR: 66, RR: 18, T: 36.7°C, Sat: 97% on RA

C. What does the patient look like?
a. Patient is comfortable, alert, and oriented.

D. Primary survey
a. Airway: speaking normally in full sentences
b. Breathing: no respiratory distress, no cyanosis
c. Circulation: skin warm and dry, pulses intact, normally capillary refill

E. Action
a. Consider oxygen via NC or nonrebreather mask
b. Obtain peripheral IV line(s)
c. Labs
    i. POC Glucose, CBC, CMP, coagulation studies, type and screen, cardiac enzymes, ABG/VBG
d. Monitor: BP: 137/64, HR: 66, RR: 18, T: 36.7°C, Sat: 97% on RA
e. Urinalysis
f. CXR
g. EKG
h. Bedside US (must be asked for): echo, normal ejection fraction, no pericardial effusion, no right ventricular dilation.

F. History
a. HPI: A 77-year-old male with a history of coronary artery disease, congestive heart failure, hypertension, and asthma presents with a 3-day history of what he thought was an asthma exacerbation. Patient additionally notes bilateral chest pain, nonradiating, improved with sitting up and worsened when lying down. No similar symptoms previously. Taking medications as prescribed. Generalized weakness, endorses not sleeping as well as he should be. He notes a 50 pack per year smoking history, no fever or cough. No swelling or pain in the legs.
b. PMHx: above, also hypothyroidism, asthma
c. PSHx: negative
d. Allergies: none

e. Meds: salmeterol-fluticasone, aspirin, levothyroxine, atorvastatin, lisinopril
f. Social: 50 pack per year tobacco history, social drinker, no drug use
g. FHx: noncontributory
h. PMD: Ryan Stapleton, MD

G. Secondary survey

a. General: alert and oriented, comfortable
b. Head: normal
c. Eyes: normal
d. Neck: normal, no jugular venous distension
e. Chest: nontender
f. Lungs: clear to auscultation bilaterally
g. Heart: 2/6 systolic murmur, no rubs or gallops
h. Abdomen: normal
i. Skin: normal
j. Back: normal
k. MSK: No pedal edema, full range of motion of all extremities
l. Neuro: normal, CN 2–12 intact, FNF normal, gait normal, strength 4/5 BUE and BLE. DTR delayed BUE and BLE.

H. Nurse

a. If no EKG obtained initially, vital signs change: HR: 45, BP: 90/60, Sat: 90% nonrebreather mask
b. EKG (Figure 10.1)
c. CXR (Figure 10.2)

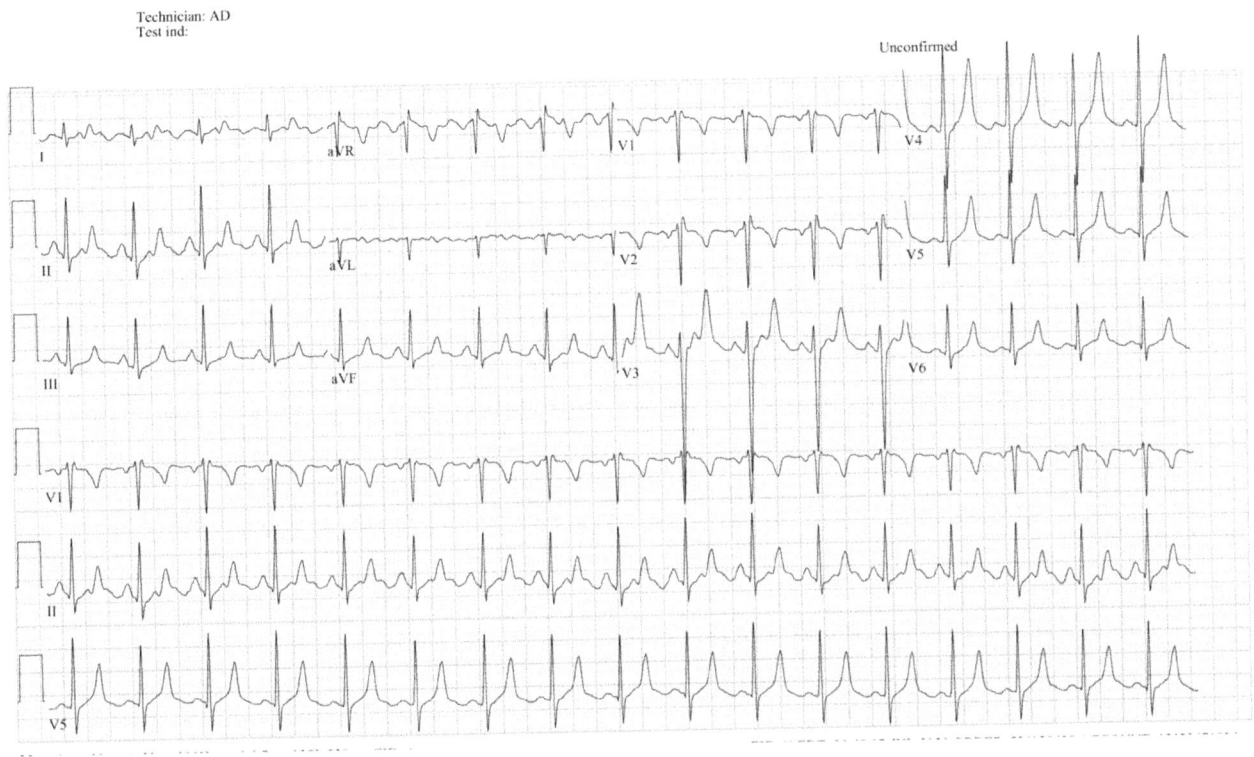

Figure 10.1

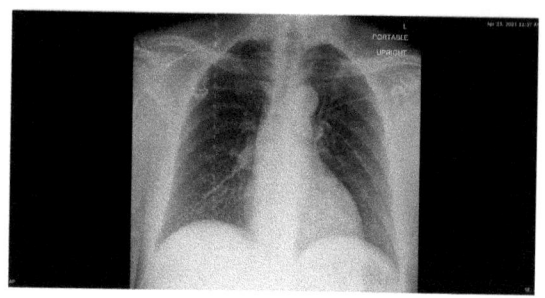

Figure 10.2

I. Action

a. Meds

    i. Calcium gluconate or calcium chloride IV 1 g

    ii. Dextrose and insulin IV

    iii. Albuterol nebulizer

    iv. Sodium bicarbonate IV

    v. Consider sodium zirconium cyclosilicate PO, furosemide IV

    vi. Consider bicarbonate and insulin continuous infusion

b. Labs

    i. STAT electrolytes

J. Results

Table 10.1 Results table

Test	Result	Test	Result
Complete blood count:		D bili	0.2 mg/dL
WBC	$10.1 \times 10^3/\mu L$	Amylase	67 U/L
Hct	35.90%	Lipase	78 U/L
Plt	$466 \times 10^3/\mu L$	Albumin	4.1 g/dL
Basic metabolic panel:		**Urinalysis:**	
Na	135 mEq/L	SG	1.030
K	6.6 mEq/L	pH	7
Cl	106 mEq/L	Prot	Neg
CO_2	18 mEq/L	Gluc	Neg
BUN	56 mEq/dL	Ketones	Neg
Cr	2.8 mg/dL	Bili	Neg
Gluc	74 mg/dL	Blood	Neg
		LE	Neg
Coagulation panel:		Nitrite	Neg
PT	12.5 sec	Color	Yellow
PTT	25.9 sec		
INR	1.1	**Arterial blood gas:**	
		pH	7.4

Table 10.1 (cont.)

Test	Result	Test	Result
Liver function panel:		pO_2	90 mmHg
AST	30 U/L	pCO_2	40 mmHg
ALT	34 U/L	HCO_3	19 mmol/L
Alk phos	44 U/L		
T bili	1.2 mg/dL	**Cardiac enzymes:**	
		Troponin	0

K. Diagnosis

a. Hyperkalemia

L. Critical actions

a. Obtain EKG
b. Note hyperkalemia (based on EKG and/or labs)
c. Immediate stabilization of cardiac membranes with calcium
d. Administration of medications that shift potassium into cells and also medications that decrease total body potassium
e. Cardiac monitoring/telemetry
f. Admission, consult to nephrology

M. Examiner instructions

a. This is a case of hyperkalemia (elevated potassium levels) due to acute renal insufficiency with possible contribution from angiotensin converting enzyme (ACE) inhibitor (lisinopril) usage. Early treatment is imperative; the candidate should obtain an EKG and potassium level rapidly. The candidate should not wait for the results of the labs before treatment. If treatment is not initiated rapidly, the patient should decompensate appropriately (become bradycardic and hypotensive). Cardiac conduction delay is the most common life-threatening manifestation associated with hyperkalemia.

N. Pearls

a. Early EKG findings of hyperkalemia include peaked T waves and PR interval prolongation. With increased potassium levels, QRS widening can occur, and ultimately the sine waves of severe hyperkalemia.
b. Other EKG abnormalities include complete heart block, ventricular fibrillation, and asystole.
c. In slowly progressive hyperkalemia, EKG findings will be evident only with higher levels of serum potassium.
d. The most common cause of hyperkalemia is a hemolyzed sample (especially in the setting of a normal creatinine level); confirm with laboratory for presence of hemolysis or recheck value.
e. Causes of hyperkalemia include renal insufficiency, medications such as potassium-sparing diuretics or ACE inhibitors; β-blockers; digoxin, hypoaldosteronism including adrenal insufficiency and type 4 renal tubular acidosis; increased intake or absorption; cellular injuries such as rhabdomyolysis or tumor lysis syndrome; pseudo-hyperkalemia such as phlebotomy-induced hemolysis; severe thrombocytosis or leukocytosis; or laboratory error.

f. Medications that redistribute potassium most rapidly include albuterol and bicarbonate followed by insulin.

g. Sodium zirconium cyclosilicate, sodium polystyrene sulfonate, and furosemide actually decrease total body potassium.

h. Although previously widely used, the safety and efficacy of utilizing sodium polystyrene sulfonate have come into question. There is a risk of colonic ischemia and necrosis with use and its efficacy is not that well proven. Sodium zirconium cyclosilicate is a reasonable alternative with a potentially better side effect profile.

i. Consider nephrology consult for emergent hemodialysis, especially in patients on dialysis and patients with acute renal failure.

O. Figure legends

a. Figure 10.1 (EKG) Hyperacute T waves; sinus tachycardia.
b. Figure 10.2 (CXR) No focal infiltrate.

P. References

a. *Tintinalli's Emergency Medicine: A Comprehensive Study Guide* (9th ed.): Chapter 17, Fluids and Electrolytes.
b. *Rosen's Emergency Medicine: Concepts and Clinical Practice* (10th ed.): Chapter 114, Electrolyte Disorders.

Headache

Wesley Pedicini, MD and Philip Bossart, MD

A. Chief complaint
a. 55-year-old female with left-sided headache and vision changes

B. Vital signs
a. BP: 152/95, HR: 95, RR: 16, T: 36°C, Sat: 100% on RA

C. What does the patient look like?
a. Patient appears uncomfortable due to pain, but is speaking normally and is alert and oriented.

D. Primary survey
a. Airway: speaking in full sentences
b. Breathing: no apparent respiratory distress, no cyanosis, clear lungs
c. Circulation: warm dry skin, regular rate and rhythm, radial pulses 2+, normal capillary refill
d. Neuro: alert and oriented, no focal sensory or motor deficits

E. Action
a. Peripheral IV line
b. Pain/nausea control: morphine/ondansetron or metoclopramide

F. History
a. HPI: This is a 55-year-old female with a history of hypertension and diabetes. She presents today with acute onset left supraorbital headache along with severely diminished vision in her left eye. Onset was 3 hours ago and she describes her left vision as very blurry. Right eye is unaffected. Patient notes nausea and one episode of vomiting. Denies trauma, prior history of similar episodes.
b. PMHx: hypertension, diabetes
c. PSHx: none
d. Allergies: none
e. Meds: metformin, lisinopril
f. Social: lives with husband, nonsmoker, drinks alcohol occasionally
g. FHx: not relevant
h. PMD: Dr. Fisher

G. Secondary survey
a. General: alert, oriented, moderate distress due to pain
b. Head: normocephalic, atraumatic, no tenderness over temporal area

c. Eyes: there is no periorbital edema, injected conjunctiva on the left. Extra-ocular motions are intact. Left globe firm compared to right; left pupil mid-dilated, nonreactive, right eye visual acuity 20/30, left eye visual acuity is 20/200.
  - Slit lamp examination: left cornea "steamy," narrow anterior chamber, no evidence of hyphema
  - Tonometer: right 15 mmHg, left 70 mm/Hg (must ask)
d. Chest: normal
e. Heart: normal
f. Abdomen: normal
g. Extremities: normal
h. Back: normal
i. Neuro: normal

I. Actions

a. Emergent ophthalmology consult (will not be available until after meds given)
b. Meds
  i. Brimonidine 0.15% or other α-2 agonist to left eye
  ii. Timolol 0.5% or other β-blocker to left eye
  iii. Mannitol IV 1–2 g/kg
  iv. Acetazolamide 500 mg IV/PO or other carbonic anhydrase inhibitor
  v. Prednisolone or other topical steroid in left eye
c. Reassess – recheck intraocular pressure and visual acuity. Re-administration of medications should be performed if pressures remain elevated.
d. Discuss with ophthalmology emergent surgical intervention if pressures remain elevated versus 24-hour follow-up if pressures have stabilized

J. Diagnosis

a. Acute angle-closure glaucoma

K. Critical actions

a. Thorough eye examination, including intraocular pressures (IOP), slit lamp, visual acuity
b. Early administration medications to lower intraocular pressure: a carbonic anhydrase inhibitor, a topical β-blocker, a topical α-agonist, and IV mannitol
c. Ophthalmology consult
d. Continued administration of meds until normalization of IOP

L. Examiner instructions

a. This is a case of acute narrow angle or angle-closure glaucoma. In this disorder, the normal flow of aqueous humor within the eye is interrupted, leading to increased ocular pressures. This results in pain, decreased blood flow, and optic nerve damage with potential for vision loss. This is an ophthalmologic emergency. Critical actions include rapid identification of the diagnosis, brisk administration of a combination of medicines aimed at decreasing IOP via different mechanisms. Ophthalmology must be consulted emergently. Any delays in diagnosis or appropriate administration of medications increase the likelihood of permanent loss of vision. Laboratory evaluation is not necessary; if sent, results will be normal.

M. Pearls

a. Acute angle-closure glaucoma commonly presents as headache in addition to eye pain and vision loss. Other presenting symptoms include nausea, vomiting, and abdominal pain. Consider migraine, temporal arteritis, subarachnoid hemorrhage, and intraabdominal emergencies in your differential diagnoses.

b. It is more common in older patients as their lenses become thicker and/or cataracts develop, causing narrower angles. Patients of Asian descent also have a higher predisposition due to narrower angles at baseline.

c. Glaucoma attacks are usually triggered by pupillary dilatation such as reading in low light. Medications that cause dilatation of the eye can precipitate an attack as well. These include parasympatholytic meds such as antihistamines and sympathomimetics such as epinephrine or pseudoephedrine. Attacks can be induced by diagnostic mydriasis in the ED, though the incidence of this is low.

d. Acute treatment seeks to reduce intraocular pressure:
   - Carbonic anhydrase inhibitors (acetazolamide), topical β-blockers (timolol), and systemic osmotic agents (mannitol) reduce aqueous humor production.
   - Topical α-agonists (phenylephrine) and steroids (prednisolone) increase outflow.

e. Remember the relative contraindications for glaucoma medications:
   i. Acetazolamide: sickle cell (encourages sickling), sulfa allergies
   ii. Mannitol: hypotension/dehydration
   iii. Timolol: caution in asthma and COPD but do not withhold this medication in this population
   iv. Pilocarpine is not recommended acutely, as it can make the anterior chamber even more shallow.

N. References

a. *Tintinalli's Emergency Medicine: A Comprehensive Study Guide* (9th ed.): Chapter 241, Eye Emergencies.

b. *Rosen's Emergency Medicine: Concepts and Clinical Practice* (10th ed.): Chapter 18, Red and Painful Eye. Chapter 16, Headache.

Abdominal Pain

Angela Chen, MD and Joseph Chiang, MD

A. Chief complaint
a. 55-year-old male with severe abdominal pain, nausea, and vomiting

B. Vital signs
a. BP: 86/57, HR: 110, RR: 20, T: 37.1°C, Sat: 99% on RA

C. What does the patient look like?
a. Patient appears uncomfortable and in pain.

D. Primary survey
a. Airway: speaking in full sentences
b. Breathing: no apparent respiratory distress
c. Circulation: peripheral pulses equal, normal capillary refill

E. History
a. HPI: A 55-year-old male presents with one day of worsening abdominal distension, pain, and two episodes of vomiting. He reports swelling and tenderness in the right groin as well. He has had swelling in the groin before, but it has gotten worse, more painful, and has become "hard." He denies fever or chest pain.
b. PMHx: hypertension, diabetes, asthma
c. PSHx: cholecystectomy
d. Allergies: penicillin
e. Meds: metformin
f. Social: lives with wife at home, denies alcohol, smoking, drugs, monogamous sex with wife
g. FHx: hypertension, diabetes
h. PMD: Dr. Chang

F. Nurse
a. EKG: sinus tachycardia, left ventricular hypertrophy

G. Secondary survey
a. General: alert and oriented, tachycardic, moderate distress due to pain
b. HEENT: normal, oral mucosa dry
c. Neck: normal
d. Chest: normal
e. Heart: tachycardic

f. Abdomen: distended, diffusely tender, bowel sounds absent, no pulsatile masses, no masses, positive rebound, positive guarding
g. Rectal: hemoccult negative, normal tone, no masses
h. GU: large right inguinal hernia, not reducible, overlying skin is dusky, no testicular tenderness or swelling
i. Extremities: normal
j. Back: normal, no costovertebral angle tenderness
k. Neuro: normal
l. Skin: pale, no rashes, no edema
m. Lymph: normal

H. Action

a. Two large-bore peripheral IV lines
b. Labs
   i. CBC, BMP, LFT, PT/PTT, blood type and screen, VBG/ABG with lactate
c. 1 L bolus of crystalloid
d. Monitor: BP: 86/57, HR: 110, RR: 20, T: 37.1°C, Sat: 99% on RA
e. EKG
f. Consult
   i. Surgery
g. Imaging
   i. Upright CXR
   ii. CT abdomen pelvis with IV and PO contrast
h. Meds
   i. NS 1 L bolus
   ii. IV antiemetic
   iii. IV analgesia
   iv. IV antibiotics

I. Results

Table 12.1 Results table

Test	Result	Test	Result
Complete blood count:		T bili	1.6 mg/dL
WBC	$18.4 \times 10^3/\mu L$	D bili	0.5 mg/dL
Hct	52.00%	Amylase	123 U/L
Plt	$288 \times 10^3/\mu L$	Lipase	140 U/L
		Albumin	3.9 g/dL
Basic metabolic panel:			
Na	139 mEq/L	**Urinalysis**	
K	4.6 mEq/L	SG	1.030
Cl	92 mEq/L	pH	6
CO_2	31 mEq/L	Prot	Neg

Table 12.1 (cont.)

Test	Result	Test	Result
BUN	18 mEq/dL	Gluc	Neg
Cr	1.2 mg/dL	Ketones	Neg
Gluc	160 mg/dL	Bili	Neg
		Blood	Neg
Coagulation panel:		LE	Neg
PT	12.9 sec	Nitrite	Neg
PTT	31.2 sec	Color	Yellow
INR	1.1		
		Arterial blood gas:	
Liver function panel:		pH	7.4
AST	40 U/L	pO_2	86 mmHg
ALT	23 U/L	pCO_2	40 mmHg
Alk phos	107 U/L	HCO_3	27 mmol/L

a. Lactate: 1.9 mmol/L
b. EKG (Figure 12.1)
c. CXR (Figure 12.2)
d. CTAP (Figure 12.3)

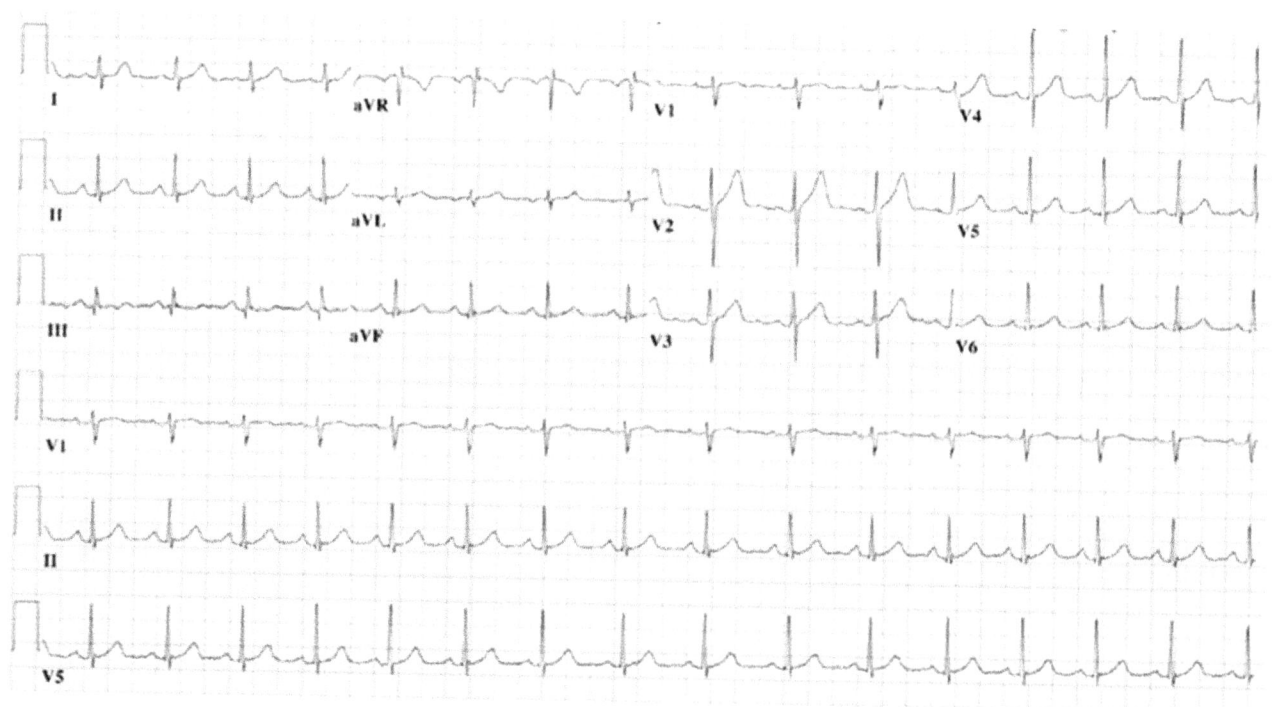

Figure 12.1

CASE 12: Abdominal Pain

A

B

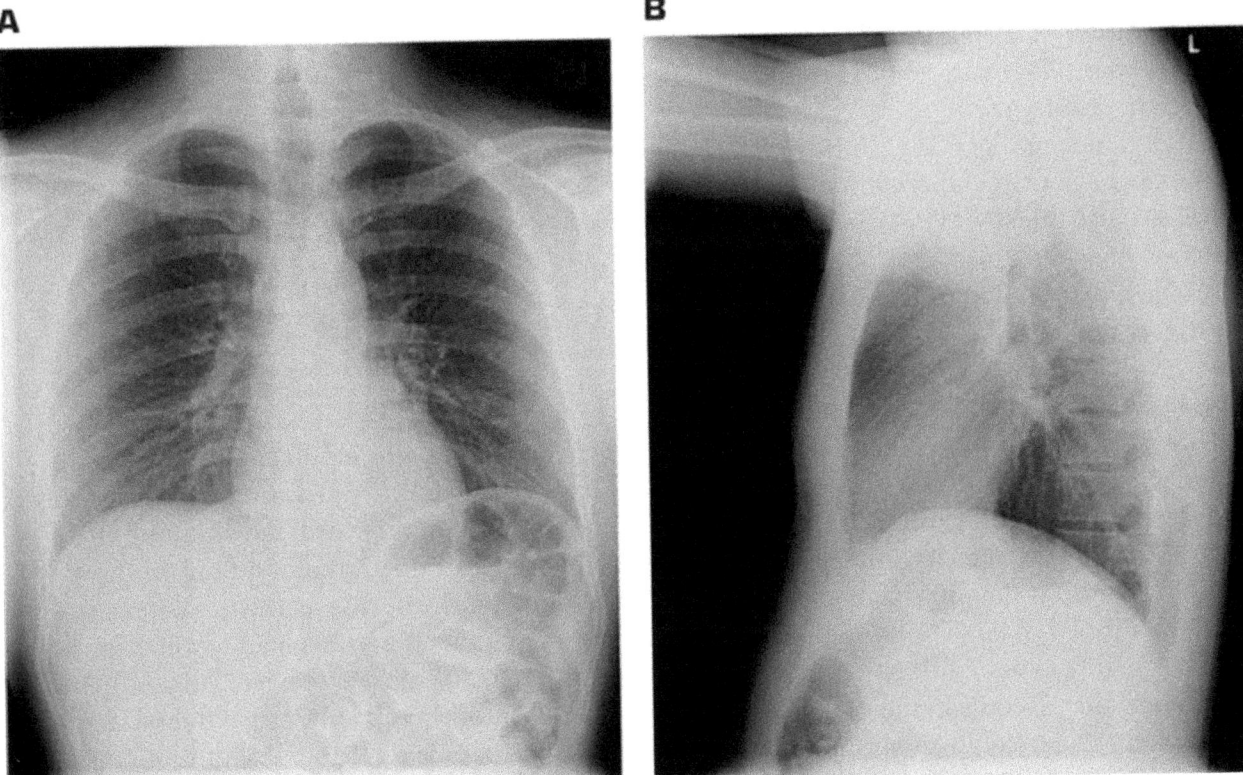

Figure 12.2

Figure 12.3

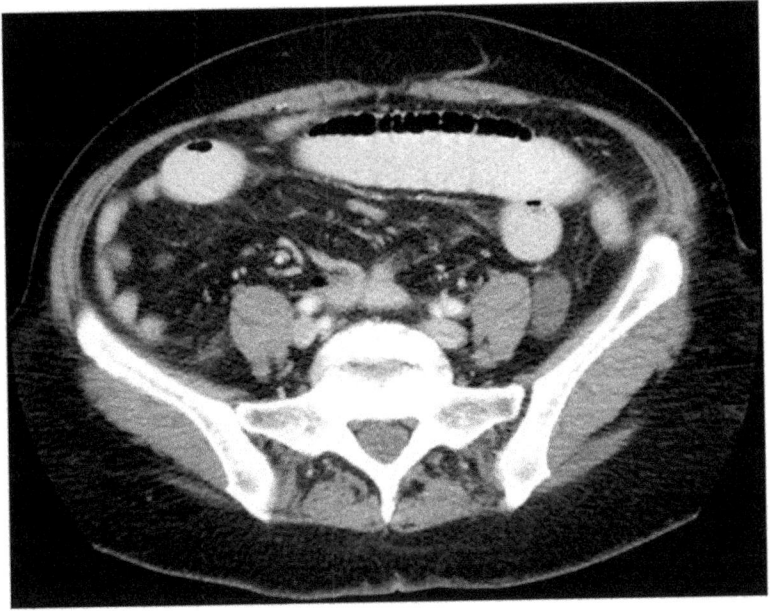

J. Action

a. Surgery consult
    i. Patient taken to OR for repair of incarcerated hernia.

K. Diagnosis

a. Incarcerated hernia with bowel obstruction

L. Critical actions
a. Recognition of hernia
b. Large-bore IV access and fluid bolus
c. Upright chest x-ray
d. CT abdomen and pelvis with IV contrast
e. Pain management and antiemetics
f. Nasogastric tube (NGT) placement if symptoms not controlled
g. Pain management
h. Broad-spectrum antibiotics
i. Surgery consult

M. Examiner instructions
a. This is a case of a strangulated hernia. The patient's bowel has slipped from the abdominal cavity into a defect in the inguinal wall where it has become trapped. An incarcerated hernia is firm, painful, and cannot be reduced with direct pressure. In this case, the skin findings over the site of the hernia suggest the hernia is strangulated, with impaired blood flow. In the event of skin findings the physician should refrain from reducing the hernia as this may increase the likelihood of bowel perforation. Incarcerated or strangulated hernias lead to obstruction of normal digestion with pain, distension of the abdomen, and tissue damage. Dilated loops of bowel on CT confirm the diagnosis of obstruction. IV fluids are used to treat dehydration and correct electrolyte abnormalities caused by the continuous vomiting. IV antibiotics are indicated in patients who are planned for surgery or in which perforation is suspected. Patients should be hospitalized for monitoring and treatment; surgery is often indicated.

N. Pearls
a. Upright chest x-ray is more sensitive than KUB for free air.
b. X-ray findings are estimated to be diagnostic in approximately 50–60% of cases of small bowel obstruction (SBO). CT has been shown to detect SBO with a high degree of sensitivity and specificity and can also provide information on the cause of obstruction and has largely replaced the obstruction series.
c. Peritoneal signs are ominous in cases of obstruction, and often suggest a surgical emergency. Consider fluids, broad-spectrum antibiotics, and surgical consultation immediately.
d. Do not attempt reduction of a strangulated hernia, this can lead to perforation and sepsis.
e. There is little evidence to support nasogastric decompression in decreasing the duration of SBO. If the patient's nausea and vomiting can be controlled with antiemetics, it is reasonable to delay NGT placement.
f. A high white blood cell count may be seen with bowel gangrene, abscess, or peritonitis.

O. Figure legends
a. Figure 12.1 (EKG) Sinus tachycardia.
b. Figure 12.2 (CXR) Normal chest x-ray.
c. Figure 12.3 (CT abdomen and pelvis) CT abdomen and pelvis with air fluid levels and dilated bowel suggestive of SBO.

P. References
a. *Tintinalli's Emergency Medicine: A Comprehensive Study Guide* (9th ed.): Chapter 86, Bowel Obstruction and Volvulus. Chapter 87, Hernias in Adults.
b. *Rosen's Emergency Medicine: Concepts and Clinical Practice* (10th ed.): Chapter 78, Small Intestine.

Ringing in the Ears

Taryn Webb, MD, Michelle N. Marin, MD, and Joseph Chiang, MD

A. Chief complaint
a. 17-year-old female with nausea, tremor, and ringing in the ears

B. Vital signs
a. BP: 107/56, HR: 117, RR: 22, T: 37.2°C, Sat: 97% on RA

C. What does the patient look like?
a. Patient appears stated age, comfortable, in no acute distress while lying in stretcher, alert, and oriented.

D. Primary survey
a. Airway: speaking in full sentences
b. Breathing: no apparent respiratory distress, slightly tachypneic
c. Circulation: warm skin, good pulses bilaterally

E. History
a. HPI: A 17-year-old female notes headache last night for which she took aspirin. Headache improved, and she went to sleep soon after. Woke up in the morning and felt nauseated, tremulous, and had ringing in her ears. No cough, fever, or chills. Reports a total dose of six 325 mg tablets of aspirin (only if asked).
b. PMHx: none
c. PSHx: none
d. Allergies: none
e. Meds: none
f. Social: lives with family, nonsmoker, occasional alcohol use
g. FHx: diabetes

F. Secondary survey
a. General: alert and oriented, afebrile, tachycardic, and tachypneic
b. HEENT: normal, tympanic membranes clear
c. Neck: normal
d. Chest: normal
e. Heart: normal
f. Abdomen: bowel sounds normal; no distension or peritoneal signs; mild tenderness in right upper and lower quadrants

g. Extremities: normal
h. Back: normal
i. Neuro: normal
j. Skin: warm, dry, normal color
k. Psychiatric: normal affect; judgment and insight normal; remote and recent memory normal; no suicidal or homicidal ideation

G. Action

a. Peripheral IV line
b. Monitor: BP: 107/56, HR: 117, RR: 22, T: 37.2°C, Sat: 97% on RA
c. Labs
   i. Finger stick, VBG, CBC, BMP, LFT, lipase and amylase, PT/PTT, salicylate, acetaminophen, and alcohol levels
d. EKG
e. CXR
f. Urinalysis
g. Urine pregnancy test

H. Nurse

a. Patient: remains symptomatic
b. EKG (Figure 13.1)
c. CXR (Figure 13.2)

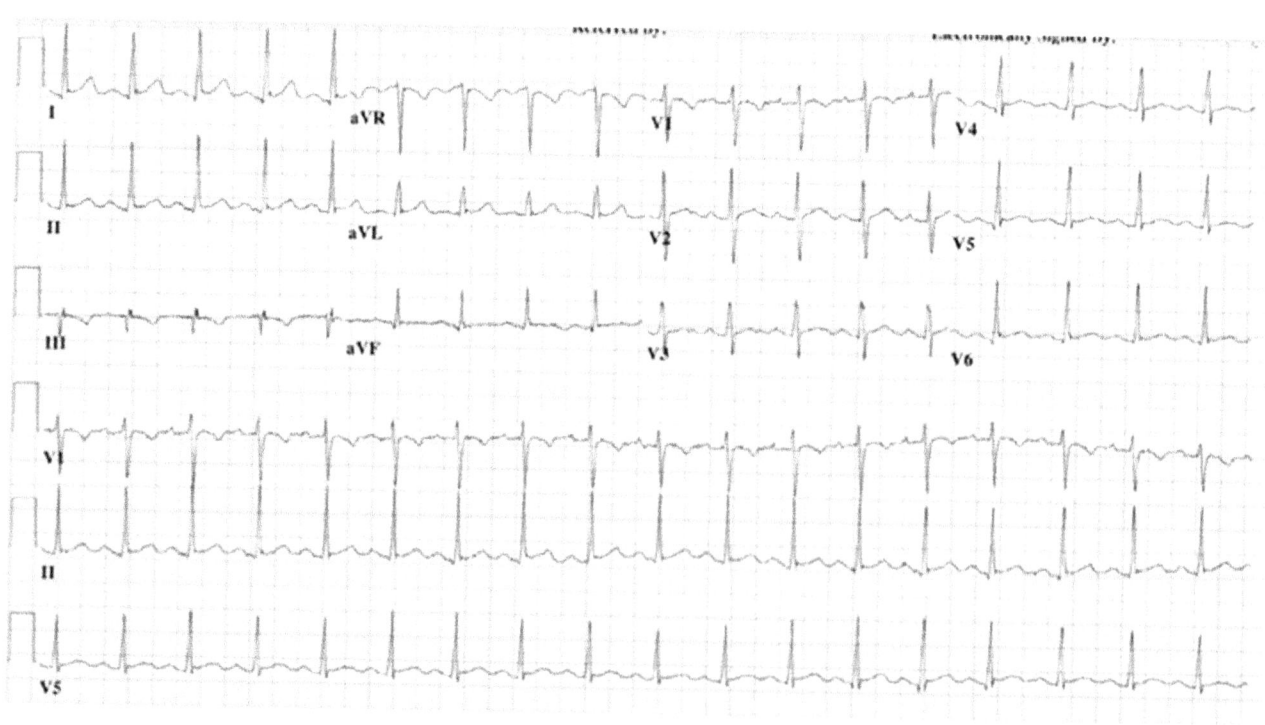

Figure 13.1

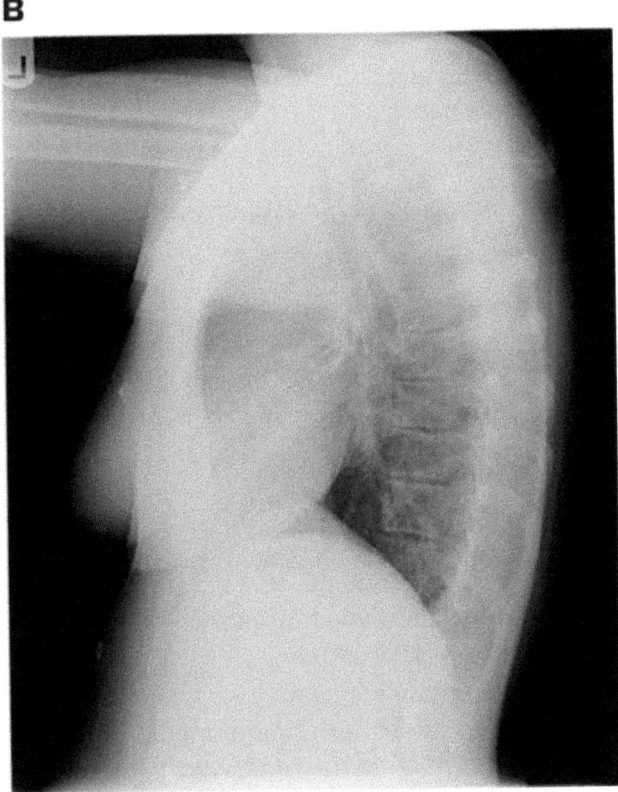

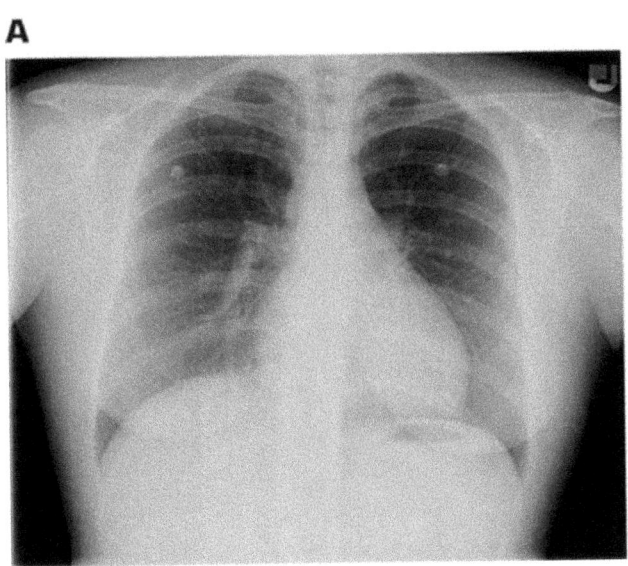

Figure 13.2

I. Results

Table 13.1 Results table

Test	Result	Test	Result
Complete blood count:		T bili	0.5 mg/dL
WBC	$12.3 \times 10^3/\mu L$	D bili	0.1 mg/dL
Hct	36.60%	Amylase	153 U/L
Plt	$300 \times 10^3/\mu L$	Lipase	35 U/L
		Albumin	4.4 g/dL
Basic metabolic panel:			
Na	146 mEq/L	**Urinalysis**	
K	3.1 mEq/L	SG	1.020
Cl	117 mEq/L	pH	6
CO_2	17 mEq/L	Prot	Neg
BUN	10 mEq/dL	Gluc	Neg
Cr	0.8 mg/dL	Ketones	Neg
Gluc	105 mg/dL	Bili	Neg
		Blood	Neg

Table 13.1 (cont.)

Test	Result		Test	Result
Coagulation panel:			LE	Neg
PT	12.7 sec		Nitrite	Neg
PTT	25.9 sec		Color	Yellow
INR	1.1			
			Arterial blood gas:	
Liver function panel:			pH	7.54
AST	21 U/L		pO_2	90 mmHg
ALT	16 U/L		pCO_2	21 mmHg
Alk phos	68 U/L		HCO_3	17 mmol/L

a. Salicylate level: 60 mg/dL
b. Acetaminophen level: negative
c. Alcohol level: negative
d. Urine pregnancy: negative
e. Urinalysis (after initiation of medication)
   i. pH: 8.0
   ii. All other values: normal

J. Action
a. ICU consult
   i. Admission for close monitoring
b. Discussion with patient and family regarding acute overdose of aspirin and its presentation and treatments
c. Meds
   i. Metoclopramide IV (for nausea)
   ii. Bicarbonate drip
   iii. Multiple doses of activated charcoal (first dose with sorbitol)
d. Add 20–40 mEq of potassium chloride to bicarbonate infusion for hypokalemia promoting alkalinization of the urine
e. Repeat salicylate levels 2 hours after bicarbonate was initiated
f. Continued monitoring of vital signs
g. Poison Control Center contacted – recommends frequent labs and continued treatment until salicylate level falls below 20 mg/dL

K. Diagnosis
a. Aspirin toxicity

L. Critical actions
a. Large-bore IV access
b. Pregnancy test
c. Obtain history of salicylate use
d. Alkalinization of urine with sodium bicarbonate
e. Close monitoring of patient and salicylate levels
f. ICU admission

M. Examiner instructions

a. This is a case of acute salicylate overdose. Her presentation is classic: nausea, tremor, tinnitus, tachycardia, and tachypnea. Cardiac and pulmonary causes of shortness of breath should be sought (through careful physical examination, EKG, CXR). The patient should not disclose the headache initially. She won't connect last night's headache with today's symptoms unless specifically asked about other recent illnesses or medications.

N. Pearls

a. Multiple dose activated charcoal can be used for any patients who present symptomatically and is initially with sorbitol then independently until salicylate level falls <40 mg/dL.

b. Salicylate blood levels may peak in less than 1 hour or after more than 6 hours, depending on the type of tablets ingested.

c. Urinary salicylate clearance can be increased by the administration of sodium bicarbonate bolus followed by maintenance doses until salicylate levels fall below 20 mg/dL and clinical improvement is noted.

d. Avoid intubation, as the increased minute ventilation keeps salicylates from crossing the blood–brain barrier into the central nervous system.

e. Patients present initially with respiratory alkalosis due to direct stimulation of the medulla leading to tachypnea and hyperpnea. Later, increased anion gap metabolic acidosis develops. Patients usually remain alkalemic with a pH >7.4.

f. Development of acidemia is an ominous sign. A decrease in pH is a poor prognostic marker and is often a preterminal event.

g. Early consultation with the ICU and a toxicologist is prudent.

h. Worsening of patient symptoms manifesting in end-organ damage will require emergent hemodialysis.

i. Hypokalemia interferes with urine alkalinization; potassium levels should be monitored and hypokalemia corrected.

O. Figure legends

a. Figure 13.1 Normal sinus rhythm, minimal voltage criteria for LVH.

b. Figure 13.2 Normal chest x-ray.

P. References

a. *Tintinalli's Emergency Medicine: A Comprehensive Study Guide* (9th ed.): Chapter 189, Salicylates.

b. *Rosen's Emergency Medicine: Concepts and Clinical Practice* (10th ed.): Chapter 139, Aspirin and Nonsteroidal Agents.

Vomiting Child

Temima Waltuch, MD and Joseph Chiang, MD

A. Chief complaint
a. 7 year-old boy with vomiting for 1 day

B. Vital signs
a. BP: 96/63, HR: 136, RR: 28, T: 36.1°C, Sat: 98%, Wt: 23 kg

C. What does the patient look like?
a. Patient appears uncomfortable due to pain; lying supine on the stretcher.

D. Primary survey
a. Airway: speaking in full sentences
b. Breathing: no respiratory distress, no cyanosis
c. Circulation: warm and well perfused, good peripheral pulses

E. History
a. HPI: 7-year-old boy presents with 1 day of diffuse colicky abdominal pain, several episodes of emesis, 1 episode of bloody diarrhea, and decreased oral intake. He is also complaining of leg pain while walking. He has been afebrile. Denies dysuria or hematuria. Patient was seen at PMD last week and diagnosed with URI. Denies sick contacts or recent travel.
b. PMHx: intermittent asthma, seasonal allergies
c. PSHx: none
d. Meds: none
e. Allergies: none
f. Social: lives with parents and 4-year-old sister
g. FHx: unknown

F. Secondary survey
a. General: awake, alert, uncomfortable-appearing but NAD
b. HEENT: pupils equal, round, reactive; no conjunctival erythema; tympanic membranes normal; 2+ tonsils without erythema or exudate; dry lips and tongue
c. Neck: supple, FROM
d. Lungs: clear to auscultation bilaterally; no wheezes, rhonchi, or rales
e. Heart: tachycardic, no murmurs
f. Abdomen: soft, mild distension, diffuse abdominal tenderness, decreased bowel sounds, no rebound, voluntary guarding
g. Rectal: hemoccult positive, no fissures
h. GU: normal Tanner 1 male

i. Extremities: bilateral knees and ankles with periarticular swelling and tenderness with no overlying erythema or warmth, 2+ dorsalis pedis pulses
j. Back: normal, no CVA tenderness
k. Neuro: normal
l. Skin: palpable purpura on bilateral lower extremities and buttocks; warm well perfused with normal skin turgor
m. Lymph: normal

G. Action
a. Monitor: BP: 96/63, HR: 136, RR: 28, Sat: 98%
b. Peripheral IV
c. Labs
   i. CBC, BMP, LFT, PT/PTT/INR, type and screen and urinalysis
d. 20 mL/kg NS bolus intravenously
e. NPO
f. Imaging
   i. Abdominal x-ray, obstructive series
   ii. Abdominal ultrasound (Figure 14.1)

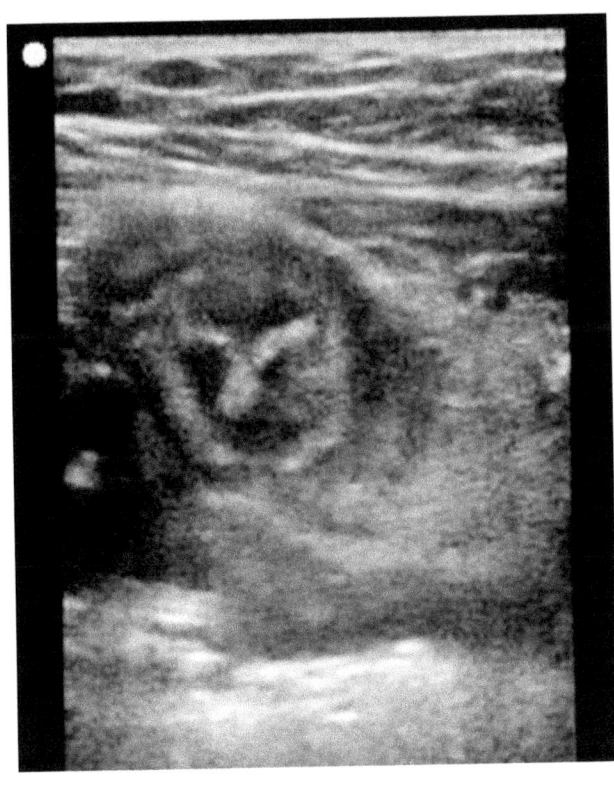

Figure 14.1

g. Consults
   i. Consider surgery consult
   ii. Consider pediatric nephrology consult, based on labs/urine results
h. Meds
   i. 20 mL/kg NS bolus
   ii. Continue D5 NS at maintenance rate thereafter (63 mL/hr)

iii. NSAIDs for management of arthritis if renal function is normal

iv. Consider corticosteroids to reduce symptoms of severe abdominal pain or joint pain

i. Additional labs

    i. Consider IgA

    ii. Consider VBG with lactate

H. Results

Table 14.1 Results table

Test	Result	Test	Result
Complete blood count:		**Liver function panel:**	
WBC	$15.3 \times 10^3/\mu L$	AST	21 U/L
Hct	37%	ALT	43 U/L
Hgb	12 g/dL	Alk phos	179 U/L
Plt	$495 \times 10^3/\mu L$	T bili	1.3 mg/dL
		D bili	0.2 mg/dL
Basic metabolic panel:		Amylase	61 U/L
Na	138 mEq/L	Lipase	100 U/L
K	3.8 mEq/L	Albumin	3.9 g/dL
Cl	100 mEq/L		
CO_2	18 mEq/L	**Urinalysis:**	
BUN	15 mg/dL	SG	1.025
Cr	0.6 mg/dL	pH	6
Gluc	71 mg/dL	Prot	+
		Gluc	Neg
Coagulation panel:		Ketones	+
PT	13 sec	Bili	Neg
PTT	27 sec	Blood	Neg
INR	0.9	LE	Neg
		Nitrite	Neg
		Color	Yellow

a. IgA: 299 mg/dL (normal = 124 ± 45)

b. AXR: dilated loops of bowel with paucity of colonic gas. No free air.

c. US abdomen (Figure 14.1)

I. Action

a. Surgery consult to determine monitoring for spontaneous reduction vs. surgical reduction.

b. Continue hydration and NPO.

J. Diagnosis

a. Henoch–Schönlein purpura with jejuno-ileal intussusception

K. Critical actions

a. Fluid resuscitation
b. Laboratory and urine testing to evaluate for renal injury
c. Abdominal x-ray
d. Abdominal ultrasound
e. Pain management
f. Surgery consult

L. Examiner instructions

a. This child is suffering from Henoch–Schönlein purpura (HSP), complicated by intussusception, which occurs in about 3.5% of cases. HSP is a small-vessel vasculitis with immune complex deposition with immunoglobulin A. It is most common in children between the ages of 2 and 11 years old and is characterized by a triad of palpable purpuric rash, arthritis, and acute abdominal pain. Renal involvement including hematuria, edema, and proteinuria may also occur and can be the most significant long-term consequence. The cause of HSP is largely unknown, but often follows a viral illness or Group A *Streptococcus* infection and is immunologically mediated. (When prompted, the mother will describe a rash on the lower extremity and buttocks for a few days.)

M. Pearls

a. HSP is a clinical diagnosis.
b. The rash occurs in all cases; it may begin as maculopapular or urticarial, but then progresses to the classic palpable purpura. The rash is typically found on the extensor surfaces of the lower extremities and buttocks, but may also occur on the upper extremities and ears.
c. Severe, colicky abdominal pain may indicate possible intussusception, bowel obstruction, or gastrointestinal hemorrhage brought on by damage to the GI vasculature. Abdominal radiographs and/or ultrasound will aid in the diagnosis of intussusception. Stool guaiac may be positive in 50% of cases (in the absence of intussusception) and does not require further evaluation.
d. In children younger than 2 years old, most cases of intussusception are idiopathic, occurring in healthy children involving the ileocolic region. In older children, however, approximately 75% of cases of intussusception have a pathologic lead point from causes including HSP vasculitis, lymphoma, duplication cyst, postsurgical scars, and intestinal polyps. Intussusception may occur at any point in the GI tract, but in HSP it is most frequently a small bowel–small bowel intussusception.
e. In cases of intussusception, therapeutic intervention depends on the location of the intussusception, the condition of the patient, and the resources available. When involving the ileocolic region, in a stable child without any evidence of pneumoperitoneum or peritonitis, nonoperative reduction using air or contrast enema is attempted first, with a success rate approaching 90%. If enema reduction is unsuccessful, surgical reduction is performed. In cases of small bowel–small bowel intussusception, the intussusception will often reduce spontaneously. If persistent despite medical management or there is a resultant ileus, it may be managed surgically. Air enema reduction is usually unsuccessful in small bowel–small bowel intussusception and therefore not attempted.

f. Management of HSP with glucocorticoids is controversial. It has been shown to help with severe pain symptoms, but has no effect on renal complications.

g. The overall prognosis of HSP is excellent for the vast majority of children. Long-term sequelae can occur in children with bowel perforation or those with more extensive renal involvement (gross hematuria or proteinuria).

h. Admission to the hospital may be appropriate in children who are ill-appearing, dehydrated, unable to ambulate, or have concerning renal, GU, and/or abdominal symptoms. Well-appearing children with classic HSP may be safely managed as outpatients with supportive care and close PMD follow-up for repeat urinalysis and blood pressure measurement.

N. Figure legends

a. Figure 14.1 (US) Jejuno-ileal intussusception (courtesy of Dr. James W. Tsung).

O. References

a. *Tintinalli's Emergency Medicine: A Comprehensive Study Guide* (9th ed.): Chapter 133, Acute Abdominal Pain in Infants and Children. Chapter 137, Renal Emergencies in Children.

b. *Rosen's Emergency Medicine: Concepts and Clinical Practice* (10th ed.): Chapter 166, Pediatric Gastrointestinal Disorders.

Snake Bite

Matthew Harris, MD and Joseph Chiang, MD

A. Chief complaint
a. "My son was bitten by a snake!"

B. Vital signs
a. BP: 101/57, HR: 97, RR: 20, T: 36.0°C, Sat: 98% on RA
b. No pain

C. What does the patient look like?
a. Patient appears comfortable.

D. Primary survey
a. Airway: speaking in full sentences, playful
b. Breathing: no apparent respiratory distress, no cyanosis
c. Circulation: peripheral pulses equal

E. History
a. HPI: A 10-year-old male was bitten on the right leg by a snake while on a hike with his family in the Blue Ridge Mountains of North Carolina. They were on a trail when he felt a sharp pain in his leg before anyone realized there was a snake on the side of the trail. The family briefly saw a brown and white snake and heard it make a rattling noise after the incident. Rattlesnakes are known to be found in this area. A tourniquet was placed above the wound by the family, who drove immediately to the emergency department. The injury occurred 25 minutes ago. The patient is unable to give further description and currently complains only of pain at the site of the bite.
b. PMHx: none, immunizations up-to-date
c. PSHx: none
d. Allergies: none
e. Meds: none
f. Social: lives with family
g. FHx: none
h. PMD: Dr. Torres

F. Secondary survey
a. General: alert and oriented, no acute distress
b. HEENT: normal
c. Neck: normal
d. Chest: normal

e. Heart: normal
f. Abdomen: soft, nontender
g. Extremities: right lateral lower leg with two puncture wounds, with no active bleeding or discharge. The wounds are 1–2 mm in diameter, 2 cm apart. Tourniquet in place proximal to wound. Delayed capillary refill. Full range of motion, motor and sensory intact, no erythema, no edema, no induration; otherwise unremarkable examination
h. Back: normal, no marks
i. Neuro: normal, appropriate for age
j. Lymph: normal

G. Action

a. Place on monitor
b. EKG
c. Labs
   i. CBC, BMP, PT/PTT, CK, UA, fibrinogen, fibrin split products, blood type and crossmatch
d. Normal saline bolus 20 cc/kg
e. Remove tourniquet (constriction band may be placed instead).
f. Immobilize the affected limb (sling for upper extremity and splint for lower extremity); keep the affected extremity below the level of the heart.
g. Contact hospital pharmacy to ensure rattlesnake antivenom is available. If antivenom is not immediately available, consider transport to another hospital.
h. Observe patient for 12 hours (symptoms will not progress during this time).

H. Results

Table 15.1 Results table

Test	Result	Test	Result
Complete blood count:		**Coagulation panel:**	
WBC	$9.1 \times 10^3/\mu L$	PT	12.3 sec
Hct	36.20%	PTT	25.4 sec
Plt	$462 \times 10^3/\mu L$	INR	0.9
Basic metabolic panel:		**Urinalysis:**	
Na	135 mEq/L	SG	1.022
K	3.7 mEq/L	pH	6
Cl	101 mEq/L	Prot	Neg
CO_2	22 mEq/L	Gluc	Neg
BUN	14 mEq/dL	Ketones	Neg
Cr	0.5 mg/dL	Bili	Neg
Gluc	93 mg/dL	Blood	Neg
		LE	Neg
		Nitrite	Neg
		Color	Yellow

a. Fibrinogen, fibrin split products: normal
b. CK: normal

J. Diagnosis
a. Pit viper bite without envenomation ("dry bite")

K. Critical actions
a. Assess ABCs
b. Assess wound
c. Identify snake, risk for venom exposure
d. Evaluate for laboratory signs of envenomation
e. Observe for physical signs of envenomation
f. Thorough history and examination, including total exposure
g. Remove tourniquet and immobilize affected extremity
h. Contact nearby Poison Control Center

L. Examiner instructions
a. This is a case of a snake bite. The most important intervention is to assess the patient's respiratory and cardiovascular status. The candidate should determine if airway management or cardiovascular resuscitation with fluids or vasopressors is needed. Identification of the snake is paramount. The local Poison Control Center can provide invaluable assistance. If possible, collect the snake in question (local animal control authorities may be contacted). Meanwhile, assess bite marks for local progression and expose the patient to visualize any other possible bites. Luckily for the child in this case, the snake did not envenomate the wound.

M. Pearls
a. Antivenom specific for each group of snakes; the local Poison Control Center may be helpful in determining the need. The majority of snakes are nonvenomous, but two major groups do pose a threat: crotalids (pit vipers, including rattlesnakes and cottonmouths) and elapids (coral snakes, cobras). Venom effects may not develop in up to 25% of cases; these are referred to as "dry bites."
b. Crotalid venom is predominantly cytolytic and may cause edema, hemorrhage, and necrosis close to and far away from the bite. Systemic signs and symptoms may include hemolysis, thrombocytopenia, disseminated intravascular coagulopathy, vomiting, and cardiovascular and respiratory failure.
c. Elapids tend to have neurotoxic venom, producing neurological symptoms (diplopia, ptosis, respiratory depression, paresthesia). These symptoms tend to be delayed.
d. Surgery consult is warranted if compartment syndrome is suspected.
e. Tetanus should be updated and antibiotics administered in severe bites if there are concerns for infection.
f. Patients requiring antivenom therapy should be admitted to an ICU for monitoring.
g. Note that first-aid treatments such as suction and incision along with tourniquets are contraindicated. Application of a constriction band with an elastic bandage or Penrose drain, rope, or clothing wrapped proximal to the bite may retard venom absorption without compromising arterial flow. Constriction bands are only indicated for patients with hemodynamic instability; if applied, the band should be loose enough to fit the examiner's finger within it.

N. References

a. *Tintinalli's Emergency Medicine: A Comprehensive Study Guide* (9th ed.): Chapter 212, Snakebite.

b. *Rosen's Emergency Medicine: Concepts and Clinical Practice* (10th ed.): Chapter 53, Venomous Animal Injuries.

Visual Impairment

Joseph Chiang, MD and Wirachin Hoonpongsimanont, MD

A. Chief complaint
a. 70-year-old female with decreased vision in right eye

B. Vital signs
a. BP: 146/74, HR: 84, RR: 20, T: 36.9°C, Sat: 98% on RA

C. What does the patient look like?
a. Patient appears well and is in no acute distress.

D. Primary survey
a. Airway: speaking in full sentences
b. Breathing: no apparent respiratory distress, no cyanosis
c. Circulation: peripheral pulses equal

E. History
a. HPI: A 70-year-old female presents with acute, sudden-onset loss of vision in the right eye for the past 4 days. She also complains of mild dizziness. No fever, chills, nausea, vomiting, chest pain, shortness of breath, trauma, numbness, tingling, weakness, or headache noted. No eye pain, tearing, or sensation of a curtain coming down over her eyes.
b. PMHx: hypertension, diabetes, asthma, hypercholesterolemia, atrial fibrillation
c. PSHx: cataract extraction
d. Allergies: none
e. Meds: metformin, hydrochlorothiazide, albuterol, simvastatin, coumadin
f. Social: denies smoking, alcohol, drugs
g. FHx: not relevant

F. Secondary survey
a. General: alert and oriented, well appearing, has mild pain
b. HEENT: [Examiner: Make sure the candidate asks for specific portions of the eye exam, including the visual acuity.] Head is atraumatic, normal cephalic; visual acuity: 20/30 left eye, no light perception in right eye; no nystagmus; right pupil has no response to light but dilates and constricts when light is directed into unaffected eye. No fluorescein uptake in either eye. Right eye fundoscopic examination demonstrates pale, less transparent, and edematous retina with macular sparring, intraocular pressures are 15 in both eyes.
c. Neck: normal, no carotid bruit
d. Chest: normal
e. Heart: regular rate rhythm, normal s1, s2

f. Abdomen: normal
g. Extremities: normal
h. Neuro: alert and oriented, no focal motor, sensory deficits; no neglect with left eye; no facial asymmetry; normal memory; gait normal
i. Skin: pale, no rashes, no edema
j. Lymph: normal

G. Action

a. Oxygen via NC or nonrebreather mask
b. Peripheral IV line
c. Perform ocular massage, breathing in paper bag
d. Administer acetazolamide 500 mg IV or PO
e. Administer topical β-blocker
f. Labs
    i. CBC, BMP, PT/PTT
g. Monitor: BP: 146/74, HR: 84, RR: 20, Sat: 98% on RA
h. EKG
i. Consult
    i. Ophthalmology consult
j. Imaging
    i. Head CT

H. Results

Table 16.1 Results table

Test	Result	Test	Result
Complete blood count:		**Coagulation panel:**	
WBC	$5.3 \times 10^3/\mu L$	PT	14 sec
Hct	35.10%	PTT	26 sec
Plt	$265 \times 10^3/\mu L$	INR	2.1
Basic metabolic panel:		**Urinalysis:**	
Na	136 mEq/L	SG	1.03
K	3.9 mEq/L	pH	6
Cl	99 mEq/L	Prot	Neg
CO_2	33 mEq/L	Gluc	Neg
BUN	26 mEq/dL	Ketones	Neg
Cr	1.3 mg/dL	Bili	Neg
Gluc	146 mg/dL	Blood	Neg
		LE	Neg
		Nitrite	Neg
		Color	Yellow

a. Lactate: 0.8 mmol/L
b. EKG atrial fibrillation rate: 75
c. Head CT without contrast (Figure 16.1)

Figure 16.1

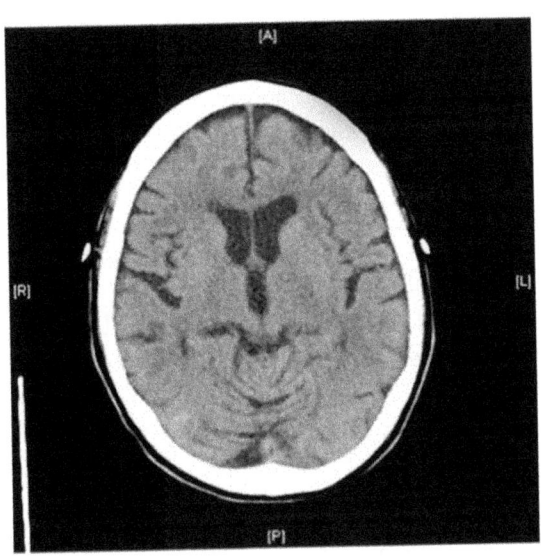

I. Action
a. Ophthalmology consult
   i. Examination demonstrates unremarkable sclera, conjunctiva, and anterior chamber in both eyes. Right eye has pale, less transparent, and edematous retina with macular sparring. Findings consistent with central retinal artery occlusion.

J. Diagnosis
a. Central retinal artery occlusion

K. Critical actions
a. Ocular examination
b. Ophthalmology consult
c. Decrease IOP methods and vasodilate retinal artery

L. Examiner instructions
a. This is a case of central retinal artery occlusion or blockage of blood supply to the eye. This causes acute onset unilateral painless loss of vision. This pathology occurs most commonly in the elderly with diabetes, hypertension, hypercholesterolemia, and atrial fibrillation. Careful history and ocular examination are important to establish the diagnosis. While there is no single, efficacious treatment for central retinal artery occlusion, the goals of treatment are to move the emboli to the peripheral artery by decreasing intraocular pressure and vasodilation, or to lyse the clot in centers where this modality is used. CT scan is unnecessary, but should be normal if obtained. If neurology consultation is attempted, the consultant will defer to the ophthalmologist's recommendations. Patients should be evaluated by an ophthalmologist emergently.

M. Pearls
a. Pale, less transparent, and edematous retina with macular sparring, "cherry red spot" is pathognomonic for central retinal artery occlusion.

b. Ophthalmoscopic examination reveals pale, less transparent, and edematous retina with macular sparing due to infarcted retina. The red color at the macula is from the intact choroidal circulation that is still visible through this thinnest part of the retina. An afferent pupillary defect may be noted in the affected eye – loss of vision in that eye prevents light information from being relayed to the brain. Thus, light shone in the affected eye will not be perceived, and the pupils dilate. When light is directed into the unaffected eye, the information is transmitted to the brain normally, and both pupils receive a signal to constrict.

c. The majority of cases are caused by emboli. Treatment is directed at moving the emboli to the periphery via massage or vasodilation, and in some centers intravenous or intraarterial tissue plasminogen activator (tPA) is used. The infarcted retina could be saved if appropriate management is provided within 90 minutes after the onset.

d. Emergency management in addition to immediate ophthalmology consultation is:

   i.   Ocular massage: Apply firm, steady digital pressure to the affected eye for 15 seconds then suddenly release to move the emboli to peripheral artery. Peripheral retinal artery occlusion will affect a smaller area of the retina.

   ii. Having the patient breathe into a paper bag to increase $PaCO_2$ and administering topical β-blocker eyedrops could help vasodilate the artery.

   iii. Administer acetazolamide IV or PO to decrease IOP while awaiting the ophthalmologist to determine whether an IOP-lowering anterior chamber paracentesis is necessary.

N. Figure legends
a. Figure 16.1 (CT) Normal head CT.

O. References
a. *Tintinalli's Emergency Medicine: A Comprehensive Study Guide* (9th ed.): Chapter 235, Eye Emergencies.
b. *Rosen's Emergency Medicine: Concepts and Clinical Practice* (10th ed.): Chapter 57, Ophthalmology.

Syncope

Maneesha Agarwal, MD and Christopher Strother, MD

A. Chief complaint
a. 14-year-old male brought in by EMS after passing out at pool

B. Vital signs
a. BP: 100/70, HR: 96, RR: 18, T: 37.2°C, Sat: 99% on RA, FS: 115 mg/dL, Wt: 60 kg

C. What does the patient look like?
a. Patient appears stated age, no distress, sitting in stretcher.

D. Primary survey
a. Airway: speaking in full sentences
b. Breathing: no apparent respiratory distress, no cyanosis
c. Circulation: warm pink skin, normal capillary refill

E. Action
a. Labs
   i. VBG/ABG, CBC, CMP, coagulation panel
b. Monitor: orthostatic vital signs (normal)
c. EKG

F. History
a. HPI: a 14-year-old male with no past medical history in usual state of health until pool party today. After jumping into the pool, he complained of chest pain and shortness of breath; then he passed out. He received CPR while an AED was applied. A shock was delivered and he woke up at baseline. Symptoms now resolved except some residual fatigue and "weakness."
b. PMHx: behavioral disorder
c. PSHx: none
d. Allergies: none
e. Meds: olanzapine
f. Social: lives with parents at home, denies alcohol use, smoking, drugs, or sexual activity
g. FHx: cousin drowned at 10 years old when swimming alone
h. PMD: Dr. Godwin

G. Nurse
a. BP: 100/75, HR: 90, RR: 18, Sat: 99% on RA
b. EKG (Figure 17.1)

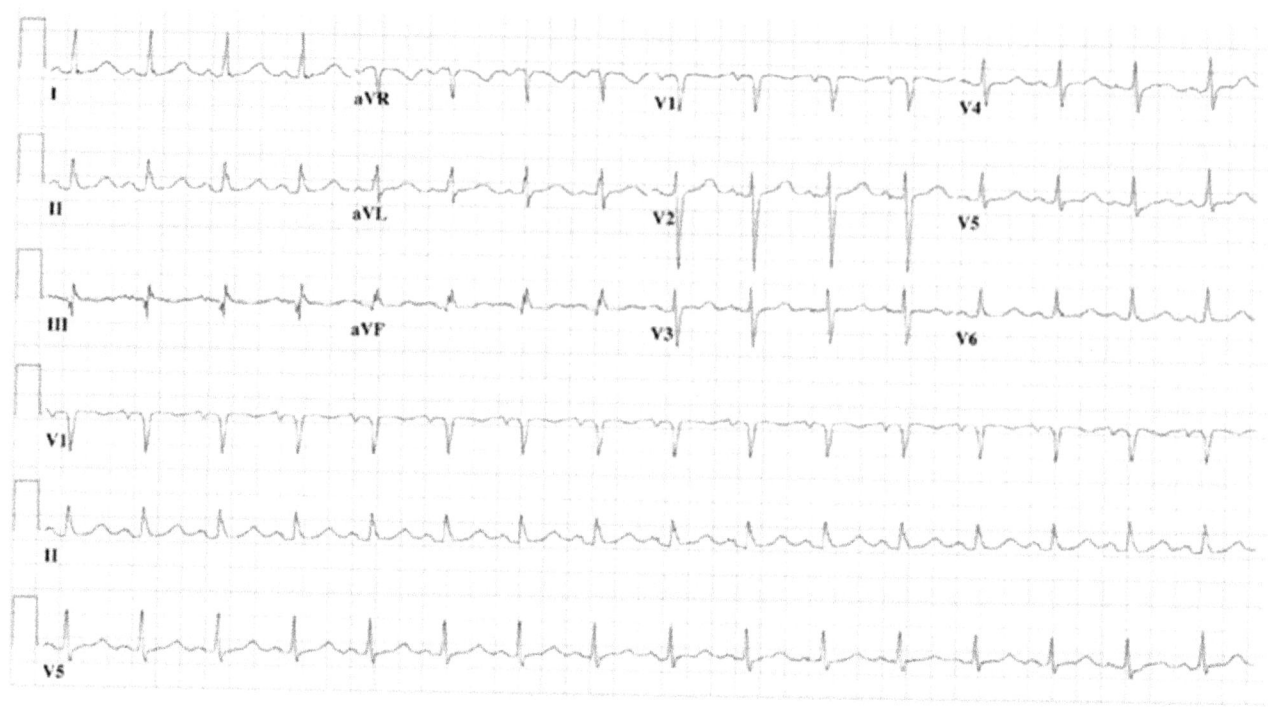

Figure 17.1

H. Secondary survey
a. General: alert and oriented, fatigued but nontoxic
b. HEENT: mildly dry mucous membranes, otherwise normal
c. Neck: normal
d. Chest: normal
e. Heart: normal, no murmur, rub, or gallops
f. Abdomen: normal
g. GU: normal
h. Extremities: normal
i. Back: normal
j. Neuro: normal
k. Skin: normal
l. Lymph: normal

I. Status change
a. Patient complains of chest pain, shortness of breath, then lapses into unconsciousness.

J. Primary survey
a. Airway: clear, normal
b. Breathing: apneic
c. Circulation: pulseless

K. Action
a. Bag-valve-mask ventilation ± intubation or supraglottic airway
b. Chest compressions
c. Monitor (Figure 17.2)

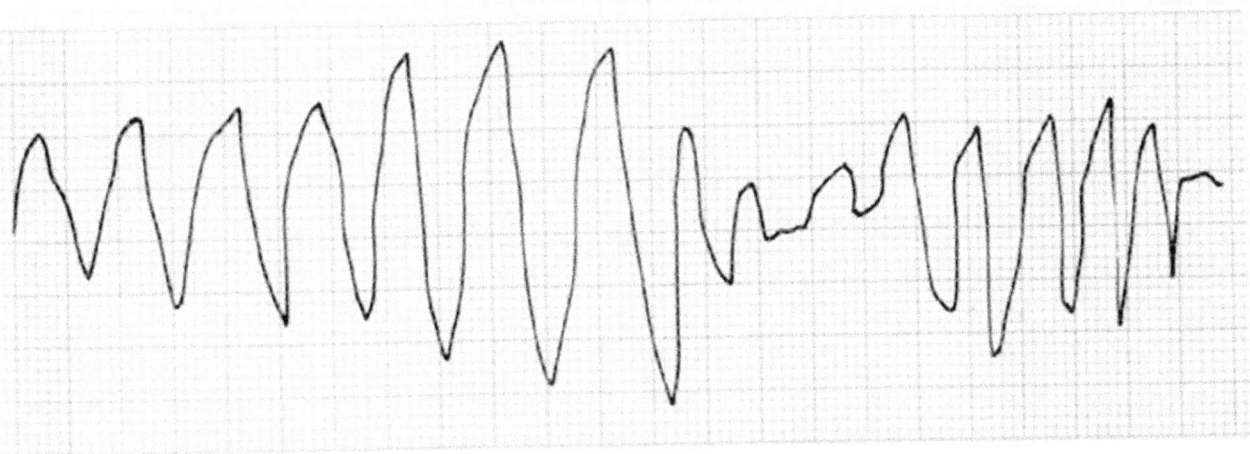

Figure 17.2

d. Defibrillate
   i. Start with 2 J/kg, then 4 J/kg (effective on second attempt)
e. Meds
   i. Epinephrine (no effect clinically)
   ii. Magnesium sulfate (no effect clinically)
f. Reassess
   i. Patient remains in ventricular fibrillation/torsades until two shocks *and* magnesium are administered.
   ii. Post-resuscitation care includes antiarrhythmic drip, labs, endotracheal tube intubation/ventilator setup, and ICU consult and transfer.
g. Imaging
   i. CXR (Figure 17.3)

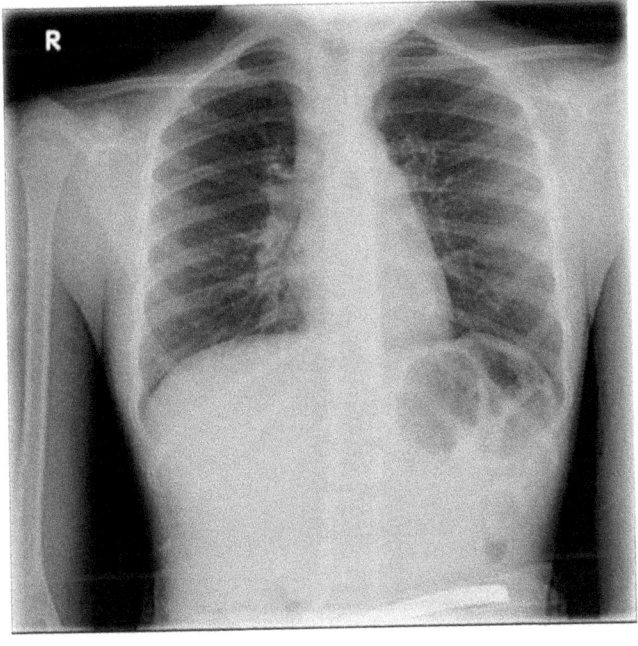

Figure 17.3

h. Access
i. IV access if not previously obtained

L. Results

Table 17.1 Results table

Test	Result	Test	Result
Complete blood count:		T bili	0.6 mg/dL
WBC	$10.7 \times 10^3/\mu L$	D bili	0.1 mg/dL
Hct	37.10%	Amylase	42 U/L
Plt	$300 \times 10^3/\mu L$	Lipase	30 U/L
		Albumin	4.0 g/dL
Basic metabolic panel:			
Na	140 mEq/L	**Urinalysis:**	
K	4.1 mEq/L	SG	1.018
Cl	108 mEq/L	pH	6
CO_2	22 mEq/L	Prot	Neg
BUN	3 mEq/dL	Gluc	Neg
Cr	0.6 mg/dL	Ketones	Neg
Gluc	120 mg/dL	Bili	Neg
		Blood	Neg
Coagulation panel:		LE	Neg
PT	11.1 sec	Nitrite	Neg
PTT	35.2 sec	Color	Yellow
INR	1.0		
		Arterial blood gas:	
Liver function panel:		pH	7.4
AST	15 U/L	pO_2	100 mmHg
ALT	12 U/L	pCO_2	40 mmHg
Alk phos	260 U/L	HCO_3	22 mmol/L

a. Lactate: 0.9 mmol/L

M. Action
a. Telemetry monitoring
b. ICU consult
c. Cardiology consult
d. Discussion with family and PMD on need for ICU and cardiology evaluation
e. Discussion of prolonged QT syndrome with cardiology or ICU staff
f. Meds
    i. Lidocaine drip – avoid amiodarone and procainamide

N. Diagnosis
a. Prolonged QT syndrome
b. Torsades de pointes

O. Critical actions
a. Order EKG, look for prolonged QT syndrome
b. Recognition of torsades after decompensation
c. Resuscitation per pediatric advanced life support (PALS) guidelines, including infusion of magnesium
d. Cardiology consultation

P. Examiner instructions
a. This is a case of a prolonged QT syndrome (an abnormal electrical conduction within the heart) leading to intermittent torsades de pointes arrhythmia. Prolonged QT can be associated with syncope and sudden death from ventricular arrhythmias. Torsades de pointes (French for "twisting of the points") is classically associated with prolonged QT syndrome; the QRS complex alternates between low and high amplitude, as if it were twisting around the baseline. Episodes can be triggered by physical activity, emotional stress, swimming/diving reflex, and startle reflex. Additionally, certain medications, such as macrolides and antipsychotics, can further prolong the QT interval. Any child with unexplained syncope should have an EKG checked for prolonged QT syndrome. Once torsades occurs as in this patient, magnesium sulfate is the drug of choice for conversion, but unstable patients need defibrillation. Post-arrest care includes an antiarrhythmic such as lidocaine. Correct hypokalemia and hypocalcemia. Additional magnesium may be warranted to push levels above 3 mg/dL to prevent additional episodes of torsades.

Q. Pearls
a. Prolonged QT is one of the more dangerous diagnoses that need to be excluded in a young patient with syncope.
b. Prolonged QT syndrome has the potential to decompensate into fatal ventricular arrhythmias, classically torsades de pointes.
c. Treatment of choice for torsades is magnesium and defibrillation.

R. Figure legends
a. Figure 17.1 EKG demonstrating sinus rhythm with prolonged QT intervals.
b. Figure 17.2 Rhythm strip demonstrating torsades de pointes.
c. Figure 17.3 Normal chest x-ray.

S. References
a. *Tintinalli's Emergency Medicine: A Comprehensive Study Guide* (9th ed.): Chapter 18, Cardiac Rhythm Disturbances.
b. *Rosen's Emergency Medicine: Concepts and Clinical Practice* (10th ed.): Chapter 65, Dysrhythmias.

Sore Throat

Ian Kane, MD and Lisa Zahn, MD

A. Chief complaint
a. 3-year-old boy brought in for sore throat and fever

B. Vital signs
a. BP: 114/80, HR: 150, RR: 28, T: 39.1°C, Sat: 98% on RA, Wt: 15 kg

C. What does the patient look like?
a. Uncomfortable-appearing male, drooling slightly and sitting upright, holding head and neck still.

D. Primary survey
a. Airway: speaking in short sentences, does not want to open mouth fully, drooling
b. Breathing: no apparent respiratory distress, no cyanosis or stridor
c. Circulation: moves all extremities, skin color within normal limits

E. Action
a. Peripheral IV line
b. Labs
    i. CBC, BMP, blood culture
c. 20 ml/kg (300 ml) NS bolus
e. Monitor: BP: 114/80, HR: 140, RR: 28, T: 39.1°C, Sat: 100% on O_2
f. Consult
    i. Otolaryngology consult
g. Meds
    i. Ibuprofen or acetaminophen

F. History
a. HPI: A 3-year-old male with no past medical history presents with 3 days of sore throat, now with drooling and increasing reluctance to move neck. Patient accompanied by grandmother. No cough, congestion, vomiting, or diarrhea.
b. PMHx: immunizations up to date, no past medical history, normal spontaneous vaginal delivery at 40 weeks, uncomplicated pregnancy
c. PSHx: none
d. Allergies: none
e. Meds: none
f. Social: lives with grandmother

g. FHx: noncontributory
h. PMD: Dr. Davis

G. Nurse

a. BP: 114/80, HR: 145, RR: 28, T: 39.1°C, Sat: 98% on O_2

H. Secondary survey

a. General: alert, oriented × 3, sitting upright in stretcher, holding head and neck in a fixed position, drooling slightly
b. Head: normocephalic, atraumatic
c. Eyes: extraocular movement intact, pupils equal, reactive to light
d. Ears: normal tympanic membranes
e. Nose: no discharge
f. Neck: no stridor, no anterior cervical lymphadenopathy, +pain with extension of neck
g. Pharynx: will not open mouth fully; grossly normal dentition, no lesions, no tonsillar exudates, or edema; uvula appears midline
h. Chest: nontender
i. Lungs: clear bilaterally
j. Heart: tachycardic, rhythm regular, no murmurs, rubs, or gallops
k. Abdomen: normal bowel sounds, soft, nontender, and non-distended
l. Extremities: full range of motion, no deformity, normal pulses
m. Back: nontender
n. Neuro: cranial nerves II to XII intact; normal sensation, strength; normal reflexes and gait
o. Skin: warm and dry
p. Lymph: no lymphadenopathy

I. Action

a. Have intubation equipment available
b. Meds
   i. Ampicillin/sulbactam or clindamycin
   ii. Ibuprofen/acetaminophen
c. Reassess
   i. Patient condition is same as at presentation, child remains febrile and tachycardic.
d. Consult
   i. Otolaryngology assessment shows swelling in soft tissue around the posterior pharynx, normal vocal cords without edema, patent airway. Recommends imaging, admission, and observation with IV antibiotics.
e. Imaging
   i. Lateral neck soft tissue x-ray
   ii. CT neck with contrast

J. Nurse

a. Antipyretic
   i. BP: 114/80, HR: 125, RR: 28, T: 38.2°C, Sat: 98%
b. No antipyretic
   i. BP: 114/80, HR: 160, RR: 28, T: 39.6, Sat: 98%

K. Results

Table 18.1 Results table

Test	Result	Test	Result
Complete blood count:		**Liver function panel:**	
WBC	$10.0 \times 10^3/\mu L$	AST	23 U/L
Hct	33.30%	ALT	26 U/L
Plt	$191 \times 10^3/\mu L$	Alk phos	42 U/L
		T bili	1.0 mg/dL
Basic metabolic panel:		D bili	0.3 mg/dL
Na	138 mEq/L	Amylase	50 U/L
K	4.3 mEq/L	Lipase	25 U/L
Cl	105 mEq/L	Albumin	4.7 g/dL
CO_2	25 mEq/L		
BUN	18 mEq/dL	**Urinalysis:**	
Cr	0.6 mg/dL	SG	1.020
Gluc	100 mg/dL	pH	7
		Prot	Neg
Coagulation panel:		Gluc	Neg
PT	12.6 sec	Ketones	Neg
PTT	26.0 sec	Bili	Neg
INR	1.0	Blood	Neg
		LE	Neg
		Nitrite	Neg
		Color	Yellow

a. Lateral soft tissue neck radiograph (Figure 18.1)
   i. 1.5 cm prevertebral widening
b. CT of the neck with contrast (Figure 18.2)

L. Action

a. Surgery – otolaryngology consult
   i. Admit to PICU
   ii. Possible surgery in the morning pending response to IV antibiotics
b. Discussion with family for admission and possible OR

M. Diagnosis

a. Retropharyngeal abscess

N. Critical actions

a. Consideration of the need for possible intubation
b. Antibiotics

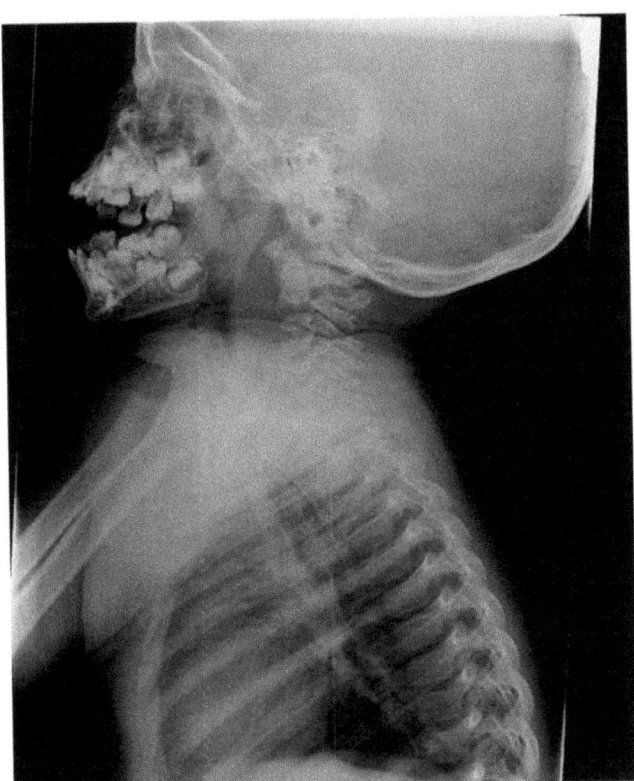

Figure 18.1

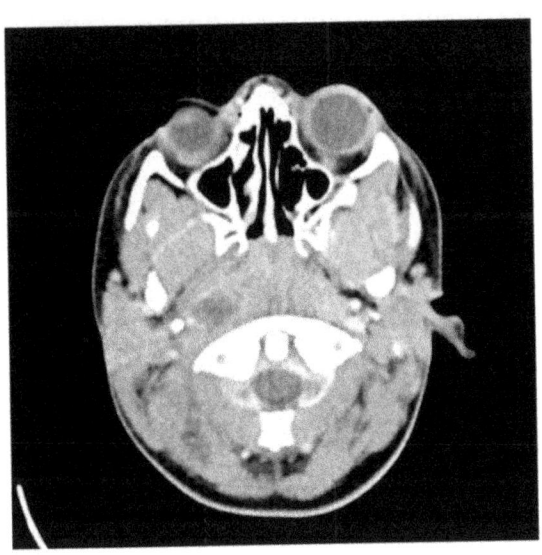

Figure 18.2

c. Soft tissue neck radiograph or CT of the neck with IV contrast
d. Otolaryngology consult
e. ICU admission

O. Examiner instructions:
a. This is a case of retropharyngeal abscess, a serious infection of the soft tissue behind the pharynx, which can in severe circumstances lead to airway obstruction or sepsis. The patient's symptoms of drooling, fever, sore throat, trismus, and neck stiffness with extension are key findings. Important early actions include airway evaluation, obtaining IV access, administering antibiotics and intravenous fluids, obtaining radiographs or CT scan, consulting

otolaryngology, and admitting the patient to an ICU setting. If the candidate does not order antibiotics, the patient will have increased difficulty in breathing and agitation. In unstable patients, CT should be deferred until the patient is stabilized or the airway is protected with intubation.

P. Pearls

a. In the setting of an acutely toxic-appearing child with airway compromise, rapid evaluation and airway assessment by a provider with advanced airway is critical. An ill-appearing child who is maintaining their airway should be kept comfortable with a minimum of painful interventions until this can be arranged.

b. Retropharyngeal abscess most commonly affects young children between the ages of 2 and 4 years, because the lymph nodes of the retropharyngeal space atrophy prior to puberty.

c. History and physical examination are crucial for diagnosis. On physical examination, extension of the neck will be particularly painful. It may be difficult in some cases to differentiate retropharyngeal abscess from meningitis due to the degree of neck stiffness and the young age of the patient. Visual inspection of the oropharynx is frequently unremarkable and is often limited by trismus and patient cooperation. Presence of stridor is worrisome for impending airway compromise. Alternative diagnoses, such as epiglottitis and peritonsillar abscess, must be considered as well. In this case, the gradual clinical progression, pain with neck extension, and full immunization status made epiglottitis and meningitis less likely.

d. Although a lateral soft tissue neck radiograph may be a good initial imaging study, it requires patient cooperation, which can be difficult in pediatric patients. The film must be taken as a perfect lateral, with the patient in inspiration. Improper patient positioning and crying can both cause a falsely widened prevertebral space. The prevertebral space is widened if it is greater than 7 mm at C2 or 14 mm at C6. For these technical reasons, further imaging with a CT of the neck with contrast is often necessary for diagnosis.

e. Broad-spectrum antibiotics must be administered early. Retropharyngeal abscesses are polymicrobial. The most common organisms are gram positives, specifically group A *Streptococcus* and *Staphylococcus aureus*. Respiratory anaerobic species have been implicated as well.

f. Early surgical consultation by ENT should be obtained because surgical drainage of the abscess may be necessary.

g. Late findings include extension into the mediastinum, airway compromise from abscess rupture, or sepsis.

Q. Figure legends

a. Figure 18.1 (XR) Lateral soft tissue neck radiograph.

b. Figure 18.2 (CT) Para- and retropharyngeal abscess (photo courtesy of Dr. Richard Jones).

R. References

a. *Tintinalli's Emergency Medicine: A Comprehensive Study Guide* (9th ed.): Chapter 119, Stridor and Drooling.

b. *Rosen's Emergency Medicine: Concepts and Clinical Practice* (10th ed.): Chapter 168, Pediatric Respiratory Emergencies.

Knee Pain

Jennifer M. Bellis, MD, MPH and Edward R. Melnick, MD, MHS

A. Chief complaint
a. 13-year-old male presents with right knee pain

B. Vital signs
a. BP: 118/77, HR: 84, RR: 16, T: 36.8°C, Sat: 99% on RA

C. What does the patient look like?
a. Patient appears stated age, is obese, and limps into the examination room from the waiting room.

D. Primary survey
a. Airway: speaking in full sentences
b. Breathing: no apparent respiratory distress, no cyanosis
c. Circulation: warm and well-perfused, normal capillary refill

E. History
a. HPI: A 13-year-old male with a history of obesity is brought in by his mother, complaining of right knee pain and limp. The pain started about 2 months ago but was a mild dull ache until yesterday after playing basketball in gym class. Since yesterday he has had a limp, and the pain became more severe. He tried one dose of ibuprofen last night and ice, but continued to have pain with bearing weight on his right lower extremity. He denies any falls or trauma. He has been well otherwise recently without fever, respiratory symptoms, swelling, or decreased range of motion. He has had no pains in his other joints.
b. PMHx: obesity, otherwise none; immunizations up to date
c. PSHx: none
d. Allergies: none
e. Meds: ibuprofen prn
f. Social: lives with parents and two younger siblings; denies alcohol, drugs, smoking; he has never been sexually active
g. FHx: no relevant history
h. PMD: Dr. Smith

F. Secondary survey
a. General: alert and oriented, comfortable sitting on stretcher, pleasant, cooperative
b. HEENT: normal
c. Neck: normal

    d. Chest: normal

    e. Heart: normal

    f. Abdomen: normal

    g. Back: normal

    h. Extremities

       i. Normal knee and ankle examination bilaterally, nontender, no effusion, full range of motion, knees stable to anterior drawer and Lachman test, 2+ dorsalis pedis and posterior tibial pulses bilaterally, normal capillary refill

      ii. Left hip examination normal; right hip externally rotated with limited range of motion in internal rotation

    i. Neuro: antalgic gait with slight external rotation of right leg while walking but otherwise intact motor, sensory, and deep tendon reflexes in lower extremities bilaterally

    j. Skin: warm and dry, no rashes, no edema, no cellulitis

    k. Lymph: normal

G. Action

    a. Meds: ibuprofen PO

    b. Reassess

       i. Right knee pain and limp persist

    c. Imaging

       i. Bilateral hip x-ray, including frog-leg view

      ii. Consider knee x-ray

H. Nurse

    a. Bilateral hip x-ray including frog-leg lateral view (Figures 19.1 and 19.2)

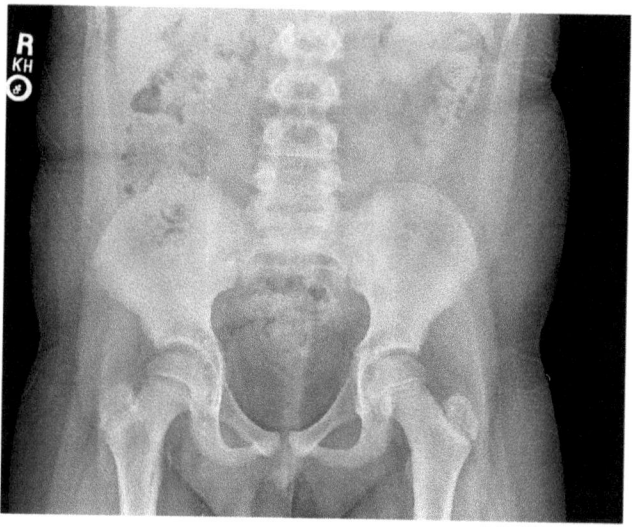

Figure 19.1

I. Action

    a. Strict nonweight-bearing on right lower extremity

    b. Orthopedic consult

       i. To OR for percutaneous pinning

    c. Discussion with family and PMD explaining slipped capital femoral epiphysis; need for prompt surgical management

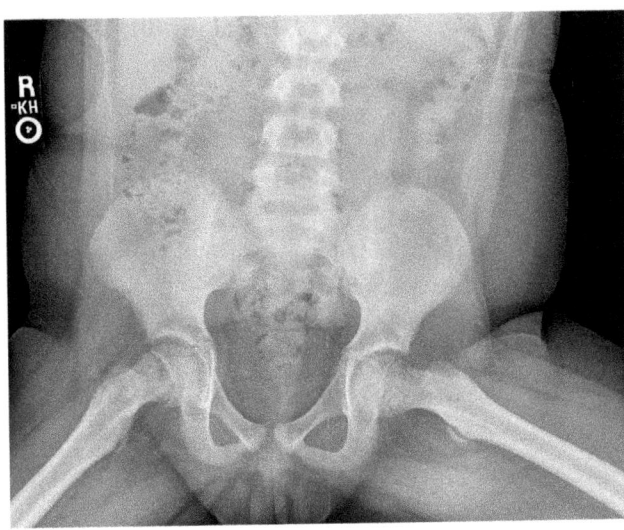

Figure 19.2

J. Diagnosis
a. Slipped capital femoral epiphysis (SCFE)

K. Critical actions
a. Physical examination of hips bilaterally
b. Bilateral hip x-ray with lateral views
c. Orthopedic consult for SCFE
d. Pain medication

L. Examiner instructions
a. This is a case of slipped capital femoral epiphysis, the most common cause of hip disability in adolescents. In this injury, the growth plate near the end of the femur becomes disrupted, and the end of the bone "slips" out of place, usually posteriorly and inferiorly. Important early actions include physical examination of the hips and x-ray imaging of the hips bilaterally, including lateral and frog-leg views. Early SCFE may only be seen with a frog-leg view. If the hips are not examined, the right knee pain and limp will persist. If the patient is discharged without a hip examination or x-ray, the patient will return 2 days later unable to walk.

M. Pearls
a. SCFE most commonly occurs in obese adolescents since the hips are exposed to repetitive minor trauma.
b. It may be acute, chronic, or acute on chronic. Newer classifications also consider stable versus unstable. SCFE may manifest as pain in the hip or referred to the knee or thigh. One should examine the hip in any child complaining of knee pain.
c. SCFE may become bilateral in 80% of cases.
d. It is three times more common in males, with an average age of 12–16 years old in males and 10–14 years old in females. This corresponds to the peak adolescent growth spurt.
e. On exam, the child may be holding the leg in flexion and external rotation. More advanced cases may lose the ability to internally rotate.
f. X-ray findings may only be apparent on lateral/frog-leg radiographic view. A line drawn along the superior aspect of the femoral neck (Klein's line) should transect the lateral quarter of the femoral head. In SCFE, no part of the femoral head is above Klein's line.

g. A modified Klein's line may identify additional cases of early SCFE. The modified line compares the amount of the epiphysis lateral to Klein's line on the affected side compared to the unaffected side. A 2 mm difference is considered positive.

h. Delay in diagnosis can lead to significant disability due to avascular necrosis of the femoral head. Other complications of unrepaired SCFE include chondrolysis, nonunion, premature closure of epiphyseal plate, and degenerative changes.

i. Inability to ambulate is ominous and is a sign of unstable SCFE. These cases are at much higher risk of developing complications than stable (ambulatory) SCFE cases. Stable SCFE are usually associated with chronic pain. Unstable are often the result of acute injury, though an acute injury may exacerbate a previously stable SCFE.

N. Figure legends

a. Figure 19.1 Right femoral head with growth plate widening (courtesy of Kathleen Maguire, MD).

b. Figure 19.2 Slippage of the capital femoral epiphysis (courtesy of Kathleen Maguire, MD).

O. References

a. *Tintinalli's Emergency Medicine: A Comprehensive Study Guide* (9th ed.): Chapter 141, Pediatric Orthopedic Emergencies.

b. *Rosen's Emergency Medicine: Concepts and Clinical Practice* (10th ed.): Chapter 170, Pediatric Musculoskeletal Disorders.

Abdominal Pain

Peter Gutierrez, MD

A. Chief complaint
a. 6-year-old male with abdominal pain

B. Vital signs
a. BP: 99/64, HR: 110, RR: 24, T: 37.3°C, Sat: 99% on RA, Wt: 20 kg

C. What does the patient look like?
a. Patient appears stated age. Uncomfortable due to pain; lying curled up on the stretcher, holding his abdomen.

D. Primary survey
a. Airway: whimpering and crying; airway patent
b. Breathing: no obvious respiratory distress, but breathing fast due to pain, no cyanosis
c. Circulation: warm and well-perfused extremities

E. History
a. HPI: A 6-year-old male with acute onset of lower abdominal pain and vomiting. When asked, he points to his right lower quadrant. Pain started 5 hours prior to presentation while playing with toys at home. Had two bouts of nonbloody, nonbilious emesis. No known trauma, fevers, dysuria, or diarrhea. No prior similar episodes of pain. Had been tolerating oral intake normally prior to the onset of pain, but hasn't wanted to eat since. Mom tried to alleviate the pain by giving acetaminophen and a laxative at home. Denies any history of hard or painful stools.
b. PMHx: healthy; born at term via spontaneous vaginal delivery
c. PSHx: none
d. Allergies: none
e. Meds: none
f. Social: lives at home with mom and 3-year-old brother; no pets in the home; immunizations are up to date
g. FHx: not relevant
h. PMD: Dr. Meeks

F. Nurse
a. IV access

G. Secondary survey

a. General: alert, oriented, answers questions while in obvious pain
b. HEENT: normal
c. Neck: normal
d. Chest: normal
e. Heart: normal
f. Abdomen: soft, nondistended; normal bowel sounds; mild suprapubic tenderness to palpation; negative Rovsing, obturator, and psoas signs (must ask)
g. Rectal: normal rectal tone; no hard stool palpated in the rectal vault
h. Urogenital: enlarged and tender left hemiscrotum; left testicle is elevated in the scrotum and has a horizontal lie; the cremasteric reflex is present on the right and absent on the left (must ask); no penile discharge
i. Extremities: normal
j. Back: normal, no CVA tenderness
k. Neuro: normal
l. Skin: warm and well perfused without rashes
m. Lymph: normal

H. Action

a. Meds
    i.   Morphine (0.1 mg/kg) IV
    ii. NS bolus (20 cc/kg) over 30 minutes
b. Labs
    i.   CBC
    ii.   BMP
    iii. CRP
    iv.   Urinalysis
    v.   Urine culture
c. Imaging
    i.   Bedside testicular ultrasound – no flow (Figure 20.1)
    ii. Testicular ultrasound with Doppler (ultrasound tech unavailable)
d. Action
    i. Consult pediatric urology or surgery (depending on resources available).
        • Is in the operating room and can come down in 30–60 minutes.
        • Requests obtaining an ultrasound (if not already asked for).
e. Procedure
    i. Attempt manual detorsion.
        a. Performed in a medial to lateral rotation ("outwards" or "opening the book")
        b. Successful if performed

I. Nurse

a. If no morphine given and manual detorsion not performed: vital signs are unchanged; in 10/10 pain.
b. If morphine given but manual detorsion not performed:
    BP: 91/53, HR: 99, RR: 22, Sat: 99% on RA; pain has improved from a 10/10 to 4/10
c. If manual detorsion is performed
    BP: 89/52, HR: 90, RR: 18, Sat: 99% on RA; pain has resolved

J. Results

Table 20.1 Results table

Test	Result	Test	Result
Complete blood count:		**Urinalysis:**	
WBC	$7.2 \times 10^3/\mu L$	SG	1.020
Hgb	$13.4 \times 10^3/\mu L$	pH	6
Hct	45.90%	Prot	Neg
Plt	$190 \times 10^3/\mu L$	Gluc	Neg
		Ketones	Neg
		Bili	Neg
Basic metabolic panel:		Blood	Neg
Na	142 mEq/L	LE	Neg
K	3.9 mEq/L	Nitrite	Neg
Cl	109 mEq/L	Color	Yellow
CO_2	24 mEq/L		
BUN	22 mEq/dL		
Cr	0.8 mg/dL		
Gluc	93 mg/dL		

a. Testicular ultrasound (Figure 20.1)

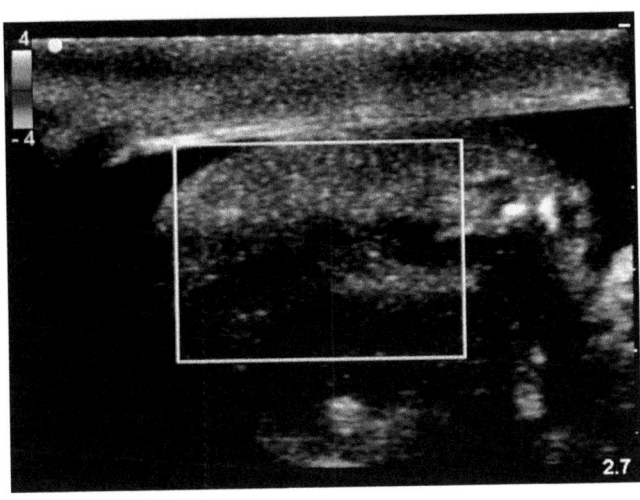

Figure 20.1

K. Action

a. Pediatric urology or surgery consult (initial consult if not called before; update if spoken to previously)
   i. Manual detorsion performed: admit to floor for urgent repair
   ii. No manual detorsion performed: admit to the OR for emergent repair
b. Discussion with family and PMD regarding the need for emergent surgical repair

L. Diagnosis

a. Testicular torsion

M. Critical actions

a. Testicular ultrasound
b. Pediatric urology or surgery consult
c. Manual detorsion attempt (if any delay in definitive care anticipated)
d. Pain management

N. Examiner instructions

a. This is a case of testicular torsion, where the testicle twists within the scrotum, causing it to cut off its own blood supply. The onset of pain is typically quick, and there is limited time to get to the operating room to maximize the chance that the testicle can be salvaged. In young children, the presenting symptom could be abdominal pain without reporting any testicular symptoms. Bedside ultrasound can show decreased blood flow, but can't adequately rule out the condition, which is why a comprehensive testicular ultrasound with Doppler is often needed. If the condition is recognized and a manual detorsion (trying to untwist the testicle) is performed, pain will resolve soon afterwards. Because there is a high chance of recurrence, surgical repair is still needed, even if detorsion is successfully performed. Urinalysis is useful in assessing for infection such as UTIs, STIs (in older patients), or epididymitis, which can also can testicular pain and swelling. If a urology consult is asked for before a testicular ultrasound with Doppler is obtained, the consultant will ask if there is confirmatory imaging.

O. Pearls

a. Consider torsion with acute onset of testicular pain, especially with nausea or vomiting, but know that it can also present with isolated abdominal pain.
b. Signs of testicular torsion can include testicular tenderness, swollen hemiscrotum/testicle, loss of cremasteric reflex, and horizontal lie of the testicle.
c. Optimal rates of testicular salvage occur when blood flow is restored within 6 hours of onset of ischemia.
d. Bedside ultrasound is specific, but not sensitive enough to exclude diagnosis of testicular torsion.
e. Manual testicular detorsion can be performed, especially when the time until corrective surgery will be prolonged. Two-thirds of torsion occur medially.
f. Definitive treatment is detorsion with orchiopexy by a pediatric urologist or surgeon.

P. Figure legends

a. Figure 20.1 (US) Testicle with no Doppler flow and reactive hydrocele (courtesy of Dr. Peter Gutierrez).

Q. References

a. *Tintinalli's Emergency Medicine: A Comprehensive Study Guide* (9th ed.): Chapter 136, Pediatric Urologic and Gynecologic Disorders.
b. *Rosen's Emergency Medicine: Concepts and Clinical Practice* (10th ed.): Chapter 168, Pediatric Genitourinary and Renal Tract Disorders.

Abdominal Pain

Yasuharu Okuda, MD

A. Chief complaint
a. 79-year-old female brought in by her husband with the complaint of worsening abdominal pain for the past 4 hours

B. Vital signs
a. BP: 85/63, HR: 96, RR: 18, T: 36.2°C, Sat: 98% on RA, FS: 110 mg/dL

C. What does the patient look like?
a. Patient appears stated age, uncomfortable secondary to pain in mild distress, lying still in stretcher.

D. Primary survey
a. Airway: speaking in full sentences
b. Breathing: no apparent respiratory distress, no cyanosis
c. Circulation: pale and cool skin, normal capillary refill

E. Action
a. Two large-bore peripheral IV lines
b. Labs
   i. CBC, Chem 7, LFT, PT/PTT, type and crossmatch 2 units, lactate
c. 1 L NS bolus
d. Monitor: BP: 92/68, HR: 96, RR: 18, Sat: 100% on RA
e. EKG

F. History
a. HPI: A 79-year-old female with a history of hypertension and hypercholesterolemia states that she has been constipated for the past few days. Today she was finally able to have a large "explosive" bowel movement which was brown and nonbloody. Since then over the past 4 hours she has developed progressive abdominal pain. The pain started in the epigastrium but now has become diffuse. The patient thought it might be indigestion. She rode a taxi to the hospital and the pain was exacerbated with shaking of the taxi. Pain also worsened with shaking of the stretcher. The patient notes nausea, but denies vomiting, fever, chills, chest pain, shortness of breath, headache, back pain, urinary symptoms, or vaginal discharge; last meal was breakfast.
b. PMHx: hypertension and hypercholesterolemia
c. PSHx: none
d. Allergies: none

    e. Meds: simvastatin, aspirin, metoprolol
    f. Social: lives with husband at home, denies alcohol, smoking, drugs, not sexually active
    g. FHx: not relevant
    h. PMD: Dr. Richardson

G. Nurse
    a. EKG (Figure 21.1)
    b. 1 L NS
        i. BP: 98/59, HR: 90, RR: 18, Sat: 98% on O_2
    c. No fluids
        i. BP: 70/45, HR: 118, RR: 20, Sat: 98% on O_2

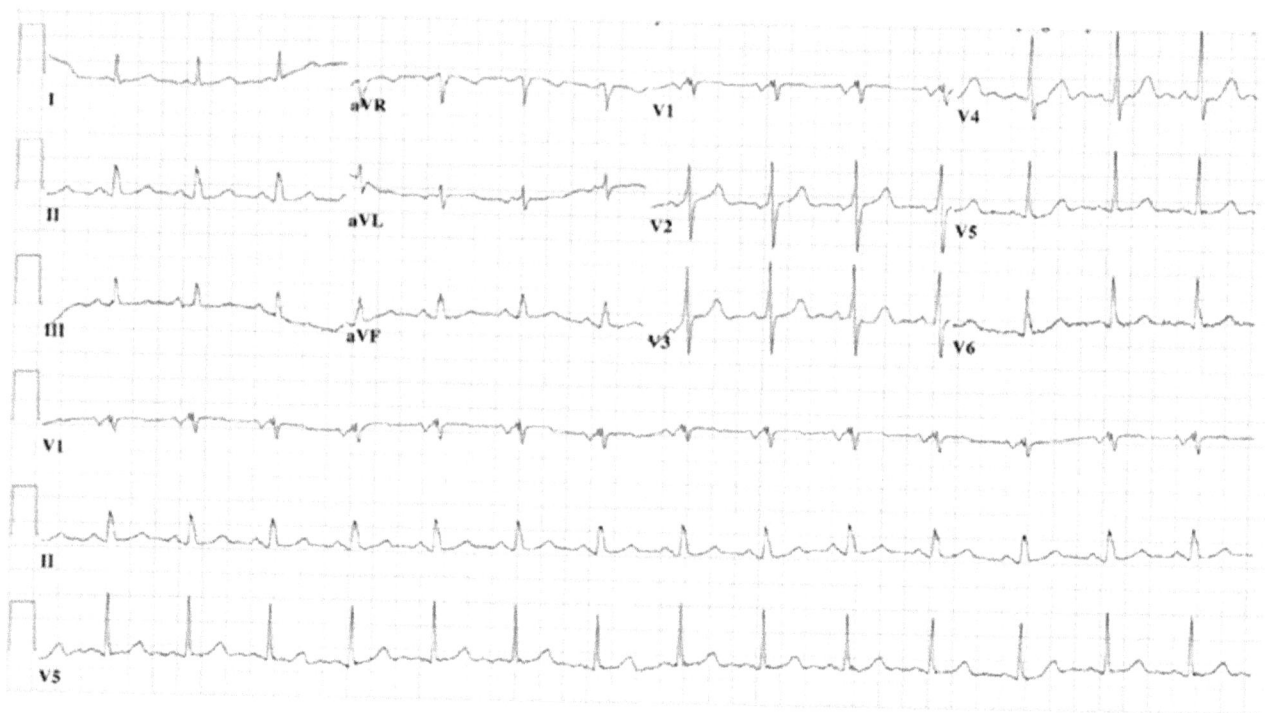

Figure 21.1

H. Secondary survey
    a. General: alert, oriented × 3, moderate distress secondary to pain
    b. Head: normocephalic, atraumatic
    c. Eyes: mildly pale conjunctiva, extraocular movement intact, pupils equal, reactive to light
    d. Ears: normal tympanic membranes
    e. Nose: no discharge
    f. Neck: full range of motion, no jugular vein distension, no stridor
    g. Pharynx: normal dentition, no lesions, no swelling
    h. Chest: nontender
    i. Lungs: clear bilaterally
    j. Heart: rate and rhythm regular, no murmurs, rubs, or gallops
    k. Abdomen: distended, diffusely tender, bowel sounds absent, no masses, no hernias, nontender at McBurney's point, negative Murphy's sign, + rebound, + guarding, no rigidity
    l. Rectal: normal tone, brown stool, occult blood positive
    m. Urogenital: normal external genitalia

n. Extremities: full range of motion, no deformity, normal pulses
o. Back: nontender
p. Neuro: cranial nerves II to XII intact; normal sensation, strength; normal reflexes and gait
q. Skin: warm and dry
r. Lymph: no lymphadenopathy

I. Action

a. Meds
    i.   Ciprofloxacin or ceftriaxone plus metronidazole or piperacillin–tazobactam
b. Reassess
    i.   Patient still reports significant discomfort, worsening pain
c. Consult
    i.   Surgery
d. Imaging
    i.   Upright CXR (if supine CXR, inconclusive results)
    ii. Obstructive series
    iii. Analgesia (e.g., morphine)

J. Nurse

a. BP: 98/59, HR: 90, RR: 18, Sat: 98% on RA (after 1 L)
b. Patient still with significant pain

K. Results

Table 21.1 Results table

Test	Result	Test	Result
Complete blood count:		**Liver function panel:**	
WBC	$12.1 \times 10^3/\mu L$	AST	23 U/L
Hct	41.50%	ALT	26 U/L
Plt	$253 \times 10^3/\mu L$	Alk phos	42 U/L
		T bili	1.0 mg/dL
		D bili	0.3 mg/dL
Basic metabolic panel:		Amylase	50 U/L
Na	138 mEq/L	Lipase	25 U/L
K	4.3 mEq/L	Albumin	4.7 g/dL
Cl	105 mEq/L		
CO_2	30 mEq/L	**Urinalysis:**	
BUN	52 mEq/dL	SG	1.020
Cr	1.2 mg/dL	pH	7
Gluc	110 mg/dL	Prot	Neg
		Gluc	Neg
		Ketones	Neg

Table 21.1 (cont.)

Test	Result	Test	Result
Coagulation panel:		Bili	Neg
PT	12.6 sec	Blood	Neg
PTT	26.0 sec	LE	Neg
INR	1.0	Nitrite	Neg
		Color	Yellow

a. Lactate: 2.2 mmol/L
b. Upright CXR (Figure 21.2)
c. Obstructive series (Figures 21.3 and 21.4)

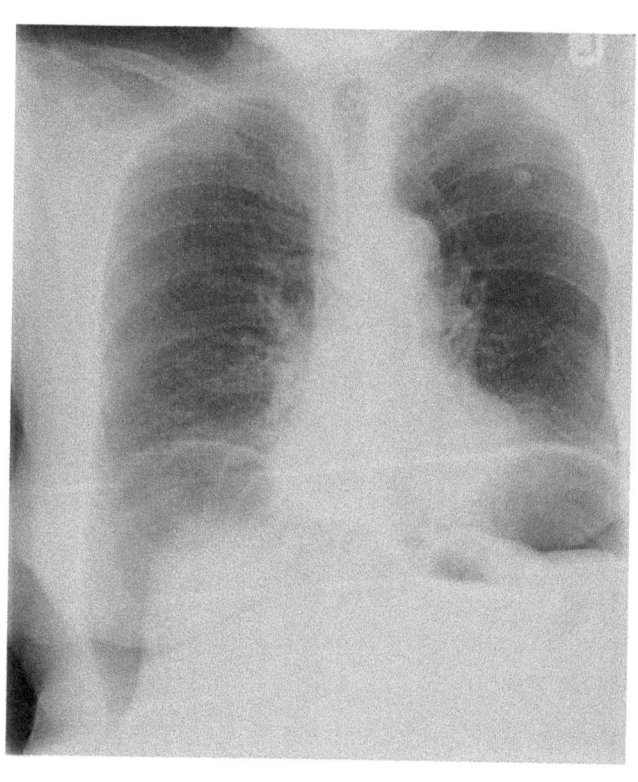

Figure 21.2

L. Action
a. Surgery consult
  i.   To OR for laparotomy
b. Discussion with family and PMD on need for emergent OR and suspicion for perforated viscus
c. Meds
  i.   Morphine

M. Diagnosis
a. Visceral perforation

N. Critical actions
a. Large-bore IV access and fluid bolus
b. Upright CXR

Figure 21.3

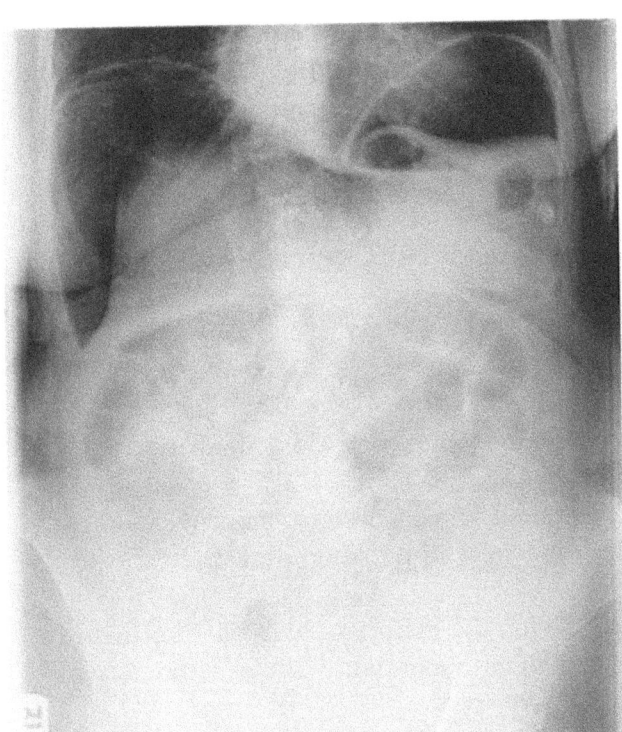

Figure 21.4

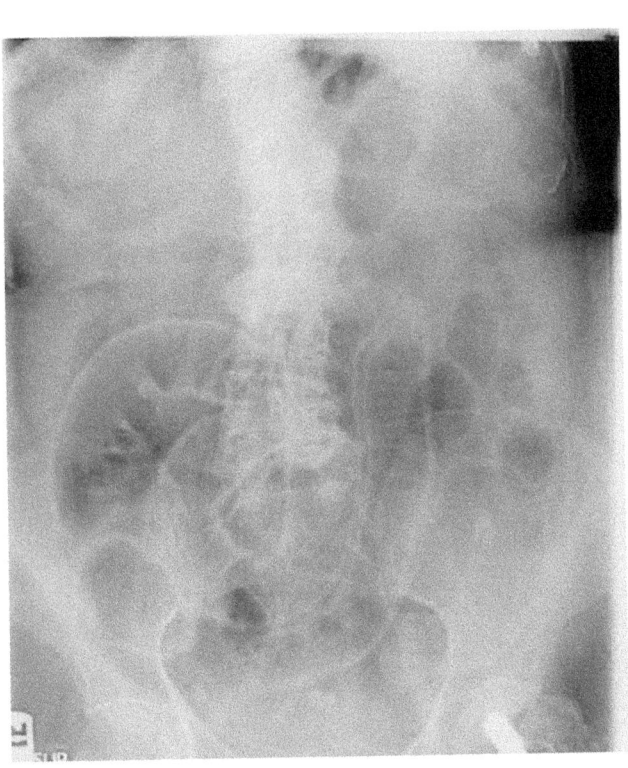

c. Pain management
d. Surgery consult
e. Antibiotics in setting of perforation

O. Examiner instructions

a. This is a case of a perforated viscus, likely from a small bowel obstruction. In this patient, an obstruction within the intestinal system caused a backup of pressure leading to rupturing of the stomach or intestinal wall. The patient's symptoms of abdominal pain began fairly abruptly and her symptoms are significantly worsened with movement of any kind due to peritoneal irritation. Important early actions include administering IV fluids, consulting surgery, starting antibiotics, and advocating for the patient to go to the OR. If fluids are not administered, the patient's blood pressure will begin to drop. Her pain will continue to increase until an opioid medication (e.g., morphine) is administered. An obstructive series with upright CXR can be readily obtained; if a CT scan is ordered, note that the scanner is busy and it will "be a while" before the test can be performed.

P. Pearls
a. Upright CXR is more sensitive than KUB for free air.
b. Peritoneal signs are ominous, and often suggest a surgical emergency. Consider early antibiotics, fluids, and surgical consultation.
c. Elderly patients with epigastric pain should be evaluated for coronary ischemia. Non–chest pain presentations are common in this age group, especially upper abdominal pain and/or shortness of breath.
d. Note that the patient has a "relative" hypotension. Given the history of high blood pressure, a systolic blood pressure in the 90s is more ominous than in a patient with baseline normal blood pressure.

Q. Figure legends
a. Figure 21.1 (EKG) Normal sinus rhythm.
b. Figure 21.2 (Upright CXR) Free air beneath diaphragm bilaterally, dilated bowel loops.
c. Figures 21.3 and 21.4 (Obstructive series) Dilated bowel loops

R. References
a. *Tintinalli's Emergency Medicine: A Comprehensive Study Guide* (9th ed.): Chapter 83, Bowel Obstruction.
b. *Rosen's Emergency Medicine: Concepts and Clinical Practice* (10th ed.): Chapter 78, Small Intestine.

Cough

Elysha Pifko, MD

A. Chief complaint
a. 5 month-old-female who presents with a cough

B. Vital signs
a. BP: 80/50, HR: 170, RR: 30, T: 37.8°C, Sat: 99% on RA, Wt: 7 kg

C. What does the patient look like?
a. Patient appears stated age. Fussy but consolable by family.

D. Primary survey
a. Airway: patient crying
b. Breathing: no increased work of breathing or cyanosis
c. Circulation: normal pulses and capillary refill

E. History
a. HPI: 5-month-old female who presents with a 3-week history of a cough. Parents report that the patient initially had a runny nose and red eyes as well. Her runny nose improved but she continues to have a persistent cough that wakes her at night. Family described multiple "coughing fits" throughout the day with post-tussive emesis. She initially had low-grade fevers, which have now improved.
b. PMHx: born full-term without complications
c. PSHx: none
d. Allergies: none
e. Meds: none
f. Social history: lives at home with parents and two older siblings, attends daycare
g. FHx: noncontributory
h. PMD: Dr. Russell

F. Secondary survey
a. General: no acute distress, smiling, multiple coughing episodes throughout exam
b. HEENT: bilateral eye injection with left subconjunctival hemorrhage
c. Neck: supple, full range of motion; no lymphadenopathy
d. Chest: diffuse rhonchi but no wheezing, crackles, or stridor; no tachypnea or retractions
e. Heart: regular rate and rhythm without murmurs
f. Abdomen: soft, nondistended, nontender; no hepatosplenomegaly

g. Urogenital: normal
h. Extremities: full range of motion of all extremities
i. Back: normal
j. Neuro: normal
k. Skin: petechial rash over bilateral cheeks and chest
l. Lymph: normal

G. Action

a. Monitor
b. Labs
    i. CBC
c. Imaging
    i. CXR
d. NS bolus

H. Nurse

a. Repeat vital signs if NS bolus given
    i. BP: 82/50, HR: 130, RR: 32, T :37.8°C, Sat: 98%
b. Repeat vital signs unchanged if NS bolus not given

I. Results

Table 22.1 Complete blood count results table

Test	Result
WBC	$30 \times 10^3/\mu L$
Hct	39.40%
Plt	$300 \times 10^3/\mu L$

a. CXR (Figure 22.1)

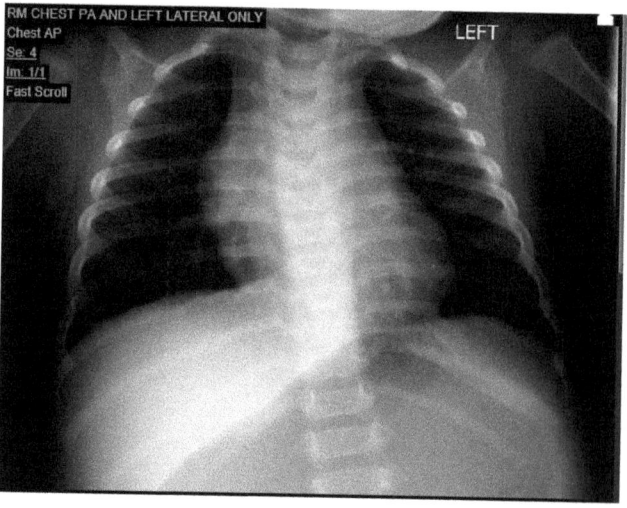

Figure 22.1

J. Action

a. Reassess
  i. Patient had a 20 second episode of apnea with associated cyanosis after a coughing episode that resolved without intervention
b. NC O_2 started
c. Admission to pediatric ward
  i. Respiratory precautions
d. Antibiotics for patient and close contacts
  i. Azithromycin PO
e. Further diagnostic testing
  i. Culture
  ii. PCR

K. Diagnosis

a. Pertussis

L. Critical actions

a. Insert peripheral IV
b. NC O_2
c. CXR
d. Antibiotics for patient and prophylaxis for close contacts
e. Admission with respiratory precautions

M. Examiner instructions

a. This is a case of pertussis in an infant. Pertussis is caused by the gram-negative bacteria *Bordetella pertussis*. Patients with this condition typically present with cough paroxysms followed by a characteristic "whoop" and vomiting. Diagnosis is based on clinical criteria as well as confirmatory labs such as a culture isolate of *B. pertussis* obtained from a throat swab or aspirate or a positive PCR. Treatment is typically a 5-day course of azithromycin and is most effective early in the course of the disease.

N. Pearls

a. The course of pertussis has three phases:
  i. The catarrhal phase
    1. Low-grade fevers
    2. Cough
    3. Coryza
  ii. The paroxysmal phase
    1. Characteristic cough paroxysms
    2. Can last up to 10 weeks
  iii. The convalescent phase
    1. Gradual recovery from symptoms
b. Children less than 6 months old can have an atypical course and often lack a "whoop" with their cough paroxysm. These young children can present with apnea, bradycardia, gagging, and gasping.
c. Complications in children less than 1 year of age include pneumonia, pulmonary hypertension, apnea, encephalopathy, and death.

d. Complications in teens and adults include weight loss, incontinence, rib fractures, and syncope.
e. Patients often have significant lymphocytosis. Infants with a leukocytosis $>30 \times 10^3/\mu L$ are at higher risk for mortality.
f. Treatment is only effective at shortening the course of disease if given during the initial catarrhal phase, but can still limit the spread of bacteria to other people if given during a later phase.

O. Figure legends
a. Figure 22.1 (CXR) Normal chest x-ray.

P. References
a. *Tintinalli's Emergency Medicine: A Comprehensive Study Guide* (9th ed.): Chapter 64, Acute Bronchitis and Upper Respiratory Tract Infections.
b. *Rosen's Emergency Medicine: Concepts and Clinical Practice* (10th ed.): Chapter 164, Pediatric Lung Disease.

Flank Pain

Dhara Amin, MD

A. Chief complaint
a. 77-year-old male with flank pain

B. Vital signs
a. BP: 100/63, HR: 94, RR: 18, T: 36.9°C, Sat: 99% on RA

C. What does the patient look like?
a. Patient appears stated age, uncomfortable due to pain, in mild distress; lying supine in stretcher.

D. Primary survey
a. Airway: speaking in full sentences
b. Breathing: no apparent respiratory distress, no cyanosis
c. Circulation: pale and cool skin, normal capillary refill

E. Action
a. Peripheral IV line
b. Labs
   i. CBC, BMP, LFT, INR/PT/PTT, blood type and crossmatch, lactate, urinalysis
c. 1 L crystalloid bolus
d. Analgesia for abdominal pain
e. Monitor: BP: 95/64, HR: 93, RR: 18, Sat: 100% on O_2
f. EKG

F. History
a. HPI: A 77-year-old male with a history of hypertension, diabetes, and hypercholesterolemia states that a few hours after he woke up today, he developed left-sided flank pain radiating to the groin. The pain is described as sharp, ripping, and constant. Over the past few hours, the pain has intensified. The patient also states he might have seen some blood in his urine. He denies any syncope, nausea, vomiting, diarrhea, melena, fever, headache, chest pain, shortness of breath, or dysuria.
b. PMHx: hypertension, hypercholesterolemia, diabetes
c. PSHx: none
d. Allergies: none
e. Meds: simvastatin, metoprolol
f. Social: lives with wife at home, smokes one pack a day for 50 years, social drinker, denies drug use, not sexually active

g. FHx: not relevant

h. PMD: switched doctors, has not seen one in over a year

G. Nurse

a. EKG (Figure 23.1)

b. If fluids given:
   i. vitals: BP: 98/62, HR: 91, RR: 18, Sat: 98% on O_2

c. If no fluids given:
   i. vitals: BP: 73/42, HR: 115, RR: 20, Sat 98% on O_2

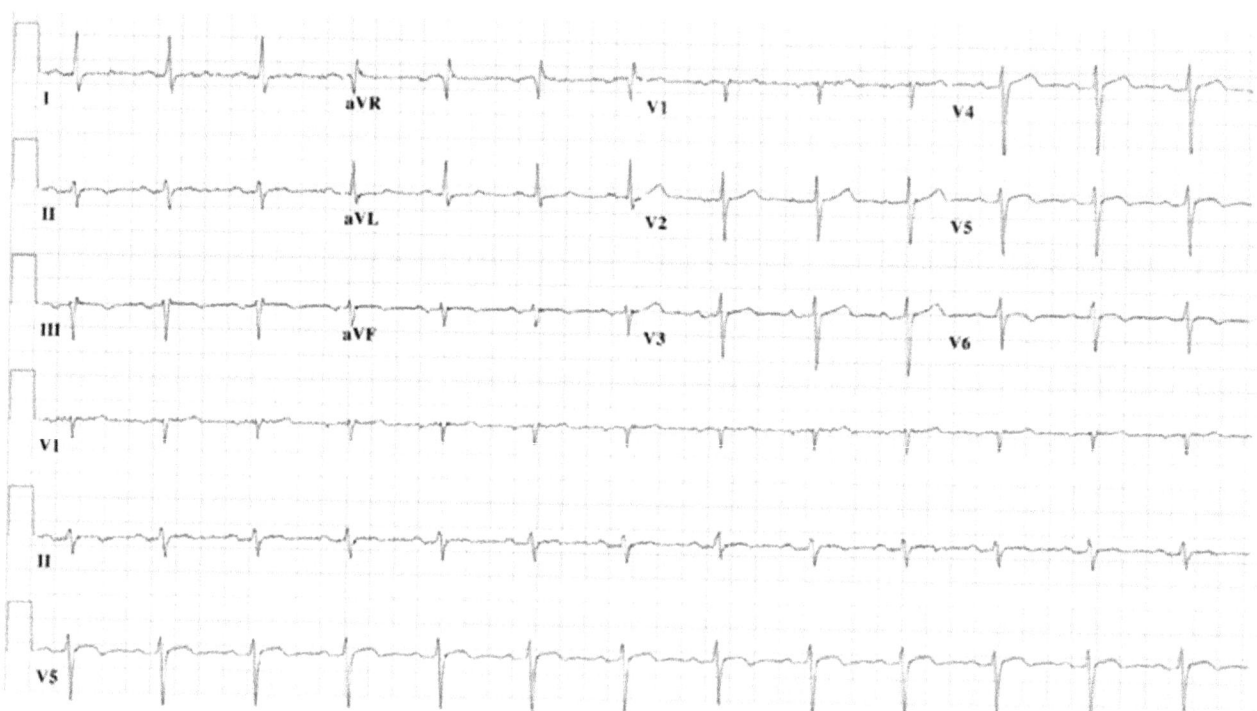

Figure 23.1

H. Secondary survey

a. General: alert, oriented, moderate distress due to pain

b. HEENT: mildly pale conjunctivae, otherwise normal

c. Neck: normal

d. Chest: normal

e. Heart: normal

f. Abdomen: obese, tender, bowel sounds present, no hernias, no rebound, no guarding, no rigidity, pulsatile mass palpated (must ask for this)

g. Rectal: hemoccult negative brown stool, normal rectal tone

h. Urogenital: normal

i. Extremities: normal

j. Back: left costovertebral angle tenderness

k. Neuro: normal

l. Skin: pale, faint bilateral flank ecchymoses

m. Lymph: normal

I. Action

a. Meds:
   i. morphine IV
b. Reassess
   i. Patient still with significant discomfort, worsening pain
c. Imaging
   i. Bedside ultrasound (Figure 23.2)
d. Consult
   i. Surgery

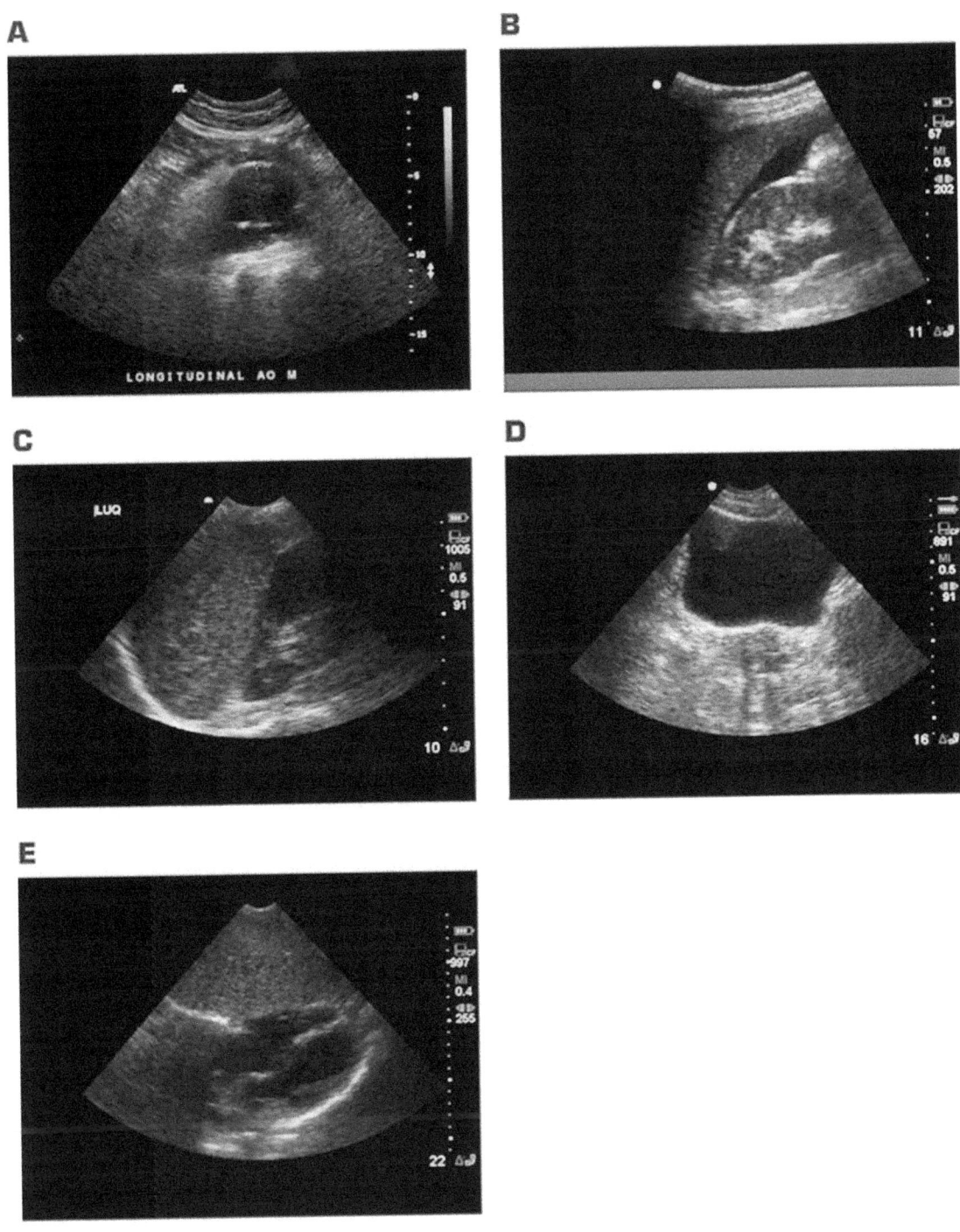

Figure 23.2

J. Nurse

a. If IV fluids or blood given, repeat vitals: BP: 98/59, HR: 90, RR: 18, Sat: 98% on O_2
b. If no IV fluids or blood given, repeat vitals: BP: 89/50, HR: 100, RR: 18, Sat: 98% on O_2
c. Patient: still with significant pain

K. Results

Table 23.1 Results table

Test	Result	Test	Result
Complete blood count:		T bili	0.7 mg/dL
WBC	$9.1 \times 10^3/\mu L$	D bili	0.1 mg/dL
Hct	22.90%	Amylase	240 U/L
Plt	$213 \times 10^3/\mu L$	Lipase	220 U/L
		Albumin	4.1 g/dL
Basic metabolic panel:			
Na	139 mEq/L	**Urinalysis:**	
K	4.1 mEq/L	SG	1.020
Cl	101 mEq/L	pH	6
CO_2	19 mEq/L	Prot	Neg
BUN	40 mEq/dL	Gluc	Neg
Cr	1.4 mg/dL	Ketones	Neg
Gluc	202 mg/dL	Bili	Neg
		Blood	+
Coagulation panel:		LE	Neg
PT	13.1 sec	Nitrite	Neg
PTT	26 sec	Color	Yellow
INR	1.0		
		Arterial blood gas:	
Liver function panel:		pH	7.33
AST	23 U/L	pO_2	92 mmHg
ALT	19 U/L	pCO_2	25 mmHg
Alk phos	87 U/L	HCO_3	19 mmol/L

a. Lactate: 2.9 mmol/L
b. CXR (Figure 23.3)

L. Action

a. Surgery consult
    i.   To OR for emergent surgical repair

Figure 23.3

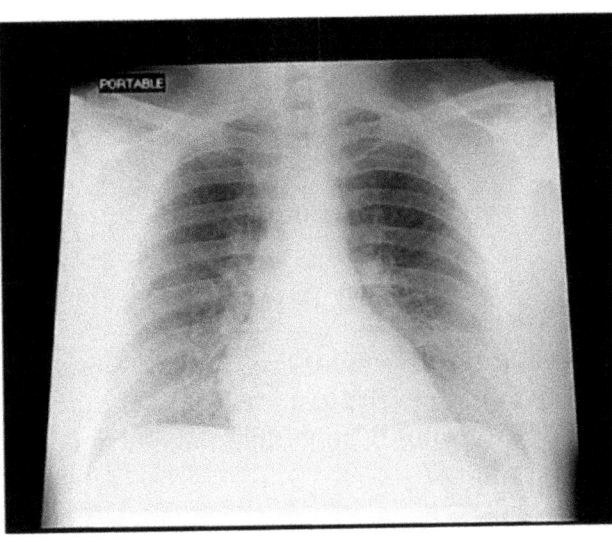

b. Discussion with patient and family regarding the diagnosis of aortic aneurysm and need for emergent surgical repair

c. Meds
   i. Initiate massive transfusion protocol or two units of uncrossmatched blood.
   ii. Call blood blank to make sure additional blood products will be available for the ED and/or OR.

M. Diagnosis
a. Abdominal aortic aneurysm (AAA)

N. Critical actions
a. Large-bore IV access
b. Fluid bolus
c. Bedside ultrasound
d. Surgery consult
e. Blood transfusion

O. Examiner instructions
a. This is a case of a leaking abdominal aortic aneurysm (AAA). Weakness in the wall of the aorta causes dilation of the vessel, which causes increased pressure at the wall, increasing the rate of stretch until a leak occurs. This condition tends to progress slowly (over years) and the risk of rupture increases with the diameter of the vessel. This patient has several risk factors for AAA, such as male gender and a significant smoking history. Important early actions include administering IV blood if hypotensive, obtaining a bedside US, consulting surgery, and advocating for the patient to go to the OR. If fluids are not administered, the patient's blood pressure will begin to drop. If the patient is still hypotensive then two units of uncrossed blood should be administered while multiple units of crossmatched blood are readied. A bedside US can readily be obtained; if a CT scan is ordered, note that the scanner is busy and it will "be a while" before the test can be performed.

P. Pearls
a. Bedside ultrasound that is technically adequate has close to 100% sensitivity for demonstrating an AAA.

b. Once a ruptured AAA is suspected, all efforts should be concentrated on stabilizing the patient and transferring the patient to the OR.

c. Elderly patients with back or flank pain should be evaluated for AAA. Hematuria is also common in patients with ruptured AAA, which can lead to the incorrect diagnosis of nephrolithiasis.

d. Flank ecchymosis (Grey–Turner's sign) is a sign of retroperitoneal hematoma.

Q. Figure legends

a. Figure 23.1 (EKG) Normal sinus rhythm; biphasic T waves V5–6.

b. Figure 23.2A (a) (Ultrasound) Enlarged aortic diameter. (b) (Ultrasound) Free fluid in Morison's pouch (right upper quadrant). (c) (Ultrasound) No free fluid in perisplenic space (left upper quadrant). (d) (Ultrasound) No free fluid in pelvis. (e) (Ultrasound) No pericardial effusion.

c. Figure 23.3 (CXR) Normal chest x-ray.

R. References

a. *Tintinalli's Emergency Medicine: A Comprehensive Study Guide* (9th ed.): Chapter 60, Aneurysmal Disease.

b. *Rosen's Emergency Medicine: Concepts and Clinical Practice* (10th ed.): Chapter 72, Abdominal Aortic Aneurysm.

S. Acknowledgements

a. We would like to acknowledge Raghu Seethala for their contribution to this chapter in the previous edition of this book, which has been updated by Dhara Amin.

Weakness

Ryan Marino, MD, and Lauren Porter, DO

A. Chief complaint
a. 57-year-old male with weakness

B. Vital signs
a. BP: 157/89, HR: 108, RR: 16, T: 36.5°C, Sat: 98% on RA

C. What does the patient look like?
a. Patient appears stated age, somnolent but responds to verbal stimuli, lying supine on the stretcher.

D. Primary survey
a. Airway: speaking in full sentences
b. Breathing: no signs of respiratory distress; no cyanosis; bilateral breath sounds
c. Circulation: warm skin, normal capillary refill, normal pulses in all extremities
d. Neuro: awake, groggy, responding to verbal stimuli, confused

E. Action
a. Two large-bore peripheral IV lines
b. Oxygen via nasal cannula as needed to maintain >95% saturation
c. Labs
   i. Fingerstick glucose (105 mg/dL, must ask for value)
   ii. CBC, BMP, LFT, INR/PT/PTT, lactate
d. Cardiac monitor
e. EKG

F. History
a. HPI: A 57-year-old male is brought to the ED by EMS after reportedly being found by his son, weak and lethargic at home. The son told EMS he last saw the patient well when he had been working on his vintage car earlier in the day. The patient states that while working on his car, he developed fatigue and weakness. He attempted to nap and has been sleeping all day. The patient's son reportedly found the patient lying on the couch with generalized weakness and the inability to ambulate. The son felt he was not acting appropriately. EMS was called and placed the patient on a cardiac monitor and oxygen, and brought the patient to the ED. The patient is currently complaining of a headache and generalized weakness. He denies any chest pain, shortness of breath, syncope, seizures, nausea, vomiting, numbness, or tingling.
b. PMHx: essential HTN
c. PSHx: laparoscopic cholecystectomy

   d. Allergies: none
   e. Meds: lisinopril
   f. Social: lives at home alone, social alcohol use, denies tobacco or drug use
   g. FHx: mother with HTN
   h. PMD: Dr. Miller

G. Nurse
   a. EKG (Figure 24.1)

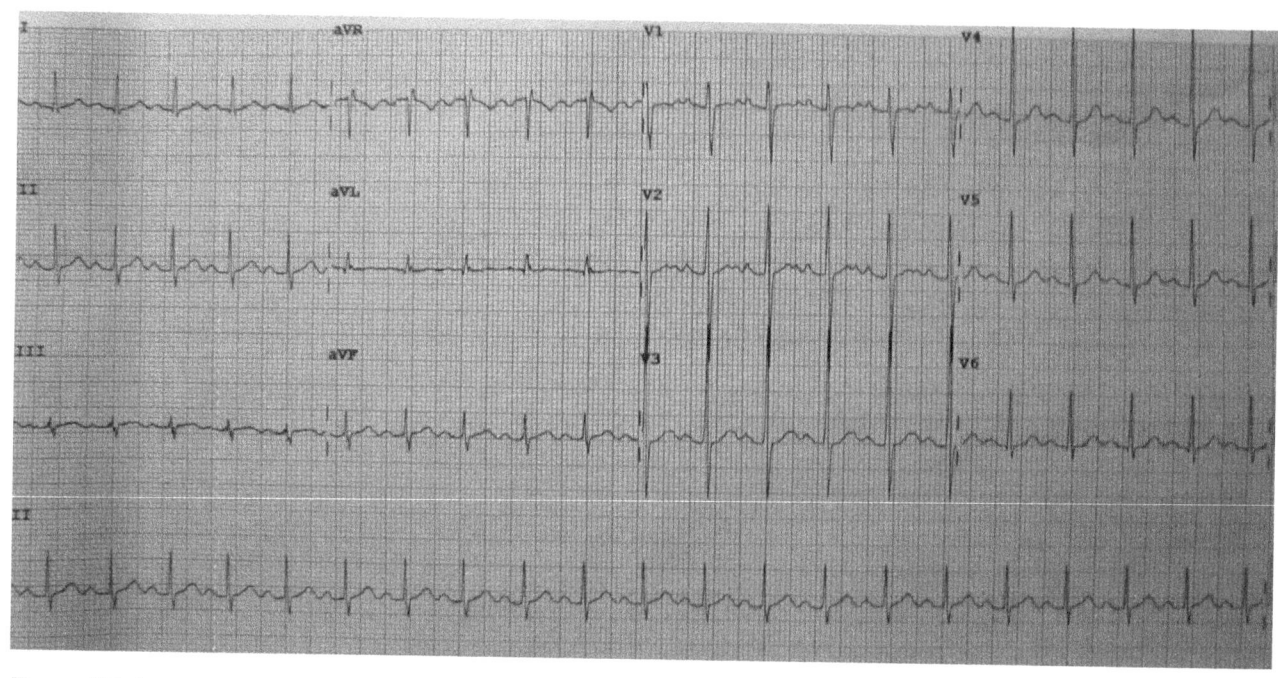

Figure 24.1

H. Secondary survey
   a. General: groggy but responds to verbal stimuli, oriented to self and location
   b. HEENT: pupils 3 mm and reactive bilaterally
   c. Neck: supple, no jugular vein distension, no nuchal rigidity
   d. Chest/pulmonary: no chest wall tenderness to palpation; symmetrical expansion; lungs are clear to auscultation bilaterally
   e. Heart: regular rate and rhythm, normal S1/S2; no murmurs, rubs, or gallops; no lower extremity edema or calf swelling
   f. Abdomen: soft, nontender, nondistended. No guarding, rebound, or rigidity
   g. Urogenital: normal
   h. Extremities: no edema, rashes, or deformities
   i. Back: no midlines spinal tenderness to palpation
   j. Neuro: groggy but responds to verbal stimuli, oriented to self and place; follows all commands; moves all extremities equally with generalized weakness; normal sensory exam, normal reflexes; gait was unsteady
   k. Skin: no rashes or edema
   l. Lymph: normal
   m. Psych: poor concentration, groggy, forgetful

Case 24: Weakness

I. Further history

a. Son later arrives at the bedside and is self-reporting a headache and states that the family cat is very sick and unresponsive. Son reports that the car's engine was running in a closed garage in the lower level of the house.

J. Action

a. Additional labs: obtain carboxyhemoglobin (COHb) and arterial blood gas
b. Reassess
   i. Patient feeling improved with oxygen
   ii. If not placed on NRB, the patient will not have improvement.
c. Imaging
   i. CT head (Figure 24.2)
   ii. CXR (Figure 24.3)

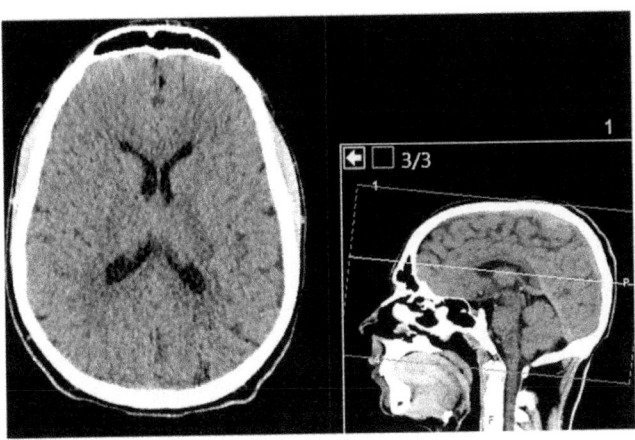

Figure 24.2

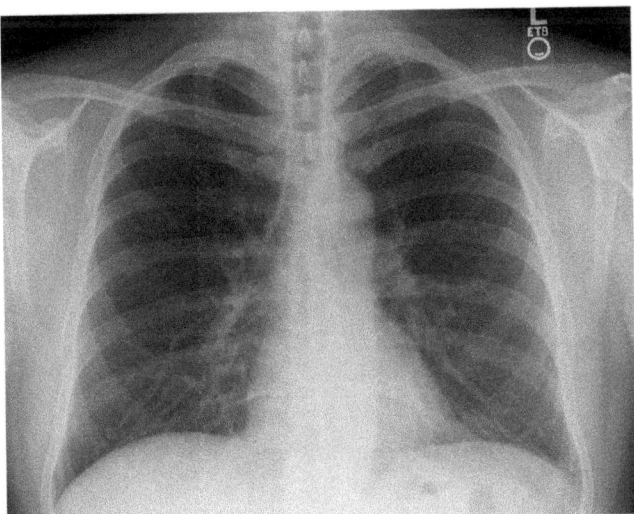

Figure 24.3

K. Results

Table 24.1 Results table

Test	Result	Test	Result
Complete blood count:		D bili	0.3 mg/dL
WBC	$10.1 \times 10^3/\mu L$	Amylase	200 U/L
Hct	39.50%	Lipase	47 U/L
Plt	$253 \times 10^3/\mu L$	Albumin	4.1 g/dL
Basic metabolic panel:		**Urinalysis:**	
Na	135 mEq/L	SG	1.019
K	3.5 mEq/L	pH	7
Cl	101 mEq/L	Prot	Neg
CO_2	21 mEq/L	Gluc	Neg
BUN	19 mEq/dL	Ketones	Neg
Cr	1.1 mg/dL	bili	Neg
Gluc	202 mg/dL	Blood	Neg
		LE	Neg
Coagulation panel:		Nitrite	Neg
PT	15.1 sec	Color	Yellow
PTT	30 sec		
INR	1.0	**Arterial blood gas:**	
		pH	7.31
Liver function panel:		PO_2	399 mmHg
AST	30 U/L	PCO_2	40 mmHg
ALT	25 U/L	HCO_2	20 mmol/L
Alk phos	88 U/L	O_2 Sat	72%
T bili	0.9 mg/dL		

a. Lactate: 2.6 mmol/L
b. COHb: 24%

L. Action
a. Notify the local poison center to assist in notifying the local health and fire departments.
b. Call the local hyperbaric center to discuss possible transfer for hyperbaric oxygen therapy.
c. Discuss diagnosis with the patient and family and need for possible transfer.

M. Diagnosis
a. Carbon monoxide poisoning

N. Critical actions

a. Apply 100% nonrebreather mask.

b. Obtain fingerstick blood glucose.

c. Obtain history consistent with carbon monoxide poisoning.

d. Obtain carboxyhemoglobin (COHb) level.

e. Discuss case with hyperbaric treatment facility for possible transfer.

O. Examiner instructions

a. This is a case of carbon monoxide (CO) poisoning. Carbon monoxide is a gas that is colorless and odorless. It is formed through incomplete combustion and methylene chloride exposure. Carbon monoxide is classified as a chemical asphyxiant and is the most common cause of fire-related death. Structural fires, generators, and space heaters being used indoors are all potential sources of exposure. The pathophysiology of the disease comes from the interaction with deoxyhemoglobin to form carboxyhemoglobin (COHb). Carbon monoxide will bind to hemoglobin more tightly than oxygen will, leading to a reduction in oxygen-carrying capacity. The history of leaving a car running, along with the patient's son and cat also having symptoms, is helpful in identifying the cause of the patient's altered mental status. Pets can also be affected, generally earlier on and more severely than humans. Early actions, including placing the patient on oxygen, obtaining the COHb level, and discussing the case for possible transfer, are all critical. Additional testing including CXR, CT of head, and additional labs including an EKG should be done to evaluate for signs of end-organ dysfunction related to CO toxicity and to evaluate other causes of altered mental status.

P. Pearls

a. Early fingerstick glucose and EKG are critical in any patient presenting with altered mental status.

b. Pulse oximetry cannot be used to determine arterial oxygenation due to the device's inability to differentiate carboxyhemoglobin from oxyhemoglobin.

c. Noninvasive carboxyhemoglobin (COHb) measurement (co-oximetry) cannot be used to accurately diagnose CO toxicity, and blood level should be obtained.

d. COHb levels do not correlate with symptoms or prognosis.

e. Symptoms of CO poisoning can be subtle and easily missed, and may mimic other conditions. When multiple family members or patients present with similar symptoms, an environmental exposure should be considered.

f. Symptoms of CO poisoning can include, but are not limited to: cardiac dysrhythmias, chest pain, myocardial ischemia, nausea, syncope, tachypnea, confusion, dizziness, dyspnea, headache, blurry vision, vomiting, and generalized weakness.

g. Hyperbaric treatment is recommended in certain cases to help prevent the development of delayed neurologic sequelae.

h. Indications for hyperbaric treatment include abnormal neurologic examination including altered mental status, coma, syncope, or seizures. Other indications are COHb level >25%, age ≥36, prolonged exposure (≥24 hours), or fetal distress in pregnancy.

   i. While patients with significant exposure should be discussed with your local hyperbaric treatment center, American College of Emergency Physicians' (ACEP) policy states that risks versus benefits should be discussed and not every exposure necessitates hyperbaric therapy. It remains unclear whether hyperbaric therapy is superior to normobaric oxygen therapy for improving long-term neurocognitive outcomes.

Q. Figure legends

a. Figure 24.1 (EKG) Sinus tachycardia.
b. Figure 24.2 (Head CT) Normal head CT.
c. Figure 24.3 (CXR) Normal chest x-ray.

R. References

a. *Rosen's Emergency Medicine: Concepts and Clinical Practice* (10th ed.): Chapter 148, Inhaled Toxins.
b. *Tintinalli's Emergency Medicine: A Comprehensive Study Guide* (9th ed.): Chapter 222, Carbon Monoxide.

Facial Trauma

Ryan McKenna, DO

A. Chief complaint
a. 55-year-old intoxicated male who presents via EMS with facial swelling and bleeding after trauma.

B. Vital signs
a. BP: 118/59, HR: 111, RR: 22, T: 36.7°C, Sat: 98% on RA

C. What does the patient look like?
a. Patient appears stated age, in mild distress, with significant facial swelling, ecchymosis, multiple missing teeth, and bleeding from the mouth. C-collar is in place.

D. Primary survey
a. Airway: patient has garbled, unintelligible speech
b. Breathing: tachypneic, frequently coughing, no cyanosis
c. Circulation: symmetric pulses throughout, capillary refill <2 seconds; active, brisk bleeding from the mouth

E. Action
a. Suction oropharynx, reposition patient, open airway with jaw thrust, administer supplemental oxygen, grasp tongue and pull anteriorly
b. Reassess
   i. No change. Bleeding from oropharynx persists. The patient will begin to desaturate if supplemental oxygen is not administered.
c. Two large-bore peripheral IV lines
d. Intubate using facilitated or awake look technique (describe procedure)
   i. If the candidate attempts to intubate using rapid sequence technique, the patient will rapidly desaturate.
   ii. The candidate should request a cricothyrotomy kit to be brought to bedside as backup.
   iii. Post-intubation management (sedation and ventilator settings)
e. Attempt to localize the bleeding. Pack the oropharynx with Kerlix or gauze if unsuccessful.
f. Labs
   i. CBC, BMP, INR/PT/PTT, type and crossmatch two units of packed red blood cells, ethanol level
g. Fingerstick glucose: 104 mg/dL
h. 1 L bolus of lactated Ringer's or normal saline

    i.   Complete trauma primary survey: assess neurologic status, expose patient, look for other trauma

    j.   Activate trauma team

    k.   Repeat vitals after intubation: BP: 110/75, HR: 120, RR: per vent settings, Sat: 100% on vent

F. History

    a.   HPI: A 55-year-old intoxicated male presents via EMS in police custody with facial trauma and bleeding. He was reportedly being arrested for public intoxication and was found urinating on a wall when police arrested him. The patient became combative and assaulted a police officer. The patient's face struck the curb when police attempted to restrain him. There was no loss of consciousness reported by police. Upon EMS arrival, the patient was intoxicated and bleeding from the mouth, but was able to speak. During transport, the patient became progressively more agitated, and the bleeding from the oropharynx worsened.

    b.   PMHx: none

    c.   PSHx: none

    d.   Allergies: none

    e.   Social: undomiciled, drinks alcohol every day, one pack per day smoker, denies drug use

    f.   FHx: none

    g.   PMD: none

G. Nurse

    a.   If 1 L bolus of lactated Ringer's or normal saline administered, repeat vitals:

        i.   BP: 130/80, HR: 95, RR: per vent settings, Sat: 100% on vent

    b.   If no fluids administered, repeat vitals:

        ii.   BP: 105/60, HR: 120, RR: per vent settings, Sat: 100% on vent

H. Secondary survey

    a.   General: patient is intubated

    b.   HEENT: marked right-sided facial swelling with crepitus and ecchymosis. Zygomatic arch is depressed bilaterally. Midface is unstable. When the hard palate is gently rocked while stabilizing the forehead, the maxilla moves independently of the face. There are multiple missing teeth. Blood briskly fills the oropharynx posteriorly, but the source is unable to be visualized. Blood in the bilateral nares and ears limits exam. Eye exam is remarkable for the right eye with periorbital ecchymosis, and is swollen shut. Retractors will be needed to open the eye. There is right subconjunctival hemorrhage and the remainder of the exam is otherwise normal, including intraocular pressures.

    c.   Neck: in cervical collar, normal

    d.   Chest: normal

    e.   Heart: tachycardic, otherwise normal

    f.   Abdomen: normal

    g.   Rectal: normal tone, no gross blood; hemoccult negative

    h.   Urogenital: normal

    i.   Extremities: abrasions to bilateral knees, arms, no deformities, no ecchymosis

    j.   Back: normal

    k.   Neuro: sedated. Prior to intubation, no obvious focal deficits, including equal, round, and reactive pupils bilaterally

    l.   Skin: pale

    m. Lymph: normal

I. Action
a. Pack the oropharynx
b. Meds:
  i. Tetanus toxoid IM
c. Imaging:
  i. FAST examination: normal
  ii. Chest x-ray, pelvis x-ray
  iii. CT head, CT C-spine, CT facial bones without contrast

J. Nurse
a. If post-intubation sedation was not verbalized, the vent will begin to alarm and the patient will begin to gag and move arms.
b. Repeat vitals: BP: 100/65, HR 115, RR per vent settings, Sat: 100% on vent

K. Results

Table 25.1 Results table

Test	Result	Test	Result
Complete blood count:		**Urinalysis:**	
WBC	$5.3 \times 10^3/\mu L$	SG	1.015
Hct	41.50%	pH	7
Plt	$350 \times 10^3/\mu L$	Prot	Neg
		Gluc	Neg
		Ketones	Neg
Basic metabolic panel:		Bili	Neg
Na	130 mEq/L	Blood	Neg
K	3.5 mEq/L	LE	Neg
Cl	101 mEq/L	Nitrite	Neg
CO_2	18 mEq/L	Color	Yellow
BUN	18 mEq/dL		
Cr	0.8 mg/dL		
Gluc	110 mg/dL	**Arterial blood gas:**	
		pH	7.35
		pO_2	155 mmHg
Coagulation panel:		pCO_2	36 mmHg
PT	14.1 sec	HCO_3	22 mmol/L
PTT	22.0 sec		
INR	1.1		

a. Ethanol level: 410 mg/dL
b. Chest x-ray (Figure 25.1)
c. Pelvis x-ray (Figure 25.2)
d. CT head – normal

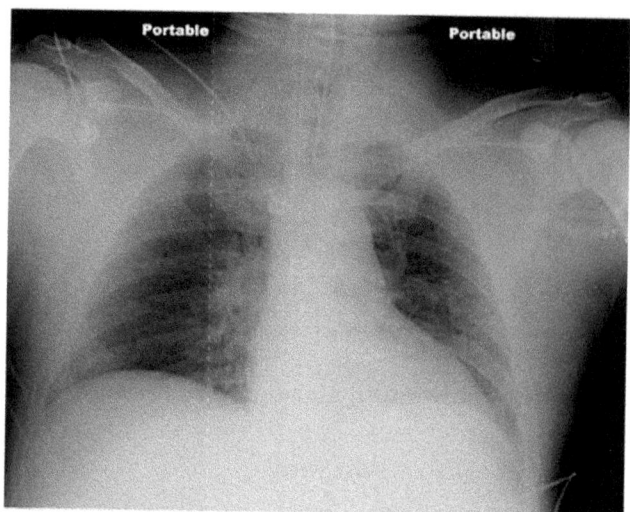

Figure 25.1

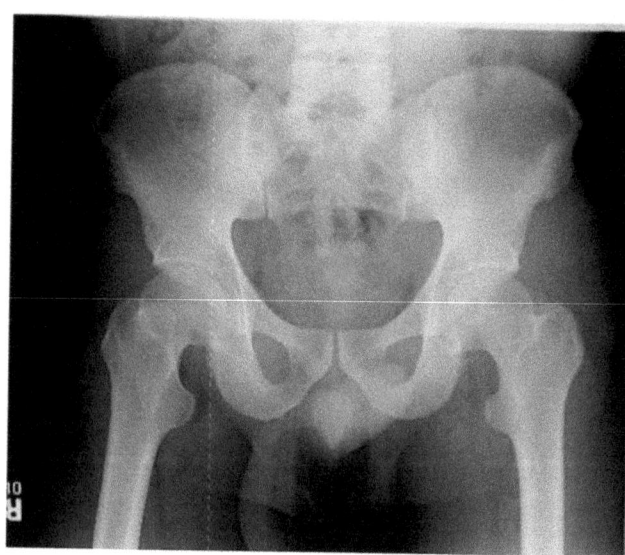

Figure 25.2

e. CT face – Le Fort III fracture, subcutaneous gas throughout face
f. CT C-spine – normal

L. Action
a. Consult oral/maxillofacial surgery or otolaryngology
    i. Operative intervention to control bleeding
b. Consult trauma
    i. Admit patient to ICU

M. Diagnosis
a. Maxillofacial trauma with Le Fort III fracture and facial hemorrhage

N. Critical actions
a. Early intubation using an awake or facilitated look with cricothyrotomy setup at bedside
b. Packing of the oropharynx to control bleeding
c. Maintain C-spine immobilization
d. CT head, C-spine, facial bones
e. ENT or oral/maxillofacial surgery consultation

O. Examiner instructions

a. This is a case of midface trauma with airway compromise. Early airway management using advanced techniques such as awake or facilitated look intubation with a double setup (preparation for cricothyrotomy) is critical. If the airway is anticipated to be difficult, or if the patient is anticipated to be difficult to ventilate using bag-valve mask, then neuromuscular blockade (rapid sequence intubation) should be avoided. Applying direct pressure or packing of the oropharynx to control hemorrhage may be necessary. Clamping vessels should be avoided due to the possibility of damaging adjacent structures.

P. Pearls

a. Maintain inline stabilization of the C-spine when attempting intubation.
b. When using video laryngoscopy, suction the oropharynx first and lead with the suction catheter to avoid soiling the camera with blood. A direct laryngoscope with a second endotracheal tube and standard, non-hyper-angulated stylet should be available as a backup.
c. Waveform capnography allows for immediately recognition of successful tracheal (versus esophageal) intubation.
d. Arterial embolization with interventional radiology may be necessary to control hemorrhage.
e. If teeth are missing, attention to aspirated foreign body should be given on post-intubation CXR.

Q. Figure legends

a. Figure 25.1 (CXR) Endotracheal tube and nasogastric tube in place; no focal infiltrate.
b. Figure 25.2 (Pelvis x-ray) Normal pelvis x-ray.

R. References

a. *Tintinalli's Emergency Medicine: A Comprehensive Study Guide* (9th ed.): Chapter 259, Trauma to the Face.
b. *Rosen's Emergency Medicine: Concepts and Clinical Practice* (10th ed.): Chapter 45, Facial Trauma.

Burn

Suzanne K. Bentley, MD, MPH

A. Chief complaint

a. 42-year-old male with burns

B. Vital signs

a. BP: 136/73, HR: 132, RR: 22, T: 37.2°C, Sat: 98% on RA

C. What does the patient look like?

a. Patient appears stated age. Burns and soot are present on patient's face and mouth. Burns and blistering are present on neck and chest. Patient cries out in pain when moved during exam and is in evident pain lying supine in stretcher.

D. Primary survey

a. Airway: speaking in full sentences; soot in nares and mouth; burns and blistering over face and mouth
b. Breathing: mild tachypnea, otherwise no apparent respiratory distress, no cyanosis
c. Circulation: normal pulses, normal capillary refill

E. Action

a. Oxygen via nonrebreather mask
b. Two large-bore peripheral IVs
c. Completely expose and examine patient to determine extent of burns
d. Obtain point of care co-oximetry if available
e. Labs
   i.   CBC, BMP, LFT, INR/PT/PTT, carboxyhemoglobin, lactate, ABG
f. 1 L NS bolus
g. Monitor: BP: 139/79, HR: 128, RR: 20, Sat: 100% on O_2
h. EKG
i. Meds
   i.   Morphine 6 mg IV (be sure to inquire about allergies before giving medications, even in emergent cases).
   ii. Consider starting treatment for carbon monoxide (CO) poisoning empirically.

F. History

a. HPI: A 42-year-old male with no significant past medical history reports he was roasting s'mores on a charcoal grill with open flame, conducted indoors at a friend's cabin because of snow and ice outside. Patient notes he remembers he developed a headache and states he lost his balance and fell face first into the fire. Friends were able to pull the patient out.

He currently complains of intense pain all over his face, neck, arms, and torso. He is unable to recall when his last tetanus shot was.

b. PMHx: none
c. PSHx: none
d. Allergies: none
e. Meds: none
f. Social: social use of alcohol, smoker, denies drug use
g. FHx: not relevant
h. PMD: none

G. Nurse

a. EKG (Figure 26.1)
b. If 1 L NS given, repeat vitals: BP: 130/79, HR: 90, RR: 24, Sat: 98% on O_2

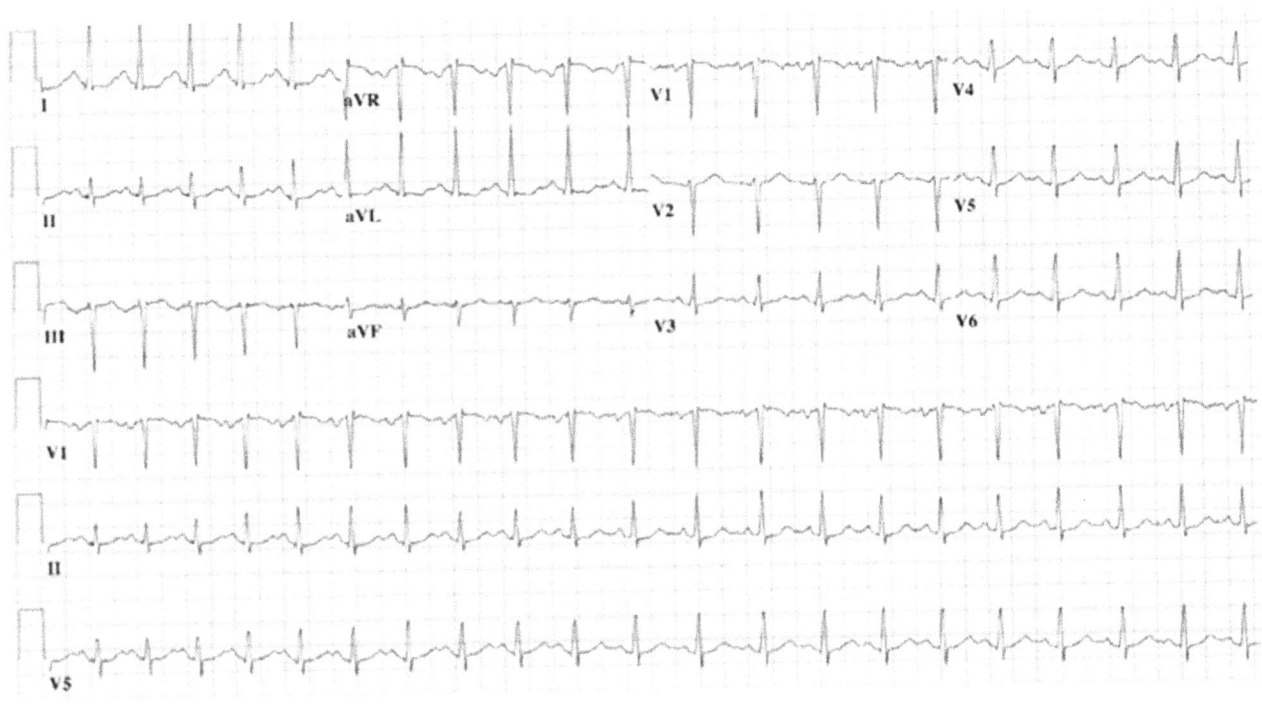

Figure 26.1

H. Secondary survey

a. General: arousable to name and touch. Oriented × 3 but is somewhat somnolent. Continually verbalizing significant pain.
b. HEENT: painful, blistered burns to face, lips; soot on face, in nares, and mouth
c. Neck: painful, blistered burn to anterior neck, significant soft tissue swelling of neck, no stridor
d. Chest: painful, blistered burn involving entire anterior chest; breath sounds clear bilaterally
e. Heart: tachycardic, no murmur
f. Abdomen: painful, blistered burn to anterior abdomen, no guarding, no rebound
g. Urogenital: normal
h. Extremities: circumferential burn to left forearm – skin thickened and white with superficial charring, with minimal sensation; decreased distal pulses
i. Back: normal
j. Neuro: normal

k. Skin: burns as described earlier
l. Lymph: normal

I. Action

a. Identify suspected carbon monoxide (CO) poisoning and treat, if not done earlier
    i. 100% oxygen via nonrebreather mask or 100% FiO_2 if patient intubated
    ii. May consider sodium thiosulfate or hydroxocobalamin for possible concomitant cyanide (CN) poisoning, awaiting lab results
b. Intubate
    i. Rapid sequence intubation
c. Fluid administration
    i. Use Parkland formula to calculate fluid requirements for the first 24 hours; one-half of total fluids should be administered within 8 hours of the burn and the other half over the next 16 hours.
d. Nursing
    i. Place Foley catheter
e. Perform escharotomy of left forearm
f. Imaging
    i. CXR
g. Meds
    i. Tetanus toxoid IM
h. Reassess
    i. Patient is intubated and requires ongoing sedation and analgesia.

J. Nurse

a. Repeat vitals: BP: 107/80, HR: 106, RR: 16, Sat: 98% on 100% FiO_2

K. Results

Table 26.1 Results table

Test	Result	Test	Result
Complete blood count:		D bili	0.6 mg/dL
WBC	$14.1 \times 10^3/\mu L$	Amylase	25 U/L
Hct	44.50%	Lipase	34 U/L
Plt	$295 \times 10^3/\mu L$	Albumin	4.0 g/dL
Basic metabolic panel:		Urinalysis:	
Na	138 mEq/L	SG	1.030
K	4.2 mEq/L	pH	6
Cl	101 mEq/L	Prot	Neg
CO_2	18 mEq/L	Gluc	Neg
BUN	38 mEq/dL	Ketones	Neg
Cr	1.6 mg/dL	Bili	Neg

Table 26.1 (cont.)

Test	Result	Test	Result
Gluc	102 mg/dL	Blood	Neg
		LE	Neg
		Nitrite	Neg
Coagulation panel:		Color	Yellow
PT	13.1 sec		
PTT	26.0 sec		
INR	1.0	**Arterial blood gas:**	
		pH	7
		pCO_2	25 mmHg
Liver function panel:		pO_2	120 mmHg
AST	32 U/L	HCO_3	18 mmol/L
ALT	20 U/L		
Alk phos	89 U/L		
T bili	1.5 mg/dL		

a. Lactate: 11 mmol/L
b. Carboxyhemoglobin: 40%
c. CXR (Figure 26.2)

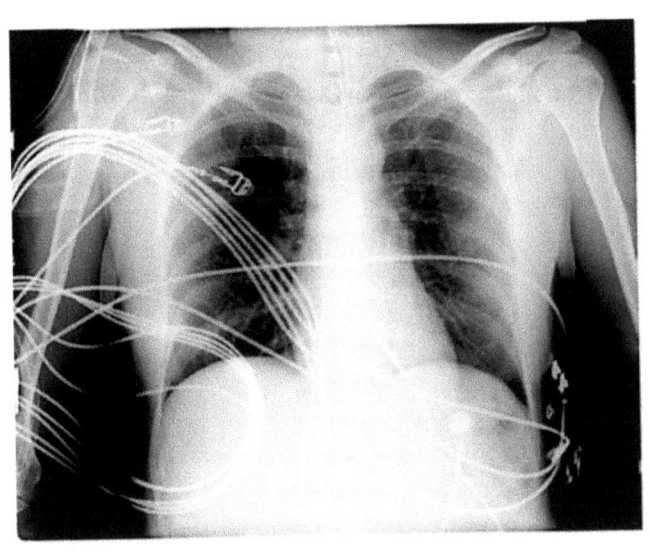

Figure 26.2

L. Action
a. Consult local toxicology service.
b. Identify elevated carboxyhemoglobin level and ensure oxygen delivery is maximized.
c. Identify lactic acidosis suggestive of cyanide toxicity and start sodium thiosulfate or hydroxocobalamin, per local protocols.
d. Contact burn unit and inform of need for hyperbaric treatment.
   i. Transfer patient to burn unit.
e. Discussion with family regarding the need for emergent transfer of the patient to the burn unit and for hyperbaric treatment.

f. Meds
  i. Morphine (or other opioid) boluses or infusion

M. Diagnosis
a. Thermal burn with carbon monoxide and cyanide toxicity

N. Critical actions
a. Large-bore IV access and fluid resuscitation (following Parkland formula)
b. Analgesia
c. Intubation
d. Carbon monoxide toxicity identification and management
e. Cyanide toxicity identification and management
f. Escharotomy for circumferential third-degree burn to extremity
g. Tetanus administration
h. Transfer to burn unit/ICU

O. Examiner instructions
a. Important early actions in this case include obtaining large-bore IV access, initiating fluid resuscitation, intubating the patient, recognizing carbon monoxide and cyanide poisoning, and transferring the patient to a burn center. Although the patient did not exhibit stridor or any respiratory distress upon arrival to the ED, it is critical to intubate burn patients presenting with significant swelling of the neck or lower face. If the patient is not intubated before ICU transfer, he will develop significant difficulty breathing due to throat swelling, and intubation will become very difficult. If this occurs, advanced airway techniques (such as fiberoptic intubation or cricothyrotomy) will be required for successful intubation. If anesthesia or ENT consultants are called to manage the airway early in the case, they will argue that the patient appears well, has a normal oxygen level, and does not require intubation. If consulted once the patient becomes symptomatic, they will be out of the hospital and unavailable for 20 minutes (necessitating the candidate to manage the airway themselves). If CO/CN poisoning is not recognized, the toxicology consult may prompt the examinee to order/interpret appropriate related laboratory tests and medications.

P. Pearls
a. Early intubation is warranted if impending airway compromise is suspected in burn patients. Stridor, hoarseness, hypoxia, and blood gas abnormalities are often late signs of airway compromise, and signify that airway edema has already become critical.
b. Appropriate fluid resuscitation (following the Parkland formula) requires administration of half the total fluid requirement within the first 8 hours of the injury, not presentation to the ED. For example, if the patient presents to the ED 2 hours after injury, half of the total fluid requirement needs to be administered within the next 6 hours.
c. Assess for carbon monoxide and cyanide poisoning in all burn patients and consider empiric treatment based on patient history (in this case: open fire of charcoal grill in enclosed space of a cabin, patient noting headache preceding fall into the fire, decreased responsiveness on exam).
d. Note that this patient had deep circumferential burns to the left forearm and required escharotomy. Loss of distal pulses is a late finding and patients with deep circumferential burns require escharotomy to prevent compartment syndrome.

Q. Figure legends
a. Figure 26.1 (EKG) Sinus tachycardia.
b. Figure 26.2 (XR) ET and NGT in place; no focal infiltrate.

R. References
a. *Tintinalli's Emergency Medicine: A Comprehensive Study Guide* (9th ed.): Chapter 217, Thermal Burns. Chapter 222, Carbon Monoxide.
b. *Rosen's Emergency Medicine: Concepts and Clinical Practice* (10th ed.): Chapter 54, Thermal Injuries. Chapter 148, Inhaled Toxins.

S. Acknowledgements
a. We would like to acknowledge Raghu Seethala for their contribution to this chapter in the previous edition of this book, which has been updated by Suzanne K. Bentley

Vomiting Blood

Gregory Podolej, MD

A. Chief complaint

a. 56-year-old female vomiting blood

B. Vital signs

a. BP: 90/60, HR: 128, RR: 20, T: 37.0°C, Sat: 96% on RA

C. What does the patient look like?

a. Patient appears pale and lethargic

D. Primary survey

a. Airway: patent, able to speak
b. Breathing: no apparent respiratory distress, no cyanosis
c. Circulation: pale and cool skin, prolonged capillary refill

E. Action

a. Two large-bore IV lines
b. Oxygen via nasal cannula or nonrebreather mask as needed to maintain >95% saturation
c. Monitor: BP: 90/60, HR: 128, RR: 20, T: 37.0°C, Sat: 99% on O_2
d. Labs
   i. CBC, BMP, LFT, lipase, INR/PT/PTT, type and cross-match (prepare ≥2 units), lactate, urinalysis
e. Transfuse two units of uncrossed blood
f. EKG
g. CXR
h. Glucose: 125 mg/dL

F. History

a. HPI: A 56-year-old female with a history of diabetes, hypertension, hepatitis C, and cirrhosis presents via EMS with three episodes of vomiting bright red blood just prior to arrival. She reports that she was nauseous during the day and started vomiting prior to arrival. She notes the blood was bright red. Her spouse noted there was "a lot" of blood and blood clots in the toilet, for which they called EMS. The patient had two further episodes of hematemesis enroute. She denies recent trauma, diarrhea, dark stools, or blood in the urine. No passing out. She denies fevers, chills, chest pain, cough, trouble breathing, leg swelling, or recent surgeries. She does endorse worsening abdominal swelling in the past few weeks.
b. PMHx: diabetes, hypertension, hepatitis C, cirrhosis with paracentesis 3 months ago
c. PSHx: none

d. Allergies: azithromycin (causes hives)
e. Meds: metformin, amlodipine, ribavirin
f. Social: lives with wife at home, smokes one pack a day for 50 years, social alcohol drinker, denies drug use. Not sexually active. Hepatitis C was contracted after a blood transfusion in the 1980s (if asked).
g. FHx: not relevant
h. PMD: Dr. Gala

G. Nurse
a. EKG (Figure 27.1)
b. Repeat vitals:
    i. If blood or 1 L NS given: BP: 98/62, HR: 118, RR: 22, Sat: 99% on O$_2$
    ii. If no blood or fluids given: BP: 73/42, HR: 135, RR: 26, Sat 98% on O$_2$

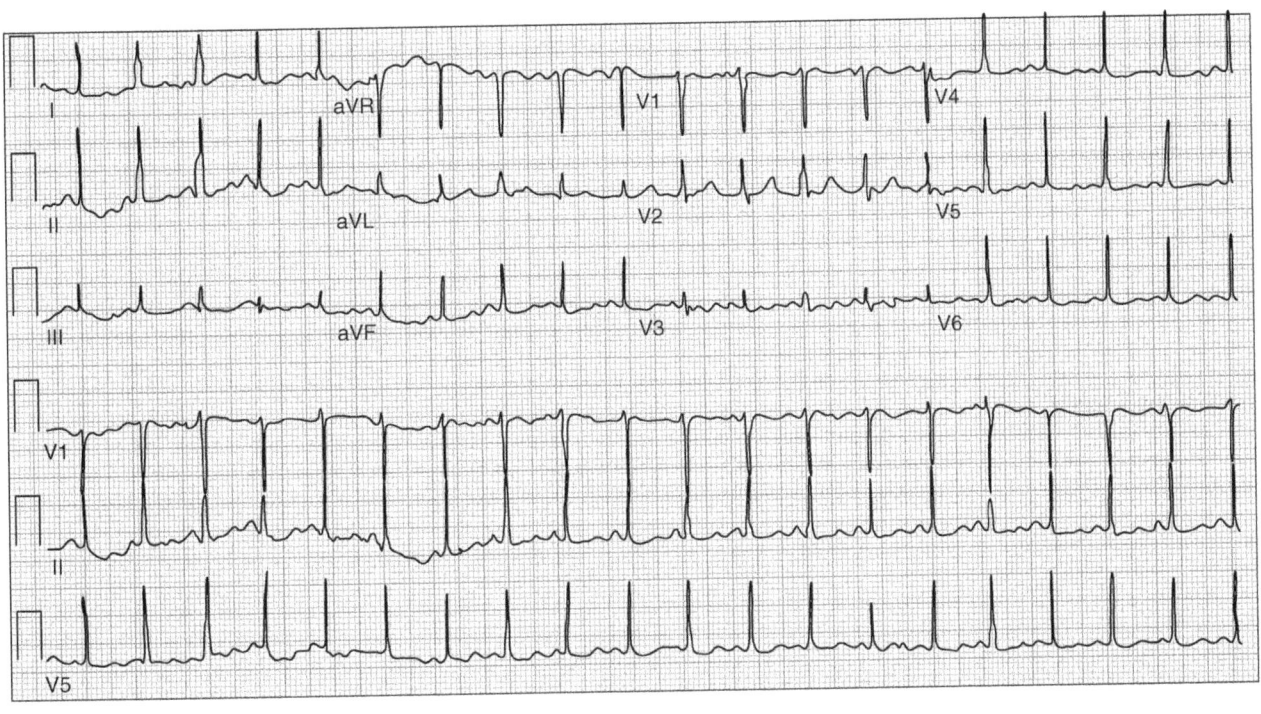

Figure 27.1

H. Secondary survey
a. General: alert, anxious appearing, moderate distress
b. HEENT: dried blood around mouth; scleral icterus; pale conjunctivae noted
c. Neck: normal
d. Chest: normal
e. Heart: tachycardic; no rubs, murmurs, or gallops
f. Abdomen: protuberant, nontender. Hyperactive bowel sounds present. No masses, no hernias, no rebound, no guarding, no rigidity. Ascites present with positive fluid wave (must ask for this) and caput medusae present (must ask for this).
g. Rectal: hemoccult positive brown stool, normal rectal tone
h. Urogenital: normal
i. Extremities: normal

j.   Back: normal
k.   Neuro: normal
l.   Skin: pale, scattered ecchymoses
m.   Lymph: normal

I. Action
a.   1 L IV fluid bolus
b.   Give antiemetic medication
c.   IV proton-pump inhibitor
d.   IV octreotide bolus of 50 mcg followed by octreotide infusion at 25–50 mcg/hr
e.   Blood transfusion (pRBCs and platelets) after consent obtained from patient
f.   IV antibiotics: ciprofloxacin 400 mg IV or ceftriaxone 1 g IV
g.   Have materials for intubation as well as balloon tamponade devices such as a Sengstaken–
     Blakemore or Minnesota tube at bedside as a precautionary measure
h.   Emergent gastroenterology (GI) consult

J. Nurse
a.   Repeat vitals: BP: 100/70, HR: 110, RR: 22, Sat: 99% on O_2
b.   Patient still appears ill and with nausea (unless antiemetic given)

K. Results

Table 27.1 Results table

Test	Result	Test	Result
Complete blood count:		D bili	2.8 mg/dL
WBC	$9.1 \times 10^3/\mu L$	Lipase	60 U/L
Hgb	6.7 g/dL	Albumin	2.1 g/dL
Hct	22.90%		
Plt	$24 \times 10^3/\mu L$	Lactate	3.4 mmol/L
Basic metabolic panel:		**Urinalysis:**	
Na	132 mEq/L	SG	1.020
K	4.1 mEq/L	pH	6
Cl	101 mEq/L	Prot	Neg
CO_2	18 mEq/L	Gluc	Neg
BUN	40 mEq/dL	Ketones	Neg
Cr	1.7 mEq/dL	Bili	Neg
Gluc	127 mEq/dL	Blood	+
		Leuk Esterase	Neg
Coagulation panel:		Nitrite	Neg
PT	13.1 sec	Color	Yellow

Table 27.1 (cont.)

Test	Result	Test	Result
PTT	40 sec	Urine preg.	Neg
INR	3.7		
		Arterial blood gas:	
Liver function panel:		pH	7.33
AST	23 U/L	pO_2	92 mmHg
ALT	19 U/L	pCO_2	25 mmHg
Alk phos	87 U/L	HCO_3	19 mmol/L
T bili	4.2 mg/dL		

a. CXR (Figure 27.2)

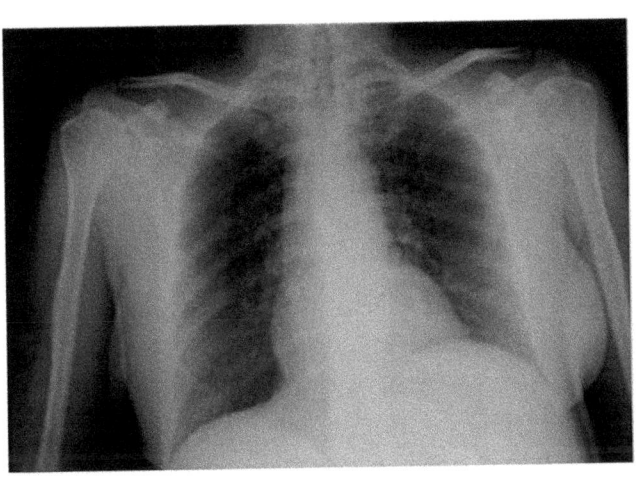

Figure 27.2

L. Action
a. GI consult
   i. Emergent endoscopy for variceal source control
b. Discussion with patient, family, and PMD regarding need for emergent endoscopy and diagnosis of variceal bleeding.
c. Meds
   i. Transfuse two units of pRBCs, as well as platelets.
   ii. Call blood bank to make sure 10–16 units of blood and fresh frozen plasma will be available (massive transfusion protocol).
d. Reverse coagulopathy (vitamin K, FFP, or 4-factor prothrombin complex concentrate [PCC]).

M. Diagnosis
a. Variceal upper GI bleed

N. Critical actions
a. Large-bore IV access and fluid bolus
b. Blood product administration
c. Antibiotic administration

    d. GI consult

    e. ICU admission

O. Examiner instructions

a. This is a case of a variceal upper GI bleed in a patient with worsening cirrhosis and portal hypertension as evidenced by her ascites and caput medusae on exam. Variceal bleeding should be suspected in patients presenting with hematemesis who have a history of advanced liver disease or those with known esophageal varices. Critical steps in managing this patient include obtaining large-bore IV access, fluid and blood resuscitation, antibiotic administration, and emergent GI consultation. If the patient does not receive crystalloid or blood early in the resuscitation, she will become hypotensive and obtunded, requiring a technically difficult intubation. If no blood is given and the coagulopathy is not addressed, the patient will have worsening hematemesis and hemodynamic compromise. Initially the gastroenterologist will be reluctant to perform the procedure, stating "It will be too bloody for me to see anything," and will request that she be given medications and observed until the morning. The candidate should advocate for emergent endoscopy given concern for variceal bleeding.

P. Pearls

a. Suspect variceal bleeding in patients presenting with signs of upper GI bleeding and history of liver disease.

b. Octreotide is a somatostatin analog that causes splanchnic vasoconstriction and should be considered in cases of known or suspected variceal bleeding.

c. Overly aggressive fluid resuscitation leads to increased central venous pressure which can dislodge variceal clots and worsen bleeding. Therefore, early administration of blood products (especially platelets) is recommended.

d. Patients with cirrhosis are immunocompromised and require antibiotics for GI bleeding.

e. Coagulopathy in cirrhosis and advanced liver disease is complicated, and the INR alone does not adequately reflect coagulation. Some experts recommend a thromboelastogram (TEG) in these patients to adequately characterize bleeding risk. Consensus guidelines state that coagulopathy should be reversed in cases of nonvariceal upper GI bleeding with elevated INR or with thrombocytopenia.

Figure legends

Figure 27.1 (EKG) Sinus tachycardia.

Figure 27.2 (CXR) Normal chest X-ray.

Q. References

a. *Tintinalli's Emergency Medicine: A Comprehensive Study Guide* (9th ed.): Chapter 75, Upper Gastrointestinal Bleeding.

b. *Rosen's Emergency Medicine: Concepts and Clinical Practice* (10th ed.): Chapter 26, Gastrointestinal Bleeding.

Lightheadedness

Kendra Amico, MD

A. Chief complaint
a. 82-year-old female brought in with lightheadedness and syncope

B. Vital signs
a. BP: 69/43, HR: 42, RR: 20, T: 36.1°C, Sat: 94% on RA

C. What does the patient look like?
a. Patient appears pale, lying supine in bed, with decreased alertness.

D. Primary survey
a. Airway: patent, able to mumble her name
b. Breathing: breathing spontaneously, no apparent respiratory distress
c. Circulation: pale, cool distal extremities, 1+ femoral pulses

E. Action
a. Oxygen via nasal cannula or nonrebreather mask
b. Finger-stick blood glucose (354 mg/dL; must ask for this)
c. Two large-bore peripheral IV lines
d. Cardiac monitor
e. Labs
   i. CBC, BMP, troponin, INR/PT/PTT, lactate, blood cultures, blood type and hold
f. Obtain EKG
g. 1 L NS bolus
h. Portable CXR

F. History
a. HPI: An 82-year-old female was found by family in bed. She was reportedly pale with decreased responsiveness and rushed to the ED. While getting her out of bed, the family reports the patient had a brief atraumatic syncopal event with subsequent return of consciousness. Patient is unable to provide any additional history. Family denies any known chest pain, shortness of breath, nausea, vomiting, fever, chills, or neurologic complaints. They report the patient was acting like her normal self yesterday. She reportedly takes her medications as prescribed.
b. PMHx: diabetes mellitus, hypertension, prior stroke/TIA without residual deficits
c. PSHx: none
d. Allergies: penicillin, morphine
e. Meds: aspirin, amlodipine, lisinopril, metformin, metoprolol, omeprazole

f.   Social: remote smoker, denies alcohol or drug use, lives with family

g.   FHx: hypertension, diabetes

G. Nurse

a.   EKG (Figure 28.1)

b.   Repeat vitals:

i.   If 1 L NS given: BP: 75/52, HR: 44, RR: 20, Sat: 94% on 4 L O_2

ii.   If no fluids given: BP: 65/40, HR: 44, RR: 20, Sat 94% on O_2

c.   Place transcutaneous pacing pads on patient's chest (must ask for this)

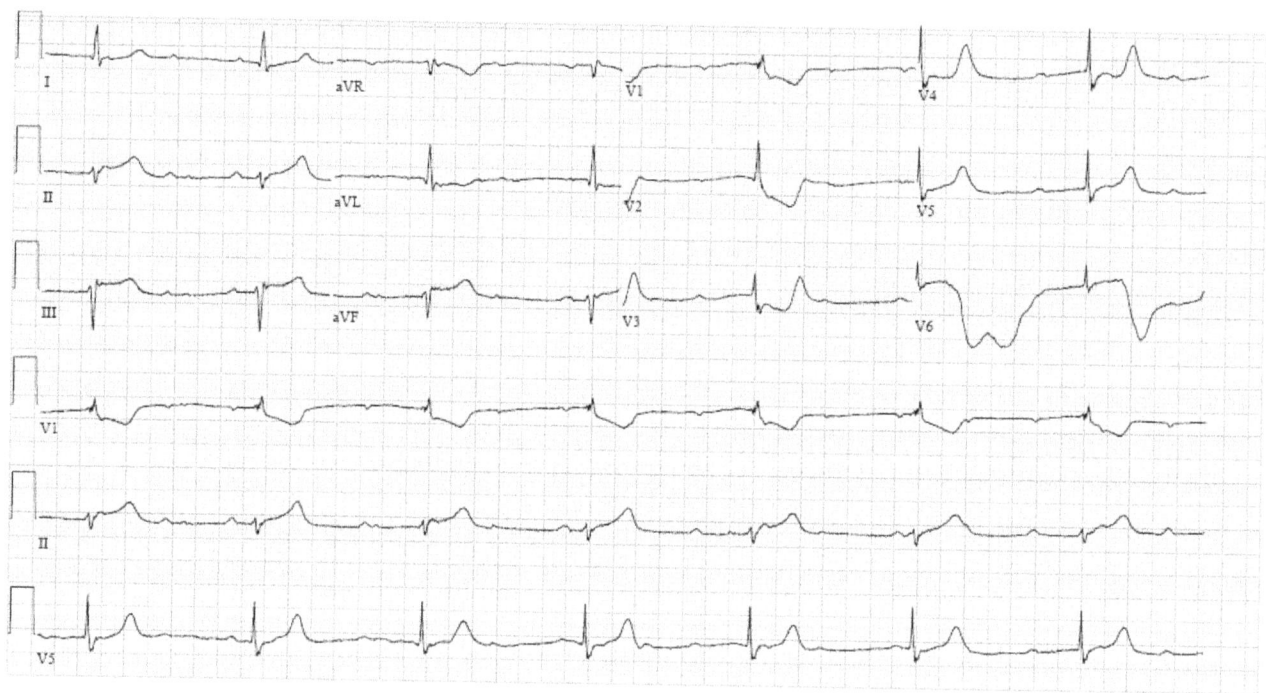

Figure 28.1

H. Secondary survey

a.   General: alert to self, appears fatigued

b.   HEENT: dry mucous membranes, no secretions; gag intact

c.   Neck: supple, no jugular venous distension

d.   Chest: normal spontaneous respiratory movement, clear and equal breath sounds bilaterally

e.   Heart: bradycardic, no murmurs, 1+ femoral pulses bilaterally, capillary refill time >3 seconds

f.   Abdomen: normal

g.   Rectal: incontinent of brown stool; hemoccult negative

h.   Extremities: no deformity, radial pulses not palpable; 1+ femoral pulses bilaterally

i.   Back: normal

j.   Neuro: alert to self, localizes painful stimuli, no obvious focal deficits

k.   Skin: cool, delayed capillary refill

I. Action

a.   NS bolus IV

b.   Atropine 1 mg IV initially, repeat every 3–5 minutes for total of 3 mg (do not allow medication administration to delay pacing)

c. Aspirin
d. Consult interventional cardiology

J. Nurse

a. No response to atropine; heart rate remains in low 40s; blood pressure is unchanged

K. Action

a. Initiate temporary cardiac pacing – place pads and start pacing transcutaneously (ask candidate to explain procedures)
b. Activate catheterization lab in consultation with cardiology
c. Consider dopamine (start at 3 mcg/kg/min)

L. Results

Table 28.1 Results table

Test	Result	Test	Result
Complete blood count:		Cr	0.7 mg/dL
WBC	$13 \times 10^3/\mu L$	Gluc	354 mg/dL
Hct	36.30%	Troponin	0.06 ng/mL
Plt	$399 \times 10^3/\mu L$	Lactate	7 mg/dL
Basic metabolic panel:		**Coagulation panel:**	
Na	140 mEq/L	PT	12 sec
K	3.4 mEq/L	PTT	38 sec
Cl	108 mEq/L	INR	2.1
CO_2	16 mEq/L	Magnesium	2.3 mg/dL
BUN	24 mEq/dL		

a. CXR (Figure 28.2)
b. Repeat EKG: now paced at 70

Figure 28.2

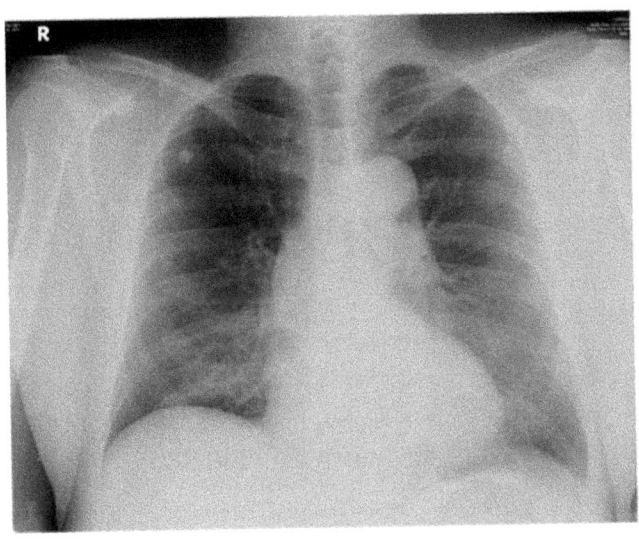

M. Action

a. If poor capture, prepare for transvenous pacing (in ED or cardiac catheterization laboratory).
b. Discuss heparin and platelet receptor inhibitor (i.e., clopidogrel or ticagrelor) administration with interventional cardiologist.
c. Admission to ICU.

N. Diagnosis

a. Symptomatic bradycardia; inferior myocardial infarction (MI) with third-degree AV block (AVB)

O. Critical actions

a. EKG
b. Atropine 1 mg IV (may repeat up to total 3 mg)
c. Pacing (transcutaneous or transvenous)
d. Aspirin
e. Interventional cardiology consultation for catheterization lab activation
f. Admission to ICU or directly to catheterization laboratory

P. Examiner instructions

a. This is a case of symptomatic bradycardia in the setting of myocardial infarction. The patient's EKG demonstrates an inferior and lateral myocardial infarction from a fully occluded left circumflex artery, which has led to pronounced bradycardia with associated third-degree AVB. The EKG shows a junctional escape rhythm as well. The patient's low heart rate is not able to sustain adequate cardiac output, leading to hypotension and causing her symptoms of dizziness and syncope, as well as diminished alertness from poor cerebral perfusion. Immediate recognition of patient's hemodynamic instability and EKG findings is essential. Important management steps include immediate cardiac monitoring including EKG, transcutaneous pacing, and cardiology consultation in order to facilitate prompt revascularization as well as rhythm stabilization. Continual reassessment is needed to determine response to medications and transcutaneous pacing. Pacing should not be delayed by medication administration. If the candidate attempts to treat a possible β-blocker overdose with glucagon, this strategy will be ineffective.
b. Curveball: Transcutaneous pacing becomes ineffective due to poor capture, forcing the candidate to place a transvenous pacemaker in the ED. Have the candidate describe the procedure.

Q. Pearls

a. For symptomatic or unstable bradycardic patients, transcutaneous pacing should be initiated immediately. If the external pacer fails to capture, a transvenous pacer should be inserted emergently.
b. In patients with inferior MI, provide adequate volume resuscitation as this type of MI will diminish preload.
c. A trial of atropine is still indicated for bradycardia in patients with hypotension or other signs of poor perfusion (decreased alertness, poor peripheral perfusion, etc.). Atropine is ineffective in patients with a deinnervated heart (i.e., heart transplant). Look for the cause of third-degree AVB, including prior and progressive conduction disease, hyperkalemia, thyroid disease, medications, or – as in this case – inferior MI (which can develop in up to 8% of acute inferior MIs).

d. Consider dopamine initiation in the setting of hemodynamic instability, starting at 3 mcg/kg/minute and titrating up to 20 mcg/kg/minute. Dobutamine is preferred in the setting of congestive heart failure associated with complete heart block. Norepinephrine has become the preferred pressor in patients with hypotension from myocardial infarction without complete heart block.

e. In this patient population, prompt revascularization is the goal and often corrects the arrhythmia without need for a permanent pacemaker.

R. Figure legends
a. Figure 28.1 (EKG) Bradycardia, third degree block; anterior ST depressions and lateral ST elevation, consistent with acute inferolateral myocardial infarction.
b. Figure 28.2 (CXR) Normal chest x-ray.

S. References
a. *Tintinalli's Emergency Medicine: A Comprehensive Study Guide* (9th ed.): Chapter 18, Cardiac Rhythm Disturbances. Chapter 49, Acute Coronary Syndromes.
b. *Rosen's Emergency Medicine: Concepts and Clinical Practice* (9th ed.): Chapter 69, Dysrhythmias.

Shortness of Breath

Abraham Feshazion, MD, PharmD, MPH, and Linda Katirji, MD

A. Chief complaint
a. 46-year-old female with shortness of breath

B. Vital signs
a. BP: 110/77, HR: 130, RR: 34, T: 36.5°C, Sat: 91% on RA

C. What does the patient look like?
a. Patient is obese and appears older than stated age, sitting up in hospital bed and appears to be in moderate respiratory distress.

D. Primary survey
a. Airway: speaking 2–3 words at a time with gasping in between
b. Breathing: moderate respiratory distress, using accessory muscles, bilateral wheezing with long expiratory phase
c. Circulation: warm, normal capillary refill

E. Action
a. Supplemental oxygen via nonrebreather mask as needed to maintain >95% saturation or nebulizer treatments
b. Two large-bore IV lines
c. 1 L NS bolus
d. EKG
f. Labs
i. CBC, BMP, LFT, troponin, BNP, INR/PT/PTT, type and screen, ABG/VBG, lactate
g. Portable CXR

F. History
a. HPI: A 46-year-old female with a history of hypertension and asthma reports that 1 hour prior to arrival she developed progressively worsening shortness of breath while at home watching television. She used several puffs of her albuterol MDI with no improvement of symptoms. In the last 45 minutes, her wheezing worsened and she reports difficulty speaking. Associated symptoms include dry cough and central nonradiating chest pain. The chest pain is described as tight and increases with cough. She denies headache, lightheadedness, fever, chills, diaphoresis, nausea, vomiting, abdominal pain, weakness, or leg swelling.
b. PMHx: asthma (two previous intubations and ICU admissions in the last three years – must ask for this), hypertension, obesity
c. PSHx: none

d. Allergies: ibuprofen
e. Meds: ranitidine, aspirin, metoprolol, montelukast, albuterol, fluticasone/salmeterol
f. Social: former smoker, denies alcohol or recreational drug use.
g. FHx: not relevant
h. PMD: Dr. Tesfa
i. Patient reports lack of reliable transportation to appointments or to pharmacy.

G. Action
a. Albuterol–ipratropium nebulizer solution inhaled every 20 minutes × 3 doses or continuous
b. Methylprednisolone 125 mg IV
c. Albuterol nebulizers inhaled continuously for 1 hour
d. Magnesium 2 g IV

H. Secondary survey
a. General: alert, oriented, moderate respiratory distress, speaking 2–3 words at a time, obese
b. HEENT: normal
c. Neck: normal, no jugular vein distension
d. Chest: tachypneic with diffuse wheezing in all lung fields, using accessory respiratory muscles
e. Heart: tachycardic with regular rhythm; normal S1/S2; no murmur
f. Abdomen: normal
g. Extremities: no edema, 2+ pulses throughout, capillary refill <2 seconds
h. Back: normal
i. Neuro: normal
j. Skin: normal
k. Rectal: normal, hemoccult negative
l. GU: normal
m. Lymph: normal

I. Nurse
a. Patient is still tachypneic and tachycardic after oxygen and medication therapy.
b. Repeat vitals: BP: 112/78, HR: 121, RR: 40, T: 36.5°C, Sat: 95% on O_2
c. EKG (Figure 29.1)
d. CXR (Figure 29.2)

J. Action
a. Meds:
   i. Administer terbutaline 0.25 mg SQ every 20 minutes × 3 doses, or epinephrine 0.3 mg SQ every 20 minutes × 3 doses
b. Trial of bilevel positive airway pressure (BiPAP) with in-line continuous nebulized albuterol
c. Reassess
   i. If BiPAP started, the patient maintains oxygen saturation but begins to appear tired.
   ii. If BiPAP not started, the patient begins to desaturate to 85% and appears sleepy and confused.

K. Nurse
a. Patient is still tachypneic and appears sleepy and exhausted, slower to respond to questioning
b. Repeat vitals: BP: 170/100, HR: 125, RR: 30, Sat: 98% on BiPAP (Sat: 89% if not on NIPPV)

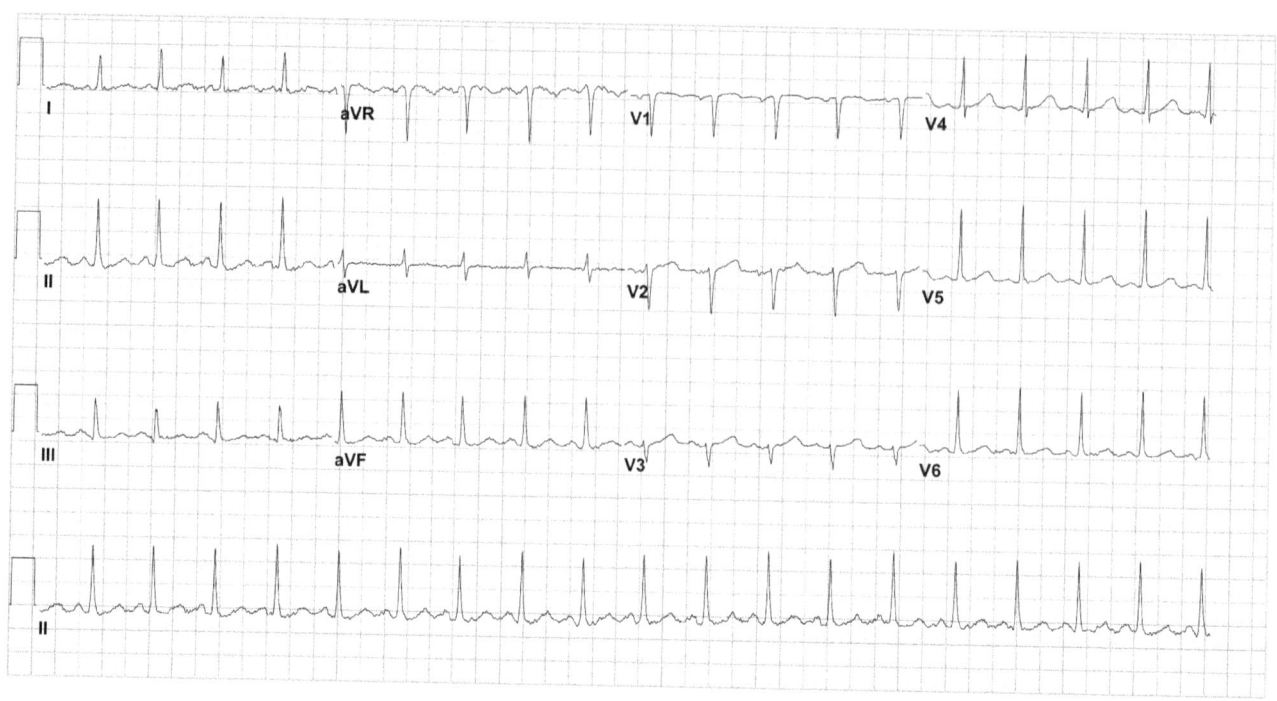

Figure 29.1

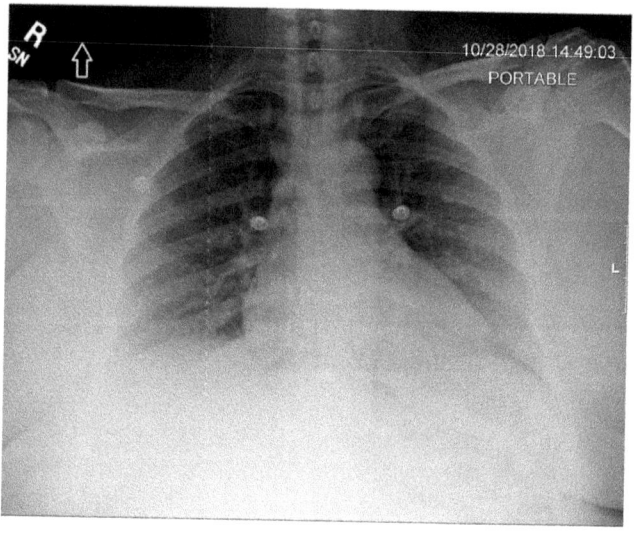

Figure 29.2

L. Action

a. Discuss need for intubation with patient.
b. Perform RSI intubation.
    i.   Induction with ketamine 1.5 mg/kg
    ii. Paralysis with rocuronium 1 mg/kg
    iii. Post-intubation sedation with propofol drip
c. Post-intubation portable CXR (Figure 29.3) and VBG/ABG
d. Nasogastric tube placement for decompression
e. ICU admission

Figure 29.3

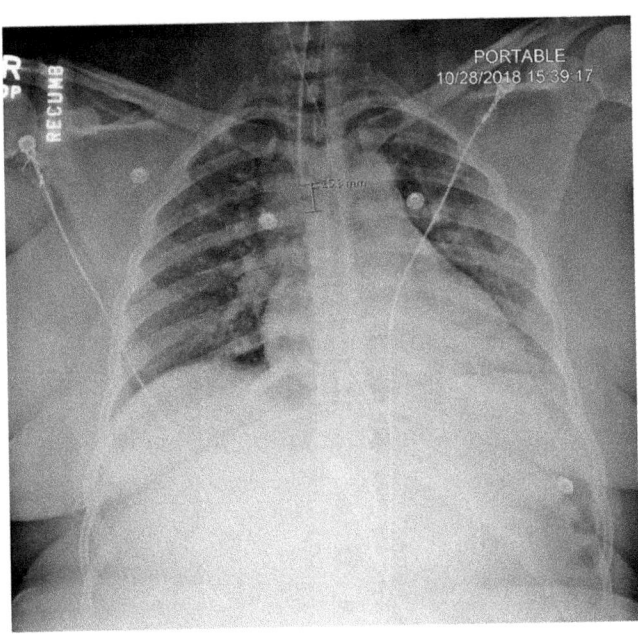

M. Results

Table 29.1 Results table

Test	Result	Test	Result
Complete blood count:		**Liver function panel:**	
WBC	$11.1 \times 10^3/\mu L$	AST	16 U/L
Hct	34.10%	ALT	11 U/L
Plt	$358 \times 10^3/\mu L$	Alk phos	65 U/L
		T bili	0.3 mg/dL
		D bili	0.1 mg/dL
Basic metabolic panel:		Albumin	4.2 g/dL
Na	141 mEq/L		
K	4.0 mEq/L		
Cl	106 mEq/L	Troponin	<0.02 ng/mL
CO_2	23 mEq/L	BNP	63 pg/mL
BUN	11 mEq/dL		
Cr	0.94 mg/dL	**Arterial blood gas:**	
Gluc	106 mg/dL	pH	7.42
		pO_2	60 mmHg
		pCO_2	32 mmHg
Coagulation panel:		HCO_3	20.8 mmol/L
PT	13.0 sec		
PTT	24.0 sec		
INR	1.0		

a. Lactate: 2.4 mmol/L

N. Nurse

a. Repeat vitals after patient is intubated: BP: 114/71, HR: 104, RR: 18, Sat: 99% on vent

O. Diagnosis

a. Acute asthma exacerbation (status asthmaticus)

P. Critical actions

a. Large-bore IV access
b. Patient placed on monitor with continuous pulse oximetry
c. Supplemental oxygen administration
d. Administration of bronchodilators and steroids
e. Adjunctive therapies for severe asthma (e.g., magnesium, terbutaline or epinephrine, BiPAP) prior to intubation
f. Intubation when all other medical therapies fail
g. Disposition to ICU

Q. Examiner instructions

a. This is a case of a severe acute asthma exacerbation (status asthmaticus) in a patient with a history of multiple intubations and ICU admissions for disease refractory to standard treatment of inhaled bronchodilators and steroids. Asthma is an obstructive airway disease that can be caused by many environmental insults. These insults cause airway smooth muscle contraction, bronchial wall edema, and copious secretions that result in increased airway resistance. This increased resistance increases the work of breathing for the patient, which if not alleviated quickly enough will cause hemodynamic instability. The patient will develop hypoxia, hypercarbia, acidosis, confusion, and eventual respiratory fatigue leading to respiratory arrest.
b. Patients suffering from asthma are generally treated as outpatients with regularly scheduled dosing of inhaled long-acting β-agonists and steroids to reduce the quantity and severity of acute exacerbations. As-needed inhaled short-acting β-agonists are used when acute exacerbations do occur. Patients with poor ability to follow up with their regular physician appointments and/or with barriers to acquisition of medications are at higher risk for more frequent and severe asthma attacks.
c. The assessment of acute asthma exacerbations includes grading the severity of the episode using a peak flow meter in order to objectively measure the effectiveness of subsequent therapy. Standard management of acute asthma exacerbations includes supplemental oxygen, a series of nebulized β-agonists and anticholinergics, and oral or systemic steroids.
d. Status asthmaticus is defined as a severe asthma exacerbation refractory to standard asthma management. When a patient is considered in "status," adjunct therapy is initiated which usually consists of a combination of intravenous magnesium, terbutaline, or epinephrine. A trial of noninvasive positive pressure ventilation such as BiPAP should be attempted prior to considering endotracheal intubation.
e. Generally, intubation of the patient experiencing an acute asthma exacerbation is to be avoided. The risks of barotrauma from high plateau pressures in breath-stacking must be balanced against the risk of acidosis from hypoventilation, and managing that balance can be very challenging for even the most experienced clinicians. However, if a patient such as the one presented in this case develops one or more of the indications for intubation (worsening hypoxia, hypercarbia, acidosis, confusion, or respiratory fatigue after administration of maximal standard and adjunct therapy), invasive airway protection and external breathing

control via endotracheal intubation and mechanical ventilation is a critical and necessary action. Keep in mind that optimal medical management may help avoid intubation in most cases, but optimize patient for intubation in the remaining cases. Therefore it is as critical as airway management.

R. Pearls

a. Asthma disproportionally affects children, women, African Americans, smokers, and those who live in urban environments.

b. It is important to note the number of times a patient has been hospitalized and intubated from refractory asthma exacerbations in the past as a history of severe disease is directly related to future intubations and ICU admissions.

c. Initial and repeat peak flow measurements are sufficient in guiding management in mild to moderate asthma exacerbations. Serial arterial blood gas measurements can be used in severe cases, but the patient's clinical status (including work of breathing, diaphoresis, mental status, and other signs of acuity) is paramount.

d. The initial presentation of an asthma exacerbation in the ED is variable and may not include audible wheezing. Wheezing requires a certain amount of airflow which is significantly reduced in severe cases. Patients often complain of cough and chest tightness. Allow the medical history to aid in your assessment and treatment decisions.

e. Common mimics of asthma exacerbation include: acute heart failure, upper airway obstruction, pulmonary embolism, aspiration of foreign body, severe GERD, tumors causing endobronchial obstruction, interstitial lung disease, or vocal cord dysfunction.

f. A chest radiograph is of little value in most acute asthma exacerbations and should be restricted to patients with a suspected complicating cardiopulmonary process, such as pneumonia, pneumothorax, pneumomediastinum, subcutaneous emphysema, or congestive heart failure.

g. Agents that have uncertain or no benefit in the treatment of acute asthma exacerbations include: supplemental heliox (80% helium and 20% oxygen), methylxanthines such as aminophylline, and mast cell/leukotriene modifiers such as montelukast.

h. Magnesium has proven benefit as an adjunct to albuterol administration, but diligent blood pressure monitoring is prudent as it may decrease blood pressure.

i. Ketamine decreases catecholamine reuptake, which aids in alleviation of asthma symptoms and has the added benefit of dissociative effects in higher doses, which may be used for induction prior to intubation.

j. The decision to intubate should be made clinically as hypercapnia (secondary to airway obstruction and respiratory fatigue) is a late manifestation.

k. Intubation of asthmatics is reserved as a last resort as this cohort is notorious for complications stemming from increased pulmonary pressures caused by air trapping. If a patient in status asthmaticus is intubated, ventilator settings should be set to allow for low tidal volumes and longer expiratory phase ventilation (1:3 I:E ratio) to reduce the incidence of barotrauma. Post-intubation deep sedation is advised as it mitigates the need for continued paralytics. Often blood pressure drops with deep sedation but is usually corrected with IV fluids.

S. Figure legends

a. Figure 29.1 (EKG) Sinus tachycardia.

b. Figure 29.2 (CXR) Normal chest x-ray.

c. Figure 29.3 (CXR) ET in place; mild to moderate interstitial edema.

T. References

a. *Tintinalli's Emergency Medicine: A Comprehensive Study Guide* (9th ed.): Chapter 69, Acute Asthma and Status Asthmaticus.

b. *Rosen's Emergency Medicine: Concepts and Clinical Practice* (10th ed.): Chapter 59, Asthma.

Rash and Fever

Nikolas Sekoulopoulos, MD, Stephanie Gaines, MD, and Jessica Berrios, MD

A. Chief complaint
a. 35-year-old male with rash and fever

B. Vital signs
a. BP: 100/62, HR: 96, RR: 20, T: 38.5°C, Sat: 98% on RA

C. What does the patient look like?
a. Patient appears stated age, alert, in mild distress from pain.

D. Primary survey
a. Airway: patent, able to speak in full sentences
b. Breathing: clear to auscultation bilaterally, no wheezing, no apparent respiratory distress
c. Circulation: good radial pulses, normal capillary refill

E. Action
a. IV access
b. Labs
    i. CBC, BMP, urinalysis, blood and urine cultures, lactate
c. Monitor
d. EKG
e. CXR
f. Administer ibuprofen or acetaminophen for fever
g. 1 L NS bolus

F. History
a. HPI: A 35-year-old male presents with fever, fatigue, and malaise that started 3 days ago. He noted a red rash yesterday to his upper chest and neck area that has now spread to his abdomen and arms. The rash is painful to touch but not pruritic. He has also developed ulcers in his mouth and is having burning with urination. He is HIV positive and has never had a similar rash. He is compliant with his HAART medications. No sick contacts with a similar rash. Patient recently started on an antibiotic 6 days ago after an I&D of an abscess. He has not missed any doses of his antibiotic. He has not taken anything for fever at home.
b. PMHx: HIV, abscesses, gynecomastia
c. PSHx: incision and drainages
d. Allergies: penicillins (causes anaphylaxis)

e. Meds: HAART triple therapy, started on sulfamethoxazole and trimethoprim for abscess 6 days ago
f. Social: no tobacco, occasional alcohol, occasional marijuana; monogamous with a single male partner
g. FHx: not relevant
h. PMD: none

G. Secondary survey

a. General: alert and oriented, obese, comfortable after antipyretic administered
b. HEENT: small oral erosions to bilateral buccal mucosa, lips with crusting, no drainage; injected conjunctiva bilaterally; tympanic membranes clear, nares clear
c. Neck: supple, no lymphadenopathy
d. Chest: mild gynecomastia noted, not tender to palpation
e. Heart: normal
f. Abdomen: normal
g. Urogenital: normal
h. Extremities: no edema; normal pulses, moves with normal ROM
i. Back: normal
j. Neuro: normal
k. Skin: symmetric red, purpuric macules and plaques over neck and chest that are tender to palpation, some with sloughing and necrosis of larger plaques; extensor surfaces of arms (~9%) with vesicles and bullae; bullae spread with pressure, some appear like target lesions

H. Nurse

a. EKG (Figure 30.1)
b. Repeat vitals:
    i. If antipyretic and 1 L IV fluids given: BP: 101/67, HR: 93, RR: 18, T: 37.6°C, Sat: 98% on RA
    ii. If no antipyretic or fluids given: BP: 95/58, HR: 102, RR: 20, T: 38.9°C, Sat: 98% on RA

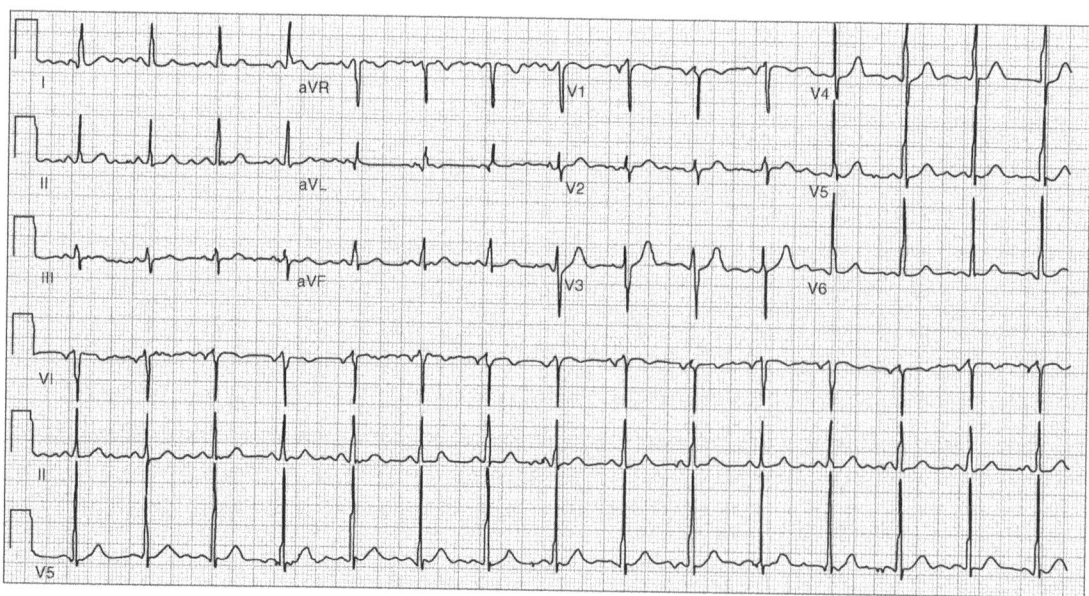

Figure 30.1

I. Results

Table 30.1 Results table

Test	Result	Test	Result
Complete blood count:		T bili	0.7 mg/dL
WBC	$4.0 \times 10^3/\mu L$	D bili	0.1 mg/dL
Hct	32.00%	Amylase	30 U/L
Plt	$250 \times 10^3/\mu L$	Lipase	45 U/L
		Albumin	3.9 g/dL
Basic metabolic panel:			
Na	141 mEq/L	**Urinalysis:**	
K	3.8 mEq/L	SG	1.015
Cl	102 mEq/L	pH	6
CO_2	22 mEq/L	Prot	Neg
BUN	14 mEq/dL	Gluc	Neg
Cr	0.65 mg/dL	Ketones	Trace
Gluc	100 mg/dL	Bili	Neg
		Blood	Trace
		LE	Neg
Coagulation panel:		Nitrite	Neg
PT	15 sec	Color	Yellow
PTT	28.0 sec		
INR	1.0	**Arterial blood gas:**	
		pH	7.35
Liver function panel:		pO_2	88 mmHg
AST	19 U/L	pCO_2	44 mmHg
ALT	25 U/L	HCO_3	25 mmol/L
Alk phos	69 U/L		

a. Lactate: 1.2 mmol/L
b. CXR (Figure 30.2)

J. Action

a. Dermatology consultation
b. NS bolus
c. Discontinue use of sulfamethoxazole and trimethoprim
d. ICU or burn unit admission

K. Diagnosis

a. Stevens–Johnson syndrome

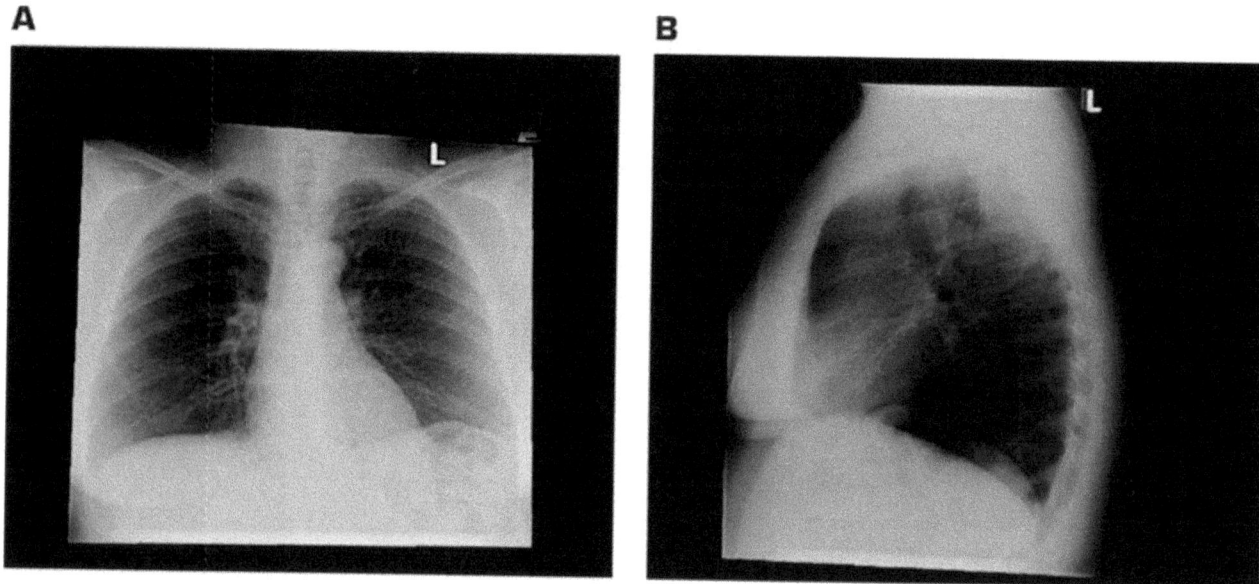

Figure 30.2

L. Critical actions

a. Obtain history of recent antibiotic use
b. Skin examination
c. Establish diagnosis of Stevens–Johnson syndrome
d. Stop the offending agent
e. Fluid administration
f. Dermatology consultation
g. ICU or burn unit admission

M. Examiner instructions

a. This is a case of Stevens–Johnson syndrome (SJS), a vesiculobullous disease with acute inflammatory reaction in the skin and mucosa. It is one of three diseases on a spectrum defined by the amount of epidermal detachment present. Erythema multiforme has no epidermal detachment. SJS has <10% involvement. Toxic epidermal necrolysis (TEN) has >30% involvement. SJS also characteristically has mucous membrane involvement. Although the exact pathophysiology is not well known, this syndrome is often associated with medication reactions and infections. This patient is taking a sulfur-containing antibiotic for his abscess, which is likely the culprit. Important actions include making the diagnosis on the basis of history and physical examination, consulting dermatology, and admitting the patient to a burn unit. When consulted, the dermatologist will not be able to provide any additional assistance beyond agreeing with the candidate's plan for admission and IV fluids. They will not be able to help make the diagnosis for the candidate. Early ophthalmology consult can prevent/treat involvement of the eyes.

N. Pearls

a. Medications are the most common trigger of SJS. Among those implicated are antibiotics (penicillins, sulfonamides, and cephalosporins), antiepileptics, NSAIDs, antipsychotics, and antigout medications.
b. Patients with HIV who take sulfamethoxazole and trimethoprim are at 40 times greater risk of developing SJS.

c. Males have 2:1 greater risk than females for developing SJS.

d. Ocular involvement is very common (70%).

e. The syndrome carries a 1–5% mortality. Sepsis is the major cause of death.

f. Prophylactic IV antibiotics are not routinely recommended – treatment includes removing the causative agent and supportive care.

g. In this case, SJS is the cause for fever and constitutional symptoms. However, it would be totally reasonable to administer empiric antibiotics to a patient with immune compromise, malaise, fever, and a rash after abscess drainage. Be sure to select an agent that is not associated with SJS, such as clindamycin.

h. IV fluids are recommended for supportive care similar to burns; however, in less quantity given only epidermal involvement.

i. Recurrence may occur with repeat exposure to the etiologic agent. Especially in children with the causative agent being herpes simplex virus (HSV), up to 75% of cases will recur with reactivation of HSV.

j. Intravenous immunoglobulins (IVIGs), steroids, and plasmapheresis have been studied, but insufficient evidence exists to recommend their use in all patients.

O. Figure legends

a. Figure 30.1 (EKG) Normal sinus rhythm.

b. Figure 30.2 (CXR) Normal chest x-ray.

P. References

a. *Tintinalli's Emergency Medicine: A Comprehensive Study Guide* (9th ed.): Chapter 249, Generalized Skin Disorders.

b. *Rosen's Emergency Medicine: Concepts and Clinical Practice* (10th ed.): Chapter 107, Dermatologic Presentations.

Weakness

Stephanie Gaines, MD

A. Chief complaint
a. 52-year-old female with dizziness and weakness

B. Vital signs
a. BP: 126/65, HR: 99, RR: 18, T: 37.6°C, Sat: 95% on RA

C. What does the patient look like?
a. Patient appears weak and fatigued, sitting in bed in no apparent distress.

D. Primary survey
a. Airway: patent, no secretions
b. Breathing: lungs clear to auscultation bilaterally and unlabored
c. Circulation: strong pulses throughout, normal capillary refill

E. History:
a. HPI: A 52-year-old female presents with dizziness and weakness. Her symptoms began about one week ago when she first noticed numbness and tingling in her feet. She then developed a bad headache and was treated with a "migraine cocktail" at an urgent care center. Since then, she has had progressively worsening symptoms. The numbness has spread up to both of her knees and hands. Now she has trouble walking and feels like it is hard for her to swallow at times. She still has a severe headache along with photophobia. She denies any recent travel or known insect bites. She notes a mild "stomach flu" 1 week prior to symptom onset, consisting of nausea, vomiting, and diarrhea. She denies any fevers. No falls.
b. PMHx: asthma
c. PSHx: none
d. Allergies: no known drug allergies, but has intolerance to shellfish
e. Meds: albuterol as needed
f. Social: denies smoking, drinks alcohol socially, denies illicit drug use
g. FHx: hypertension and asthma
h. PMD: none

F. Action
a. Oxygen via nasal cannula needed to maintain >95% saturation
b. Peripheral IV access
c. Labs
    i. CBC, CMP, ABG, urinalysis, urine pregnancy test, erythrocyte sedimentation rate (ESR)
d. Cardiac monitor

e. Finger stick blood glucose: 120 mg/dL
f. EKG
g. CXR

G. Secondary survey

a. General: awake and alert, though fatigued, in no acute distress
b. HEENT: normocephalic, atraumatic; extraocular movements intact, pupils equally round and reactive to light, 3 mm; oropharynx clear, no exudates, uvula midline
c. Neck: weakness of neck muscles; no lymphadenopathy
d. Chest: clear to auscultation bilaterally, poor effort, no wheezing or rales
e. Heart: normal
f. Abdomen: soft, nontender, nondistended, normal bowel sounds
g. Urogenital: normal
h. Extremities: no gross deformity or swelling
i. Back: normal
j. Neuro: weak gag reflex, weak CN 9 with inability to keep cheeks puffed out, remaining cranial nerves are intact; 3/5 strength in bilateral lower extremities, 4/5 strength in bilateral upper extremities, diminished deep tendon reflexes of lower extremities; sensation intact, normal sphincter tone; unable to walk, mild ataxia in the upper extremities
k. Skin: dry and warm, no lesions or rash
l. Lymph: normal

H. Action

a. Obtain bedside spirometry testing; have respiratory therapist perform negative inspiratory force (NIF) and forced vital capacity (FVC).
b. Obtain consent from patient and perform lumbar puncture.
c. Ensure second large-bore IV access.

I. Results

Table 31.1 Results table

Test	Result	Test	Result
Complete blood count:		Alk phos	77 U/L
WBC	$5.2 \times 10^3/\mu L$	T bili	0.4 mg/dL
Hct	32.80%	D bili	0.1 mg/dL
Plt	$232 \times 10^3/\mu L$		
		Urinalysis:	
Basic metabolic panel:		SG	1.020
Na	142 mEq/L	pH	5
K	4.0 mEq/L	Prot	Neg
Cl	101 mEq/L	Gluc	Neg
CO_2	22 mEq/L	Ketones	Neg
BUN	14 mEq/dL	Bili	Neg
Cr	0.7 mg/dL	Blood	Neg

Table 31.1 (cont.)

Test	Result	Test	Result
Gluc	121 mg/dL	LE	Neg
		Nitrite	Neg
Coagulation panel:		Color	Yellow
PT	12.8 sec		
PTT	25.0 sec	Urine pregnancy:	Neg
INR	1.0		
		Arterial blood gas:	
Liver function panel:		pH	7.42
AST	24 U/L	pO_2	80 mmHg
ALT	17 U/L	pCO_2	48 mmHg
		HCO_3	25 mmol/L

a. ESR: 30 mm/hr
b. CSF results from lumbar puncture: protein 400, normal cell count and glucose, Gram stain negative
c. EKG (Figure 31.1)
d. CXR: Normal lungs, no acute pulmonary process

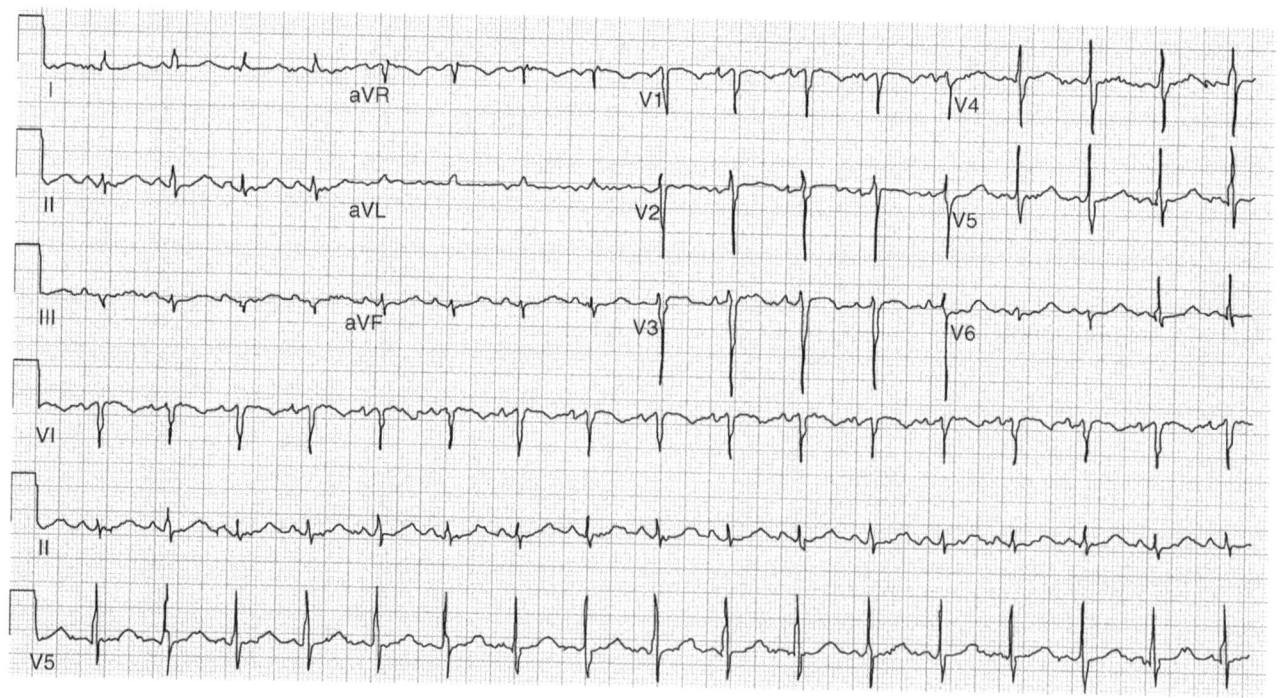

Figure 31.1

e. NIF below normal
f. FVC below normal

J. Nurse

a. Patient appears lethargic, more tachypneic, shallow breaths; O_2 sat 92% on 2 L via NC, complaining of increasing heaviness to head and now drooling.

K. Action

a. Place nonrebreather mask, prepare equipment for intubation.
b. After discussion with patient and family, perform intubation for declining respiratory status and airway protection.
c. Consult neurology.
d. Admission to ICU.
e. Administer IV immunoglobulin or plasma exchange.

L. Diagnosis

a. Guillain–Barre syndrome

M. Critical actions

a. Obtain fingerstick blood glucose.
b. Perform complete neurologic examination including motor, sensory, and reflexes.
c. Establish diagnosis of Guillain–Barre syndrome.
d. Neurology consultation.
e. Recognize worsening respiratory status, electively intubate.
f. Admission to ICU.
g. Begin plasma exchange or IV immunoglobulin.

N. Examiner instructions

a. This is a case of Guillain–Barre syndrome (GBS), an acute, immune-mediated inflammatory demyelinating polyneuropathy affecting the peripheral nerves. GBS is usually preceded by a viral illness, *Campylobacter jejuni* diarrheal infection, or recent vaccination. There are multiple variants of GBS; however, the typical presentation includes progressive ascending symmetrical weakness/paralysis with decreased or absent reflexes. There may be variable sensory findings along with autonomic dysfunction resulting in respiratory compromise requiring intubation. It is important to distinguish GBS symptoms from a central process such as stroke or spinal cord injury, metabolic disorders, or other causes of weakness. The candidate must recognize that the patient's symptoms have worsened based on clinical assessment or pulmonary function testing and intubation should be performed. A neurologist should be consulted, and the patient should be admitted to the ICU.
b. FVC < 12 mL/kg or NIF < 20 cmH_2O is an indication for intubation. If the patient is intubated using succinylcholine as a paralytic, the patient will lose pulses and demonstrate a wide-complex tachycardia (consistent with severe hyperkalemia) on the monitor. Standard ACLS protocols will be unsuccessful, unless calcium and other acute therapy for hyperkalemia are rapidly initiated.

O. Pearls

a. Initial treatment for GBS includes respiratory support, admission to a monitored setting, and neurological consultation.
b. Indications for intubation are largely clinical; however, some quantitative measures include a forced vital capacity less than 12 mL/kg, NIF less than 20 cmH_2O, aspiration, rapid progression of weakness, and autonomic instability.

c. Succinylcholine should not be used when intubating patients with GBS. As with any demyelinating disorder, acetyl cholinesterase receptors are upregulated. This can cause severe and prolonged hyperkalemia when a depolarizing neuromuscular blocker is used.

d. A lumbar puncture and/or nerve conduction study may help to diagnose GBS. The CSF analysis typically shows high protein and a normal cell count.

P. Figure legends

a. Figure 31.1 (EKG) Sinus tachycardia; prolonged QTc interval.

Q. References

a. *Tintinalli's Emergency Medicine: A Comprehensive Study Guide* (9th ed.): Chapter 172, Acute Peripheral Neurologic Disorders.

b. *Rosen's Emergency Medicine: Concepts and Clinical Practice* (10th ed.): Chapter 9, Weakness. Chapter 93, Peripheral Nerve Disorders.

Abdominal Pain and Vomiting

Linda Katirji, MD

A. Chief complaint
a. 67-year-old female with abdominal pain and vomiting

B. Vital signs
a. BP: 136/78, HR: 64, RR: 20, T: 35.9°C, Sat: 100% on RA

C. What does the patient look like?
a. Patient appears to be in severe pain, actively vomiting.

D. Primary survey
a. Airway: speaking in full sentences
b. Breathing: no apparent respiratory distress, no cyanosis
c. Circulation: dry and cool skin, normal capillary refill

E. Action
a. IV access
b. Labs
   i. CBC, BMP, LFT, lipase, INR/PT/PTT, blood type and crossmatch, lactate
c. 1 L NS bolus
d. EKG
e. Morphine IV
f. Zofran IV
g. Nothing by mouth (NPO)

F. History
a. HPI: A 67-year-old female with history of hypertension and asthma presents with lower abdominal pain for the past 2 days. The pain is intermittent, feels tight and squeezing, and has been increasing in severity. She developed nausea and vomiting within the past day and has not been able to tolerate anything by mouth. She denies diarrhea, fever, dysuria, chest pain, vaginal bleeding, or shortness of breath. Her last bowel movement was 3 days ago and normal in quality.
b. PMHx: hypertension, asthma
c. PSHx: appendectomy, tubal ligation, bladder surgery, hysterectomy
d. Allergies: none
e. Meds: esomeprazole, loratadine, gabapentin, fluticasone, zolpidem
f. Social: lives with family at home, denies alcohol, smoking, or drugs
g. FHx: not relevant

G. Nurse

a. EKG (Figure 32.1)
b. Vitals: BP: 136/78, HR: 64, RR: 20, T: 35.9°C, Sat: 100% on RA

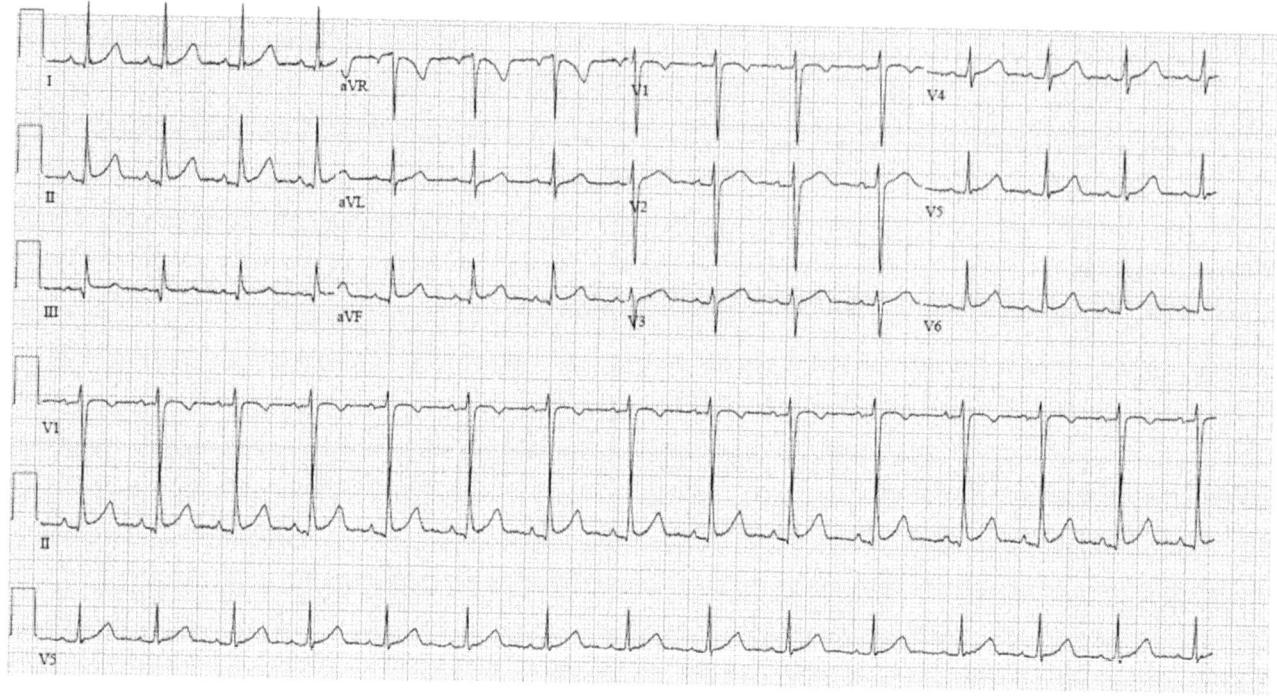

Figure 32.1

H. Secondary survey

a. General: alert and oriented, severe distress due to pain, vomiting
b. HEENT: normal
c. Neck: normal
d. Chest: normal
e. Heart: normal
f. Abdomen: bilateral lower quadrant tenderness with voluntary guarding; no rebound tenderness; bowel sounds normal, moderate distension, no masses, no hernias, nontender at McBurney's point, negative Murphy's sign
g. Rectal: hemoccult negative
h. Pelvic: normal
i. Extremities: normal
j. Back: normal
k. Neuro: normal
l. Skin: dry, no rash or induration
m. Lymph: normal

I. Action

a. Meds
    i. Morphine 4 mg IV
    ii. Zofran 4 mg IV
b. Reassess
    i. Patient continues to have significant discomfort, vomiting.

  c. Imaging
     i. Obstructive series (x-rays)
     ii. CT abdomen and pelvis with contrast
  d. Consult
     i. Surgery

J. Nurse

a. If IV fluids are given, vitals: BP: 113/65, HR: 60, RR: 18, Sat: 100% on RA
b. If fluids are not given, vitals: BP: 80/55, HR: 112, RR: 20, Sat: 100% on RA
c. Patient continues to have significant pain (until a total of 4 mg of IV morphine or equivalent is administered).

K. Results

Table 32.1 Results table

Test	Result	Test	Result
Complete blood count:		**Liver function panel:**	
WBC	$12.6 \times 10^3/\mu L$	AST	24 U/L
Hct	37.40%	ALT	22 U/L
Plt	$253 \times 10^3/\mu L$	Alk phos	181 U/L
		T bili	0.4 mg/dL
		D bili	0.2 mg/dL
Basic metabolic panel:		Amylase	71 U/L
Na	143 mEq/L	Lipase	77 U/L
K	4.1 mEq/L	Albumin	4.1 g/dL
Cl	105 mEq/L		
CO_2	25 mEq/L		
BUN	12 mEq/dL	**Urinalysis:**	
Cr	0.8 mg/dL	SG	1.022
Gluc	96 mg/dL	pH	6
		Prot	Neg
		Gluc	Neg
Coagulation panel:		Ketones	Neg
PT	11.9 sec	Bili	Neg
PTT	28 sec	Blood	Neg
INR	0.9	LE	Neg
		Nitrite	Neg
		Color	Yellow

a. Lactate: 1.9 mmol/L
b. Upright CXR and obstructive series (Figures 32.2–32.4)

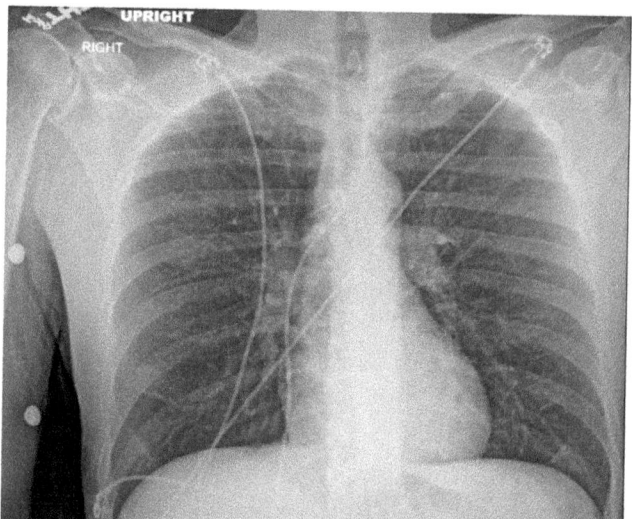

Figure 32.2

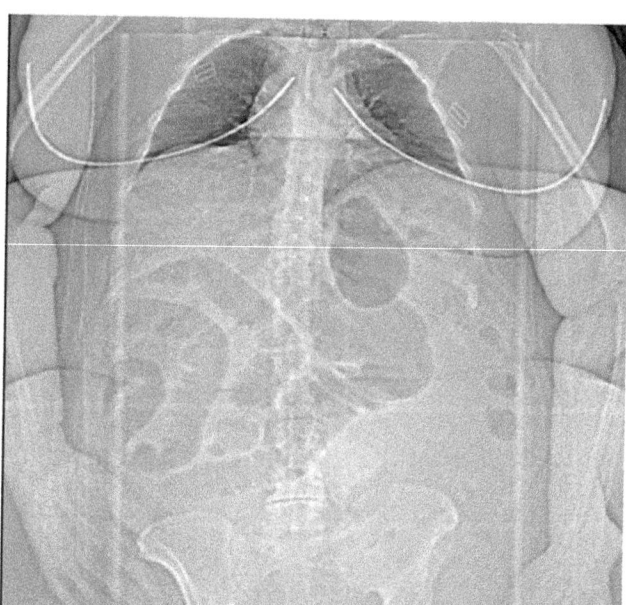

Figure 32.3

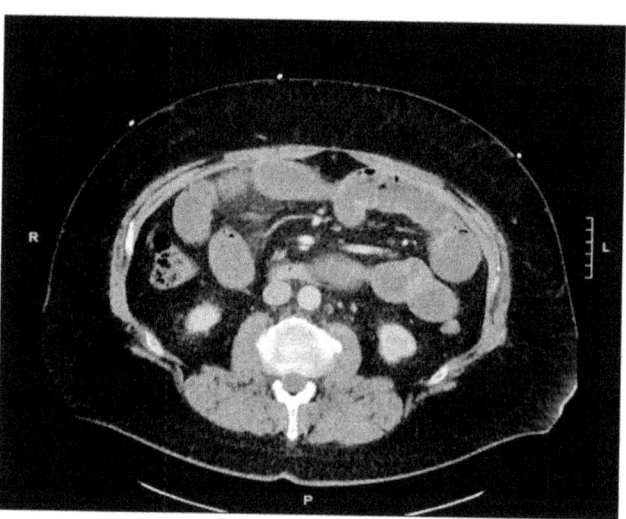

Figure 32.4

L. Action

a. Surgery consult
   i. Advocate for patient admission
b. Discuss need for admission with patient
c. Meds
   i. Morphine IV (if patient remains in significant pain)
   ii. Antiemetics IV
d. Nasogastric tube for decompression

M. Diagnosis

a. Small bowel obstruction (SBO)

N. Critical actions

a. IV access and fluid bolus
b. Obstructive series or CT scan (preferred)
c. Pain management
d. Surgery consult
e. NG tube

O. Examiner instructions

a. This is a case of small bowel obstruction (SBO). The patient is at increased risk of obstruction because of her prior abdominal surgeries, which can lead to scarring and adhesions that may block proper flow of intestinal contents. Important early actions include administering IV fluids, consulting surgery, decompressing the stomach, and pain control. If fluids are not administered, the patient may become tachycardic and hypotensive. Her pain will continue to increase until an opioid medication (e.g., morphine) is administered. If a nasogastric tube is not placed after diagnosis, the patient may continue vomiting and aspirate. If the patient is sent home, she should return to the ED in 2 hours with peritonitis.

P. Pearls

a. Obstructive series (plain abdominal films with the patient supine and then upright) with upright CXR are useful for ruling out free air, and may help localize causes and sites of obstruction. The x-rays may reveal distended loops of small bowel and the upright abdominal film may show a pattern of intestinal air–fluid levels arranged similarly to a stepladder proximal to the obstruction.
b. Abdominal CT with intravenous (and without oral) contrast is the imaging modality of choice according to the American College of Radiology Appropriateness Criteria. It may differentiate dynamic ileus from mechanical SBO, diagnose bowel strangulation (which can occur with incarcerated hernia), and may determine a specific transition point (such as a tumor) amenable to surgical intervention.
c. Middle-aged and elderly patients with epigastric pain should be evaluated for coronary ischemia. Non-chest pain presentations are common in this age group, especially upper abdominal pain and/or shortness of breath.
d. Patients should be hydrated with IV fluid to replace fluid loss (vomiting and intestinal third-spacing and lack of oral intake).
   If an immediate operation is advocated or if the patient has signs of peritonitis or ischemia, the
      ent should be given broad-spectrum antibiotics.
         G tube for gastric decompression.

g. Surgical intervention is often needed to correct obstruction, although a trial of medical management initially can be pursued for obstruction that has not been complicated by ischemia, peritonitis, or bowel perforation.

Q. Figure legends
a. Figure 32.1 (EKG) Normal sinus rhythm.
b. Figure 32.2 (Upright CXR) No free air beneath diaphragm.
c. Figure 32.3 (Abdominal XR) Dilated loops of bowel.
d. Figure 32.4 (Abdominal XR) Dilated loops of bowel and air-fluid levels.

R. References
a. *Tintinalli's Emergency Medicine: A Comprehensive Study Guide* (9th ed.): Chapter 83, Bowel Obstruction.
b. *Rosen's Emergency Medicine: Concepts and Clinical Practice* (10th ed.): Chapter 78, Small Intestine.

S. Acknowledgements
a. We would like to acknowledge Natasha Spencer for their contribution to this chapter in the previous edition of this book, which has been updated by Linda Katirji.

Chest Pain

Robert M. Hughes, DO

A. Chief complaint
a. 44-year-old male with chest pain

B. Vital signs
a. BP: 172/100, HR: 105, RR: 20, T: 36.1°C, Sat: 98% on RA

C. What does the patient look like?
a. Patient is clutching his chest and appears uncomfortable.

D. Primary survey
a. Airway: speaking in full sentences
b. Breathing: clear to auscultation bilaterally, no apparent respiratory distress, no cyanosis
c. Circulation: tachycardic, radial pulses 2+ bilaterally and are symmetric, capillary refill < 2 seconds

E. Action
a. Oxygen via nasal cannula or nonrebreather mask as needed to maintain >95% saturation
b. Two large-bore peripheral IV lines
c. Labs
    i. CBC, BMP, PT/PTT, troponin, type and screen
d. Cardiac monitor
e. Pulse oximetry
f. EKG
g. CXR – portable

F. History
a. HPI: A 44-year-old male with history of hypertension, diet-controlled diabetes, polysubstance use disorder, and schizophrenia presents with chest pain with onset 1 hour prior to arrival after smoking crack-cocaine. He describes the pain as crushing, radiating to the left neck and jaw as well as the left arm. He endorses shortness of breath, nausea, and diaphoresis. He denies radiation to the back or abdomen. He denies trauma. He has a history of similar events, but has not sought treatment as they were self-limited.
b. PMHx: hypertension, diet-controlled diabetes, schizophrenia
c. PSHx: none
d. Allergies: none
e. Meds: hydrochlorothiazide
f. Social: 1 pack per day tobacco use, crack-cocaine use disorder, alcohol use disorder, endorsing 3–6 12-ounce beers daily
g. FHx: no history of early cardiac disease in mother or father

G. Nurse
a. Vital signs
  i. BP: 170/95, HR: 108, RR: 20, Sat: 97% on RA
b. EKG (Figure 33.1)

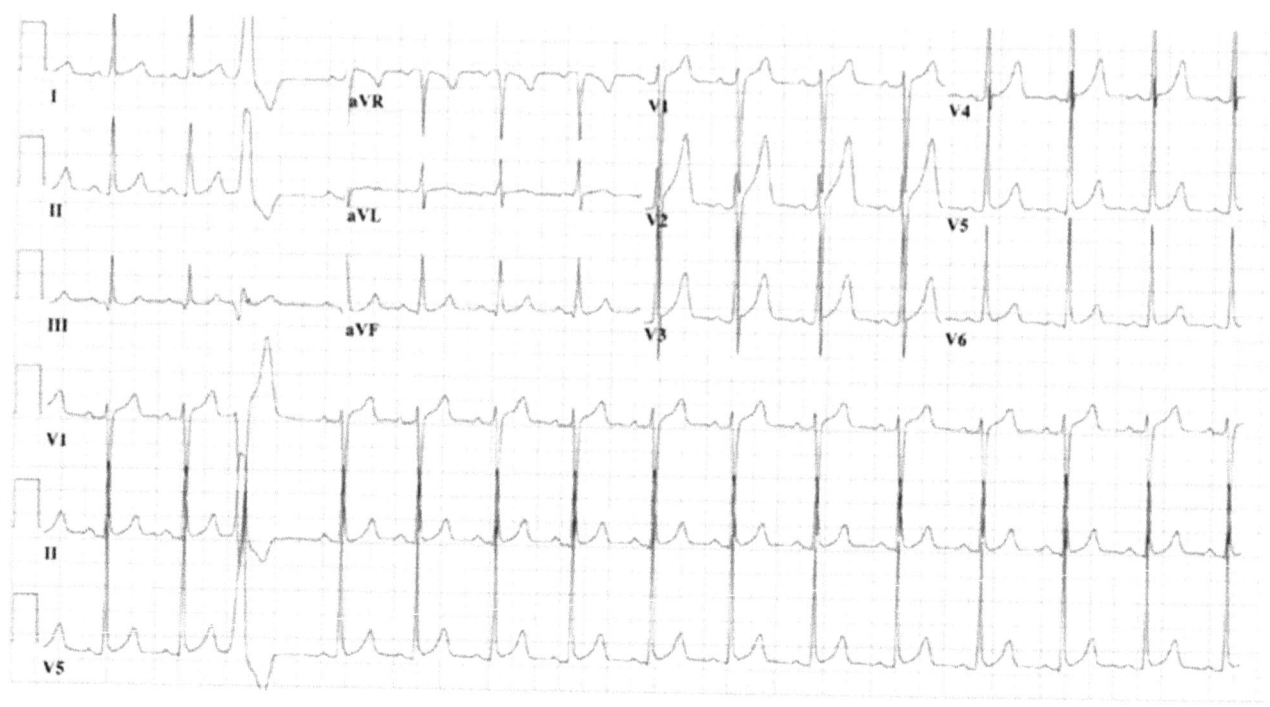

Figure 33.1

H. Secondary survey
a. General: alert and oriented to person, place and self, slightly agitated and uncomfortable due to chest pain
b. HEENT: pupils dilated bilaterally
c. Neck: supple, no tender thyromegaly, no jugular vein distension
d. Chest: breath sounds equal and without adventitious sounds; no respiratory distress; no chest tenderness
e. Heart: tachycardic, normal S1/S2, no murmur or rub; heart sounds clear and unmuffled
f. Abdomen: soft, nontender, and nondistended; no masses; bowel sounds normal; no guarding, no rebound
g. Extremities: no cyanosis, clubbing, or edema; joints without erythema or warmth
h. Back: no gross abnormalities, no bruising, no tenderness to palpation to entire spine
i. Neuro: normal gait; face symmetric; strength equal in upper and lower extremities; sensation intact and symmetric
j. Skin: warm, diaphoretic
k. Vascular: no carotid bruit; pulses 2+ and symmetric at radial, femoral, dorsalis pedis, and posterior tibial bilaterally

I. Action
a. Meds
  i. Lorazepam IV
  ii. Aspirin PO
  iii. Nitroglycerin sublingual

b. Reassess
   i. Patient less agitated; chest pain improved but still present
   ii. Repeat EKG – unchanged
   iii. Vital signs: BP: 138/81, HR: 90, RR: 16, Sat: 99% on NC O_2
c. Imaging
   i. Portable CXR (Figure 33.2)

J. Results

Table 33.1 Results table

Test	Result	Test	Result
Complete blood count:		Cr	1.0 mg/dL
WBC	$11.3 \times 10^3/\mu L$	Gluc	102 mg/dL
Hct	45.10%		
Plt	$401 \times 10^3/\mu L$	**Coagulation panel:**	
		PT	13.0 sec
Basic metabolic panel:		PTT	31.2 sec
Cl	97 mEq/L	INR	0.9
CO_2	21 mEq/L		
BUN	12 mEq/dL		

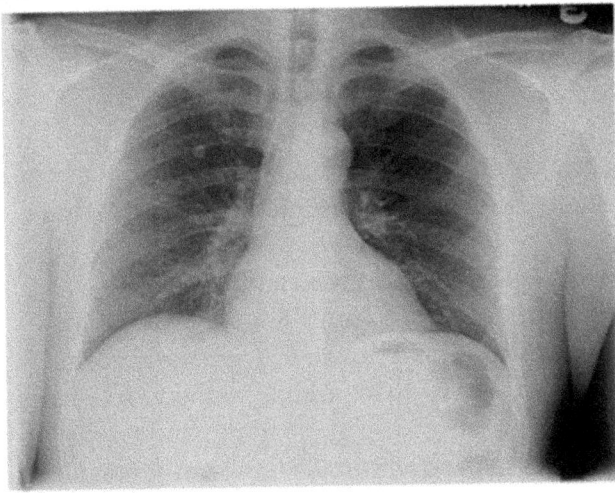

Figure 33.2

a. Type and screen: A+
b. Troponin: <0.02 ng/ml

K. Action
a. Patient admitted to observation unit for monitoring and serial troponins, given cocaine chest pain

L. Diagnosis

a. Cocaine-induced chest pain

M. Critical actions

a. EKG and monitor vital signs
b. Benzodiazepines
c. Nitrates
d. Aspirin
e. Troponin
f. CXR
g. Telemetry (hospital or observation unit admission) for cocaine-induced chest pain

N. Examiner instructions

a. This is a case of chest pain in the setting of cocaine use disorder. The patient's symptoms may be due to cocaine-induced vasoconstriction of the coronary arteries coupled with increased myocardial oxygen demand. Early critical actions include obtaining an EKG, administering nitrates for coronary vasodilation, giving aspirin, and giving benzodiazepines to control tachycardia and hypertension. Benzodiazepines are the recommended first-line agent for cocaine chest pain. If benzodiazepines are not administered, the patient will become more tachycardic and hypertensive. A CXR is important to rule out pulmonary etiologies that may result from cocaine-induced barotrauma, such as pneumothorax. If the patient is sent home before standard acute coronary syndrome workup, the patient should return to the ED in 2 hours with signs/symptoms of acute coronary syndrome.

O. Pearls

a. Chest pain in the context of cocaine use may be caused by etiologies that are cardiovascular (e.g., myocardial ischemia/infarction, aortic dissection, or endocarditis with septic pulmonary emboli) or noncardiac (e.g., those from inhalation-related barotraumas including pneumomediastinum, pneumothorax, pneumopericardium, pulmonary hemorrhage/infarction).
b. Cocaine itself can cause coronary vasospasm, secondary increased myocardial oxygen demand, and resultant ischemic pain. Long-term use of cocaine can serve as an independent risk factor for coronary artery disease and resultant acute coronary syndromes.
c. Benzodiazepines (e.g., lorazepam or diazepam) are useful to treat hypertension and tachycardia and thus reduce myocardial oxygen demand. Avoid haloperidol, droperidol, and chlorpromazine, as they may contribute to hyperthermia and may lower the seizure threshold.
d. Treat potential ischemia or acute coronary syndrome according to standard protocol, including nitrates (unless you suspect a right-sided or posterior infarction and preload dependence), morphine, supplemental oxygen (as needed, titrate to a saturation of >92%), aspirin, and possible heparin and stress test and/or cardiac catheterization.
e. Use morphine with caution in acute ST-elevation myocardial infarction (STEMI). It may precipitate hypotension in preload-dependent lesions (such as a right-sided or posterior STEMI) due to peripheral vasodilation and decreased venous return. It may also impair gastrointestinal absorption of secondary antiplatelet agents, such as clopidogrel or ticagrelor.
f. Traditionally, β-adrenergic antagonists have been avoided because of concern that unopposed α-adrenergic stimulation may exacerbate symptoms. Consider IV phentolamine for patients with ischemic EKG changes and persistent hypertension and chest pain that have not responded to first-line medications.

g. Tachydysrhythmias or QRS-complex prolongation can be treated with sodium bicarbonate in order to alkalinize the serum to a target pH of 7.45–7.5.

P. Figure legends
a. Figure 33.1 (EKG) Normal sinus rhythm with PVC.
b. Figure 33.2 (CXR) Normal chest x-ray.

Q. References
a. *Tintinalli's Emergency Medicine: A Comprehensive Study Guide* (9th ed.): Chapter 187, Cocaine and Amphetamines.
b. *Rosen's Emergency Medicine: Concepts and Clinical Practice* (10th ed.): Chapter 144, Cocaine and Other Sympathomimetics.

R. Acknowledgements
a. We would like to acknowledge Natasha Spencer for their contribution to this chapter in the previous edition of this book, which has been updated by Robert M. Hughes.

Seizure

Sylvia E. Garcia, MD

A. Chief complaint
a. 22-month-old female with generalized shaking

B. Vital signs
a. HR: 135, RR: 35, BP: 98/54, T: 38.5°C, Sat: 98% on RA

C. What does the patient look like?
a. Patient appears well, but is crying, yet easily consoled by parents.

D. Primary survey
a. Airway: crying
b. Breathing: clear lungs bilaterally, no nasal flaring, no retractions, no cyanosis
c. Circulation: normal capillary refill, warm extremities

E. History
a. HPI: A 22-month-old female with no past medical history, developmentally normal, presents after a generalized shaking episode 45 minutes ago. An hour ago, the patient was noted to have a tactile fever and was given ibuprofen. Fifteen minutes later, while lying in bed watching TV with her mother, she was noted to have generalized, rhythmic shaking of all extremities with eyes rolling back. The episode lasted for 5 minutes, after which the patient was sleepy. No incontinence was noted. The patient has had rhinorrhea for the past 2 days, but no cough, vomiting, diarrhea, or fever before today. The patient had a recent normal well-child check.
b. PMHx: none; born at term; immunizations up-to-date
c. PSHx: none
d. Allergies: none
e. Meds: ibuprofen
f. Social: lives with family at home
g. FHx: none

F. Action
a. Acetaminophen PO or PR

G. Nurse
a. Vital signs
    i. HR: 135, RR: 35, BP: 98/54, T: 38.5°C, Sat: 98% on RA, Wt: 24.5 kg
b. Finger stick glucose: 85 mg/dL (must ask)

H. Secondary survey

a. General: well-appearing, alert, active, in no apparent distress
b. HEENT: normocephalic, atraumatic; normal tympanic membrane; oropharynx is clear
c. Neck: shotty LAD, supple
d. Chest: normal
e. Heart: normal
f. Abdomen: normal
g. Extremities: normal
h. Back: normal
i. Neuro: awake, alert, appropriate for age; gait normal for age; can reach, grab, and hold onto objects with each hand
j. Skin: warm and dry, no rash or induration, no petechiae
k. Lymph: normal

I. Action

a. Reassess
   i. Patient in no apparent distress, playing with blocks
b. Discussion with patient's parents about diagnosis, prevention, precautions, and follow-up
c. Discharge patient home with outpatient pediatrician follow-up

J. Results

Table 34.1 Results table

Test	Result	Test	Result
Complete blood count:		**Urinalysis:**	
WBC	$11.5 \times 10^3/\mu L$	SG	1.010
Hct	33.90%	pH	5.5
Plt	$350 \times 10^3/\mu L$	Prot	Neg
		Gluc	Neg
		Ketones	Neg
Basic metabolic panel:		Bili	Neg
Na	134 mEq/L	Blood	Neg
K	4.2 mEq/L	LE	Neg
Cl	101 mEq/L	Nitrite	Neg
CO_2	24 mEq/L	Color	Yellow
BUN	13 mEq/dL		
Cr	0.4 mg/dL		
Gluc	90 mg/dL		

K. Diagnosis

a. Simple febrile seizure

L. Critical actions

a. Detailed history and physical examination to assess risk for meningitis or serious bacterial infection, and identify any symptoms or focal findings to direct workup.

b. Acetaminophen administered every 4 hours and/or ibuprofen every 6 hours to reduce fever.
c. Counsel parents about simple febrile seizures and follow-up.

M. Examiner instructions

a. This is a case of a simple febrile seizure, typically lasting <15 minutes and generalized in nature, occurring in children aged 6 months to 5 years. This patient's seizure is unlikely due to central nervous system (CNS) infection. Important early actions include a careful history and physical examination. If acetaminophen or ibuprofen has not been given, the fever will persist and the patient may seize again. If labs are drawn, the WBC count will be slightly elevated. If a lumbar puncture (LP) is performed, it will be normal. If a neurological consult is called, they will suggest sending the child home without blood work or an LP.

N. Pearls

a. Any child who is actively seizing in the ED should be presumed to be in status epilepticus and treated accordingly (oxygen, monitor, medication to stop seizure, identification and treatment of triggers, and further evaluation/treatment of etiology).
b. A simple febrile seizure can be presumed in children aged 5 months to 5 years with a normal neurological examination after a generalized seizure lasting less than 15 minutes in the setting of fever (≥100.4°F or 38°C by any method).
c. Laboratory evaluation (beside a glucose finger stick), neuroimaging, lumbar puncture, and hospitalization are almost never needed for children with a simple febrile seizure. Any workup or treatment should be aimed at identifying the infectious etiology based on concerning symptoms and/or focal physical findings on exam.
d. A lumbar puncture, however, is recommended for the ill-appearing child or those with concerning signs and symptoms suggesting meningitis or an intracranial infection. It should also be considered in patients between 6 and 12 months of age who have not received *Haemophilus influenzae* type b (Hib) or *Streptococcus pneumoniae* immunizations appropriate for their age or if immunization status cannot be confirmed; for children 12 months and older with a first-time focal seizure; for toxic-appearing patients who have not returned to baseline in the postictal period; or if the patient had already been receiving antibiotic treatment.
e. Treatment of simple febrile seizure is aimed at its etiology; acetaminophen or ibuprofen should be given to treat fevers.
f. Hospitalization for children with a simple febrile seizure is not needed unless the seizure recurs within several hours to 1 day and/or if the fever has a complicated etiology not easily treated at home.

O. References

a. *Tintinalli's Emergency Medicine: A Comprehensive Study Guide* (9th ed.): Chapter 138, Seizures in Infants and Children.
b. *Rosen's Emergency Medicine: Concepts and Clinical Practice* (10th ed.): Chapter 161, Pediatric Fever.

P. Acknowledgements

a. We would like to acknowledge Natasha Spencer for their contribution to this chapter in the previous edition of this book, which has been updated by Sylvia E. Garcia.

Chest Pain

Sean Abraham, DO

A. Chief complaint
a. 45-year-old female with chest pain

B. Vital signs
a. BP: 125/79, HR: 122, RR: 18, T: 37.3°C, Sat: 98% on RA

C. What does the patient look like?
a. She appears comfortable, in no significant distress.

D. Primary survey
a. Airway: speaking in full sentences
b. Breathing: no apparent respiratory distress, no cyanosis; clear lungs bilaterally
c. Circulation: radial pulses 2+ bilaterally, normal capillary refill

E. Action
a. EKG
b. Place on a cardiac monitor
c. Obtain IV access

F. History
a. HPI: A 45-year-old female presents with chest pain for 1 day. The pain is located in the right chest under the breast, is stabbing, radiates to her back, and is worse with breathing. The pain is accompanied by shortness of breath. She denies cough, fever, or trauma.
b. PMHx: obesity
c. PSHx: tonsillectomy
d. Allergies: none
e. Meds: none
f. Social: denies alcohol, smoking, or drugs
g. FHx: hypertension, high cholesterol

G. Nurse
a. EKG (Figure 35.1)

H. Secondary survey
a. General: alert and oriented, no apparent distress
b. HEENT: normal
c. Neck: normal
d. Chest: chest is nontender; breath sounds normal; no respiratory distress

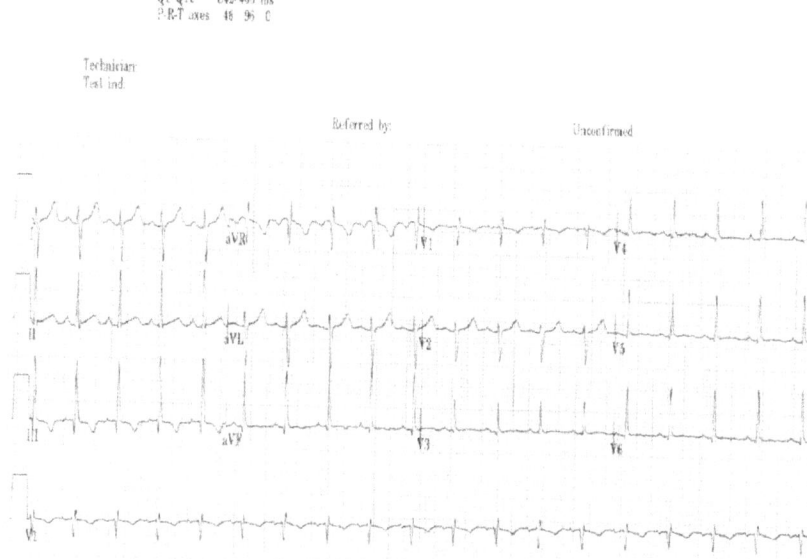

Figure 35.1

e. Heart: tachycardic and regular; normal S1/S2; no murmurs, gallops, or rub; no lower extremity edema
f. Abdomen: soft and nontender to palpation, bowel sounds present
g. Rectal: hemoccult negative
h. Extremities: no edema; normal capillary refill; no calf tenderness; 2+ pulses in all four extremities
i. Back: normal
j. Neuro: normal
k. Skin: warm and dry; no rash, erythema, or induration
l. Lymph: normal

I. Action
a. Two large-bore peripheral IV lines
b. Labs
   i.   CBC, BMP, troponin, INR/PT/PTT, urine or serum hCG, consider BNP, consider D-dimer
c. Monitor
d. Analgesia (acetaminophen PO or morphine IV)

J. Action
a. Monitor: BP: 116/78, HR: 120, RR: 18, Sat: 98% on RA
b. Reassess
   i.   If analgesia is given, the patient is without pain; comfortable
c. Imaging
   i.   CXR (Figure 35.2)

Case 35: Chest Pain

K. Nurse
a.   Repeat vitals: BP: 114/55, HR: 115, RR: 20, Sat: 99% on RA

L. Results

Table 35.1 Results table

Test	Result	Test	Result
Complete blood count:		**Coagulation panel:**	
WBC	$5 \times 10^3/\mu L$	PT	13.5 sec
Hgb	11.3 g/dL	PTT	30 sec
Hct	35.70%	INR	1.0
Plt	$339 \times 10^3/\mu L$		
		Troponin	0.12 ng/ml*
Basic metabolic panel:		HCG	<2 mIU/mL
Na	142 mEq/L	D-dimer	1290 ng/mL
K	4.1 mEq/L	BNP	16 pg/mL
Cl	104 mEq/L		
CO_2	25 mEq/L		
BUN	10 mEq/dL		
Cr	0.7 mg/dL		
Gluc	84 mg/dL		

*normal < 0.04 ng/ml

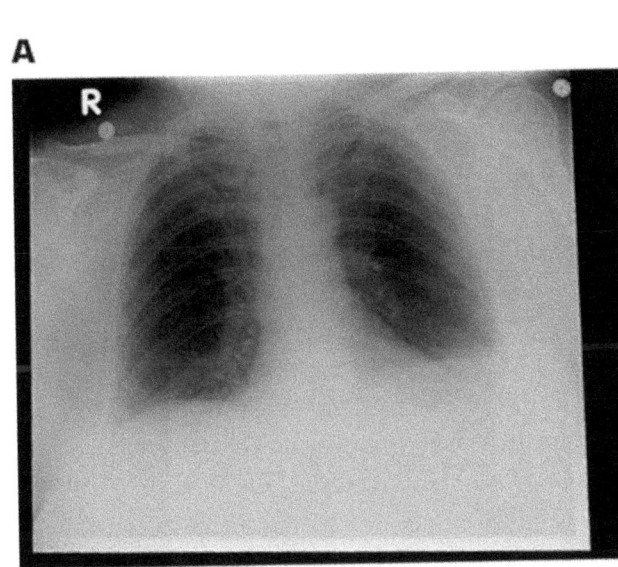

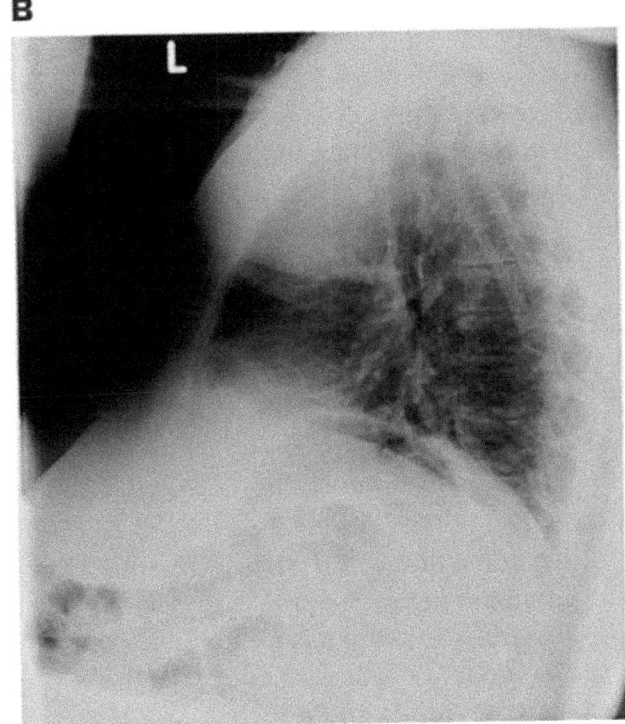

Figure 35.2

a. (If requested) bedside transthoracic echocardiogram shows right ventricular dilation with apical hyperkinesis, normal left ventricular ejection fraction, and no pericardial effusion.

M. Action
a. Chest CT angiogram with IV contrast – multiple segmental emboli in right pulmonary vasculature
b. Ventilation-perfusion scan (VQ scan) (if ordered instead of CT) – high probability of PE

N. Action
a. Discussion with patient regarding findings, need for treatment, and admission
b. Admit patient to medicine service for continued anticoagulation
c. Medications
   i. Heparin sodium bolus and drip or low-molecular-weight heparin or novel oral anticoagulant
   ii. Analgesics as needed for pain (avoid nonaspirin NSAIDS, given need for anticoagulation)
   iii. Consider giving aspirin due to elevated troponin

O. Diagnosis
a. Pulmonary embolism (PE)

P. Critical actions
a. EKG
b. CXR
c. Chest CT angiogram or VQ scan
d. Initiation of anticoagulation
e. Admit patient for anticoagulation and monitoring

Q. Examiner instructions
a. Although this is a case of pulmonary embolism (PE), the candidate should demonstrate the ability to evaluate undifferentiated chest pain. Early EKG (to evaluate for cardiac ischemia) is essential for expedient diagnosis of STEMI and the need for time-sensitive interventions. Chest x-ray in PE is most commonly normal, but may demonstrate pleural effusion, wedge-shaped peripheral infarction (Hampton's hump) or abrupt cutoff of the pulmonary vasculature (Westermark sign). If a D-dimer is ordered, it is elevated and definitive imaging should be ordered.
b. If the patient is discharged home without diagnosing the PE, they will collapse and experience cardiac arrest in the parking lot. While there is growing evidence that some patients with PE can be safely treated as outpatients, this patient is a poor candidate for outpatient treatment given her persistent tachycardia. If the candidate considers discharge, the patient will have no insurance and no primary care doctor for follow-up, thus making outpatient treatment impractical.

R. Pearls
a. Estimating the pretest probability for PE is useful to guide workup of chest pain. The PERC (pulmonary embolism rule-out criteria) rule is often used. When the clinician's pretest probability of pulmonary embolism is less than 15% and all clinical criteria are present, there is less than a 2% chance of PE.
b. Low-risk criteria for PE include

    i. Age < 50 years

    ii. Pulse rate < 100 bpm

    iii. O_2 sat > 94%

    iv. No history of hemoptysis, unilateral leg swelling, recent major surgery or trauma, prior PE or DVT, or exogenous estrogen use

c. Obtaining a D-dimer is most useful among patients with a low level of suspicion for PE, as PE can be ruled out with a negative quantitative D-dimer assay. If the D-dimer is positive in such patients, however, either a negative CT or a normal VQ scan can rule out the diagnosis.

d. ABG and CXR are nonspecific for PE, but may show hypoxemia or basilar atelectasis, respectively. These studies may also be helpful when evaluating alternative diagnoses. EKG is also nonspecific for PE, but may show a pattern consistent with right heart strain (tachycardia, T wave inversions in V1–4, S1Q3T3 pattern, and/or right bundle branch block).

e. PE is treated with anticoagulation. Traditionally, unfractionated heparin or low-molecular-weight heparin (LMWH) have been used. If a major contraindication to heparin is present (e.g., recent large cerebral infarction or major trauma), consider emergent inferior vena cava filter placement. Consider thrombolysis (e.g., with alteplase) for patients with cardiorespiratory collapse due to PE. Newer oral anticoagulants have been introduced that may also be used in lieu of "bridging" heparin to warfarin.

f. In clinical practice, while it may be reasonable to consider outpatient treatment for select patients with pulmonary emboli, this is still somewhat controversial. Doing so would be unadvisable on an oral board examination.

S. Figure legends

a. Figure 35.1 (EKG) Sinus rhythm with S1Q3T3 pattern, suggestive of right ventricular strain.

b. Figure 35.2 (X-ray) No pulmonary infiltrates, small left pleural effusion.

T. References

a. *Tintinalli's Emergency Medicine: A Comprehensive Study Guide* (9th ed.): Chapter 56, Venous Thromboembolism Including Pulmonary Embolism.

b. *Rosen's Emergency Medicine: Concepts and Clinical Practice* (10th ed.): Chapter 74, Pulmonary Embolism and Deep Vein Thrombosis.

U. Acknowledgements

a. We would like to acknowledge Natasha Spencer for their contribution to this chapter in the previous edition of this book, which has been updated by Sean Abraham.

Throat Swelling

Nicole Gerber, MD

A. Chief complaint
a. 5-year-old male with funny feeling in his throat

B. Vital signs
a. BP: 82/50, HR: 170, RR: 30, T: 36.5°C, Sat: 93% on RA, Wt: 18.4 kg

C. What does the patient look like?
a. Sitting up in bed, intermittently coughing, erythematous skin, anxious appearing

D. Primary survey
a. Airway: answering questions in short sentences
b. Breathing: intermittent coughing, diffuse inspiratory wheezing bilaterally, no accessory muscle use or retractions
c. Circulation: tachycardic, normal capillary refill

E. Action
a. Oxygen via NC as needed to maintain >95% saturation
b. Two large-bore peripheral IV lines
c. Monitor

F. History
a. HPI: A 5-year-old male with known peanut allergy and asthma presents with coughing, rash, and anxiety after eating a cookie at a birthday party. About 20 minutes after eating it, he developed a rash with itching as well as some abdominal pain. He had one episode of emesis and was reporting some difficulty breathing and a funny feeling in his throat. Mom called a taxi to take him to the ED.
b. PMHx: asthma – no history of intubations or PICU admission
c. PSHx: none
d. Allergies: peanuts – no prior history of anaphylaxis
e. Meds: albuterol prn
f. Social: lives at home with family
g. FHx: not relevant

G. Action
a. Epinephrine (0.01 mg/kg of 1 mg/mL concentration, or 0.15 mg) IM
b. NS 360 mL (20 mL/kg) IV bolus

   c. Albuterol nebulizer
   d. Diphenhydramine IV
   e. Ranitidine IV
   f. Methylprednisolone IV

H. Nurse
   a. Reassess vital signs
      a. BP: 85/50, HR: 140, RR: 28, T: 36.6°C, Sat: 100% while receiving albuterol

II. Secondary survey
   a. General: alert, sitting up in bed, uncomfortable appearing
   b. HEENT: no tongue or lip swelling, no uvular swelling, airway grossly patent
   c. Neck: normal, no stridor
   d. Chest: occasional cough; diffuse expiratory wheezing bilaterally; no accessory muscle use or retractions
   e. Heart: tachycardic, no murmurs
   f. Abdomen: soft, mild tenderness is epigastrium, no masses, bowel sounds normal, no distension, no peritoneal signs
   g. Pelvic: deferred
   h. Extremities: normal
   i. Back: normal
   j. Neuro: awake, alert, appropriate for age
   k. Skin: diffuse erythema with scattered raised urticarial lesions
   l. Lymph: normal

J. Action
   a. Reassess after medications administered
      i. Patient able to speak in full sentences, erythema improving
      ii. BP: 94/58, HR: 110, RR: 24, T: 36.0°C, Sat: 97% on RA
   b. Observation for 6 hours in the ED
      i. Patient not coughing; is speaking in full sentences, rash resolved
      ii. BP: 96/52, HR: 100, RR: 24, Sat: 98% on RA
   c. Counsel parents about avoiding allergen
   d. Give parents prescription for two epinephrine autoinjectors
   e. Discharge patient home with pediatrician and allergist outpatient follow-up

K. Diagnosis
   a. Anaphylaxis

L. Critical actions
   a. Airway assessment
   b. Oxygen
   c. Epinephrine IM
   d. NS (20 mg/kg) IV bolus
   e. Observation for at least 6 hours
   f. If discharged, should be given a prescription for two epinephrine autoinjectors and told to avoid the allergic trigger

M. Examiner instructions

a. This is a case of anaphylaxis, a severe multiorgan system type 1 allergic reaction. If epinephrine is not given, respiratory distress should worsen. If ENT or anesthesia are consulted, they should say they are at another emergency and will be down after about 30 minutes. If the patient is monitored for less than 4 hours, the patient will have a relapse of respiratory distress. Any labs requested will be normal.

N. Pearls

a. Anaphylaxis is characterized by acute onset of involvement of two or more organ symptoms including skin, respiratory, GI, and vascular, or by reduced BP after a known allergen exposure.

b. Half of fatalities from anaphylaxis happen within the first hour. Fatalities occur from bronchospasm, laryngoedema, and/or cardiovascular collapse.

c. Epinephrine is the mainstay of therapy. Epinephrine should be administered via IM injection into the lateral thigh, and can be given every 5–10 minutes and there are no absolute contraindications to administering it. If refractory or hemodynamically unstable, the drug should be administered intravenously via infusion. Hypotensive patients who are not responding to IV fluids and epinephrine can be given additional vasopressors.

d. Fluid resuscitation is critical in anaphylaxis. Multiple fluid boluses may be required, as this is a cause of distributive shock.

e. Second-line therapy for anaphylaxis includes diphenhydramine, H2 receptor blockers like ranitidine, inhaled β-agonists, and corticosteroids.

f. Consider early endotracheal intubation for severe bronchospasm or angioedema as delay may result in complete airway obstruction. When preparing for intubation, consider adjuncts such as video laryngoscopy, gum elastic bougie, or other tools, as intubation may be difficult.

g. The risk of biphasic reaction may be as high as 20%, and typically occurs within the first 8 hours. Patients who remain without symptoms after treatment can be discharged home after 4–6 hours of observation. Patients who require ongoing treatment despite initial therapy should be admitted to an ICU.

O. References

a. *Tintinalli's Emergency Medicine: A Comprehensive Study Guide* (9th ed.): Chapter 27, Anaphylaxis, Acute Allergic Reactions and Angioedema.

b. *Rosen's Emergency Medicine: Concepts and Clinical Practice* (10th ed.): Chapter 106, Allergy, Anaphylaxis, and Angioedema.

P. Acknowledgements

a. We would like to acknowledge Natasha Spencer for their contribution to this chapter in the previous edition of this book, which has been updated by Nicole Gerber.

Abdominal Pain

Ani Aydin, MD

A. Chief complaint
a. 24-year-old female with nausea, vomiting, and abdominal pain

B. Vital signs
a. BP: 120/80, HR: 90, RR: 12, T: 38.2°C, Sat: 98% on RA

C. What does the patient look like?
a. The patient appears as her stated age. She is uncomfortable and is lying supine and still in the stretcher.

D. Primary survey
a. Airway: speaking in full sentences
b. Breathing: no apparent respiratory distress, no cyanosis, clear lungs
c. Circulation: regular rate and rhythm, pale and cool skin, radial pulses 2+ bilaterally, normal capillary refill

E. Action
a. IV access
b. Labs
   i. CBC, BMP, pregnancy test, type and screen, urinalysis
c. Place the patient on the monitor
d. Nothing by mouth (NPO)
e. Analgesia as needed
f. Antiemetics as needed
g. Hydration as needed

F. Nurse.
a. Pain assessment after opioids: 6/10

G. History
a. HPI: A 24-year-old female presents with abdominal pain, nausea, vomiting, and decreased oral intake for 1 day, now with worsened abdominal pain for the past 3 hours. The abdominal pain started acutely yesterday, initially in her lower abdomen, and is now localized to the right lower quadrant. She states that the pain is now more severe. She complains of nausea and vomiting (nonbloody) today. She complains of a subjective fever, but did not take her temperature at home. Her last menstrual period was 2 weeks ago. The patient denies any diarrhea, dysuria, or hematuria, vaginal bleeding or discharge, chest pain, shortness of

breath, rectal bleeding, history of sexually transmitted diseases, or other pertinent history of gynecologic problems.
b. PMHx: none.
c. P OB/Gyn Hx: nulliparous.
d. PSHx: none
e. Allergies: none
f. Meds: none
g. Social: lives with husband at home; denies alcohol, smoking, or drugs; sexually active only with her husband, no condom use
h. FHx: not relevant
i. PMD: Dr. Miller

H. Secondary survey
a. General: alert and oriented, moderate distress due to pain in her abdomen
b. HEENT: normal
c. Neck: normal
d. Chest: normal
e. Heart: normal
f. Abdomen: tender to palpation in right lower quadrant, with voluntary guarding, no rebound tenderness, bowel sounds present, no pulsatile masses, no masses, no hernia, negative Murphy's sign, tenderness at McBurney's point, positive Rovsing sign, negative psoas and obturator signs
g. Rectal: no rectal mass, no gross blood, hemoccult negative brown stool
h. Pelvic:
    i.   External vagina: normal
    ii. Speculum: no blood or lesions in vaginal vault, cervix normal
    iii. BME: no suprapubic tenderness to palpation (TTP), no cervical motion tenderness (CMT), no ovarian masses or TTP, internal os closed
i. Extremities: normal
j. Back: normal
k. Neuro: normal
l. Skin: normal
m. Lymph: normal

I. Action
a. Meds
    i.   Analgesia as needed (e.g., morphine IV)
    ii. Antiemetics as needed
    iii. Hydration as needed
b. Reassess
    i.   Serial abdominal examination – unchanged from prior
c. Imaging
    i.   CT abdomen/pelvis with oral contrast
        1. Some institutions may perform the CT imaging studies without oral contrast, depending on the generation of CT scanner and/or expertise of the radiologist.
        2. Alternatively, given the patient's young age, an RLQ ultrasound would be a good initial examination, with the understanding that an equivocal study with a high-risk probability should prompt additional CT imaging.

Case 37: Abdominal Pain

   d. Surgery consultation
      i. Appendicitis is a clinical diagnosis and surgical consultation should be obtained in cases of high suspicion prior to imaging results.

J. Nurse
   a. BP: 120/80, HR: 90, RR: 12, T: 38.2°C, Sat: 100% on RA
   b. Patient still with significant pain

K. Results

Table 37.1 Results table

Test	Result	Test	Result
Complete blood count:		**Coagulation panel:**	
WBC	$15.1 \times 10^3/\mu L$	PT	14 sec
Hct	40.50%	PTT	31 sec
Plt	$253 \times 10^3/\mu L$	INR	1.0
Basic metabolic panel:		**Urinalysis:**	
Na	139 mEq/L	SG	1.022
K	4.2 mEq/L	pH	6
Cl	101 mEq/L	Prot	Neg
CO_2	23 mEq/L	Gluc	Neg
BUN	10 mEq/dL	Ketones	Neg
Cr	1.0 mg/dL	Bili	Neg
Gluc	90 mg/dL	Blood	Neg
		LE	Neg
		Nitrite	Neg
		Color	Yellow

   a. Urine pregnancy test: negative
   b. CT abdomen/pelvis: acute appendicitis

L. Action
   a. Surgery consultation
      i. To OR for appendectomy
   b. Discussion with family and PMD need for emergent OR and diagnosis of appendicitis
   c. Blood cultures
   d. IV fluids: 20–30 cc/kg crystalloid bolus
   e. Medications
      i. Antibiotics IV
         1. ciprofloxacin IV and metronidazole IV, or
         2. ampicillin–sulbactam IV, or
         3. piperacillin-tazobactam

    ii. Antiemetics, as needed

    iii. Analgesics, as needed

M. Diagnosis

a. Acute appendicitis

N. Critical actions

a. Urine pregnancy test
b. Urinalysis
c. Pelvic examination in woman of child-bearing age with lower abdominal pain and tenderness
d. Pain management
e. Antibiotics preoperatively
f. Serial abdominal examination
g. CT abdomen/pelvis or RLQ US
h. Surgery consultation for operative management

O. Examiner instructions

a. This is a case of acute appendicitis in a young woman of child-bearing age. Important early actions include administration of pain medication and antiemetics as needed, and obtaining an appropriate imaging study to evaluate the etiology of her RLQ abdominal pain. A urine pregnancy test and pelvic examination should be performed in this patient to evaluate for an alternative etiology of her RLQ abdominal pain. A CT abdomen/pelvis should be obtained, but an ultrasound can be considered as a first step in a younger patient to avoid excess radiation exposure.

P. Pearls

a. Appendicitis is a clinical diagnosis – early actions (such as surgical consultation) should be undertaken before imaging results in patient with a high pretest probability. If perforation is suspected, antibiotics should be administered and surgery consulted early in the examination.
b. Vital signs are often normal, especially early in appendicitis; the patient may have a low-grade fever.
c. CT abdomen/pelvis (with or without enteric contrast) should be performed in males and women of nonchild-bearing age with equivocal signs.
d. An ultrasound can be used as a first step in children, pregnant women, and women of child-bearing age with a possible pelvic etiology of pain. However, this is often operator- and institution-dependent, and the sensitivity of the test is not sufficient to rule out appendicitis. An MRI should be considered in pregnant women, with early OB consultation as well.
e. Pregnant women have the same risk of appendicitis as the general population; appendicitis is most common during the second trimester.
f. Perforation is more likely at the extremes of age.
g. It is unlikely that pain medication will mask the abdominal findings of appendicitis, so there is no clinical benefit to withholding analgesia when needed.
h. Peritoneal signs are ominous, and often suggest a surgical emergency; rebound tenderness is a late finding.
i. Uncomplicated appendicitis has a 0.1% mortality; this rate rises to 3–4% with perforation.

Q. References

a. *Tintinalli's Emergency Medicine: A Comprehensive Study Guide* (9th ed.): Chapter 81, Acute Appendicitis.

b. *Rosen's Emergency Medicine: Concepts and Clinical Practice* (10th ed.): Chapter 79, Acute Appendicitis.

Altered Mental Status

Ani Aydin, MD

A. Chief complaint
a. 85-year-old male with altered mental status

B. Vital signs
a. BP: 135/70, HR: 88, RR: 13, T: 36°C, Sat: 97% on RA

C. What does the patient look like?
a. Patient appears older than stated age, sleeping on stretcher but arousable and cooperative.

D. Primary survey
a. Airway: speaking in full sentences
b. Breathing: no apparent respiratory distress, no cyanosis, clear lungs
c. Circulation: pale and cool skin, regular rate and rhythm, radial pulses 2+, normal capillary refill
d. Neuro: alert and oriented to name and place only, follows simple commands, confused

E. Action
a. Peripheral IV line
b. Finger stick blood glucose (107 mg/dL; must ask)
c. Labs
   i. CBC, Chem 7, LFT, UA/urine culture, PT/PTT/INR
d. Cardiac monitor
e. EKG
f. CXR

F. History
a. HPI: An 85-year-old male was brought from home via ambulance with complaints of increased confusion. As per the patient's wife, he has been increasingly confused over the last 2 days. His wife relays that today he had difficulty recalling his address or phone number. Of note, the patient tripped and fell in his bathroom 3 days ago, no known loss of consciousness, with complaints of a headache since that time. He complains of a frontal headache, no radiation, constant, no alleviating or aggravating factors. He denies neck pain, photophobia or phonophobia, changes in vision or hearing, arm or leg weakness or numbness, nausea or vomiting, lightheadedness or dizziness. He also denies any shortness of breath, chest pain, abdominal pain, dysuria, hematuria, blood per rectum, fever, or chills. There have been no changes in his appetite.
b. PMHx: hypertension, hypercholesterolemia
c. PSHx: umbilical hernia repair 20 years ago
d. Allergies: none

Case 38: Altered Mental Status

e. Meds: metoprolol, simvastatin, aspirin 81 mg
f. Social: lives with wife (80 years old with multiple medical problems); drinks beer one to two times per month, denies any cigarette or drug use; at baseline able to perform all activities of daily living well
g. FHx: not relevant
h. PMD: Dr. Stern

G. Nurse
a. EKG (Figure 38.1)
b. CXR (Figure 38.2)

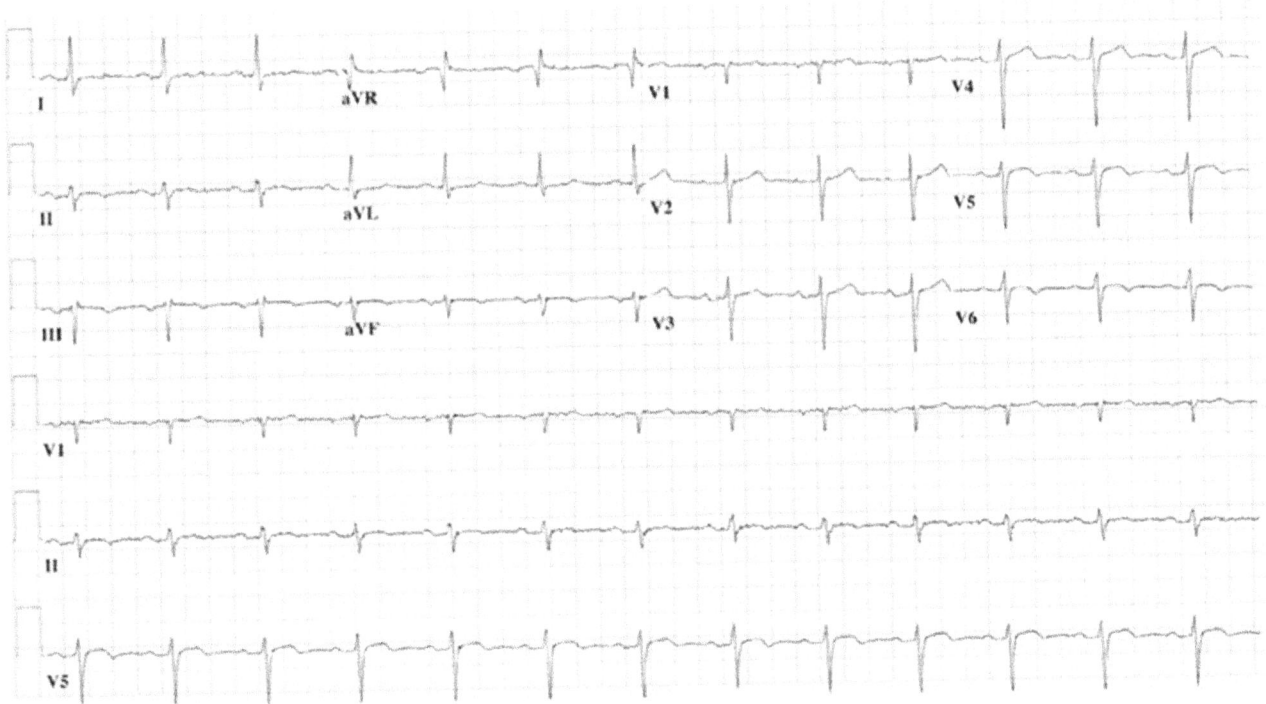

Figure 38.1

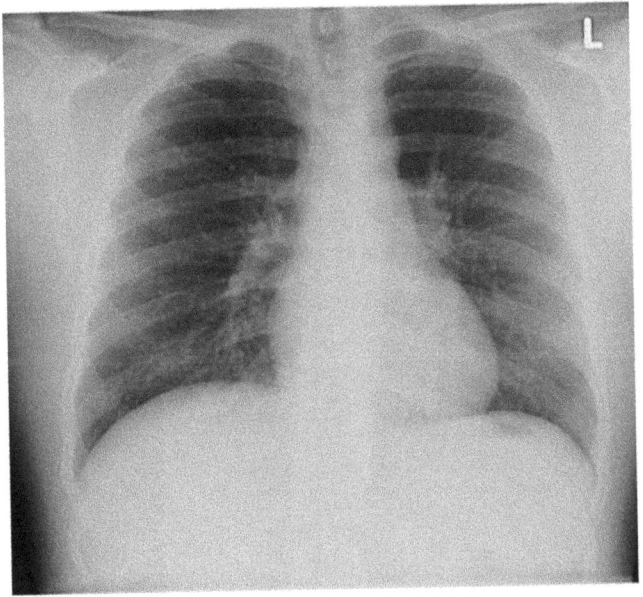

Figure 38.2

H. Secondary survey
a. General: alert, oriented to person and place; unsure of date, appears comfortable on stretcher
b. HEENT: no ecchymoses or lacerations noted; tympanic membranes normal bilaterally; extraocular movements intact; pupils equal, round, reactive; conjunctiva normal; fundoscopic examination normal; no septal deviation; palate normal; uvula midline
c. Neck: normal
d. Chest: normal
e. Heart: normal
f. Abdomen: normal
g. Rectal: hemoccult negative brown stool, normal tone
h. Extremities: normal
i. Back: normal
j. Neuro: alert, oriented to self and place only (does not know the date), cooperative; 5/5 strength bilateral upper and lower extremities; sensation grossly intact; cranial nerves II to XII intact; reflexes 2/2 and symmetric bilaterally; normal gait
k. Skin: no ecchymoses, lacerations, or abrasions noted
l. Lymph: normal

I. Action
a. Meds
    i.   Acetaminophen PO for pain
b. Imaging
    i.   Noncontrast CT head

J. Nurse
a. BP: 135/70, HR: 88, RR: 13, T: 36°C, Sat: 98% on RA
b. Patient: no change in neurological examination, no apparent distress

K. Results

Table 38.1 Results table

Test	Result	Test	Result
Complete blood count:		Liver function panel:	
WBC	$9.2 \times 10^3/\mu L$	AST	24 U/L
Hct	41.50%	ALT	33 U/L
Plt	$223 \times 10^3/\mu L$	Alk phos	120 U/L
		T bili	0.9 mg/dL
Basic metabolic panel:		D bili	0.1 mg/dL
Na	137 mEq/L	Amylase	60 U/L
K	4.2 mEq/L	Lipase	104 U/L
Cl	108 mEq/L	Albumin	3.1 g/dL
CO_2	23 mEq/L		
BUN	20 mEq/dL		
Cr	0.6 mg/dL		

Case 38: Altered Mental Status

Table 38.1 (cont.)

Test	Result	Test	Result
Gluc	110 mg/dL	Urinalysis:	
		SG	1.020
		pH	7
Coagulation panel:		Prot	Neg
PT	13.0 sec	Gluc	Neg
PTT	29 sec	Ketones	Neg
INR	1.1	Bili	Neg
		Blood	Neg
		LE	Neg
		Nitrite	Neg
		Color	Yellow

a. CT scan head (Figure 38.3)

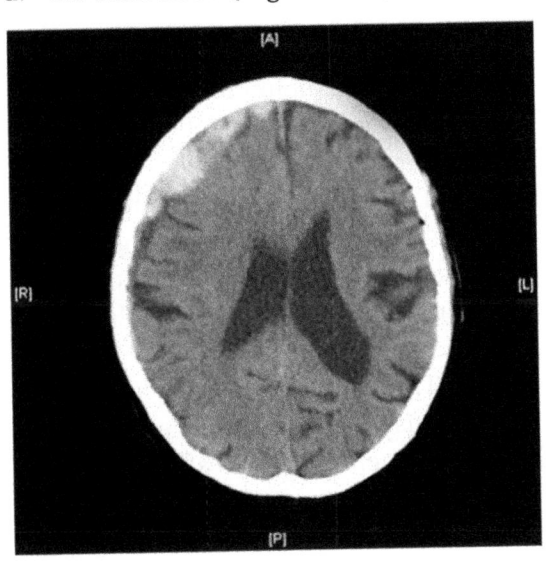

Figure 38.3

L. Action
a. Consult neurosurgery (for drainage).
b. Discussion with family and PMD regarding need for admission to neurosurgical service for drainage of his subdural hematoma.
c. Discussion with neurosurgery about aspirin reversal with platelets.
d. Discussion with neurosurgery about the need for antiepileptic medications for seizure prophylaxis.

M. Diagnosis
a. Subdural hematoma with midline shift

N. Critical actions
a. Early finger stick blood glucose
b. Obtain history of recent fall
c. Noncontrast head CT

   d. Discuss possible aspirin reversal with platelet transfusion
   e. Discuss possible antiepileptic medications for seizure prophylaxis
   f. Laboratory evaluation
   g. Pain management – avoid NSAID medications which could make bleeding worse
   h. Neurosurgery consultation
   i. Admission to ICU

O. Examiner instructions

   a. This is a case of an acute–subacute subdural hematoma (bleeding around the brain) with a
       midline shift. This can occur after relatively minor head trauma in elderly patients, and leads
       to worsening mental status or even focal neurologic findings. There are many processes that
       can cause confusion in the elderly; a rapid assessment of blood glucose levels, EKG, and a
       thorough history and physical examination are key steps in the patient's early management.

P. Pearls

   a. The most common complaint after head trauma is a headache. A careful history and physical
       examination will reveal more subtle findings, including neurologic and mental status changes.
   b. The noncontrast head CT can differentiate between acute intracranial and extracranial
       bleeding, subarachnoid hemorrhage, brain swelling, and large stroke.
   c. Patients at the extremes of age (greater than 60 or less than 2) should be considered high risk
       for intracranial injury, despite only having sustained minor head trauma.
   d. Patients with moderate to severe head trauma or with high clinical suspicion for bleeding may
       require observation, even those with an initial normal noncontrast head CT, especially those
       patients on antiplatelet or anticoagulant medications.
   e. Subdural hematomas (SDHs) occur between the dura and brain. In elderly patients and those
       with a history of alcoholism, brain atrophy causes stretching of the superficial bridging veins
       between the dura and brain. Thus, these patients are at increased risk for SDHs. Since this
       venous bleeding is slow, signs and symptoms may not develop rapidly and extensive damage
       may occur before the time the patient becomes symptomatic.
   f. In epidural hematomas, the bleeding occurs outside the dura. The majority are associated with
       skull fractures. Since the bleeding is arterial, signs and symptoms usually develop earlier than
       in subdural hematomas. However, these patients can develop a "lucid interval" after an initial
       episode of loss of consciousness.
   g. Traumatic subarachnoid hemorrhages (SAHs) result in blood within the meninges and spinal
       fluid. Up to two-thirds of patients with subarachnoid hemorrhage may have no bleeding noted
       on their initial noncontrast head CT, though this is time-dependent. The sooner the head CT is
       performed in relation to the onset of symptoms, the more likely SAH will be observed on CT
       brain imaging. One of the most severe complications of SAH is vasospasm, which can result in
       significant ischemia.
   h. Patients who are anticoagulated require special consideration, and often reversal of their
       anticoagulation. Treatments can include intravenous vitamin K, 3-factor or 4-factor prothrombin
       complex concentrate, or fresh frozen plasma. Although there is little evidence of benefit for the
       administration of platelets in patients on aspirin or clopidogrel, it is still a common practice.

Q. Figure legends

   a. Figure 38.1 (EKG) Normal sinus rhythm; biphasic T waves V5–6.
   b. Figure 38.2 (CXR) Normal chest x-ray.
   c. Figure 38.3 (Head CT) Acute right subdural hematoma with slight midline shift.

R. References
a. *Tintinalli's Emergency Medicine: A Comprehensive Study Guide* (9th ed.): Chapter 168, Altered Mental Status and Coma. Chapter 257, Head Trauma.
b. *Rosen's Emergency Medicine: Concepts and Clinical Practice* (10th ed.): Chapter 13, Depressed Consciousness and Coma. Chapter 33, Head Trauma.

Rectal Pain

Ani Aydin, MD

A. Chief complaint
a. 28-year-old male with pain in anal region

B. Vital signs
a. BP: 120/80, HR: 80 RR: 12, T: 37°C, Sat: 100% on RA

C. What does the patient look like?
a. Patient lying prone on the stretcher due to pain in his anal region.

D. Primary survey
a. Airway: speaking in full sentences
b. Breathing: no apparent respiratory distress, no cyanosis
c. Circulation: pale and cool skin, normal capillary refill

E. History
a. HPI: A 28-year-old male with a history of Crohn's disease presents with pain in the anal region for 1 week. The pain is severe, located in the anal area without radiation. It has been progressively worsening, dull, constant, worse with defecation and sitting, better with warm baths. The patient also noted some stains on his underwear this morning but denies any rectal bleeding. He had a prior similar episode as a teenager, and required a "surgery" in the ED. He denies any fever or chills, changes in his appetite, nausea, vomiting, blood per rectum, or weight loss.
b. PMHx: Crohn's disease
c. PSHx: "surgery" in ED 10 years ago
d. Allergies: none
e. Meds: mesalamine; no steroids at this time
f. Social: lives alone, single. Denies alcohol use, smoking, drugs. Sexually active with women, compliant with condom use
g. FHx: brother with Crohn's disease
h. PMD: Dr. Langan

F. Action
a. IV access
b. Pain medication, as needed
c. Labs
    i. CBC, BMP
d. Monitor: BP: 120/80, HR: 80, RR: 12, T: 37°C, Sat: 100% on RA

G. Nurse

a. Reassess pain score

H. Secondary survey

a. General: alert and oriented, moderate distress secondary to pain
b. HEENT: normal
c. Neck: normal
d. Chest: normal
e. Heart: normal
f. Abdomen: normal
g. Rectal: 2 × 2 cm fluctuant, indurated mass with some serous drainage near anal verge. No purulence. No surrounding erythema or edema or warmth. No hemorrhoids or lesions noted on anoscope examination. No lesions, no focal tenderness or fluctuance, and no palpable mass on rectal examination. No gross blood, hemoccult negative brown stool.
h. Urogenital: normal
i. Extremities: normal
j. Back: normal
k. Neuro: normal
l. Skin: normal
m. Lymph: normal

I. Action

a. Meds
   i. Pain medication (e.g., morphine) as needed
   ii. Consider antibiotics
b. Reassess
   i. Patient with some improvements in pain symptoms after analgesia, but continues to complain of anal pain
c. Consult
   i. None at this time
d. Imaging
   i. None needed (in this case the lesion is superficial and the remainder of the thorough exam does not reveal any deeper areas affected or systemic process)
   ii. It would be very reasonable to obtain a CT scan of the pelvis in any case where it was not clear that the infection was an isolated and uncomplicated perianal abscess.

J. Nurse

a. BP: 120/80, HR: 80, RR: 12, T: 37°C, Sat: 100% on RA
b. Patient: lying prone with pain in anal region, somewhat improved with pain medication

K. Results

Table 39.1 Results table

Test	Result	Test	Result
Complete blood count:		**Basic metabolic panel:**	
WBC	$8.2 \times 10^3/\mu L$	Na	137 mEq/L
Hct	41.50%	K	3.9 mEq/L
Plt	$253 \times 10^3/\mu L$	Cl	102 mEq/L
		CO_2	28 mEq/L
		BUN	19 mEq/dL
		Cr	0.9 mg/dL
		Gluc	100 mg/dL

L. Action
a. Incision and drainage, packing
b. Discussion with patient and PMD regarding the need for follow-up for wound checks and repacking. The patient should be given strict return instructions, including signs of infection or worsening symptoms.
c. Meds
 i. Systemic pain medication (e.g., morphine IV)
 ii. Local anesthesia (e.g., local infiltration with lidocaine)

M. Diagnosis
a. Uncomplicated perianal abscess

N. Critical actions
a. Pain medications
b. Thorough examination to rule out signs of fistula formation and systemic involvement
c. Incision and drainage (I&D)
d. Discuss post-incision and drainage management – sitz baths, stool softeners, frequent dressing changes until incision is healed
e. Arrange follow-up (within 24 hours to reassess for any progression, and then with GI or surgery within a week because fistula formation may occur)

O. Examiner instructions
a. This is a case of uncomplicated perianal abscess, or collection of pus, likely due to Crohn's disease. The prior "surgery" in the ED was an incision and drainage (I&D) of a similar lesion conducted 10 years prior. There are no signs of deeper involvement, fistula formation, or systemic signs on this examination. If a surgical consultation is requested, they should reply that they are in an emergency operative case and will follow-up with the patient in the morning.

P. Pearls
a. There are four types of perirectal abscesses: perianal, ischiorectal, pelvirectal, and intersphincteric. Uncomplicated perianal abscesses may be incised and drained in the ED. However, all other types of perirectal abscesses and fistulas should be managed operatively.

b. Perirectal abscesses occur more commonly in adult males but can also be found in the pediatric population.

c. They are associated with malignancies, Crohn's disease, tuberculosis, an immunocompromised host, anal fissures, foreign bodies, anorectal trauma, and actinomycosis.

d. Most cases involve mixed anaerobic and aerobic flora.

e. Consider antibiotics. They are not necessary for treating an infection as long as the I&D was performed and there is no underlying immune compromise or cellulitis. However, antibiotics may reduce the chances of developing a fistula.

Q. References

a. *Tintinalli's Emergency Medicine: A Comprehensive Study Guide* (9th ed.): Chapter 85, Anorectal Disorders.

b. *Rosen's Emergency Medicine: Concepts and Clinical Practice* (10th ed.): Chapter 82, Anorectum.

Vaginal Bleeding

Ani Aydin, MD

A. Chief complaint
a. 25-year-old female with abdominal pain and vaginal bleeding

B. Vital signs
a. BP: 95/63, HR: 96, RR: 12, T: 37°C, Sat: 100% on RA

C. What does the patient look like?
a. Patient appears stated age, anxious and uncomfortable due to pain, lying still and supine on her stretcher.

D. Primary survey
a. Airway: speaking in full sentences
b. Breathing: no apparent respiratory distress, no cyanosis
c. Circulation: pale and cool skin, normal capillary refill

E. History
a. HPI: A 25-year-old female, G2P2002, with a history of bilateral tubal ligation after her last pregnancy two years prior, presents to the ED with abdominal pain and vaginal bleeding since this morning. Her last menstrual period was about 6 weeks ago. The patient states that she soaked though five pads since this morning, which was heavier than her normal menses. The patient did not note any clots. She has been sexually active with her husband and has not been using any protection since her tubal ligation. She complains of some lightheadedness and dizziness. She denies any shortness of breath, chest pain, nausea, vomiting, fever, decreased appetite. She denies any history of sexually transmitted infections, including gonorrhea, chlamydia, HIV, or herpes.
b. PMHx: G2P2002
c. PSHx: two prior caesarean sections (2 and 3 years ago); bilateral tubal ligation after her most recent pregnancy
d. Allergies: none
e. Social: lives with husband and two children at home; denies alcohol, smoking, drugs; sexually active with husband only, not using any protection
f. FHx: not relevant
g. PMD: Dr. Johansen

F. Action
a. Two large-bore peripheral IV lines
b. Labs
   i. Urine pregnancy test, CBC, BMP, PT/PTT, type and screen, urinalysis

c. Crystalloid (lactated Ringer's or 0.9% normal saline) 1 L bolus IV
d. Monitor: BP: 95/63, HR: 96, RR: 12, T: 37°C, Sat: 100% on RA

G. Nurse

a. After 1 L crystalloid bolus: BP: 105/70, HR: 85, RR: 12, Sat: 100% on RA
   i. If no fluids are administered: BP: 85/60, HR: 118, RR: 15, Sat: 98% on RA
b. Urine pregnancy test positive

H. Secondary survey

a. General: alert and oriented, moderate distress due to abdominal pain, nervous
b. HEENT: mildly pale conjunctiva, otherwise normal
c. Neck: normal
d. Chest: normal
e. Heart: normal
f. Abdomen: soft, nondistended, normal bowel sounds; mild tenderness in the hypogastrium; some voluntary guarding, no rebound, no rigidity; no palpable masses
g. Pelvic:
   i. External vagina: normal
   ii. Speculum exam: bright red blood in vaginal vault, no clots; no vaginal lesions or lacerations or abrasions noted; no discharge noted
   iii. Bimanual examination: internal cervical os closed; no suprapubic tenderness to palpation; mild tenderness bilateral adnexa; no cervical motion tenderness
h. Rectal: hemoccult negative brown stool
i. Urogenital: normal
j. Extremities: normal
k. Back: normal
l. Neuro: normal
m. Skin: normal
n. Lymph: normal

I. Action

a. Meds
   i. Pain medication as needed
b. Reassess
   i. Patient anxious about bleeding, continues to complain about abdominal pain.
c. Consult
   i. Obstetrics
d. Imaging
   i. Pelvic US
e. Serum hCG
f. Type and screen

J. Nurse

a. Vital signs: BP: 105/70, HR: 85, RR: 12, Sat: 100% on RA (after 1 L of crystalloid)
b. Patient still with significant pain

K. Results

Table 40.1 Results table

Test	Result		Test	Result
Complete blood count:			**Urinalysis:**	
WBC	$12.1 \times 10^3/\mu L$		SG	1.030
Hct	29.80%		pH	6
Plt	$253 \times 10^3/\mu L$		Prot	Neg
			Gluc	Neg
Basic metabolic panel:			Ketones	Neg
Na	139 mEq/L		Bili	Neg
K	4.2 mEq/L		Blood	Neg
Cl	111 mEq/L		LE	Neg
CO_2	23 mEq/L		Nitrite	Neg
BUN	10 mEq/dL		Color	Yellow
Cr	0.8 mg/dL			
Gluc	92 mg/dL			

a. Serum hCG: 10,500
b. Blood Type: O⁻
c. Transvaginal US (Figure 40.1)
d. FAST US (Figure 40.2)

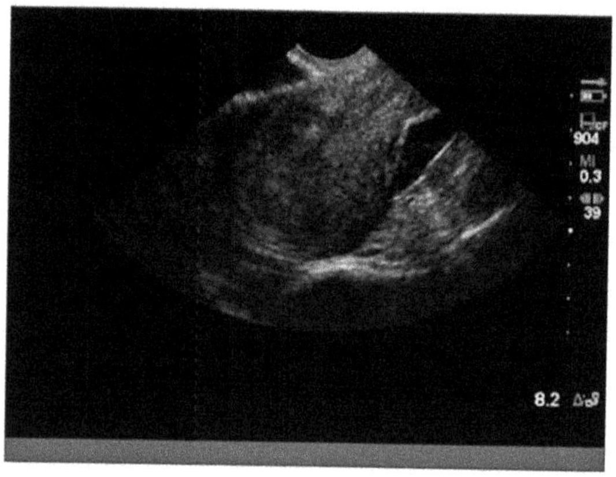

Figure 40.1

L. Action

a. Medications
    i.   Pain medication as needed (such as morphine)
    ii. Rho (D) immune globulin IM (RhoGAM)
    iii. Transfuse packed red blood cells
b. Obstetrics consultation
    i.   To OR for laparotomy
c. Discuss with patient, family, and PMD need for emergent OR and diagnosis of ectopic pregnancy

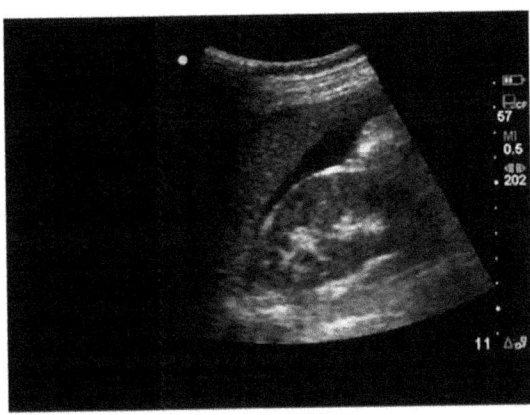

Figure 40.2

M. Diagnosis
a. Ruptured ectopic pregnancy

N. Critical actions
a. Large-bore IV access
b. Crystalloid or packed red blood cell administration
c. Blood type and crossmatch
d. Rho (D) immune globulin IM in Rh negative patients
e. hCG
f. Pelvic examination
g. Pelvic US
h. Pain management
i. Obstetrics consult

O. Examiner instructions
a. This is a case of an ectopic pregnancy, which is the abnormal implantation of the embryo outside of the uterus. Prior tubal ligations likely increased this patient's risk for ectopic pregnancy. Scarring from surgery, trauma, or pelvic infections can increase the risk as well. The patient presents with the classic triad of abdominal pain, vaginal bleeding, and amenorrhea, though only half of ectopic pregnancies present this way. Important early actions include confirmatory pregnancy testing with beta hCG, resuscitation of hypotensive patients with crystalloid or blood products depending on the amount of bleeding, and early consultation of obstetrics in patients with a high pretest probability of ectopic pregnancy or any abnormal findings on bedside examination, such as surgical abdomen in a patient early in their pregnancy or a positive bedside ultrasound examination. In stable patients, an ultrasound should be obtained to confirm the presence or absence of an intrauterine pregnancy.
b. Given the patient's hypotension in this case, crystalloid fluids or blood should have been administered while a pelvic examination was performed and confirmatory testing, including a beta hCG and hematocrit were obtained. Obstetrics should be consulted emergently for operative intervention in cases of ruptured ectopic pregnancies.

P. Pearls
a. Ectopic pregnancies are the leading cause of first-trimester pregnancy-related maternal deaths.
b. The incidence is higher in nonwhite women and teenagers.

c.   There is an increased incidence in patients with prior sexually transmitted diseases, unsuccessful tubal ligations, assisted reproduction, intrauterine devices, prior ectopic pregnancies, previous pelvic surgeries, and exposure to diethylstilbestrol.

d.   Most ectopic pregnancies occur in the fallopian tubes. Other sites include abdominal cavity, cervix, and ovary.

e.   It is critical to administer Rho (D) immune globulin IM to Rh negative mothers to reduce the risk of maternal antibody formation against fetal hemoglobin. This sensitization can lead to neonatal hemolytic anemia and fetal hydrops in future pregnancies.

f.   Peritoneal signs are ominous and suggest an obstetrical emergency.

Q. Figure legends

a.   Figure 40.1 Empty uterus without any products of conception.

b.   Figure 40.2 Free fluid in the right upper quadrant.

R. References

a.   *Tintinalli's Emergency Medicine: A Comprehensive Study Guide* (9th ed.): Chapter 98, Ectopic Pregnancy and Emergencies in the First 20 Weeks of Pregnancy.

b.   *Rosen's Emergency Medicine: Concepts and Clinical Practice* (10th ed.): Chapter 173, Complications of Pregnancy.

Agitation

Ani Aydin, MD

A. Chief complaint
a. 49-year-old male with agitation

B. Vital signs
a. BP: 110/75, HR: 96, RR: 16, T: 37°C, Sat: 98% on RA

C. What does the patient look like?
a. Patient appears older than stated age; slurring speech, eyelids drooping, disheveled, urine stains on clothing; attempting to get off the stretcher; small laceration noted on forehead.

D. Primary survey
a. Airway: slurred speech, protecting airway and saturating well on RA
b. Breathing: no apparent respiratory distress, no cyanosis
c. Circulation: pale and cool skin, normal capillary refill

E. Action
a. Large-bore peripheral IV
b. Labs
    i.   Urinalysis, urine toxicology panel, alcohol level, BMP, CBC, LFT
c. Monitor: BP: 110/75, HR: 96, RR: 16, T: 37°C, Sat: 98% on RA
d. Finger stick glucose (130 mg/dL; must ask)
e. Verbal redirection to cooperate with history and exam

F. History
a. HPI: A 49-year-old undomiciled male with a history of alcohol intoxication and hepatitis is brought in by ambulance for public intoxication and agitation. Upon presentation to the ED, the patient insists that he is fine and wants to be discharged immediately. He denies any headache, dizziness, lightheadedness, chest pain, shortness of breath, abdominal pain, nausea, vomiting, changes in vision, blurry vision, or fever. He states that he drinks approximately one pint of vodka per day, and his last drink was just before being picked up by the ambulance. He denies any other ingestion. The patient requests a sandwich and a change of clothing.
b. PMHx: alcohol abuse, hepatitis, tetanus immunization up to date
c. PSHx: none
d. Allergies: none
e. Social: undomiciled, unemployed; drinks one pint of vodka per day; he has smoked one pack of cigarettes per day for the past 35 years. He denies any cocaine, crack, heroin, marijuana, or IV drug use. He is not currently sexually active.

    f. FHx: unknown

    g. PMD: none

G. Nurse

    a. BP: 120/75, HR: 96, RR: 16, T: 37°C, Sat: 98% on RA

H. Secondary survey

    a. General: thin with a large abdomen; awake, oriented × 2 (knows his name, knows that he is in hospital); disheveled, agitated, slurred speech

    b. HEENT: erythematous conjunctiva, eyelids drooping, 1.5 cm linear laceration located on left forehead with some ecchymosis

    c. Neck: normal

    d. Chest: clear to auscultation bilaterally; spider angiomas noted

    e. Heart: normal

    f. Abdomen: soft, nontender, distended, + bowel sounds; + fluid wave; hepatomegaly; no guarding, no rebound; small umbilical hernia, reducible

    g. Rectal: hemoccult negative brown stool

    h. Urogenital: normal

    i. Extremities: asterixis

    j. Back: normal

    k. Neuro: normal

    l. Skin: forehead laceration as above

    m. Lymph: normal

I. Action

    a. Meds

        i. Thiamine

        ii. Folic acid

    b. Reassess

        i. Patient is belligerent at times, but able to be consoled. He is awake and oriented × 2, unable to ambulate unassisted.

    c. Imaging

        i. Noncontrast head CT

J. Nurse

    a. BP: 120/75, HR: 96, RR: 16, T: 37°C, Sat: 98% on RA

    b. Patient: agitated but able to be consoled; awake, slurred speech

K. Results

Table 41.1 Results table

Test	Result	Test	Result
Complete blood count:		**Liver function panel:**	
WBC	5.5 × 10³/µL	AST	65 U/L
Hct	31.4%	ALT	30 U/L
Plt	99 × 10³/µL	Alk phos	100 U/L

Table 41.1 (cont.)

Test	Result	Test	Result
		T bili	0.5 mg/dL
		D bili	0.2 mg/dL
Basic metabolic panel:		Amylase	30 U/L
Na	138 mEq/L	Lipase	23 U/L
K	4.2 mEq/L	Albumin	3.5 g/dL
Cl	107 mEq/L		
CO_2	17 mEq/L		
BUN	17 mEq/dL	**Urinalysis:**	
Cr	1.2 mg/dL	SG	1.010
Gluc	130 mg/dL	pH	6
		Prot	Neg
		Gluc	Neg
Coagulation panel:		Ketones	Neg
PT	13.1 sec	Bili	Neg
PTT	31 sec	Blood	Neg
INR	1.5	LE	Neg
		Nitrite	Neg
		Color	Yellow

a. Osmolar gap = 9
b. Urine toxicology panel negative
c. Alcohol 350 mg/dL
d. Noncontrast head CT (Figure 41.1)

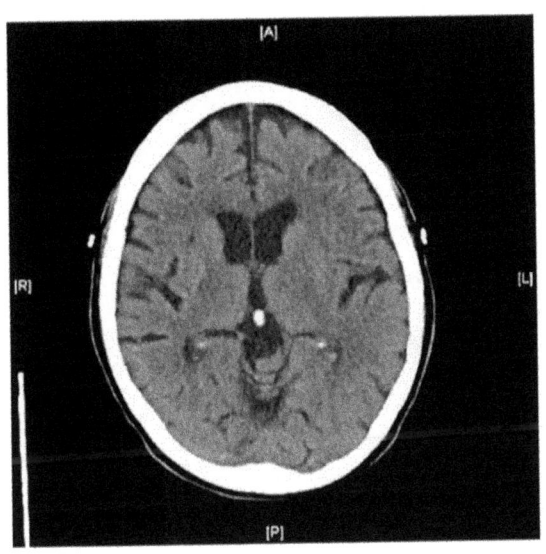

Figure 41.1

L. Action
a. Feed patient
b. Repair laceration

M. Diagnosis
a. Alcohol intoxication

N. Critical actions
a. Finger stick glucose
b. Noncontrast head CT
c. Anion gap, osmolar gap
d. Laceration repair

O. Examiner instructions
a. This is a case of alcohol intoxication. The patient is belligerent and has a head injury. Since he is not fully oriented and unable to give an accurate history, a noncontrast head CT is appropriate. Depending on resources (CT availability, staff workload), it is feasible to follow such patients with serial neurologic examinations, with the expectation they should gradually sober on repeat assessments, and any focal neurologic findings on exam should be evaluated with imaging. Should the patient become very agitated, sedatives may be used, but the patient should be redirected when appropriate.
b. Curveball: Although acute alcohol intoxication is a common ED presentation, patients often have other illnesses that may easily be missed. If the candidate does not request a finger stick glucose quickly, the patient should lose consciousness. The glucose in this scenario will be 35, and the patient will remain unresponsive until dextrose is administered intravenously.

P. Pearls
a. Alcohol intoxication contributes to 100,000 deaths per year.
b. About 2.5% of ED visits are related to alcohol use/abuse.
c. Screenings can be conducted in the ED using the "CAGE" questions and the Michigan Alcohol Screening Test.
d. In agitated patients, co-ingestions should be considered as well as head injury.
e. A noncontrast head CT is appropriate in an intoxicated patient with obvious head injury.

Q. Figure legends
a. Figure 41.1 Normal noncontrast CT of the head.

R. References
a. *Tintinalli's Emergency Medicine: A Comprehensive Study Guide* (9th ed.): Chapter 185, Alcohols.
b. *Rosen's Emergency Medicine: Concepts and Clinical Practice* (10th ed.): Chapter 137, Alcohol-Related Disease.

Abdominal Pain

Nicholas Genes, MD, PhD

A. Chief complaint
a. 45-year-old female with abdominal pain and fever

B. Vital signs
a. BP: 99/62, HR: 122, RR: 24, T: 38.4°C, Sat: 97% on RA

C. What does the patient look like?
a. Patient appears stated age, uncomfortable due to pain, in moderate distress, slowly writhing on stretcher.

D. Primary survey
a. Airway: speaking in full sentences
b. Breathing: no apparent respiratory distress, no cyanosis, increased respiratory rate
c. Circulation: warm and flushed skin, normal capillary refill

E. History
a. HPI: A 45-year-old female with severe diffuse abdominal pain for a day, fevers on and off since yesterday; persistent nausea with two episodes of vomiting today (yellowish material and food contents); no diarrhea; last menstrual period was 1 year ago.
b. PMHx: type 1 diabetes
c. PSHx: none
d. Allergies: none
e. Social: lives with husband at home, denies alcohol, smoking, or drugs; sexually active
f. FHx: aunt had type 1 diabetes, father has hypertension, mother has hyperthyroidism
g. PMD: Dr. Pomerleau

F. Action
a. Two large-bore peripheral IV lines
b. Labs
   i. CBC, BMP, LFT, arterial or venous blood gas with lactate, blood cultures, urine culture, urinalysis, urine pregnancy test
c. Monitor: BP: 99/62, HR: 122, RR: 24, T: 38.4°C, Sat: 97% on RA
d. Cardiac monitoring
e. 1 L NS bolus
f. Finger stick glucose
g. EKG

G. Nurse
a. EKG (Figure 42.1)
b. Glucose: 385 mg/dL
c. BP: 98/59, HR: 95, RR: 22, Sat: 98% on O_2

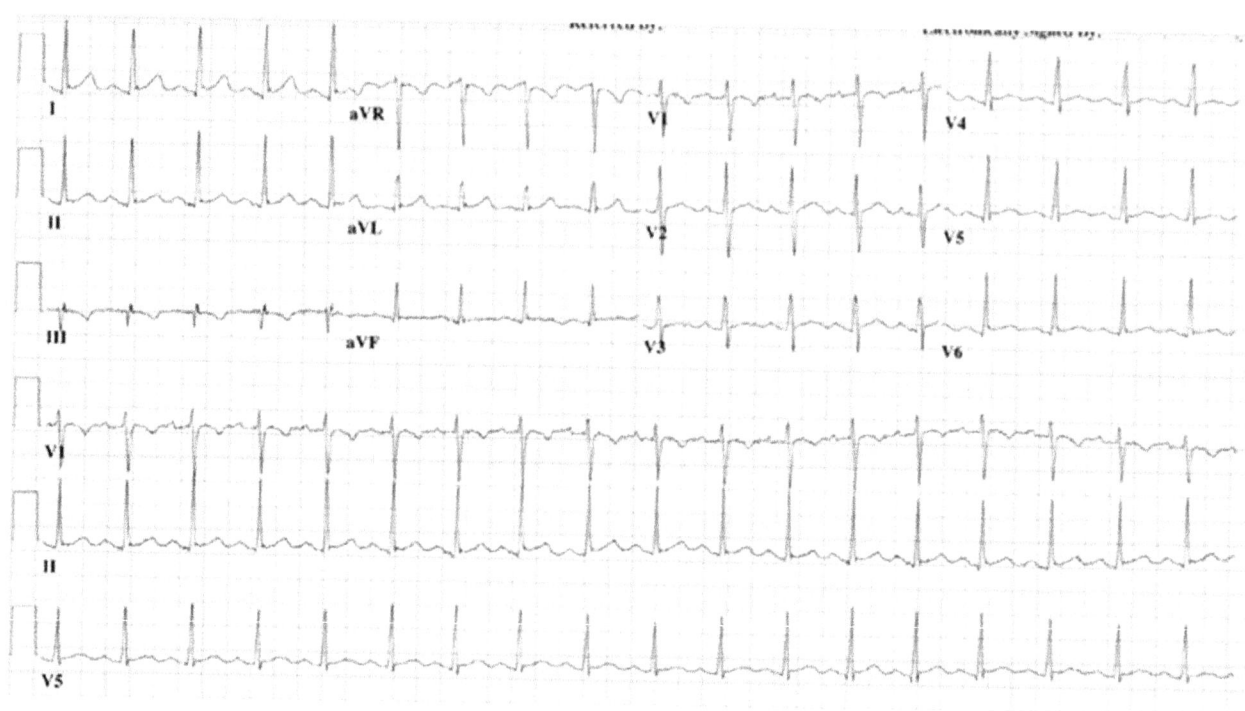

Figure 42.1

H. Secondary survey
a. General: appears dry on examination, tachycardic; alert and oriented, moderate distress due to pain
b. HEENT: mildly pale conjunctivae, otherwise normal
c. Neck: normal
d. Chest: lungs clear to auscultation bilaterally, tachypneic, no wheezes or rales
e. Heart: tachycardic, regular rate and rhythm, no murmurs or rubs
f. Abdomen: mildly distended, diffusely tender, bowel sounds decreased, no pulsatile masses, no masses, no hernias, nontender at McBurney's point, negative Murphy's sign; rebound and guarding are noted, no rigidity
g. Rectal: hemoccult negative brown stool
h. Urogenital: normal
i. Extremities: normal
j. Back: normal, no costovertebral angle tenderness
k. Neuro: normal
l. Skin: dry, poor turgor, no rashes, no edema, no cellulitis
m. Lymph: normal

I. Action
a. Second liter IV fluid bolus
b. Recheck blood glucose
c. Start insulin drip; reassess labs (especially glucose and electrolytes for anion gap) every 1–2 hours

J. Imaging

a. Upright CXR

b. Obstructive series

c. Meds
   i. Morphine IV
   ii. Metoclopramide IV

d. Reassess
   i. Patient's heart rate returning to normal, pain subsiding (if analgesia given; if not, no change in pain).

K. Nurse

a. BP: 112/69, HR: 90, RR: 18, Sat: 98% on O_2 (after 1 L)

b. Patient still complains of some abdominal pain

L. Results

Table 42.1 Results table

Test	Result	Test	Result
Complete blood count:		T bili	0.5 mg/dL
		D bili	0.2 mg/dL
WBC	$12.1 \times 10^3/\mu L$	Amylase	84 U/L
Hct	41.50%	Lipase	50 U/L
Plt	$253 \times 10^3/\mu L$	Albumin	4.2 g/dL
Basic metabolic panel:		**Urinalysis:**	
Na	135 mEq/L	SG	1.035
K	4.0 mEq/L	pH	8
Cl	100 mEq/L	Prot	Neg
CO_2	10 mEq/L	Gluc	+
BUN	34 mEq/dL	Ketones	+
Cr	1.4 mg/dL	Bili	Neg
Gluc	301 mg/dL	Blood	+
		Nitrite	+
Coagulation panel:		Color	Yellow
PT	13.1 sec		
PTT	26 sec		
INR	1.0	**Arterial blood gas:**	
		pH	7.13
		pO_2	80 mmHg
Liver function panel:		pCO_2	25 mmHg
AST	22 U/L	HCO_3	13 mmol/L
ALT	20 U/L		
Alk phos	100 U/L		

a. Lactate: 3.2 mmol/L
b. Upright CXR (Figure 42.2)
c. Abdominal x-ray (Figure 42.3)

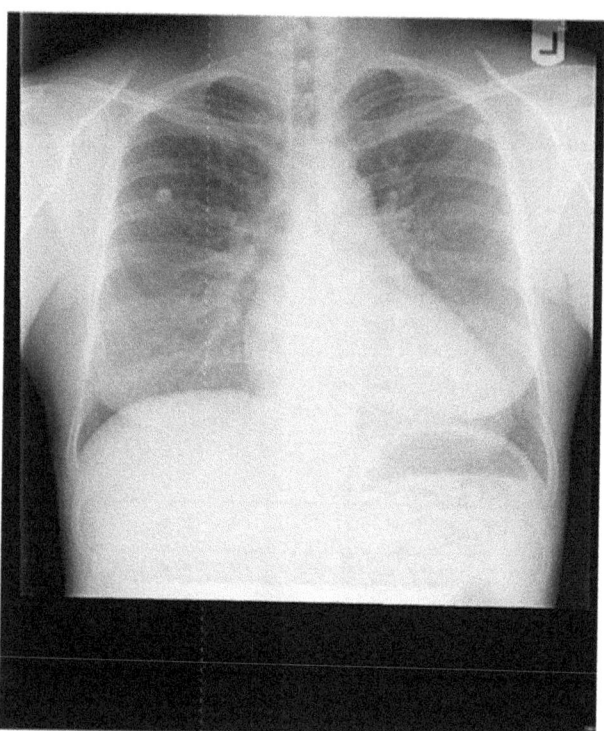

Figure 42.2

A

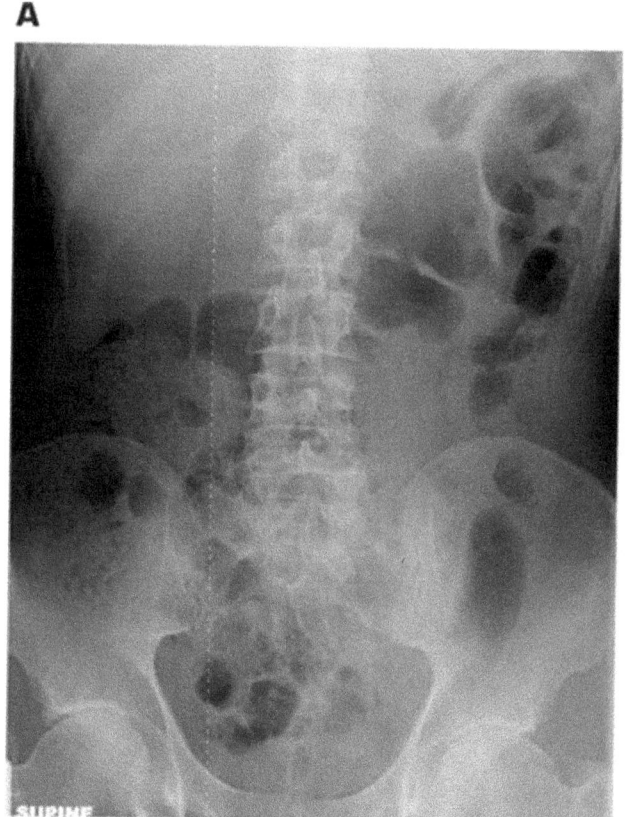

B

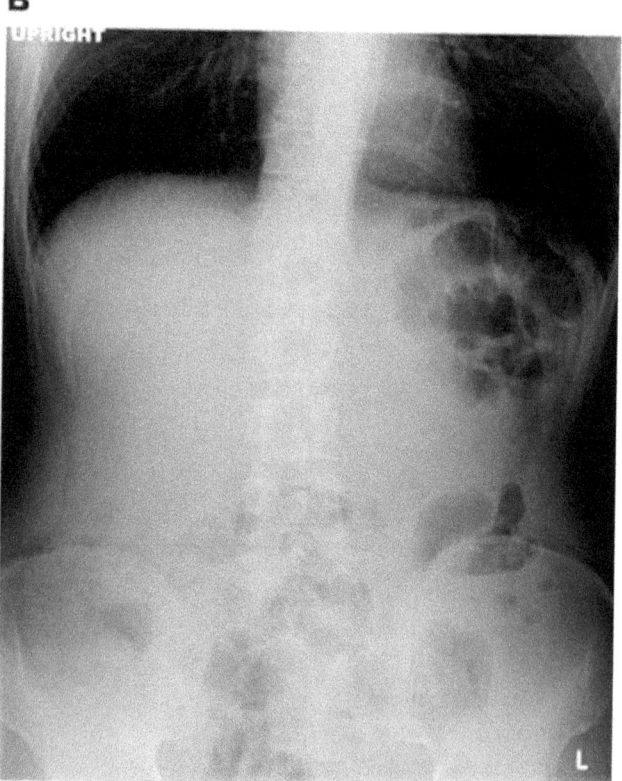

Figure 42.3

M. Action

a. IVF bolus, insulin drip, replete K, follow labs, EKG, ICU admit, antibiotics for UTI (UTI as likely precipitant of diabetic ketoacidosis)
b. Meds
   i. Antibiotics (such as fluoroquinolone or cephalosporin)
   ii. Morphine IV if pain persists
c. Discussion with family and PMD regarding need for admission, hydration, insulin drip
d. EKG: normal sinus rhythm, no U waves
e. Consider CT scan if abdominal pain persists

N. Diagnosis

a. Diabetic ketoacidosis
b. Urinary tract infection

O. Critical actions

a. Early blood glucose assessment
b. Calculation of anion gap
c. Fluid replacement
d. Insulin drip
e. Replete potassium
f. ICU admission for insulin drip and frequent laboratory monitoring
g. Antibiotics for UTI

P. Examiner instructions

a. This is a case of diabetic ketoacidosis (DKA). DKA can be a presentation of new diabetes, a result of noncompliance with insulin therapy, or due to stressors, inflammation, or infection. If a blood glucose is assessed early (finger stick or venous sample), therapy for DKA may be started much earlier. Do not reveal the patient's blood glucose level unless it is specifically requested. The most important initial therapy in adults is IV fluids, not insulin. The patient's symptoms will worsen (blood pressure will fall and heart rate will rise) until fluid is administered. As fluid and insulin are administered, the symptoms of abdominal pain will resolve. Any evaluation for surgical cause of abdominal pain (surgical consultation, CT scan, etc.) will reveal no pathology.

Q. Pearls

a. Diagnosis depends on a blood glucose of 250 mg/dL or higher, a bicarbonate level of 15 mEq/L or lower, and a pH (by arterial or venous blood gas) of 7.3 or lower with ketonuria.
b. Let the anion gap guide insulin therapy, not serum glucose or ketones.
c. Insulin should be continued until the anion gap resolves, not until the glucose normalizes. When glucose levels fall below 250 mg/dL, dextrose should be added to the IV fluid infusion to avoid hypoglycemia.
d. Be wary of potassium levels. They will drop as acidemia is corrected – begin repleting early.
e. Abdominal pain is a frequent complaint in DKA. It may be related to the precipitating cause, or it may be idiopathic. Peritoneal signs are ominous, and often suggest a surgical emergency. Consider early antibiotics, fluids, and surgical consultation.
f. There is little evidence that bicarbonate or phosphate repletion is of benefit. Giving insulin and fluids is usually ample therapy for treating the acidosis. The insulin given in DKA is not really for sugar reabsorption (insulin sometimes isn't given in mild DKA). Instead, the insulin is for ketogenesis and to overcome the acidosis.

R. Figure legends
a. Figure 42.1 (EKG) Sinus tachycardia.
b. Figure 42.2 (CXR) No acute cardiopulmonary pathology.
c. Figure 42.3 (Abdominal film series) Nonspecific bowel gas pattern.

S. References
a. *Tintinalli's Emergency Medicine: A Comprehensive Study Guide* (9th ed.): Chapter 225, Diabetic Ketoacidosis.
b. *Rosen's Emergency Medicine: Concepts and Clinical Practice* (10th ed.): Chapter 115, Diabetes Mellitus and Disorders of Glucose Homeostasis.

Abdominal Pain

Nicholas Genes, MD, PhD

A. Chief complaint
a. 61-year-old man with epigastric pain and nausea

B. Vital signs
a. BP: 122/77, HR: 62, RR: 18, T: 36.3°C, Sat: 97% on RA, FS: 183 mg/dL

C. What does the patient look like?
a. Patient appears stated age, uncomfortable due to pain, in moderate distress, looking pale and complaining of nausea.

D. Primary survey
a. Airway: speaking in full sentences
b. Breathing: no apparent respiratory distress, no cyanosis, increased respiratory rate
c. Circulation: cool and clammy skin, normal capillary refill

E. Action
a. Peripheral IV line access
b. Labs
   i. CBC, BMP, LFT, cardiac enzymes, PT/PTT, blood type and screen
c. 500 mL NS bolus
d. Cardiac monitor
e. Monitor: BP: 109/62, HR: 55, RR: 20, T: 37.3°C, Sat: 97% on 2 L NC
   i. If no fluids given: BP: 98/50, HR: 50, RR: 20, T: 37.3°C, Sat: 97% on 2 L NC
   ii. If nitroglycerin given: BP: 75/42, HR: 60, RR: 22, T: 37.3°C, Sat: 95% on 2 L NC, distended neck veins
f. EKG

F. History
a. HPI: A 61-year-old male with history of type 2 diabetes and hypertension who felt weak and nauseous several times yesterday, unrelated to exertion. Today, his stomach felt upset when walking 3 hours prior to arrival. He felt lightheaded and vomited once. The upset stomach settled into a heavy epigastric dullness; he felt weak and called 911.
b. PMHx: type 2 diabetes, hypertension, believes he has been told his cholesterol is high
c. PSHx: appendectomy, age 18
d. Allergies: none
e. Social: lives with wife, quit smoking 2 years ago, no alcohol, no drugs
f. FHx: father died of heart attack at age 50; mother has type 2 diabetes
g. PMD: Dr. Brown

G. Nurse

a. EKG (Figure 43.1)
b. Patient still has epigastric sensation described in HPI

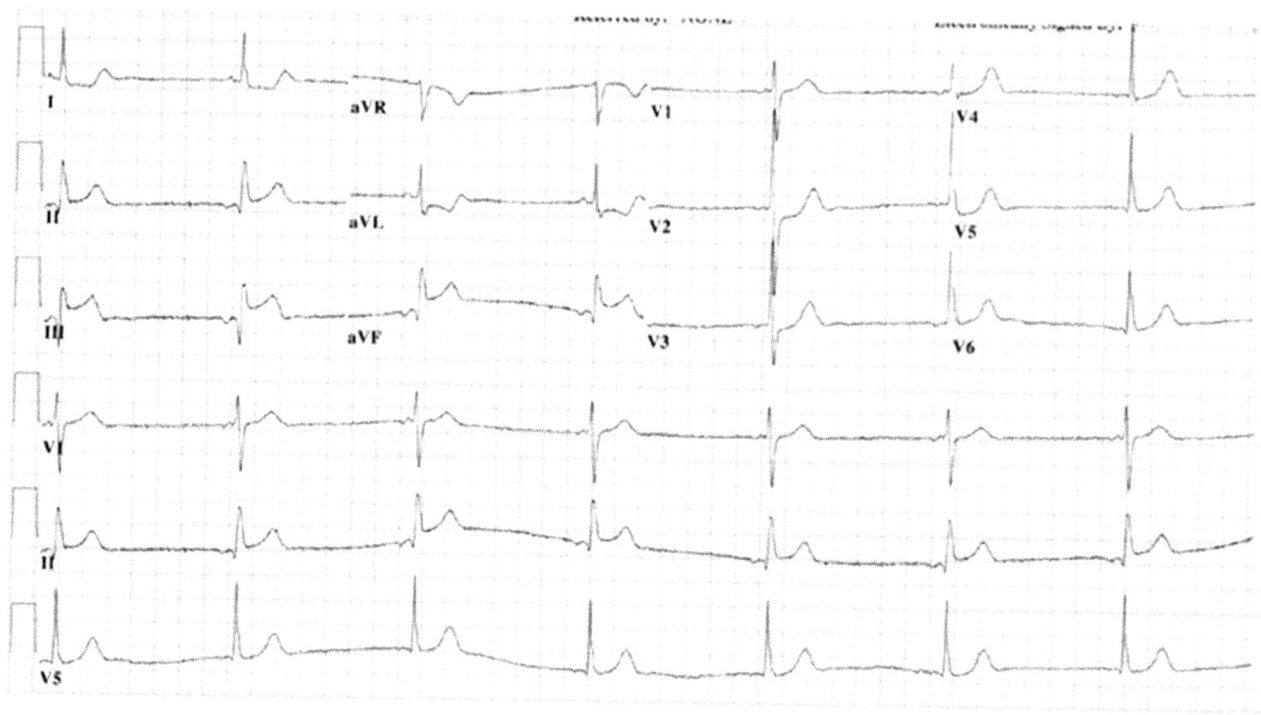

Figure 43.1

H. Actions

a. EKG with right-sided and posterior leads
b. CXR
c. 324 mg aspirin chewable

I. Secondary survey

a. General: alert and oriented, moderate distress due to pain, appears pale, clammy
b. HEENT: normal
c. Neck: normal
d. Chest: lungs clear to auscultation, no wheezes, no rales
e. Heart: bradycardic, no murmurs or rubs
f. Abdomen: soft, nontender, no distension, no hepatosplenomegaly
g. Rectal: hemoccult negative brown stool
h. Urogenital: normal
i. Extremities: normal
j. Back: normal
k. Neuro: normal
l. Skin: pale, clammy, no rashes, no edema, no clubbing
m. Lymph: normal

J. Action

a. Consult cardiology and activate cardiac catheterization lab
b. Repeat EKG (Figure 43.1)
c. If 500 mL NS given: BP: 108/59, HR: 60, RR: 18, Sat: 98% on O_2

d. If no fluids given: BP: 80/45, HR: 52, RR: 20, Sat: 95% on O_2
e. If repeated nitroglycerin or morphine is given, patient will go into shock which will require
    IV fluids and vasopressors

K. Nurse
a. CXR (Figure 43.2)

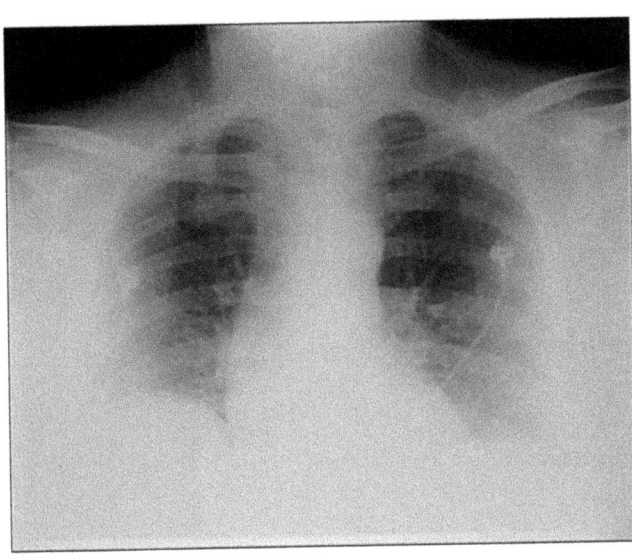

Figure 43.2

L. Results

Table **43.1** Results table

Test	Result	Test	Result
Complete blood count:		T bili	0.9 mg/dL
WBC	11.5×10^3/uL	D bili	0.2 mg/dL
Hct	40.0%	Amylase	250 U/L
Plt	206×10^3/uL	Lipase	66 U/L
		Albumin	4.1 g/dL
Basic metabolic panel:			
Na	138 mEq/L	**Urinalysis:**	
K	3.8 mEq/L	SG	1.022
Cl	103 mEq/L	pH	7.1
CO_2	25 mEq/L	Prot	Neg
BUN	28 mEq/dL	Gluc	Neg
Cr	1.2 mg/dL	Ketones	Neg
Gluc	144 mg/dL	Bili	Neg
		Blood	Neg
Coagulation panel:		LE	Neg
PT	14 sec	Nitrite	Neg

Table 43.1 (cont.)

Test	Result	Test	Result
PTT	30 sec	Color	Yellow
INR	1.1		
		Arterial blood gas:	
Liver function panel:		pH	7.4
AST	44 U/L	PO_2	90 mmHg
ALT	35 U/L	PCO_2	44 mmHg
Alk Phos	67 U/L	HCO_3	24 mmol/L

a. Troponin I: 1.2 ng/mL

M. Diagnosis
a. Inferior wall myocardial infarction with right ventricular involvement

N. Critical actions
a. Obtain EKGs – including right-sided and posterior leads
b. Recognize myocardial infarction pattern
c. IV access and fluid bolus
d. Aspirin administration
e. Avoid nitroglycerin and morphine administration
f. Cardiology consultation
g. Activate cardiac catheterization lab

O. Examiner instructions
a. This is a case of inferior wall myocardial infarction (MI) or heart attack. The patient's symptoms are vague and can suggest an abdominal process. This occurs frequently in diabetic patients or elderly patients and is more common with occluded coronary arteries overlying the diaphragm. Any delay in obtaining an EKG and diagnosing MI will result in worsening of the patient's symptoms. Treating this patient with antiemetics, antacids, and pain medications may provide temporary relief, but the astute clinician must be concerned with cardiac pathology in any diabetic patient with nausea and vomiting. Note that nitroglycerin or morphine administration will cause the patient's blood pressure to drop and their symptoms to worsen.

P. Pearls
a. About one-third of inferior wall MIs involve the right ventricle, which has been associated with higher mortality and complications, especially in the setting of arrhythmias (though prognosis is good with prompt and appropriate therapy).
b. EKGs with inferior ST elevations ought to prompt an order for a right-sided EKG. The right leads RV4–6 with elevation is highly suggestive of right coronary artery occlusion and right ventricular infarction.
c. Any drugs that decrease preload – such as nitroglycerin, morphine, and some diuretics – should be avoided. Efforts must be taken to avoid triggering vagal stimulation in the patient with right ventricular infarct. Even Foley catheter placement may cause vagal stimulation sufficient to worsen right ventricular function.

d. Several liters of IV fluids may be safely administered. If central venous pressure monitoring is in effect, a pressure of 15 mmHg is the target. Fluids above that limit are unlikely to improve hemodynamics; vasopressors may be of benefit at that point.

e. β-blockers and calcium channel blockers will slow heart rate and AV nodal conduction, and decrease contractility. Their use should be avoided in the hemodynamically unstable patient. These medications should be considered very cautiously for use in stable patients only when indicated and with careful monitoring.

f. Reperfusion therapy, either through cardiac catheterization or thrombolysis, reduces morbidity and mortality for both inferior and right ventricular MI, just as it does for anterior MI.

Q. Figure legends

a. Figure 43.1 (EKG) Sinus bradycardia, with inferior leads (II, III, and aVF) showing ST elevation, with some reciprocal ST depression in high lateral leads (I, aVL).

b. Figure 43.2 (CXR) Nonspecific findings.

R. References

a. *Tintinalli's Emergency Medicine: A Comprehensive Study Guide* (9th ed.): Chapter 49, Acute Coronary Syndromes.

b. *Rosen's Emergency Medicine: Concepts and Clinical Practice* (10th ed.): Chapter 64, Acute Coronary Syndromes.

Abdominal Pain

Nicholas Genes, MD, PhD

A. Chief complaint
a. 25-year-old female with abdominal pain

B. Vital signs
a. BP: 115/73, HR: 96, RR: 18, T: 37.2°C, Sat: 98% on RA

C. What does the patient look like?
a. Patient appears stated age, sitting upright, clutching abdomen and grimacing in pain.

D. Primary survey
a. Airway: speaking in short sentences, phonating well
b. Breathing: no apparent respiratory distress, no cyanosis
c. Circulation: warm, flushed skin, good capillary refill

E. Action
a. Large-bore peripheral IV access
b. Labs
    i. CBC, BMP, LFTs, urine pregnancy test, urinalysis, type and screen × 2, PT/PTT/INR

F. History
a. HPI: A 25-year-old female with no significant past medical history states she experienced abrupt onset of right lower quadrant aching at work, several hours prior. She describes feeling "fine" beforehand, with normal bowel movements, no urinary burning or frequency, no fevers or chills, no cough or cold symptoms. States she had been out with friends the night prior. She had a similar pain once before, she thinks on the same side, but it resolved within minutes and was not this intense. She has vomited twice since the onset of pain.
b. PMHx: none
c. PSHx: none
d. Allergies: none
e. Meds: none
f. Social: nonsmoker, drinks alcohol socially, several male sexual partners in the past year. No prior pregnancies, no history of birth control; last menstrual period was 3 weeks ago, some menses are irregular with heavy bleeding and spotting in between periods
g. FHx: father has hypertension; mother has diabetes
h. PMD: none

Case 44: Abdominal Pain

G. Nurse

a. Urine pregnancy test negative.

H. Action

a. Infuse 1 L NS IV
b. Analgesia
c. Reassess vital signs
    i. BP: 110/65, HR: 90, RR: 18, Sat: 98% on RA

I. Secondary survey

a. General: mildly obese, hirsute woman, alert and oriented, significant distress due to pain
b. HEENT: normal
c. Neck: normal
d. Chest: normal
e. Heart: normal
f. Abdomen: no distension, exquisitely tender over right lower quadrant, bowel sounds present, no masses, no hernias; negative Murphy's sign, + guarding, no rigidity
g. Rectal: hemoccult negative brown stool
h. Urogenital: no external lesions; pelvic speculum examination shows no discharge, no blood at cervix; bimanual examination shows no cervical motion tenderness, but significant tenderness is noted at right adnexa
i. Extremities: normal
j. Back: normal
k. Neuro: normal
l. Skin: normal
m. Lymph: normal

J. Action

a. Meds
    i. IV pain and nausea medication (e.g., morphine, metoclopramide)
b. Reassess
    i. Patient's discomfort improving but still present
c. Imaging
    i. Doppler US of pelvis
    ii. If CT scan of abdomen/pelvis is ordered, inform candidate test will "take some time"

K. Nurse.

a. BP: 112/69, HR: 85, RR: 18, Sat: 98% on RA

L. Results

Table 44.1 Results table

Test	Result	Test	Result
Complete blood count:		**Liver function panel:**	
WBC	$11.1 \times 10^3/\mu L$	AST	22 U/L
Hct	38.50%	ALT	50 U/L
Plt	$253 \times 10^3/\mu L$	Alk phos	55 U/L
		T bili 0.5	mg/dL
Basic metabolic panel:		D bili 0.2	mg/dL
Na	137 mEq/L	Amylase	34 U/L
K	4.1 mEq/L	Lipase	30 U/L
Cl	101 mEq/L	Albumin	4.0 g/dL
CO_2	24 mEq/L		
BUN	13 mEq/dL	**Urinalysis:**	
Cr	0.9 mg/dL	SG	1.020
Gluc	122 mg/dL	pH	6
		Prot	Neg
Coagulation panel:		Gluc	Neg
PT	13.1 sec	Ketones	Neg
PTT	26.2 sec	Bili	Neg
INR	1.0	Blood	Neg
		LE	Neg
		Nitrite	Neg
		Color	Yellow

a. Lactate: 1.2 mmol/L (if ordered)
b. Pelvic US (Figures 44.1–44.3) shows edematous polycystic right ovary with decreased blood flow on Doppler imaging

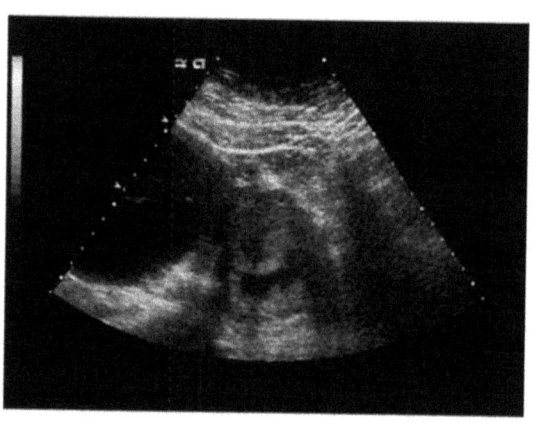

Figure 44.1

Figure 44.2

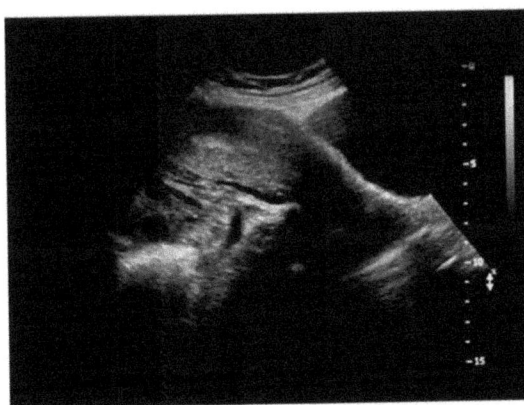

Figure 44.3

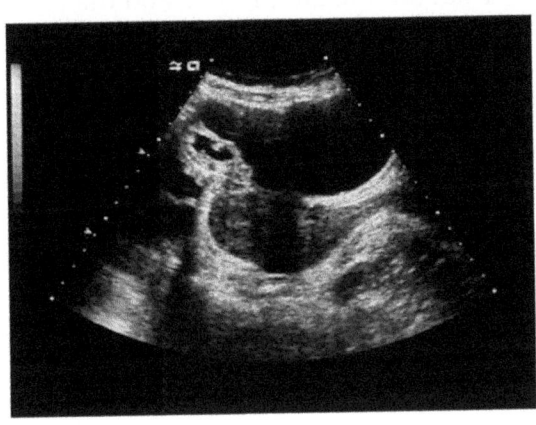

M. Action
a. Preop labs
    i. Blood type and crossmatch
b. Meds
    i. IV pain medication (opioid)
c. Gynecology consult
    i. Emergent laparoscopy for detorsion
d. Discussion with patient regarding need for emergent surgery for ovarian torsion, risk of losing ovary, and infertility
e. If US is not ordered and a course of observation is selected, patient will start to experience worsening symptoms

N. Diagnosis
a. Ovarian torsion

O. Critical actions
a. Pregnancy test
b. Pelvic examination
c. Pelvic US
d. Ob/gyn consultation for laparoscopy and detorsion
e. Analgesia and reassessment

P. Examiner instructions

a. This is a case of ovarian (adnexal) torsion. The ovary has twisted around its blood supply, causing lack of blood flow and pain, and threatening the viability of the organ. The patient's symptoms are severe, abrupt in onset, with occasional respites from a nonspecific but intense pain. Important early actions include ruling out pregnancy (and, by extension, ectopic pregnancy), identifying an enlarged ovary, and evaluating blood flow to the ovaries by Doppler US. A CT scan would show a large ovary, and could show fat stranding or other inflammatory changes. The patient's pain will be partially relieved by pain medication, and her laboratory results will not aid in diagnosis. Treatment of ovarian torsion is extremely time-sensitive; the risk of losing the ovary increases with total ischemic time. If gynecology is consulted prior to obtaining Doppler US, the consultant should be reluctant to see the patient rapidly; the candidate should explicitly describe a concern for ovarian torsion and understand the emergent need for operative intervention.

Q. Pearls

a. Adnexal torsion, a twisting of the ovary on its vascular pedicle, is a surgical emergency, responsible for approximately 3% of gynecologic emergencies. The duration of ischemia necessary to cause irreversible tissue necrosis is unknown, but a delay in diagnosis may result in the loss of the ovary and fallopian tube.

b. Torsion of a normal-sized ovary is rare; ovarian cysts greater than 5 cm and polycystic ovaries are more prone to torsion. Previous history of ovarian mass or infertility treatments have been reported as risk factors. Prior ectopic pregnancies, pelvic inflammatory disease, or endometriosis are not risk factors.

c. Laboratory findings are nonspecific in ovarian torsion, and cannot be used to assess tissue necrosis or ischemia.

d. Massive ovarian edema on imaging is suggestive of intermittently impaired blood flow.

R. Figure Legends

a. Figure 44.1 (Pelvic US) Edematous right polycystic ovary with decreased flow.

b. Figure 44.2 (Pelvic US) Edematous right polycystic ovary with decreased flow.

c. Figure 44.3 (Pelvic US) Edematous right polycystic ovary with decreased flow.

S. References

a. *Tintinalli's Emergency Medicine: A Comprehensive Study Guide* (9th ed.): Chapter 97, Abdominal and Pelvic Pain in the Nonpregnant Female.

b. *Rosen's Emergency Medicine: Concepts and Clinical Practice* (10th ed.): Chapter 86, Gynecologic Disorders.

Altered Mental Status

Nicholas Genes, MD, PhD

A. Chief complaint
a. 33-year old male found unconscious

B. Vital signs
a. BP: 95/63, HR: 66, RR: 11, T: 37.2°C, Sat: 96% on RA

C. What does the patient look like?
a. Patient appears stated age, unconscious on stretcher.

D. Primary survey
a. Airway: not speaking; no apparent obstruction or trauma
b. Breathing: no respiratory distress, no cyanosis
c. Circulation: warm skin, normal capillary refill

E. Action
a. Supplement oxygen as needed to maintain >95% saturation and/or monitor end-tidal CO_2
b. Two large-bore peripheral IV lines
c. Labs
   i. CBC, BMP, serum acetaminophen, salicylates, alcohol, creatine phosphokinase (CPK), urine toxicology screen, ± carboxyhemoglobin level
d. Monitor: BP: 96/68, HR: 71, RR: 10, Sat: 100% on O_2
e. EKG
f. Finger stick glucose (98 mg/dL; must ask)

F. History
a. HPI: A 33-year-old male recently began working as a home health aide for a client with advanced cancer. EMS reports the patient voiced no complaints, behaved normally until he went to the bathroom about 2 hours ago. Client discovered the patient collapsed by the toilet.
b. PMHx: unknown
c. PSHx: unknown
d. Allergies: unknown
e. Social: unknown
f. FHx: unknown
g. PMD: unknown

G. Nurse
a. EKG (Figure 45.1)

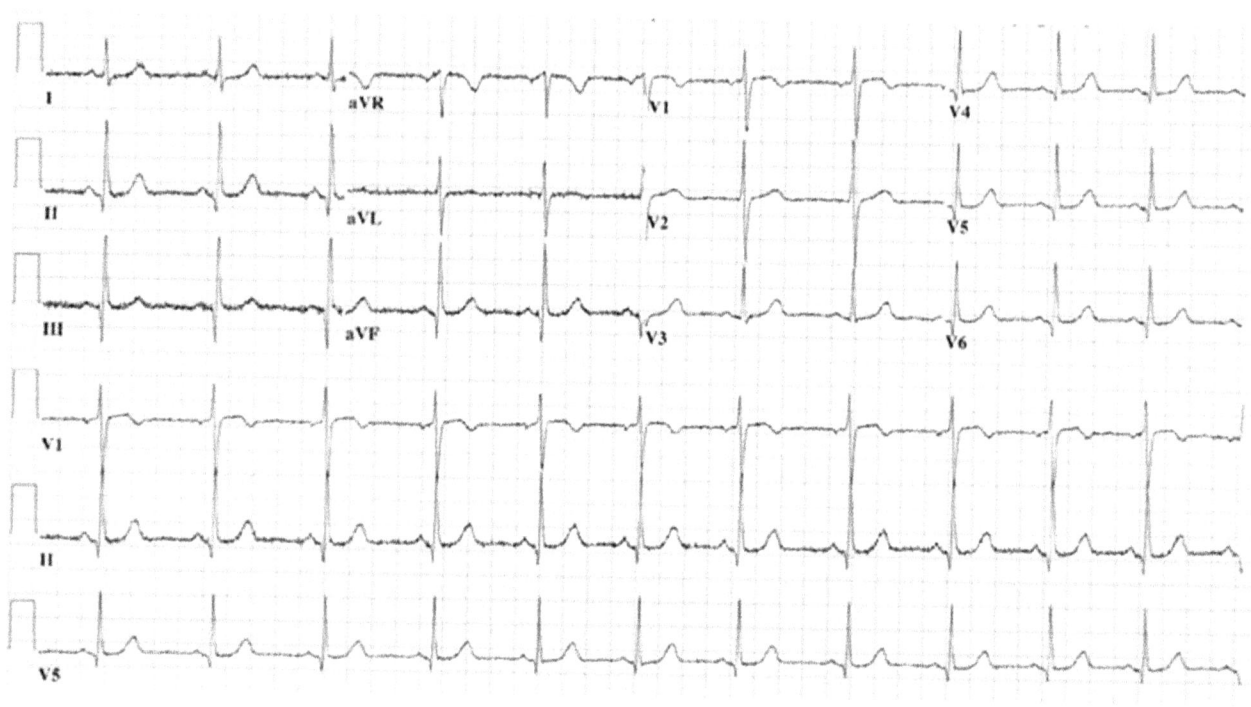

Figure 45.1

H. Secondary survey

a. General: obtunded, minimally arousable, no apparent distress
b. HEENT: pupils equal, round and reactive to light, 2 mm to 1 mm, no signs of head trauma
c. Neck: normal
d. Chest: lungs clear, normal breath sounds with no wheezes, rhonchi, or rales
e. Heart: normal, no murmurs, rubs, or gallops
f. Abdomen: soft, nontender, nondistended
g. Rectal: hemoccult negative, normal rectal tone
h. Urogenital: normal
i. Extremities: normal
j. Back: normal
k. Neuro: obtunded, barely arousable; moves all extremities, uncooperative with examination
l. Skin: pale, no rashes, edema, or cellulitis
m. Lymph: normal

I. Action

a. Meds
    i. Administer naloxone, dose 0.1–0.4 mg IV; also may give normal saline, thiamine, and folate through IV
b. Reassess
    i. Patient more easily aroused with noxious stimuli (e.g., sternal rub)
c. Imaging
    i. Portable CXR (evaluate for aspiration, radio-opaque pill fragments)
    ii. Consider head CT (not necessary if no signs of trauma, no appreciable neuro deficit, and patient rapidly improves with antidote)

J. Nurse

a. If naloxone given: BP: 98/59, HR: 80, RR: 13, Sat: 98% on O_2
b. If naloxone not given: BP: 98/59, HR: 80, RR: 8, Sat: 93% on O_2

K. Results

Table 45.1 Results table

Test	Result	Test	Result
Complete blood count:		Amylase	40 U/L
WBC	$6.1 \times 10^3/\mu L$	Lipase	53 U/L
Hct	41.50%	Albumin	4.1 g/dL
Plt	$253 \times 10^3/\mu L$		
		Urinalysis:	
Basic metabolic panel:		SG	1.020
Na	137 mEq/L	pH	6
K	4.1 mEq/L	Prot	Neg
Cl	103 mEq/L	Gluc	Neg
CO_2	25 mEq/L	Ketones	Neg
BUN	12 mEq/dL	Bili	Neg
Cr	0.8 mg/dL	Blood	Neg
Gluc	102 mg/dL	LE	Neg
		Nitrite	Neg
Liver function panel:		Color	Yellow
AST	45 U/L		
ALT	40 U/L	**Arterial blood gas:**	
Alk phos	100 U/L	pH	7.3
T bili	0.8 mg/dL	pO_2	80 mmHg
D bili	0.1 mg/dL	pCO_2	65 mmHg
		HCO_3	24 mmol/L

a. Urine toxicology results not available
b. Alcohol, acetaminophen, salicylates negative
c. CPK, carboxyhemoglobin levels normal (if ordered)
d. CXR (Figure 45.2)

I. Action

a. Meds
    i. Naloxone IV until status improves
    ii. If naloxone not given, suffers respiratory depression, requires intubation and ICU admission – or codes in the ER

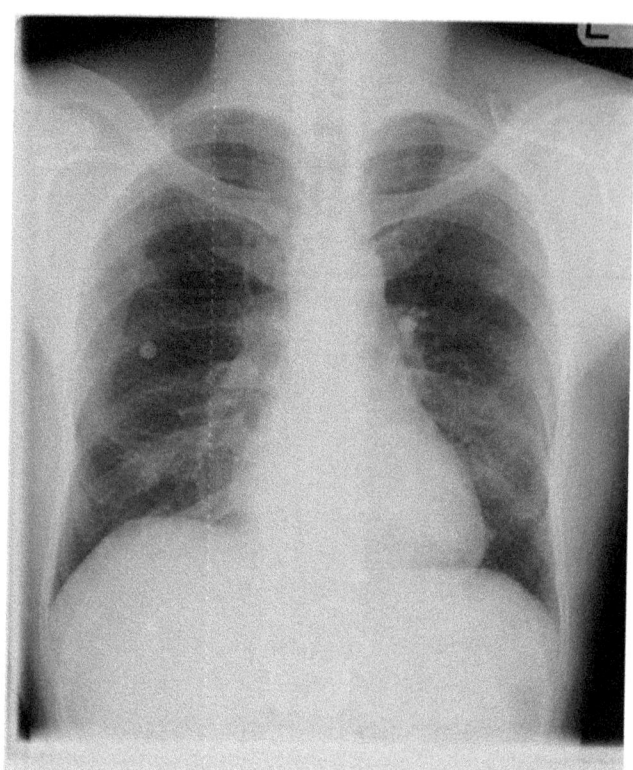

Figure 45.2

b. Observation for 12 hours if repeated doses of naloxone given; consider admission
   i. With repeated escalating doses of naloxone if mental status declines, or administer naloxone IV drip
c. Consult Poison Center and discharge with referral for substance abuse counseling

J. Diagnosis
a. Opioid overdose

K. Critical actions
a. Finger stick glucose
b. Naloxone administration
c. EKG
d. CXR
e. Reassessment after interventions
f. Observation for 6 hours after naloxone administration

L. Examiner instructions
a. This is a case of opioid (narcotic) intoxication from access to client's medications, which included fentanyl patches and oxycodone tablets. The patient presents with the "classic triad" of opioid overdose – coma, miosis (small pupils), and decreased respiratory rate. Important early actions include administering naloxone incrementally, as a large initial dose can precipitate withdrawal, vomiting, and possibly aspiration. Prolonged delay, (as if waiting for urine toxicology screen results) will result in respiratory depression and necessitate intubation to prevent death. Failure to monitor and observe for hours after naloxone administration will result in recurrence of obtundation and respiratory depression. If this patient is sent outside of the ED (for nonportable CXR or a CT scan) without intubation, inform candidate that the

"patient has stopped breathing in radiology." The patient will be found apneic, hypoxic, and bradycardic, requiring ACLS.

M. Pearls
a. While opioid withdrawal alone is not life-threatening, suddenly precipitating withdrawal with high-dose naloxone can pose significant risk. Withdrawal symptoms can be managed with clonidine, antiemetics, antidiarrheals, and methadone.
b. A titrated dose of naloxone is warranted in patients who maintain appropriate airway patency and ventilation. A naloxone dose of up to 2.0 mg IV may be necessary in patients with significant respiratory depression, and may be repeated every 3 minutes until 10 mg have been administered or respiratory depression is reversed. If no improvement, bag-valve-mask ventilation and/or endotracheal intubation is indicated.
c. The duration of action of naloxone IV is 20–60 minutes, which is shorter than most opioids. Thus, it may be necessary to re-dose, especially in the setting of sustained-release opioid ingestions.
d. Many opioid overdoses can be safely discharged after a period of observation in the ED; in this case the severe respiratory depression, need for multiple doses of naloxone, and prolonged symptoms warranted further management and admission.
e. Gastric decontamination (with activated charcoal) can be considered in toxic ingestions, particularly when less than 1 hour after ingestion (especially β-blockers, calcium channel blockers, and cyclic antidepressants). However, the risks of aspiration in a comatose patient must be balanced with potential gains. Gastric decontamination rarely affects clinical outcomes in the undifferentiated poisoned patient and should not be used routinely.
f. Urine toxicology screens are time-consuming, highly prone to false readings, and will not change emergent management of adult patients.
g. A finger stick blood sugar test is key to eliminating a common cause of altered mental status, and should be performed immediately on every altered patient.
h. Some states mandate reporting of impaired healthcare workers and reporting intoxication cases to Poison Control Centers, which can aid in management and outpatient follow-up.
i. Consider naloxone prescription for patients being discharged after opioid overdose. Many public health efforts seek to address opioid overdose mortality through increasing bystander access to naloxone, so be aware of local resources.

N. Figure legends
a. Figure 45.1 (EKG) Normal sinus rhythm (inferior Q waves suggest old infarction).
b. Figure 45.2 (CXR) Normal chest X-ray.

O. References
a. *Tintinalli's Emergency Medicine: A Comprehensive Study Guide* (9th ed.): Chapter 186, Opioids.
b. *Rosen's Emergency Medicine: Concepts and Clinical Practice* (10th ed.): Chapter 151, Opioids.

Diarrhea

Nicholas Genes, MD, PhD

A. Chief complaint
a. 34-year-old man with abdominal pain and diarrhea

B. Vital signs
a. BP: 122/77, HR: 92, RR: 18 T: 37.5°C, Sat: 99% on RA

C. What does the patient look like?
a. Patient appears stated age, comfortably lying on his stretcher.

D. Primary survey
a. Airway: speaking in full sentences
b. Breathing: no respiratory distress, no cyanosis
c. Circulation: warm and dry skin, normal capillary refill

E. History
a. HPI: A 34-year-old man with no significant past medical history presents with persistent diarrhea over the past few weeks. He denies fever. He defecates more than six times a day, producing a watery brown stool with a foul odor and no signs of blood or flecks of mucus. His abdomen feels bloated and occasionally diffusely painful. Symptoms were initially worse, then seemed to resolve, but have returned and persisted. He thinks he has lost 10 lb. since the onset of symptoms.
b. PMHx: had asthma as a teen but has "outgrown it"
c. PSHx: none
d. Allergies: none
e. Meds: none
f. Social: lives alone, consumes alcohol socially, no smoking, no IV drug use
g. FHx: father with diabetes; brother with Crohn's disease
h. PMD: none

F. Secondary survey
a. General: alert and oriented, no apparent distress
b. HEENT: mucous membranes dry
c. Neck: normal
d. Chest: lungs clear to auscultation, no wheezes
e. Heart: borderline tachycardic, no murmurs or rubs
f. Abdomen: soft, nontender, mild distension, active bowel sounds, no hepatosplenomegaly
g. Rectal: hemoccult negative brown stool

h. Urogenital: normal
i. Back: normal
j. Extremities: normal
k. Neuro: normal
l. Skin: warm, dry, no edema, no clubbing
m. Lymph: normal

G. Action

a. Further history: The patient denies recent illness and has never had unprotected sex, anal sex, or sex with high-risk partners. He has not been exposed to blood-borne pathogens. Denies antibiotic use in recent months. The patient admits to traveling outside the country about 6 weeks ago; he visited several Eastern European countries.
b. Obtain stool sample for ova and parasites, fecal leukocytes, stool culture, *Clostridium difficile* toxin, *Giardia* antigen, GI PCR testing
c. Send electrolyte panel
d. IV access

H. Nurse

a. BP: 125/73, HR: 92, RR: 18, T: 37.5°C, Sat: 99% on RA

I. Results

Table 46.1 Results table

Test	Result	Test	Result
Complete blood count:		Liver function panel:	
WBC	$10.9 \times 10^3/\mu L$	AST	44 U/L
Hct	43%	ALT	38 U/L
Plt	$220 \times 10^3/\mu L$	Alk phos	110 U/L
		T bili	0.9 mg/dL
		D bili	0.1 mg/dL
Basic metabolic panel:		Amylase	55 U/L
Na	133 mEq/L	Lipase	28 U/L
K	3.2 mEq/L	Albumin	3.9 g/dL
Cl	105 mEq/L		
CO_2	16 mEq/L		
BUN	28 mEq/dL	Urinalysis:	
Cr	1.1 mg/dL	SG	1.030
Gluc	99 mg/dL	pH	7
		Prot	Neg
		Gluc	Neg
Coagulation panel:		Ketones	Neg
PT	12.7 sec	Bili	Neg
PTT	28.3 sec	Blood	Neg
INR	1.0		

Table 46.1 (cont.)

Test	Result	Test	Result
		LE	Neg
		Nitrite	Neg
		Color	Yellow

a. Ova and parasites analysis reveal cysts and motile, pear-shaped trophozoites
b. Fecal leukocytes not seen
c. Other tests pending

J. Action
a. Oral rehydration using a glucose-containing beverage, or IV fluids such as NS with supplementary potassium
b. Prescribe antibiotics: tinidazole or metronidazole
c. Arrange for outpatient follow-up
d. Report case to the Centers for Disease Control

K. Diagnosis
a. Traveler's diarrhea – likely giardiasis.

L. Critical actions
a. Elicit social history – travel, risk factors for immune compromise, recent antibiotic use.
b. Send stool sample with ova and parasites, fecal leukocytes, *Giardia* antigen, *C. difficile* toxin and other GI immunoassay testing if available.
c. Rehydrate and replete electrolyte deficiencies.
d. Prescribe antibiotics (such as tinidazole, metronidazole, nitazoxanide).
e. Arrange for follow-up.

M. Examiner instructions
a. This is a case of traveler's diarrhea, resulting from *Giardia lamblia* infection. The patient's symptoms are vague, mild, and his clinical course in the ED is stable and unchanging. Important early actions are to elicit a travel history, risk factors for immunocompromised state, and other important causes of diarrhea and abdominal symptomatology. Critical actions include sending a stool sample for laboratory analysis, rehydrating the patient, prescribing antibiotics, and arranging for follow-up. Imaging is of no benefit in this case, and requests to consult gastroenterologists or infectious disease specialists will yield no additional information.

N. Pearls
a. Approximately 40% of Americans traveling to developing countries are affected by diarrhea or gastroenteritis in the first two weeks of travel.
b. *G. lamblia* is the most commonly identified cause of *chronic* traveler's diarrhea, as in this case (*Escherichia coli* being the most common acute cause). Giardia is a protozoan infection of the proximal gut, typically transmitted by contaminated water, commonly in Eastern Europe (though food or fecal–oral transmission is possible and accounts for occasional daycare epidemics in the United States). Infected patients are usually asymptomatic or self-limited

after an acute phase, but in some patients symptoms can persist for years. A course of metronidazole is more than 90% effective in achieving cure.

c.   *Entamoeba histolytica* amebiasis is a culprit for long-term travelers to Africa, Asia, and Latin America. Like *Giardia*, amebiasis is a protozoan infection identified by antigen or ova and parasite testing. Unlike *Giardia*, *E. histolytica* can invade the colon wall and liver, causing fevers, pain, and potentially fatal abscesses.

d.   Acute diarrheal illness (less than 2 weeks) is usually caused by bacteria or their toxins, with common organisms including *E. coli*, *Campylobacter jejuni*, *Salmonella*, *Shigella*, *Vibrio*, and *C. difficile*.

e.   *Vibrio cholera* is rarely imported into the United States, causing only 80 cases per year. It presents as a profuse, painless watery diarrhea ("rice-water stools") in tropical travelers that can result in profound dehydration and requires aggressive fluid resuscitation.

f.   The use of loperamide is discouraged in moderate to severe acute infectious diarrhea, especially in young children and diarrhea associated with abdominal pain or blood in stool.

O. References

a.   *Tintinalli's Emergency Medicine: A Comprehensive Study Guide* (9th ed.): Chapter 162, Global Travelers.

b.   *Rosen's Emergency Medicine: Concepts and Clinical Practice* (10th ed.): Chapter 167, Infectious Diarrheal Disease and Dehydration. Chapter 80, Gastroenteritis.

Seizure

Shefali Trivedi, MD

A. Chief complaint
a. 35-year-old female with seizure prior to arrival

B. Vital signs
a. BP: 122/80, HR: 102, RR: 18, T: 38.6°C, Sat: 99% on RA

C. What does the patient look like?
a. Patient appears stated age, slightly pale, sleeping comfortably on stretcher and in no acute distress.

D. Primary survey
a. Airway: patent, speaks in full sentences
b. Breathing: no apparent respiratory distress, no cyanosis
c. Circulation: warm, dry skin, normal capillary refill

E. Action
a. Oxygen via NC or nonrebreather mask as needed to maintain >95% saturation
b. Peripheral IV access
c. Labs
   i. CBC, BMP, LFT, calcium, magnesium, ± prolactin, toxicology panel, VBG/ABG with lactate
d. 1 L NS
e. Blood cultures
f. EKG and monitored bed
g. Fingerstick glucose = 112 mg/dL

F. History
a. HPI: A 35-year-old female with a past medical history of hypertension presents after a seizure witnessed by her spouse about 1 hour before arrival. According to the spouse, the seizure was generalized tonic-clonic and lasted about 30 seconds with no postictal state. There was no head trauma associated with the event. This was her first seizure. The patient does not recall the seizure, but does note that she has had subjective fever associated with generalized mild abdominal pain for the past 3 days. She denies chest pain, shortness of breath, headache, chills, upper respiratory infection symptoms, nausea, vomiting, diarrhea, urinary symptoms, trauma, sick contacts, or travel history.
b. PMHx: hypertension
c. PSHx: none
d. Allergies: none

CASE 47: Seizure

e. Meds: hydrochlorothiazide
f. Social: lives with husband and two children at home; denies smoking, alcohol, drug use; sexually active with her husband only
g. FHx: noncontributory
h. PMD: Dr. Parker, who she sees at least annually

G. Nurse
a. BP: 129/87, HR: 88, RR: 16 Sat: 100% on O$_2$, remains febrile
b. EKG

H. Secondary survey
a. General: alert and oriented, no acute distress
b. HEENT: pale conjunctivae, otherwise normal
c. Neck: normal
d. Chest: normal
e. Heart: normal
f. Abdomen: normal
g. Rectal: hemoccult negative brown stool, normal rectal tone
h. Urogenital: normal
i. Extremities: normal
j. Back: normal
k. Neuro: normal
l. Skin: petechiae and bruising noted on upper and lower extremities bilaterally
m. Lymph: normal

I. Action
a. CT head without contrast
b. Acetaminophen PO

J. Nurse
a. BP: 117/75, HR: 82, RR: 16, Sat: 100% on RA

K. Results

Table 47.1 Results table

Test	Result	Test	Result
Complete blood count:		**Liver function panel:**	
WBC	$9.9 \times 10^3/\mu L$	AST	33 U/L
Hct	19.4%	ALT	13 U/L
Plt	$20 \times 10^3/\mu L$	Alk phos	75 U/L
		T bili	1.2 mg/dL
		D bili	0.4 mg/dL
Basic metabolic panel:		Amylase	47 U/L
Na	137 mEq/L	Lipase	25 U/L
K	3.9 mEq/L		

Table 47.1 (cont.)

Test	Result	Test	Result
Cl	102 mEq/L	Albumin	4.0 g/dL
CO_2	25 mEq/L		
BUN	13 mEq/dL	**Urinalysis:**	
Cr	1.9 mg/dL	SG	1.020
Gluc	110 mg/dL	pH	6
Ca (total)	9.0 mg/dL	Prot	+
Mg	2.1 mg/dL	Gluc	Neg
		Ketones	Neg
Coagulation panel:		Bili	Neg
PT	13.8 sec	Blood	Neg
PTT	30 sec	LE	Neg
INR	1.0	Nitrite	Neg
		Color	Yellow

a. CT head
b. Urine pregnancy test negative

L. Action
a. Ask for a peripheral smear
b. Consult hematology
c. Prednisone
d. Plasma exchange

M. Diagnosis
a. Thrombotic thrombocytopenic purpura (TTP)

N. Critical actions
a. Note petechiae on physical examination
b. Obtain CBC
c. Steroids
d. Consider plasma exchange
e. Hematology consultation (noting possible diagnosis of TTP)
f. Admission to ICU

O. Examiner instructions
a. This is a case of thrombotic thrombocytopenic purpura (TTP), where platelets aggregate abnormally in small blood vessels. This may lead to bleeding complications and multiorgan system complications. A thorough search into the cause of seizure is important in this case, especially laboratory evaluation and head CT to investigate intracranial complication such as bleeding.

b. Curveball: The patient could present actively seizing, or seize during the secondary survey, requiring the candidate to alter focus on the primary survey and seizure control. Benzodiazepines (such as lorazepam, midazolam) should be the first-line agents used to treat the seizures. After two doses, the seizures should stop.

P. Pearls

a. The classic pentad of TTP includes: fever, microangiopathic hemolytic anemia, thrombocytopenia, renal impairment, and CNS impairment. Though it is uncommon to have all components of the pentad, about 90% of presentations include fever.

b. TTP is a clinical diagnosis, but characteristic laboratory findings include severe anemia (usually, Hct < 20%), thrombocytopenia (classically 10,000–50,000/mm^3), schistocytes, fragmented RBCs on the peripheral smear.

c. Neurologic findings can include headache, seizure, coma, CVA, altered mental status, or paresthesias.

d. Dialysis, anticonvulsants, or benzodiazepines may need to be ordered if the patient is suffering from severe renal impairment or seizure activity, respectively, and there is an anticipated delay before the effect of plasma exchange will take place.

e. Avoid platelet transfusions in TTP unless there is a risk of intracranial bleeding or hemorrhage, as added platelets can augment the platelet aggregation and cause worsening thrombosis and eventual ischemia. Plasma exchange with fresh frozen plasma is considered first-line treatment for severe cases, reducing mortality to about 6%. Initial therapy may also include steroids and antiplatelets.

Q. References

a. *Tintinalli's Emergency Medicine: A Comprehensive Study Guide* (9th ed.): Chapter 237, Acquired Hemolytic Anemia.

b. *Rosen's Emergency Medicine: Concepts and Clinical Practice* (10th ed.): Chapter 111, Disorders of Hemostasis.

Toothache

Shefali Trivedi, MD

A. Chief complaint
a. 36-year-old male with dental pain

B. Vital signs
a. BP: 141/79, HR: 107, RR: 18, T: 38.0°C, Sat: 99% on RA

C. What does the patient look like?
a. Patient appears stated age, sitting up in stretcher, holding left side of face, uncomfortable, mild distress due to pain.

D. Primary survey
a. Airway: patent, speaking in full sentences, difficulty opening mouth fully but protecting airway
b. Breathing: no apparent distress, no cyanosis
c. Circulation: warm, dry skin, normal capillary refill

E. History
a. HPI: A 36-year-old male with no past medical history presents with left jaw pain and left lower molar pain for 7 days and swelling associated with difficulty opening his mouth for 2 days. The patient states he was going to try to make an appointment with his dentist, but the pain was so severe that he needed to come to the emergency department first. The patient states that the swelling appears to be worsening over the past 2 days and he has noted a foul smell from his mouth. He also notes fever and chills for 2 days as well as increasing sore throat, change in his voice, and painful swallowing. He denies nausea, vomiting, diarrhea, constipation, trauma, or previous similar symptoms.
b. PMHx: none
c. PSHx: none
d. Allergies: none
e. Social: lives with his wife at home; denies smoking, drug use; drinks alcohol socially; sexually active with his wife only
f. FHx: noncontributory
g. PMD: Dr. Taylor, who he does not see regularly for routine visits

F. Secondary survey
a. General: alert and oriented, sitting up in stretcher, holding left side of face, uncomfortable, mild distress due to pain
b. HEENT: normocephalic, atraumatic, ocular examination normal, ears normal to inspection, tympanic membranes clear; nose examination normal, + left external jaw swelling, + trismus (unable to open mouth greater than 2 cm), + left submandibular area tense/indurated, swelling,

erythematous, tender to palpation, + elevation of the floor of the mouth, + mild protrusion of the tongue, + whitish discoloration of gum below left lower molars

c. Neck: normal; no crepitus
d. Chest: normal
e. Heart: normal
f. Abdomen: normal
g. Extremities: normal
h. Back: normal
i. Neuro: normal
j. Skin: normal
k. Lymph: normal

G. Action

a. Oxygen via NC or nonrebreather mask as needed to maintain >95% saturation
b. Two large-bore peripheral IV lines
c. Prepare intubation equipment (may be needed if condition worsens)
d. Labs
   i. CBC, BMP, PT/PTT, blood type and hold
e. 1 L NS bolus
f. Monitor: BP: 138/82, HR: 98, RR: 16, Sat: 100% on 2 L NC
g. Acetaminophen PO

H. Action

a. Meds
   i. Clindamycin IV (or other appropriate IV antibiotic; see below)
   ii. Morphine IV
b. Consult ear, nose, and throat (ENT) specialist or oral maxillofacial surgery (OMFS)
c. Monitor and maintain secure airway

I. Nurse

a. BP: 135/79, HR: 89, RR: 16, Sat: 99% on 2 L NC
b. Patient: symptoms improving, but pain is still present

J. Results

Table 48.1 Results table

Test	Result	Test	Result
Complete blood count:		CO_2	24 mEq/L
WBC	$24.3 \times 10^3/\mu L$	BUN	18 mEq/dL
Hct	43.50%	Cr	1.1 mg/dL
Plt	$225 \times 10^3/\mu L$	Gluc	126 mg/dL
Basic metabolic panel:		**Coagulation panel:**	
Na	138 mEq/L	PT	13.3 sec
K	3.8 mEq/L	PTT	32 sec
Cl	104 mEq/L	INR	1.1

K. Action
a. ENT or OMFS consult
b. Admission for administration of IV antibiotics and monitoring of airway patency

L. Diagnosis
a. Ludwig's angina

M. Critical actions
a. Airway management, assessment for difficult airway characteristics and anticipate advanced airway management techniques
b. Antibiotics
c. ENT or OMFS consult – should not be delayed for diagnostic imaging
d. Admission

N. Examiner instructions
a. This is a case of Ludwig's angina, which is a deep soft tissue infection in the neck, usually caused by a dental infection. Early antibiotics, airway monitoring, and surgical consultation are paramount.
b. Although diagnostic imaging such as soft tissue plain films of the neck, US, CT, or MRI may aid in the diagnosis of Ludwig's angina and its complications, Ludwig's angina is a clinical diagnosis. Unless the candidate describes a specific concern for Ludwig's angina (based on induration of the submandibular space and concerning patient presentation), the ENT consultant will simply advise that the patient should follow-up with a dentist the next day. If antibiotics are not administered in a timely manner, the patient may develop increasing airway swelling, difficulty breathing, increased heart rate and respiratory distress, and require emergency airway management.
c. The examinee should request frequent exams of the airway.
d. Curveball: This case could be used to review advanced airway management strategies. The examiner could have the patient present in more acute distress with significant airway swelling, or deteriorate rapidly during the secondary survey. Thus, the primary survey will reveal a patient in significant respiratory distress, unable to swallow his oral secretions. The candidate will have to manage the airway using advanced techniques (i.e., fiberoptic intubation, surgical airway). This should be addressed before any other intervention (in parallel with establishing IV access). If the candidate chooses rapid sequence intubation with paralysis in the setting of this significant airway edema, they will *not* be successful in viewing the vocal cords and the intubation attempt will fail.

O. Pearls
a. A recently extracted or infected lower molar tooth is often present in the history of patients with Ludwig's angina.
b. The most common physical examination findings include bilateral submandibular swelling and elevation or protrusion of the tongue.
c. Ludwig's angina is a clinical diagnosis and includes the following five criteria: cellulitis with little or no pus in the submandibular space; bilateral cellulitis; gangrene with serosanguinous putrid fluid; involvement of connective tissue, fascia, and muscles, but sparing of glandular tissue; and cellulitis spread by continuity and not by lymphatics.
d. Airway compromise can occur suddenly and especially if action is not taken immediately. Posterior displacement of the tongue often leads to obstruction of the airway and patients may

require endotracheal intubation. However, this is often difficult given the altered anatomy from the edema and infection. Fiberoptic oral intubation, nasotracheal intubation, or a surgical airway may be necessary.

e. Preferred antibiotic choices include high-dose penicillin with metronidazole, clindamycin, ticarcillin–clavulanate, or piperacillin–tazobactam.

f. Admission (consider ICU admission) may be required for IV antibiotics and close airway monitoring.

g. Incision and drainage may be indicated if the patient does not respond to antibiotics.

P. References

a. *Tintinalli's Emergency Medicine: A Comprehensive Study Guide* (9th ed.) Chapter 246, Neck and Upper Airway Disorders.

b. *Rosen's Emergency Medicine: Concepts and Clinical Practice* (10th ed.): Chapter 61, Upper Respiratory Tract Infections.

Penetrating Chest Trauma

Abiola Fasina, MD, Jodi Jones MD, and Mandy Pascual MD

A. Chief complaint
a. 24-year-old male stabbed in the chest

B. Vital signs
a. BP: 115/62, HR: 120, RR: 30, T: 97°F, Sat: 97% on RA

C. What does the patient look like?
a. Young male with pale clammy skin, supine on a stretcher. Patient is somnolent with slow speech. Large gauze is present over the left mid-chest, soaked in blood, with emergency medical technician applying pressure.

D. Primary survey
a. Airway: speaking, no stridor
b. Breathing: tachypneic, using accessory muscles in obvious distress, equal breath sounds
c. Circulation: pale, clammy skin with thready radial pulses bilaterally, which disappears while examining patient

E. Action
a. Oxygen via nonrebreather mask
b. Preparations for intubation, for airway protection and impending respiratory collapse
c. Two large-bore peripheral IV lines
d. Labs
   i. CBC, BMP, PT/PTT, blood type and crossmatch, and lactate sent
e. Monitor: BP: 90/50, HR: 135, RR: 32, Sat: 95% on nonrebreather mask
f. Intubate with appropriate RSI (e.g., etomidate and succinylcholine or rocuronium); placement confirmed with capnography
g. Order portable CXR
h. Call blood bank for massive transfusion protocol (MTP) or two units uncrossmatched O-negative blood
i. Page surgical/trauma team

F. History
a. HPI: A 24-year-old male picked up by EMS outside a bar after being stabbed in the chest with a knife during a bar brawl. Patient was found sitting on the curb clutching his chest and complaining of pain. Patient denied any medical problems but admitted to having several drinks during the course of the evening.

b. PMHx: none
c. PSHx: none
d. Allergies: none
e. Meds: none
f. Social: social alcohol use
g. FHx: noncontributory
h. PMD: none

G. Nurse
a. NS/LR wide open while waiting for blood; initiate MTP as soon as possible
b. Repeat vital signs: BP: 90/52, HR: 145, RR: 24, Sat: 100% on ventilator
c. CXR (Figure 49.1)

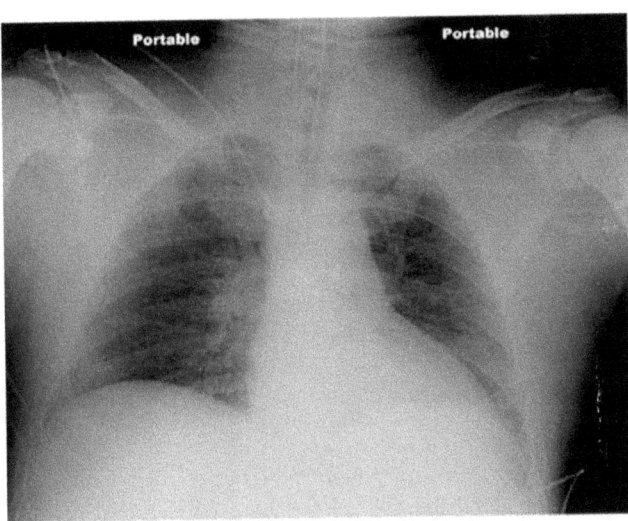

Figure 49.1

H. Secondary survey
a. General: unconscious and intubated
b. HEENT: normal; no facial lacerations or bruises are noted. Pupils equal, round, reactive and 3 mm bilaterally
c. Neck: distended neck veins
d. Chest: 2 cm wide laceration over the left anterior chest wall at approximately fifth intercostal space actively bleeding; equal breath sounds heard
e. Heart: muffled heart sounds – tachycardic
f. Abdomen: soft, nontender, no cuts, or hematomas noted
g. Rectal: normal tone with hemoccult negative stool
h. GU: normal
i. Back: normal
j. Extremities: good tone; weak radial pulses, no palpable dorsalis pedis pulses; cool clammy hands and feet
k. Neuro: withdraws to pain; unable to assess further
l. Skin: pale, no rashes or lesions
m. Lymph: normal

I. Action

a. Establish adequate IV access – two large-bore peripheral IV, intraosseous vascular access, or central venous access. Transfusion of uncrossmatched blood initiated.

b. Focused assessment with sonography in trauma (FAST) examination (Figure 49.2). Examiner may allow transient improvement if pericardiocentesis is attempted (describe procedure both with and without ultrasound), then progress to loss of vital signs.

c. CXR: heart silhouette unremarkable; endotracheal tube in correct position above the carina

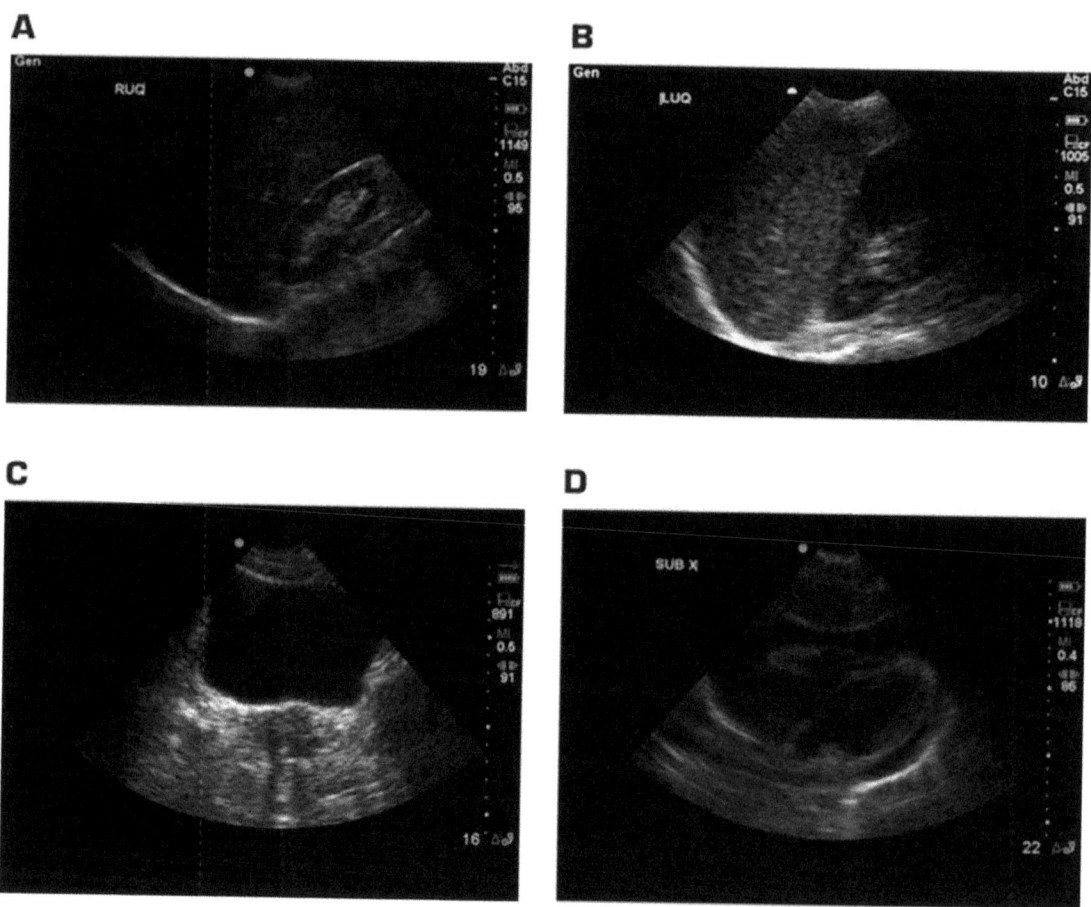

Figure 49.2

J. Nurse

a. Patient has lost vital signs, unable to palpate a pulse

K. Action

a. ED thoracotomy is performed (describe procedure) with presumptive diagnosis of acute pericardial tamponade due to penetrating chest wall injury. Once patient has lost pulses, there should be no delay for US or any imaging modality by the candidate prior to initiating this procedure

b. Tetanus shot administered, cefazolin IV

c. Surgery/trauma team arrives and prepares to take patient to OR

d. Foley catheter

L. Results

Table 49.1 Results table

Test	Result	Test	Result
Complete blood count:		**Urinalysis:**	
WBC	$12.0 \times 10^3/\mu L$	SG	1.010
Hct	24.0%	pH	5
Plt	$250 \times 10^3/\mu L$	Prot	Neg
		Gluc	Neg
Basic metabolic panel:		Ketones	Neg
Na	141 mEq/L	Bili	Neg
K	5.0 mEq/L	Blood	Neg
Cl	111 mEq/L	LE	Neg
CO_2	24 mEq/L	Nitrite	Neg
BUN	29 mEq/dL	Color	Yellow
Cr	0.9 mg/dL		
Gluc	100 mg/dL	**Arterial blood gas:**	
		pH	7.4
		pO_2	85 mmHg
Coagulation panel:		pCO_2	40 mmHg
PT	14.6 sec	HCO_3	24 mmol/L
PTT	30 sec		
INR	1.1		

M. Action

a. Thoracotomy reveals a large amount of blood and clot in pericardium, 1 cm hole in right ventricle with active bleeding.
b. Tamponade ventricular bleeding with finger, Foley catheter, or by oversewing.
c. Patient taken emergently to OR by surgical team.

N. Diagnosis

a. Acute cardiac tamponade due to penetrating chest wall trauma

O. Critical actions

a. Intubate patient for airway protection.
b. Start fluid and blood resuscitation immediately.
c. Diagnose cardiac tamponade (recognizing Beck's triad of distended neck veins, muffled heart sounds, and hypotension or by performing US).
d. Treat cardiac tamponade.
e. Surgical consultation for emergent OR repair.

P. Examiner instructions

a. This is a case of acute cardiac tamponade due to ongoing bleeding within the pericardium (fibrous sac around the heart). This constricts the heart and prevents normal pumping of blood, causing a rapid heart rate and low blood pressure. This patient's condition will rapidly deteriorate (heart rate will rise, blood pressure and oxygen saturation fall) until the pressure is relieved. Loss of vital signs is an indication for emergency thoracotomy in the ED. If pericardiocentesis is attempted, blood will be obtained but the patient's condition will only slightly improve as there is continued blood loss. Because of the volume and rate of bleeding, the fact that some of the blood is clotting, a needle is insufficient to drain enough blood to alleviate the condition. In this case, an open approach (thoracotomy) is warranted. Pericardiocentesis is not helpful in this setting because of a high incidence of false negatives, risk of further injury to the heart, and delay in definitive management.

b. Once thoracotomy is performed, the patient should be taken to the OR by trauma/surgery for surgical repair.

Q. Pearls

a. ABCs: Airway, breathing, and circulation always come first in the management of trauma patients. Securing the airway is the first step in appropriate management of this patient.

b. Beck's triad of hypotension, distended neck veins, and muffled heart sounds raise concern for pericardial effusion, though they are all present in only about one-third of cases. Beck's triad can also be seen in tension pneumothorax or systemic air embolism.

c. Initial management of cardiac tamponade is volume resuscitation to increase right-sided intracardiac pressures.

d. CXR is frequently unremarkable in pericardial effusion; do not depend on x-ray imaging to make the diagnosis. The CXR in this case served to confirm ETT tube position.

e. The cardiac view in the FAST exam will show pericardial fluid, with right ventricular collapse during diastole, which is more specific for tamponade.

f. Tamponade can also cause Kussmaul's sign (distension of neck veins during inspiration) and pulsus paradoxus (drop in systolic blood pressure of more than 10–15 mmHg during inspiration).

R. Figure legends

a. Figure 49.1 (CXR) ET and NGT in place, no focal infiltrate.

b. Figure 49.2 (US) Cardiac view, pericardial effusion with right ventricle collapse in diastole.

S. References

a. *Tintinalli's Emergency Medicine: A Comprehensive Study Guide* (9th ed.): Chapter 262, Cardiac Trauma.

b. *Rosen's Emergency Medicine: Concepts and Clinical Practice* (10th ed.): Chapter 37, Thoracic Trauma.

Animal Bite

Shefali Trivedi, MD

A. Chief complaint
a. 35-year-old male presents with cat bite to right hand 4 hours ago

B. Vital signs
a. BP: 128/82, HR: 78, RR: 16, T: 36.6°C, Sat: 98% on RA

C. What does the patient look like?
a. Patient appears stated age, comfortable, sitting on stretcher, and in no acute distress.

D. Primary survey
a. Airway: speaking in full sentences
b. Breathing: no apparent respiratory distress, no cyanosis
c. Circulation: warm, dry skin, normal capillary refill

E. History
a. HPI: A 35-year-old right-handed male with a past medical history of hypertension presents with a cat bite to the right hand 4 hours ago while playing with his neighbor's cat. The patient reports minimal bleeding and mild pain with making a fist. He denies fever, chills, nausea, vomiting, diarrhea, or constipation. He is right-hand dominant. He states that his neighbor informed him that the cat is a house cat, has received all appropriate vaccinations, and has been healthy and acting normally. He denies other injuries and his last tetanus is unknown.
b. PMHx: hypertension
c. PSHx: none
d. Allergies: none
e. Meds: amlodipine
f. Social: lives with his wife and daughter at home; denies alcohol use, smoking, or illicit drug use; sexually active with his wife only
g. FHx: no relevant history
h. PMD: Dr. Fox

F. Secondary survey
a. General: alert, oriented × 3, comfortable
b. Head: normocephalic, atraumatic
c. Eyes: extraocular movement intact, pupils equal, reactive to light
d. Ears: normal tympanic membranes
e. Nose: no discharge
f. Neck: full range of motion, no jugular vein distension, no stridor

g. Pharynx: normal dentition, no lesions, no swelling
h. Chest: nontender
i. Lungs: clear bilaterally
j. Heart: rate and rhythm regular, no murmurs, rubs, or gallops
k. Abdomen: normal bowel sounds, soft, nontender, not distended
l. Extremities: puncture wound on right index finger over the MCP joint not actively bleeding; full range of motion at all joints, mild pain with flexion at MCP joint, neurovascularly intact; no erythema, swelling, foreign body, streaking; normal capillary refill; left hand and bilateral lower extremities within normal limits
m. Back: nontender
n. Neuro: cranial nerves II to XII intact; normal sensation, strength; normal reflexes and gait, right index finger with normal flexion and extension at DIP, PIP, MCP joint with normal sensation
o. Skin: warm and dry (normal other than noted earlier)
p. Lymph: no lymphadenopathy

G. Action
a. Wound care
    i. Irrigation
b. Meds
    i. Amoxicillin/clavulanate or cefuroxime, initiated in ED
    ii. Tetanus toxoid
c. Follow-up
    i. Wound check in 48 hours in ED or with PMD
d. Discussion regarding rabies – low risk, have friend monitor for unusual behavior
e. Imaging
    i. X-ray of finger to rule out foreign body

H. Diagnosis
a. Cat bite

I. Critical actions
a. Appropriate antibiotics
b. Tetanus immunization
c. Follow-up for wound check

J. Examiner instructions
a. This is a case of cat bite from a known healthy cat, with verifiable immunization records, without evidence of neurovascular injury by exam. The candidate should ask about the cat to identify risk for rabies and perform a thorough examination to assess for tendon injury and infection. An x-ray of the finger may be helpful to evaluate for foreign bodies since it is a puncture wound and difficult to directly visualize. The candidate should also request follow-up within 24–48 hours for the patient because up to 80% of wounds caused by cat bites can become infected.

K. Pearls
a. Prophylactic antibiotics are indicated for all cat bites, as these wounds tend to be deep and difficult to adequately irrigate. Amoxicillin–clavulanate is recommended for prophylactic treatment, and therapy should be initiated in the ED for high-risk bites, such as cat bites to

the hand. Penicillin V or ampicillin may also be appropriate first-line treatment. A dose of IV antibiotic therapy may be preferable for high-risk bites.

b. Infection tends to be polymicrobial. The most common organisms isolated from cat bites include *Staphylococcus* species, *Streptococcus* species, and most often, *Pasteurella multocida*.

c. Prophylaxis is also recommended in bites in immunocompromised hosts, deep dog bite wounds, hand wounds, and any lacerations being sutured.

d. Consider rabies vaccination in all high-risk animal bites according to CDC guidelines.

L. References

a. *Tintinalli's Emergency Medicine: A Comprehensive Study Guide* (9th ed.): Chapter 46, Puncture Wounds and Bites.

b. *Rosen's Emergency Medicine: Concepts and Clinical Practice* (10th ed.): Chapter 52, Mammalian Bites.

Abdominal Pain

Shefali Trivedi, MD

A. Chief complaint

a. 24-year-old female brought in by her mother with complaint of lower abdominal pain for the past 4 days

B. Vital signs

a. BP: 110/75, HR: 110, RR: 14, T: 39.1°C, Sat: 99% on RA

C. What does the patient look like?

a. Patient appears stated age, lying supine in stretcher, in moderate discomfort due to pain.

D. Primary survey

a. Airway: speaking in full sentences
b. Breathing: no apparent respiratory distress, no cyanosis
c. Circulation: warm, dry skin, normal capillary refill

E. Action

a. Peripheral IV access
b. Labs
    i. CBC, BMP, LFTs, coagulation studies, blood type and crossmatch
    ii. Lactate, blood cultures, urinalysis, urine culture, urine pregnancy test
c. 1 L NS bolus
d. Monitor: BP: 115/76, HR: 98, RR: 16, Sat: 99% on O_2 or RA

F. History

a. Ask mother to step out of the room during the examination. Candidate may begin the interview with mother present, but should ask to conduct at least part of the interview with mother out of the room.
b. HPI: A 24-year-old female with no past medical history presents with lower abdominal pain for 4 days. Patient states that the pain is a constant, nonradiating, sharp pain in the left lower quadrant that has worsened over the past 4 days. She also notes that she has had a thick malodorous yellow/green vaginal discharge for the past 1 week for which she has not sought medical attention. She also notes fever to 102°F at home yesterday associated with chills. She is sexually active with two partners and admits that she is inconsistent with using protection. She denies urinary symptoms, nausea, vomiting, diarrhea, constipation, sick contacts, travel history, unusual food intake, trauma, or previous similar symptoms.
c. PMHx: none
d. PSHx: none

e. Allergies: none
f. Meds: oral contraceptive
g. Social: lives with her mother, father, and younger sister at home; social smoker and drinks alcohol socially; denies drug use; sexually active with two partners
h. FHx: no relevant history
i. PMD: none

G. Secondary survey
a. General: alert, oriented, mild distress secondary to pain
b. Head: normocephalic, atraumatic
c. Eyes: extraocular movement intact, pupils equal, reactive to light
d. Ears: normal tympanic membranes
e. Nose: no discharge
f. Neck: full range of motion, no jugular vein distension, no stridor
g. Pharynx: normal dentition, no lesions, no swelling
h. Chest: nontender
i. Lungs: clear bilaterally
j. Heart: rate and rhythm regular, no murmurs, rubs, or gallops
k. Abdomen: soft, positive tenderness left suprapubic area with voluntary guarding, no rebound, nontender McBurney's point, no hepatosplenomegaly, no masses, no hernias, no peritoneal signs, positive bowel sounds
l. Rectal: normal tone, brown stool, occult blood negative
m. Urogenital: normal external genitalia, moderate amount of dark yellow/green, malodorous discharge in the vaginal vault, no blood in vaginal vault; positive friable cervix, os closed, positive cervical motion tenderness, positive left adnexal tenderness, normal right adnexal examination
n. Extremities: full range of motion, no deformity, normal pulses
o. Back: nontender, no CVA tenderness
p. Neuro: cranial nerves II to XII intact; normal sensation, strength; normal reflexes and gait
q. Skin: warm and dry
r. Lymph: no lymphadenopathy

H. Nurse
a. Labs
   i. Urine pregnancy test negative

I. Action
a. Meds
   i. Cefoxitin IV
   ii. Doxycycline IV/PO
   iii. Acetaminophen
   iv. Morphine
b. Reassess
   i. Morphine: pain improved
   ii. No morphine: pain persists
c. Consult
   i. Gynecology
d. Imaging
   i. Pelvic US

e. Labs

　　i.　Gonorrhea and chlamydia culture (send specimen during pelvic examination for culture)

J. Nurse

a.　BP: 112/76, HR: 84, RR: 14, T: 37.9°C Sat: 100% on RA

b.　Patient: still with mild discomfort

c.　Pelvic US (Figure 51.1)

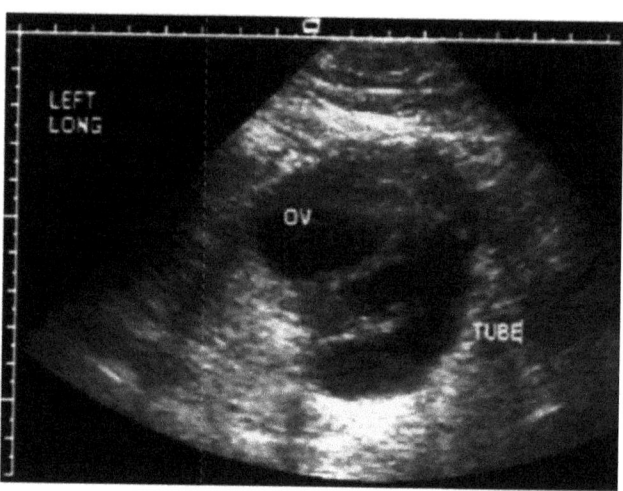

Figure 51.1

K. Results

Table 51.1 Results table

Test	Result	Test	Result
Complete blood count:		**Liver function panel:**	
WBC	$13.2 \times 10^3/\mu L$	AST	25 U/L
Hct	43.8%	ALT	23 U/L
Plt	$289 \times 10^3/\mu L$	Alk phos	56 U/L
		T bili	0.6 mg/dL
Basic metabolic panel:		D bili	0.4 mg/dL
Na	142 mEq/L	Amylase	64 U/L
K	4.2 mEq/L	Lipase	28 U/L
Cl	105 mEq/L	Albumin	4.2 g/dL
CO_2	24 mEq/L		
BUN	15 mEq/dL	**Urinalysis:**	
Cr	0.9 mg/dL	SG	1.010–1.030
Gluc	110 mg/dL	pH	5–8
		Prot	Neg
Coagulation panel:		Gluc	Neg
PT	12.2 sec	Ketones	Neg

Table 51.1 (cont.)

Test	Result	Test	Result
PTT	27.2 sec	Bili	Neg
INR	0.89	Blood	Neg
		LE	Neg
		Nitrite	Neg
		Color	Yellow

a. Lactate 2.0 mmol/L

L. Action
a. Gynecology consult
i. Discuss need for admission for IV antibiotics for tubo-ovarian abscess
b. Discussion with patient and PMD regarding need for admission for IV antibiotics

M. Diagnosis
a. Tubo-ovarian abscess

N. Critical actions
a. Urine pregnancy test
b. Urogenital examination
c. Pelvic US
d. Antibiotics
e. Gynecology consult

O. Examiner instructions
a. This is a case of tubo-ovarian abscess (TOA), a serious infection of the female upper genital tract affecting the ovaries. TOA is a type of sexually transmitted disease caused typically by *Chlamydia trachomatis* or *Neisseria gonorrhoeae* that starts from an infection of the cervix and spreads to the upper genital tract. The patient's symptoms of lower abdominal pain and fever should prompt the candidate to order urine pregnancy test early in the encounter. Important actions include urogenital examination, early antibiotics, pain control, and pelvic US. Ultimately the patient will complain of increased pain and fever if antibiotics and pain medication are not ordered. The patient should be admitted for IV antibiotics and pain control.

P. Pearls
a. TOA is part of the admission criteria for patients with pelvic inflammatory disease.
b. Most patients with TOAs improve with IV antibiotics alone, but those that do not improve may need to have drainage of the abscess laparoscopically, percutaneously, or surgically, or other pathologies need to be considered.
c. Patients may present with a bleeding pelvic mass that may be secondary to a bleeding vessel due to erosion or rupture of the abscess.
d. When considering pathologies other than TOA, the patient may require a CT abdomen/pelvis with PO and IV contrast to rule out other causes of the patient's symptoms (such

as appendicitis). The differential also includes: ovarian torsion, ruptured ovarian cyst, endometriosis, fibroids, ovarian mass.

Q. Figure legends

a. Figure 51.1 (Ultrasound) Tubo-ovarian abscess near left ovary.

R. References

a. *Tintinalli's Emergency Medicine: A Comprehensive Study Guide* (9th ed.): Chapter 103, Pelvic Inflammatory Disease.

b. *Rosen's Emergency Medicine: Concepts and Clinical Practice* (10th ed.) Chapter 29, Acute Pelvic Pain.

Headache

Bing Shen, MD and J. Mark Rendon, MD

A. Chief complaint
a. 55-year-old male brought in by wife with headache and eye pain

B. Vital signs
a. BP: 138/88, HR: 110, RR: 16, T: 38.7°C, Sat: 99% on RA, FS: 109 mg/dL

C. What does the patient look like?
a. Patient appears stated age, appears uncomfortable due to pain, in moderate distress; lying supine on stretcher.

D. Primary survey
a. Airway: speaking in full sentences
b. Breathing: no respiratory distress, no cyanosis
c. Circulation: warm skin, normal capillary refill

E. Action
a. Peripheral IV line
b. Labs
   i. CBC, BMP, LFT, PT/PTT, type and hold, lactate, urinalysis
c. 1 L NS bolus
d. Monitor: BP: 128/76, HR: 115, RR: 16, Sat: 100% on RA
e. EKG

F. History
a. HPI: A 55-year-old male states that he has had a "bad cold" over the past week. He reports experiencing yellowish-green nasal discharge and sinus pressure over this time. Over the past 2 days he has developed a gradually worsening headache and fever. Today, the headache is severe, sharp, frontal, and associated with left eye pain. His left eye is now irritated, very painful, and sensitive to light. He feels chills and has had generalized weakness from being ill. He denies any neck pain, sore throat, cough, or dysuria.
b. PMHx: hypercholesterolemia
c. PSHx: none
d. Allergies: none
e. Meds: simvastatin
f. Social: lives with wife and children at home; denies alcohol use, smoking, or illicit drug use; sexually active with wife only; no recent travel
g. PMD: switched doctors, has not followed up in about a year

G. Nurse

a. EKG (Figure 52.1)

b. If 1 L NS given:

   i. BP: 125/88, HR: 105, RR: 16, Sat: 100% on RA

c. If no fluids given:

   i. BP: 115/70, HR: 120 RR: 16, Sat: 100% on RA

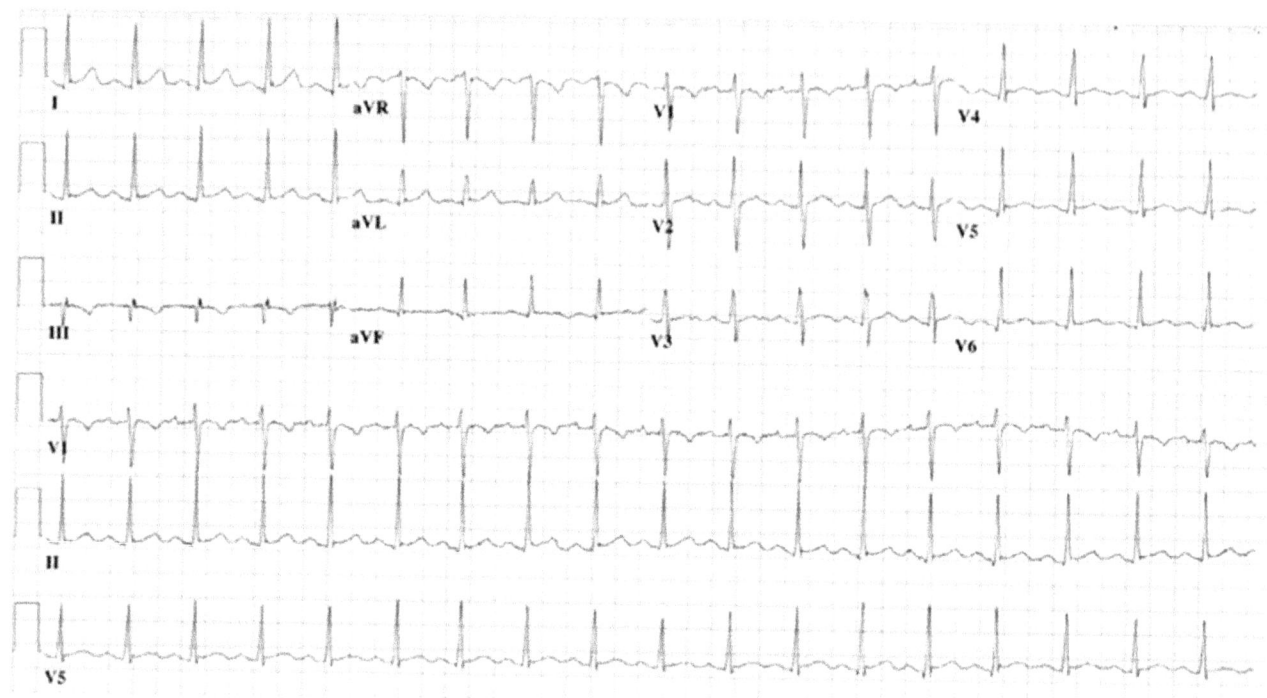

Figure 52.1

H. Secondary survey

a. General: alert, oriented, uncomfortable, ill-appearing

b. Head: normocephalic, atraumatic, no erythema on face; tenderness over the left maxillary and frontal sinuses

c. Eyes:

   i. Left eye: conjunctival injection and chemosis, slight ptosis on left, pupil 5 mm reactive, + papilledema, + photophobia

   ii. Right eye: normal examination, pupil 3 mm reactive

d. Ears: normal tympanic membranes

e. Nose: no discharge

f. Pharynx: normal

g. Neck: full range of motion, no jugular vein distension, no stridor, Brudzinski's and Kernig's negative

h. Chest: normal

i. Heart: tachycardic, no murmurs

j. Abdomen: normal

k. Rectal: normal

l. Urogenital: normal

m. Extremities: normal

n. Back: normal

o. Neuro: normal mental status; CN: visual acuity 20/40 bilaterally; decreased abduction of left eye; slightly less sensation to touch over left periorbital area; otherwise, nonfocal neurological examination with normal cerebellar function, gait, strength, reflexes, and tone

p. Skin: warm and dry

q. Lymph: no lymphadenopathy

I. Action

a. Lumbar puncture after CTH

b. Meds
   i. Ceftriaxone
   ii. Vancomycin
   iii. Metronidazole
   iv. Dexamethasone
   v. Acetaminophen
   vi. Morphine

c. Consult
   i. Neurology
   ii. Ophthalmology

d. Imaging
   i. Head CT without contrast
   ii. MRI/MRV or CT venogram of head

J. Nurse

a. BP: 115/75, HR: 110, RR: 16, T: 38.3°C, Sat: 100% on RA

b. Patient: still with significant headache, fever, and photophobia

K. Results

Table 52.1 Results table

Test	Result	Test	Result
Complete blood count:		Liver function panel:	
WBC	$16.7 \times 10^3/\mu L$	AST	20 U/L
Hct	44.40%	ALT	15 U/L
Plt	$244 \times 10^3/\mu L$	Alk phos	110 U/L
		T bili	0.7 mg/dL
		D bili	0.2 mg/dL
Basic metabolic panel:		Amylase	110 U/L
Na	140 mEq/L	Lipase	72 U/L
K	4.0 mEq/L	Albumin	4.3 g/dL
Cl	104 mEq/L		
CO_2	24 mEq/L		
BUN	30 mEq/dL	Urinalysis:	
Cr	1.2 mg/dL	SG	1.03

Table 52.1 (cont.)

Test	Result	Test	Result
Gluc	130 mg/dL	pH	6
		Prot	Neg
Coagulation panel:		Gluc	Neg
PT	13.5 sec	Ketones	Neg
PTT	27 sec	Bili	Neg
INR	1.1	Blood	Neg
		LE	Neg
		Nitrite	Neg
		Color	Yellow

a. Lactate: 2.0 mmol/L
b. LP results
    i. Opening pressure: 28 cmH$_2$O
    ii. CSF: WBC: 30, RBC: 100, protein: 35 mg/dL, glucose: 50 mg/dL, clear, Gram stain negative
c. Head CT (Figure 52.2): sinusitis bilaterally in the maxillary sinuses; no other acute intracerebral abnormality
d. MRI: signal hyperintensities within the left cavernous sinus suggestive of cavernous sinus thrombosis

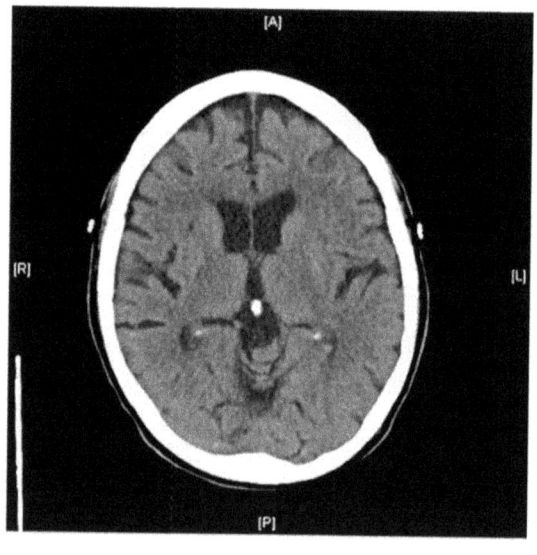

Figure 52.2

L. Action
a. Consult
    i. MICU
    ii. Neurology
    iii. Ophthalmology
b. Discussion with patient and family about severity of this illness
c. Medications

    i. IV antibiotics (if not previously given)
       1. Third- or fourth-generation cephalosporin
       2. Vancomycin or nafcillin
       3. Metronidazole
    ii. Heparin infusion, with consultation
    iii. Dexamethasone (if not given earlier)

M. Diagnosis
a. Cavernous sinus thrombosis

N. Critical actions
a. Early antibiotics
b. Lumbar puncture
c. MRI or CT venogram for diagnosis
d. ICU

O. Examiner instructions
a. This is a case of septic cavernous sinus thrombosis (CST) that likely developed from a bacterial sinus infection. This is a rare, but serious, infection of a dural venous sinus that can be life-threatening if left untreated. Prior to antibiotics, this condition was nearly always fatal. The important actions are to start antibiotics and steroids early to treat presumed meningitis. It is also important to obtain neuroimaging and perform a lumbar puncture. In this scenario, a head CT should be obtained before performing the LP due to the presence of focal neurologic deficits. The patient's severe pain should continue despite treatment; this should guide the examinee to more definitive testing, such as MRI or MRV. If the MRI is not ordered, the patient should develop worsening pain, worsening sensory changes in the trigeminal nerve distribution, and ophthalmoplegia. If the MRI is still not ordered or if the examiner feels that the candidate will not order it, the case will proceed to the neurologist/ophthalmologist's recommendation of an MRI or MRV.

P. Pearls
a. Headache is the most common chief complaint in CST. Fever, eye pain, photophobia, proptosis, ophthalmoplegia (cranial nerves III, IV, and VI) are also common. Sensory deficits in the first and second branches (ophthalmic and maxillary branches) of the trigeminal nerve may be present. Symptoms are initially unilateral but may become bilateral as infection and thrombosis spreads to the opposite eye through the communicating veins.
b. The differential diagnosis should also include orbital cellulitis, meningitis, brain abscess, and acute angle closure glaucoma.
c. A common cause of CST is sinusitis, particularly sphenoid or ethmoid. Other causes include dental infections, ear infections, or trauma.
d. LP reveals inflammatory cells in 75% of cases.
e. Aggressive antibiotic therapy is the primary treatment.
f. Anticoagulation and corticosteroids may be beneficial, but should be considered with specialist consultation.

Q. Figure legends
a. Figure 52.1 (EKG) Sinus tachycardia; minimal voltage criteria for LVH.
b. Figure 52.2 (Head CT) Normal head CT.

R. References

a. *Tintinalli's Emergency Medicine: A Comprehensive Study Guide* (9th ed.): Chapter 174, Central Nervous System and Spinal Infections.

b. *Rosen's Emergency Medicine: Concepts and Clinical Practice* (10th ed.): Chapter 89, Headache Disorders.

Pediatric Fever

Alexandria Bahan Farish, MD, Jared Senvisky, MD, Nicole Rettig, MD,
Catharine Cantrell, MD, Michelle Mendoza, MD, and Bing Shen, MD

A. Chief complaint
a. 20-month-old male brought in by a parent with the complaint of fever for 5 days

B. Vital signs
a. BP: 85/63, HR: 160, RR: 24, T: 40.2°C, Sat: 99% on RA, Wt: 10 kg

C. What does the patient look like?
a. Patient appears stated age, uncomfortable, fussy, in parent's arms.

D. Primary survey
a. Airway: able to speak words
b. Breathing: no apparent respiratory distress, no cyanosis
c. Circulation: warm skin, normal capillary refill

E. Action
a. One peripheral IV line
b. Labs
    i. CBC, BMP, LFTs
    ii. Blood cultures, urinalysis, urine culture
c. Monitor: BP: 85/63, HR: 120, RR: 24

F. History
a. HPI: A 20-month-old male is brought in by his parents for a persistent fever for 5 days. He has a new rash that was noticed earlier today. He is feeding well but is less active than normal. The fever has been as high as 103°F at home orally, minimally improved with acetaminophen; last dose was administered 12 hours ago. The child has a slight dry cough, no diarrhea, and no vomiting.
b. PMHx: normal full-term birth at 39 weeks; up-to-date vaccinations
c. PSHx: none
d. Allergies: none
e. Meds: none
f. Social: lives at home with mother and father; no siblings
g. FHx: no relevant history
h. PMD: Dr. Alvarez, who he sees regularly for routine visits

G. Secondary survey
a. General: alert, in no distress, irritable but consolable in the parent's arms
b. Head: normocephalic, atraumatic

c. Eyes: bilateral injection, extraocular movement grossly intact, pupils equal and reactive to light
d. Ears: normal tympanic membranes
e. Nose: no discharge
f. Neck: + cervical lymphadenopathy, full range of motion, no jugular vein distension, no stridor
g. Pharynx: mildly edematous, red tongue, dry, red, cracked lips
h. Chest: nontender
i. Lungs: clear bilaterally
j. Heart: tachycardic, no murmurs, rubs, or gallops
k. Abdomen: normal bowel sounds, soft, nontender, no distension
l. Rectal: normal tone, brown stool, occult blood negative
m. Urogenital: normal external genitalia
   i. Male: no discharge, normal testicular examination
n. Extremities: full range of motion, no deformity, normal pulses
o. Back: nontender
p. Neuro: moving all extremities symmetrically
q. Skin: scarlatiniform rash on perineum, erythema and mild swelling of palms and feet
r. Lymph: no lymphadenopathy

H. Action
a. Meds
   i. Initiate IV fluids: 20 mL/kg bolus or maintenance fluids
b. Imaging
   i. CXR
c. Reassess
   i. Patient still irritable
d. Testing
   i. Rapid *Strep* test, throat culture
   ii. CRP, ESR, coagulation profile, and type/screen

I. Nurse
a. BP: 85/63, HR: 125, RR: 25, T: 39.6°C, Sat: 100% on 2 L
b. Patient: still irritable

J. Results

Table 53.1 Results table

Test	Result	Test	Result
Complete blood count:		T bili	0.5 mg/dL
WBC	$14.1 \times 10^3/\mu L$	D bili	0.1 mg/dL
Hct	36.5%	Amylase	32 U/L
Plt	$410 \times 10^3/\mu L$	Lipase	53 U/L
		Albumin	3.6 g/dL
Basic metabolic panel:			
Na	139 mEq/L	**Urinalysis:**	
K	4.2 mEq/L	SG	1.010–1.030

Table 53.1 (cont.)

Test	Result	Test	Result
Cl	101 mEq/L	pH	5–8
CO_2	22 mEq/L	Prot	Neg
BUN	21 mEq/dL	Gluc	Neg
Cr	1.0 mg/dL	Ketones	Neg
Gluc	100 mg/dL	Bili	Neg
		Blood	Neg
Coagulation panel:		LE	Neg
PT	13.1 sec	Nitrite	Neg
PTT	26.0 sec	Color	Yellow
INR	1.0		
		Arterial blood gas:	
Liver function panel:		pH	7.35–7.45
AST	21 U/L	pO_2	80–100 mmHg
ALT	19 U/L	pCO_2	35–45 mmHg
Alk phos	106 U/L	HCO_3	22–26 mmol/L

a. ESR: 60 mm/hr, CRP: 5 mg/dL
b. Rapid *Strep* test: negative
c. CXR: no acute cardiopulmonary disease noted

K. Action
a. Consult
   i. Pediatric rheumatology
   ii. Infectious disease
   iii. Pediatric cardiology
b. Discussion with family regarding diagnosis and management
c. Treatment
a. Intravenous immune globulin (IVIG): 2 g/kg IV over 8–12 hours
b. Aspirin (ASA) 100 mg/kg/day divided q 6 hours

L. Diagnosis
a. Kawasaki disease (KD)

M. Critical actions
a. Treatment of KD: ASA and IVIG
b. Consultation with pediatric infectious disease or rheumatology as well as cardiology
c. Discussion with family regarding diagnosis and management

N. Examiner instructions
a. This is a case of Kawasaki disease (KD), an acute febrile vasculitis of childhood. The cause is unknown, but it affects medium-sized arteries of the body and can lead to complications

if undiagnosed and untreated. This patient presents early in the course of the disease. His clinical presentation warrants an infectious work-up. A lumbar puncture would be appropriate if there is suspicion for meningitis. Intravenous fluids and symptomatic relief may be given; however, the definitive course of therapy should be IVIG and aspirin. Antibiotics can be started if the diagnosis is not certain; however, the patient cannot be discharged without appropriate definitive treatment as KD has significant morbidity if not treated appropriately. The candidate should keep the patient's parent updated with his condition throughout the course of the encounter.

O. Pearls

a. KD is the leading cause of acquired heart disease in North American children. There are no pathognomonic laboratory findings – the diagnosis must be established clinically using the criteria listed below.

b. Diagnostic criteria
   i. Fever of at least 5 days' duration, plus
   ii. Four out of five of the following:
      1. Bilateral conjunctival injection with limbic sparing
      2. Lips and oral mucosal findings on physical exam (dry, red, fissured lips, strawberry tongue, oropharyngeal erythema)
      3. Extremity findings on physical exam (erythema of palms and soles, edema of hands and feet, periungual desquamation)
      4. Polymorphous rash
      5. Cervical lymphadenopathy (at least one node >1.5 cm)

c. Lab abnormalities:
   i. ESR and CRP may be elevated (ESR ≥40 mm/hr and CRP ≥3 mg/dL)
   ii. CBC may show elevated WBC (>15,000/mm³), left shift, anemia for age, and thrombocytosis (platelet count >450,000/mm³)
   iii. Urinalysis often shows a sterile pyuria
   iv. ALT elevation
   v. Albumin ≤3 g/dL

d. 20–25% of untreated patients develop coronary artery aneurysms. Appropriate treatment reduces this to 4–5%. Coronary artery aneurysm most commonly develops in the third or fourth week after disease onset.

e. Dysrhythmias and myocardial infarction cause sudden death in 1–2% of patients, usually in the third or fourth week from disease onset.

f. Some patients (most commonly in children aged <1 year old and >9 years old) will present with "incomplete," or "atypical" KD, which occurs when not all diagnostic criteria are met. These children are still at risk for complications and should be monitored closely. Incomplete KD should be considered in children with <4 of the clinical criteria listed above if they demonstrate prolonged fever with labs and imaging consistent with KD. This encompasses children with fever for ≥5 days with 2–3 of the clinical findings listed above or children with unexplained fever for ≥7 days. For incomplete presentations, additional lab findings can be utilized to direct further diagnosis and treatment. Further investigation can start with obtaining ESR and CRP levels. If these are normal, serial monitoring of labs and fever can be continued and echocardiogram can be obtained if the child demonstrates clinical skin findings such as peeling. If the echocardiogram is positive, then the child should be treated for KD. If the ESR and CRP are elevated, then three or more of the above lab findings indicate proceeding with treatment.

P. References

a. *Tintinalli's Emergency Medicine: A Comprehensive Study Guide* (9th ed.): Chapter 129, Congenital and Acquired Pediatric Heart Disease.

b. *Rosen's Emergency Medicine: Concepts and Clinical Practice* (10th ed.): Chapter 165, Pediatric Cardiac Disorders.

Back Pain

J. Mark Rendon, MD and Bing Shen, MD

A. Chief complaint
a. 44-year-old male with low back pain

B. Vital signs
a. BP: 137/82, HR: 94, RR: 16, T: 36.9°C, Sat: 99% on RA

C. What does the patient look like?
a. Patient appears stated age, appears uncomfortable due to pain, in moderate distress, sitting on stretcher.

D. Primary survey
a. Airway: speaking in full sentences
b. Breathing: no apparent respiratory distress, no cyanosis
c. Circulation: warm and dry skin, normal capillary refill

E. History
a. HPI: A 44-year-old male presents with severe low back pain that began 4 days ago. The pain started after reorganizing some equipment in his garage. Initially, the pain was moderate in severity and slightly improved with rest and ibuprofen. Over the past 2 days, the pain has become severe and now radiates down both legs. He reports numbness and tingling to both thighs, legs, and feet. The pain is constant, but worsens with bending, sneezing, or coughing. Today, he experienced leg weakness, left greater than right, and difficulty urinating. He denies any fevers or chills. He denies any neck, chest, or abdominal pain.
b. PMHx: hypertension
c. PSHx: none
d. Allergies: none
e. Meds: hydrochlorothiazide
f. Social: lives with wife at home, smokes one pack a day for 15 years, social drinker, denies drug use
g. FHx: not relevant
h. PMD: Dr. Abraham

F. Secondary survey
a. General: alert, answers questions appropriately, moderate distress due to pain
b. HEENT: normal
c. Neck: full range of motion
d. Chest: nontender
e. Lungs: clear to auscultation bilaterally

f. Heart: regular rate and rhythm, no murmurs
g. Abdomen: normal bowel sounds, soft, suprapubic fullness and tenderness upon palpation without rebound, guarding, or rigidity
h. Rectal: slightly decreased tone and perianal sensation, no gross blood or melena
i. Urogenital: normal external genitalia, mildly decreased perineal sensation, normal testicular exam
j. Extremities: no deformities, normal pulses; positive leg straight raise bilaterally
k. Back: tenderness to lumbar area
l. Neuro: oriented × 3, normal cranial nerves; upper extremities normal; sensory deficits to posterior thighs, lateral calves, and feet bilaterally; strength 4/5 left hip extension and abduction, 4/5 left knee flexion, 4/5 left ankle plantar flexion and dorsiflexion; strength 4+/5 throughout right lower extremity; reflexes 1+ right ankle, no response left ankle; unable to assess gait or lower extremity coordination due to pain
m. Skin: warm and dry
n. Lymph: no lymphadenopathy

G. Action
a. Peripheral IV line
b. Labs
  i. CBC, BMP, PT/PTT, type and hold, lactate, urinalysis
c. Pain control
  i. Ketorolac
  ii. Morphine
d. Foley catheter or noninvasive (ultrasound) post-void residual assessment
  e. Consult
  i. Neurosurgery
f. Imaging
  i. X-ray of lumbosacral spine
  ii. CT lumbar spine
  iii. MRI

H. Nurse
a. Vitals: BP: 130/80, HR: 85, RR: 14, Sat: 100%
b. Patient: pain improved after analgesia

I. Results

Table 54.1 Results table

Test	Result	Test	Result
Complete blood count:		**Coagulation panel:**	
WBC	$11.87 \times 10^3/\mu L$	PT	13.0 sec
Hct	43.50%	PTT	27 sec
Plt	$297 \times 10^3/\mu L$	INR	1.0

Table 54.1 (cont.)

Test	Result	Test	Result
Basic metabolic panel:		**Urinalysis:**	
Na	141 mEq/L	SG	1.034
K	4.0 mEq/L	pH	6.5
Cl	102 mEq/L	Prot	Neg
CO_2	21 mEq/L	Gluc	Neg
BUN	34 mEq/dL	Ketones	Neg
Cr	1.4 mg/dL	Bili	Neg
Gluc	132 mg/dL	Blood	Neg
		LE	Neg
		Nitrite	Neg
		Color	Yellow

a. Lactate: 1.5 mmol/L
b. Post-void residual: 625 mL
c. X-ray (Figure 54.1)
d. CT lumbar spine (if ordered): herniation of the L5–S1 intervertebral disk resulting in severe central canal stenosis
e. MRI: large L5–S1 disk herniation, causing severe thecal sac stenosis and significant compression of the adjacent cauda equina nerve roots

J. Action
a. Neurosurgical consult
   i. To operating room for emergent surgical decompression
b. Discussion with family regarding need for emergent surgical intervention and diagnosis of cauda equina syndrome
c. Meds:
   i. Consider dexamethasone IV, in consultation with neurosurgeon

K. Diagnosis
a. Cauda equina syndrome

L. Critical actions
a. Pain control
b. Complete neurological examination
c. Perform rectal and urogenital examinations
d. MRI
e. Emergent neurosurgical consultation

M. Examiner instructions
a. This is a case of cauda equina syndrome (CES), caused by a lumbar disk herniation. CES is a serious pathologic condition that occurs when the cauda equina nerve roots are compressed,

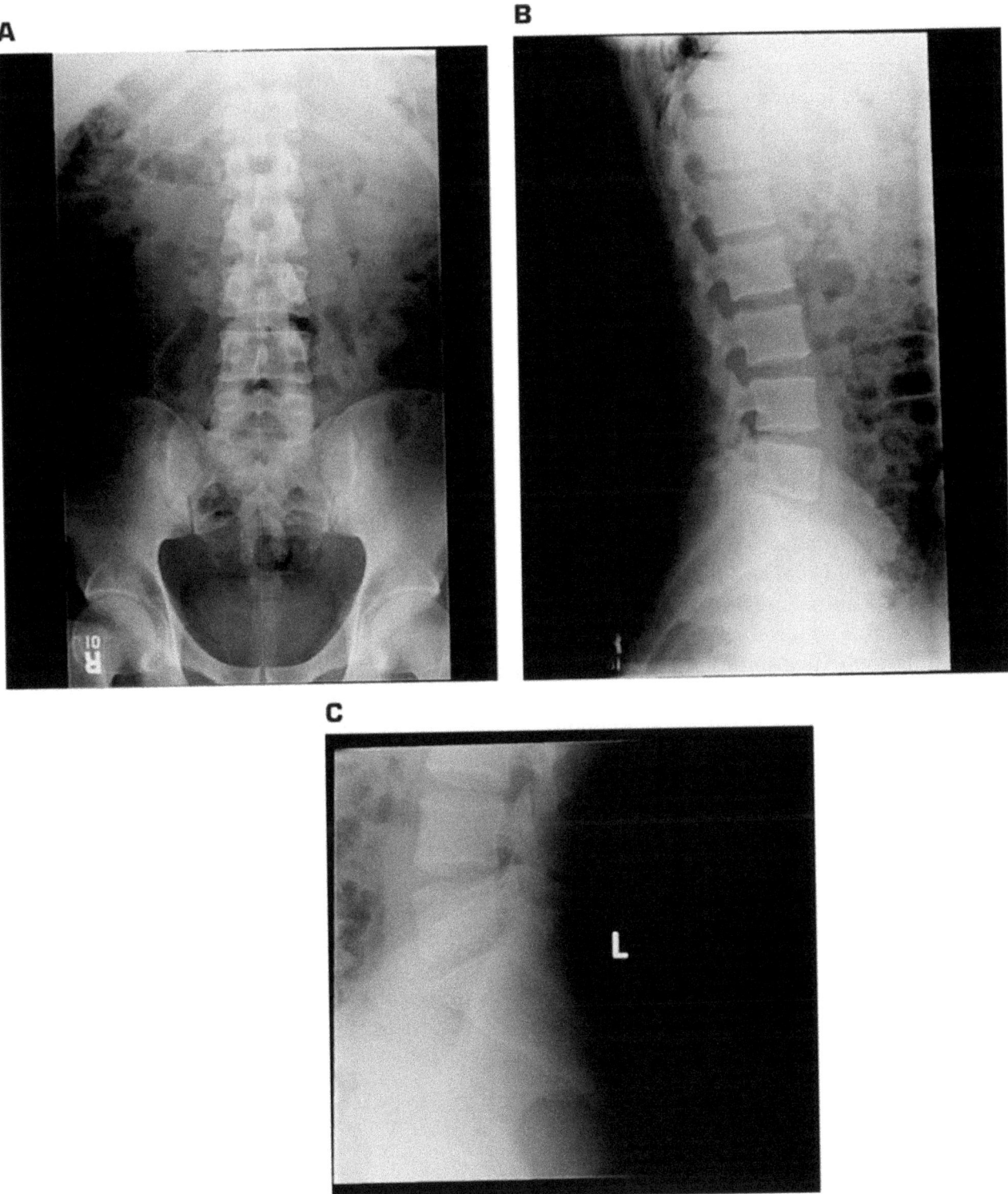

Figure 54.1

resulting in various signs and symptoms including sciatica, motor weakness, sensory loss, bladder and/or bowel dysfunction, and saddle anesthesia. Serious complications of this condition include incontinence and paralysis. The key to making this diagnosis is recognizing the concerning findings of weakness and bowel/bladder symptoms that distinguish this entity from more common presentations of uncomplicated back pain. The examiner should ask about bowel and bladder function when obtaining the HPI. The examiner should also perform a rectal exam, urogenital exam, and a thorough neurologic examination. The neurologic exam should include an evaluation of the patient's motor function, sensory function, and reflexes. Analgesics should be administered for patient comfort. An MRI should be obtained immediately, as soon as CES is suspected. Preoperative labs should be ordered, and the case is considered complete once the patient is appropriately dispositioned to the operating room under the care of a neurosurgeon.

N. Pearls

a. The cauda equina (Latin for "horse's tail") is the name given to the bundle of spinal nerves and nerve roots; it consists of the nerves L2–L5, S1–S5, and the coccygeal nerve.

b. Cauda equina syndrome is a rare and serious neurological condition due to pressure on the cauda equina. It is most often caused by lumbar disk herniation, but can also be caused by malignancy, epidural spinal abscess, localized hematoma, or vascular malformations.

c. The most common presenting symptoms are low back pain and radiculopathy. Other associated symptoms and findings include perianal sensory loss, fecal incontinence, and bladder dysfunction (urinary retention or overflow incontinence). When considering CES, urinary retention has a 90% sensitivity and 95% specificity.

d. MRI is the gold standard for diagnosis; it should be obtained urgently when history and physical examination suggest cauda equina syndrome.

e. Cauda equina syndrome is a true surgical emergency and is an indication for urgent consultation with a spine surgeon. The degree of neurologic deficits upon presentation directly correlate with functional outcomes.

f. Steroids, while traditionally recommended and often administered, do not have proven benefit.

O. Figure legends

a. Figure 54.1 (Lumbosacral x-ray) Normal lumbosacral spine film.

P. References

a. *Tintinalli's Emergency Medicine: A Comprehensive Study Guide* (9th ed.): Chapter 279, Neck and Back Pain.

b. *Rosen's Emergency Medicine: Concepts and Clinical Practice* (10th ed.): Chapter 92, Spinal Cord Disorders.

Cardiac Arrest

Bing Shen, MD and Wuya Lumeh, MD

A. Chief complaint
a. 7-month-old male is brought in by mother and EMS after noticing that the child was unresponsive, not breathing, and blue in color. EMS is delivering assisted breaths by bag-valve mask and chest compressions.

B. Vital signs
a. BP: not obtainable, HR: 0, RR: 0, T: 34.2°C (rectal), Sat: not obtainable, Wt ~8 kg, FS: 60 mg/dL

C. What does the patient look like?
a. Patient appears cyanotic, not responsive, and limp.

D. Primary survey
a. Airway: unresponsive, patent airway
b. Breathing: no spontaneous breaths
c. Circulation: no carotid, femoral, or brachial pulses; no capillary refill

E. Action
a. PALS resuscitation
  i. Advanced airway: intubation with straight laryngoscope blade, 3.5–4.0 uncuffed tube/3.0–3.5 cuffed tube (at 11–12 cm deep); verify placement via end-tidal capnography and/or bilateral auscultation/breath sounds or lung sliding on bedside ultrasonography.
  ii. Oxygen – positive pressure ventilation at 12–20 breaths/min, avoiding excessive ventilation
  iii. Chest compressions (two-thumbs-encircling hands) at 100–120/min
    1. Focus should be on high-quality compressions with minimal interruptions
    2. In children and infants, compression depth of one-third AP diameter of chest
b. Access
  i. Intraosseous (IO) lines: 18/15G at proximal tibia, distal femur, proximal humerus, or
  ii. Intravenous (IV) lines: 22G or 24G peripheral IV
c. IV fluid: 20 mL/kg (160 cc) NS bolus IV or IO
d. Rewarming (heater, warm saline, etc.)
e. Place patient on defibrillator/monitor: no pulse, rhythm remains asystole
  i. PALS cardiac arrest algorithm: 0.01 mg/kg (1:10,000) epinephrine; repeat every 3–5 minutes; continue CPR with rhythm checks at 2 minute intervals.
  ii. Address reversible causes ("Hs & Ts"): hypovolemia, hypoxia, hydrogen ion (acidosis), hypoglycemia, hypokalemia, hyperkalemia, hypothermia, tension pneumothorax, tamponade, toxins, thrombosis (coronary, pulmonary embolus).

F. History

a. HPI: A 7-month-old male with a normal full-term birth and no past medical history was found in the crib by his mother in the middle of the evening to be unresponsive and blue in color. The patient appeared well before being put to sleep. EMS was called immediately (~25 minutes ago) and child was brought immediately to the ED. CPR was initiated by EMS and no medications were given.

b. PMHx: none

c. PSHx: none

d. Allergies: none

e. Meds: none

f. Social: lives at home with mother and three siblings, ages 2, 5, and 10 years old

g. PMD: Dr. Young

G. Nurse

a. Monitor: no pulse, continued asystole; T: 35.2°C

b. Obtain health care worker (such as a social worker) to talk to mother, locate other children

H. Secondary survey

a. General: unresponsive

b. HEENT: normocephalic/atraumatic; dilated, fixed pupils; intubated

c. Neck: normal

d. Chest: no spontaneous respirations; breath sounds equal post-intubation

e. Heart: no heartbeats auscultated

f. Abdomen: normal

g. Back: normal

h. Extremities: normal

i. Neuro: no reflexes

j. Skin: cool, no signs of trauma

I. Action

a. Reassess: T: 37.2°C, no other vital signs

b. Offer family to be present during the resuscitation efforts or support family who choose not to be present in a safe area.

c. Pronounce death after significant and adequate resuscitation; do not remove tubes, lines, etc.

d. Inform family of child's death.

e. Involve clergy, social support, pediatrician, Medical Examiner's Office

f. Blood and urine collection for postmortem testing.

J. Diagnosis

a. Sudden unexpected death in infancy, in lieu of sudden infant death syndrome, which is definitively determined and diagnosed after autopsy.

K. Critical actions

a. Initiate appropriate PALS life support.

b. Assess for signs of abuse.

c. Resuscitate and ensure that the temperature is within normal limits before pronunciation of death.

d. Provide psychosocial support to the family.

e. Coordinate postmortem investigation with the Medical Examiner's Office.

L. Examiner instructions

a. This is a case of sudden unexpected death in infancy; however, that is impossible to ascertain on presentation. SIDS is a syndrome that leads to sudden death of an infant under 1 year of age without known cause. Pediatric acute life support should be initiated until futility – significant time of resuscitation (in concordance with best practices), loss of brainstem reflexes, normothermia, or definitive signs of prolonged death/down-time are identified: rigor mortis, dependent lividity, corneal clouding. Reflexes should be assessed. Warm NS and an infant heater can help rewarm the patient. The family should be offered all forms of psychosocial support. For all cases of unexpected death in a child, abuse should be considered and excluded. In this case, no evidence of abuse is found on clinical examination.

M. Pearls

a. Sudden unexpected death in infancy is the sudden death of an infant under 1 year of age, which remains unexplained after a thorough case investigation, performance of a complete autopsy, examination of the death scene, and review of the clinical history.

b. The "Back to Sleep" campaign (which instructs parents to put their infants to sleep on their backs) has reduced the rate of sudden unexpected death in infancy by greater than 40%.

c. As the cause of death is unknown, blood and urine should be sent to facilitate postmortem examination and autopsy.

d. Social and psychological support should be offered immediately to help the family come to terms with the loss and to initiate the process of grieving.

N. References

a. *Tintinalli's Emergency Medicine: A Comprehensive Study Guide* (9th ed.): Chapter 109, Resuscitation of Children.

b. *Rosen's Emergency Medicine: Concepts and Clinical Practice* (10th ed.): Chapter 158, Pediatric Resuscitation.

Knee Pain

Bing Shen, MD and Cassandra Mackey, MD

A. Chief complaint
a. 54-year-old female with right knee pain and swelling for the past 2 days

B. Vital signs
a. BP: 149/83, HR: 88, RR: 12, T: 38.4°C, Sat: 100% on RA

C. What does the patient look like?
a. Patient appears stated age, in moderate distress due to pain, and sitting on stretcher.

D. Primary survey
a. Airway: speaking in full sentences
b. Breathing: no apparent respiratory distress, no cyanosis
c. Circulation: warm and dry skin, normal capillary refill

E. Action
a. One large-bore peripheral IV line
b. Labs
    i. CBC, BMP, coagulation studies, blood type and crossmatch
    ii. ESR, CRP, blood cultures
c. Monitor: BP: 145/85, HR: 90, RR: 12, Sat: 100%

F. History
a. HPI: The patient is a 54-year-old female with a history of hypercholesterolemia, gout, and obesity. She states that she has had worsening right knee pain over the past 2 days. She has never had pain like this in the knee before but does endorse gout pain in her left big toe in the past. The pain is localized to the right knee and has steadily increased in intensity over the past few days. She denies any fevers, but states she does feel chills. She is mostly concerned about the pain, which prevents her from doing her daily activities. She took ibuprofen 800 mg × 2 every 6 hours without relief, last dose 1 hour prior to arrival. She has no other complaints; denies trauma to the knee.
b. PMHx: hypercholesterolemia, gout, and obesity
c. PSHx: none
d. Allergies: none
e. Meds: ibuprofen and acetaminophen, simvastatin, colchicine
f. Social: some alcohol use – "socially", nonsmoker, denies drugs, sexually active, lives with husband, works in computer programming

G. Secondary survey

a. General: alert, oriented, moderate distress due to pain

b. Head: normocephalic, atraumatic

c. Eyes: extraocular movement intact, pupils equal, reactive to light

d. Ears: normal tympanic membranes

e. Nose: no discharge

f. Neck: full range of motion, no jugular vein distension, no stridor

g. Pharynx: normal dentition, no lesions, no swelling

h. Chest: nontender

i. Lungs: clear bilaterally

j. Heart: rate and rhythm regular, no murmurs, rubs, or gallops

k. Abdomen: normal bowel sounds, soft, nontender or distended

l. Extremities: right knee swollen with palpable effusion; very tender to palpation and limited range of motion secondary to pain; non-erythematous but warm to the touch; patient unable to walk without extreme pain; hip and ankle both normal; distal pulses normal, equal bilaterally. Swelling localized to right knee. Normal calf. Left knee is normal.

m. Back: nontender

n. Neuro: cranial nerves II to XII intact; normal sensation, strength; normal reflexes. Gait assessment limited due to pain

o. Skin: warm and dry

p. Lymph: no lymphadenopathy

H. Action

a. Procedure

   i. Right knee arthrocentesis

      1. Informed consent with explanation of risks, benefits, and alternatives

      2. Time out to identify side, perform using sterile techniques

      3. May enter joint either medially or laterally to the patella

      4. Extend knee, insert point of needle about 1 cm inferior to patella and horizontally toward the joint space

      5. Cloudy fluid obtained – send for culture, Gram stain, cell count, crystals, protein, glucose

b. Meds

   i. Morphine (opiate) and IV antiemetic

c. Reassess

   i. Patient's pain is much improved after pain medication and arthrocentesis, but is still present

d. Imaging: x-ray right knee, two views

I. Nurse

a. BP: 130/78, HR: 88, RR: 12, Sat: 100% on O_2

b. Patient: mild distress due to pain, but improved after medication

c. X-ray right knee (Figures 56.1 and 56.2)

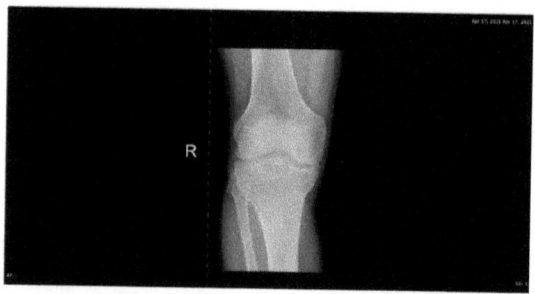

Figure 56.1

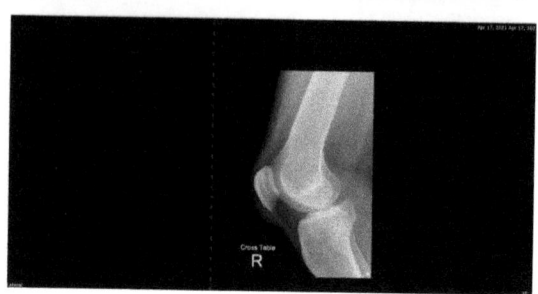

Figure 56.2

J. Results

Table 56.1 Results table

Test	Result	Test	Result
Complete blood count:		CO_2	24.2 mEq/L
WBC	$11.9 \times 10^3/\mu L$	BUN	23 mEq/dL
Diff	83.6/9.1/5.0	Cr	1.2 mg/dL
Hct	41.50%	Gluc	135 mg/dL
Plt	$553 \times 10^3/\mu L$		
		Coagulation panel:	
Basic metabolic panel:		PT	12.3–15.5 sec
Na	139 mEq/L	PTT	25.4–35.0 sec
K	4.0 mEq/L	INR	0.9–1.3
Cl	101 mEq/L		

a. ESR: if ordered – 20 mm/hr; CRP: if ordered – 18 mg/L
b. Procalcitonin: if ordered, elevated
c. Synovial fluid results
   i.   Color: cloudy, WBC: 100,000, RBC: 300, poly: 93%
   ii. Gram stain: Gram positive cocci
   iii. Crystals: crystals seen
   iv. Glucose depressed; protein elevated (if ordered)

K. Action
a. Consult
   i. Orthopedics for possible joint irrigation in OR
b. IV antibiotics (vancomycin for presumed nongonococcal septic arthritis) administered in ED, admission for IV antibiotics

L. Diagnosis

a. Septic arthritis

M. Critical actions

a. Pain management
b. Joint aspiration for Gram stain, cultures, crystals, WBC
c. Antibiotics after Gram stain, fluid results
d. X-ray to assess for osteomyelitis
e. Orthopedics consult

N. Examiner instructions

a. This is a case of septic arthritis involving the right knee; a bacterial infection that can cause severe damage to the joint if left undiagnosed and untreated. The patient is otherwise healthy and clinically appears well, so an appropriate work-up for the right knee pain and fever can be done without the concern for starting early sepsis management. IV fluids and antipyretics can be initiated as needed; however, the patient should receive pain medication. Her pain will persist until an appropriate dose of opioid, such as morphine, is given. A diagnostic arthrocentesis (joint aspiration) should be performed before all other studies (x-ray is allowable if done quickly, but should not hold up the arthrocentesis). A Gram stain should be obtained before initiating antibiotics.

O. Pearls

a. Most patients with a monoarticular arthritis, even with a history of gout, require an arthrocentesis.
b. The skin overlying the affected joint should be free of cellulitis or impetigo to avoid contamination of the joint space.
c. Proceed with caution in patients with prosthetic joints, consider discussion with orthopedics prior to joint aspiration.
d. Synovial Gram stain, cultures, and WBC are the most important studies. Serum WBC, ESR, and CRP are useful but not helpful to establish a specific diagnosis. A joint aspirate with a WBC of >50,000 with PMNs greater than 90% is 56% sensitive and 90% specific for septic arthritis.
e. An x-ray should be obtained to rule out osteomyelitis.
f. Antibiotics should be tailored to Gram stain results and patient history. Suspect gonorrheal infection in young sexually active patient and consider adding cultures of the pharynx, urogenital, and rectal areas. Ceftriaxone should be given for gonorrheal infection. Nafcillin or vancomycin should be considered for *Staphylococcus* infection. For gram-negative bacilli infection, treat with third- or fourth-generation cephalosporin with antipseudomonal coverage.
g. Lyme titers, rheumatoid factor, ANA, lupus-anticoagulant may be helpful in follow-up management of joint pain.

P. Figure legends

a. Figure 56.1 (Knee x-ray) Normal knee x-ray.
b. Figure 56.2 (Knee x-ray) Normal knee x-ray.

Q. References

a. *Tintinalli's Emergency Medicine: A Comprehensive Study Guide* (9th ed.): Chapter 284, Joints and Bursae.
b. *Rosen's Emergency Medicine: Concepts and Clinical Practice* (10th ed.): Chapter 102, Arthritis.

Rash

Angela Maxwell, MD and Braden Hexom, MD

A. Chief complaint
a. 4-year-old female presents with a complaint of fever, rash, and vomiting

B. Vital signs
a. BP: 98/52, HR: 140, RR: 20, T: 39°C, Sat: 100% on RA, Wt: 20 kg

C. What does the patient look like?
a. Patient appears her stated age. She is awake and alert. She appropriately responds to questions but is less active and uncomfortable.

D. Primary survey
a. Airway: speaking in full sentences
b. Breathing: no apparent respiratory distress
c. Circulation: warm and clammy skin, capillary refill is 2.5 seconds.

E. Action
a. Peripheral IV
b. Labs
   i. CBC, BMP, LFT, urinalysis
c. 20 mL/kg NS bolus
d. Tylenol or ibuprofen
e. Monitor: BP: 100/60, HR: 130, RR: 20, Sat: 100% on RA

F. History
a. HPI: A 4-year-old female with no past medical history presents with a fever starting 3 days ago that is now associated with vomiting, headache, and a rash. Her mother reports fevers initially up to 102°F. She started complaining of a headache in association with the fever yesterday morning. She developed a few episodes of nonbilious, nonbloody vomiting yesterday as well as a rash around her wrists and ankles. This morning she was found to have a fever of 103°F, and her mom also noticed that the rash has spread to her hands, feet, legs, and arms. The constellation of symptoms prompted the visit to the emergency department.
b. PMHx: no history, immunizations are up to date
c. PSHx: none
d. Allergies: none
e. Meds: none
f. Social: lives with parents, lives in single-family home, no indoor pets, attends daycare, no exposure to drugs, alcohol, or tobacco

g. Travel history (must ask): went camping with grandparents 1 week ago at the end of July in northeastern Arkansas. They did not report specific tick bites.
h. FHx: not relevant
i. PMD: University Medical Center Pediatric Resident Clinic

G. Nurse
a. If fluids given
   i. BP 100/50, HR 118, RR 20, T: 38.9°C, Sat: 99% on RA
b. If fluids not given
   i. BP: 95/50, HR: 148, RR: 20, T: 38.9°C, Sat: 99%
   ii. Patient will continue to have tachycardia until fluids are given
c. If Tylenol or ibuprofen given
   i. T: 37°C
d. If Tylenol or ibuprofen not given
   i. T: 39.4°C
   ii. Patient will continue to have fever until antipyretic is given

H. Secondary survey
a. General: alert, oriented appropriate for age, appears tired but not in distress
b. Head: normocephalic, atraumatic
c. Eyes: normal conjunctivae, extraocular movement intact, pupils equally reactive
d. Ears: tympanic membranes are normal
e. Nose: no rhinorrhea
f. Throat: dry mucosa, normal dentition, no lesions, no swelling
g. Neck: supple neck, full range of motion, no jugular venous distension, trachea midline
h. Chest: normal
i. Heart: tachycardia, no murmurs, rubs, or gallops
j. Lungs: clear bilaterally, nonlabored
k. Abdomen: soft, nondistended, nontender, no rebound, no guarding
l. Urogenital: normal external female genitalia
m. Extremities: full range of motion to all joints, no joint swelling or erythema
n. Back: normal, no costovertebral angle tenderness
o. Skin (must ask): warm and dry, blanching maculopapular rash to bilateral upper and lower extremities including palms of hands and soles of feet (Figure 57.1)

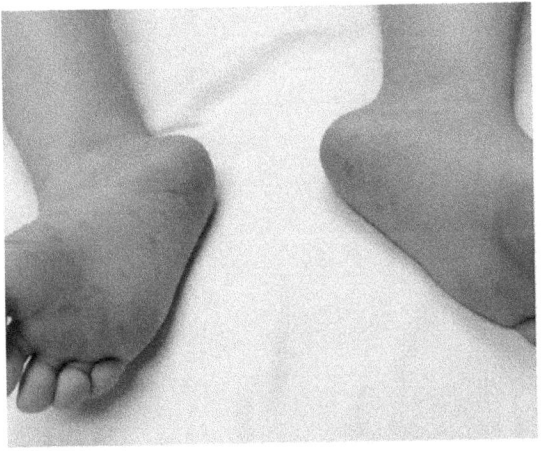

Figure 57.1

p. Neuro: cranial nerves II to XII intact; normal sensation, strength; normal reflexes and gait, negative Kernig's and Brudzinski's test

q. Lymph: mild cervical and inguinal adenopathy, no supraclavicular adenopathy

I. Action

a. Meds:
   i. Doxycycline
   ii. Chloramphenicol (not as widely available, can cause aplastic anemia)

b. Reassess
   i. Alert, refill improved and brisk (if fluids given)
   ii. Alert, refill improved and brisk, more interactive and active (if fluids and antipyretics given)
   iii. Alert, refill delayed 3 seconds, less active, tired (if no fluids, no antipyretics given)
   iv. Alert, refill improved and brisk, less active, tired (if no antipyretics given)

c. Consult
   i. Dermatology for evaluation and punch biopsy of the skin

d. Imaging
   i. Chest x-ray
   ii. Abdomen x-ray

e. Labs
   i. Antibody titer for Rocky Mountain spotted fever (usually not elevated in acute phase)

J. Nurse

a. BP: 100/60, HR: 118, RR: 18, T: 37°C, Sat: 98% on RA

K. Results

Table 57.1 Results table

Test	Result		Test	Result
Complete blood count:			Alk phos	200 U/L
WBC	$10.9 \times 10^3/\mu L$		T bili	0.3 mg/dL
Hgb	12 g/dL		D bili	0.1 mg/dL
Hct	40.00%		Albumin	3.8 g/dL
Plt	$80 \times 10^3/\mu L$			
			Urinalysis:	
Basic metabolic panel:			SG	1.020
Na	125 mEq/L		pH	6
K	3.4 mEq/L		Prot	Neg
Cl	98 mEq/L		Gluc	Neg
CO_2	20 mEq/L		Blood	Neg
BUN	20 mEq/dL		LE	Neg
Cr	0.6 mg/dL		Nitrite	Neg
Gluc	100 mg/dL		WBC	Neg
			Bacteria	Neg

Table 57.1 (cont.)

Test	Result	Test	Result
Liver function panel:			
AST	130 U/L		
ALT	120 U/L		

a. Chest x-ray (Figure 57.2)
b. Abdominal x-ray (Figure 57.3)

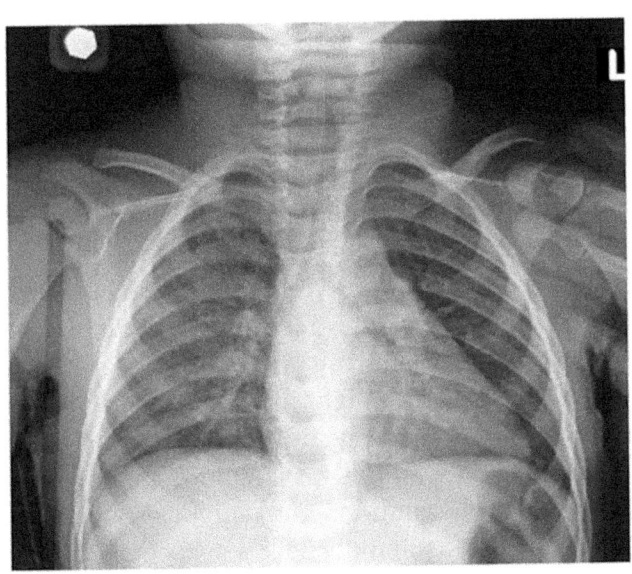

Figure 57.2

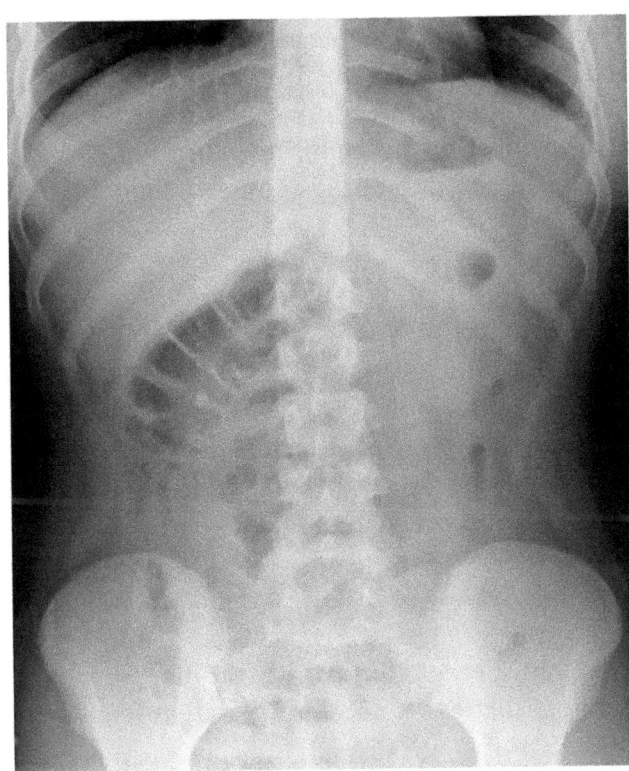

Figure 57.3

   c. Skin punch biopsy: results will not be available today

   d. Antibody titers: send out test that will not be available this week

L. Diagnosis

   a. Rocky Mountain spotted fever (RMSF)

N. Critical actions

   a. History: travel and camping in endemic area

   b. Physical examination: maculopapular rash

   c. Lab testing: CBC, BMP, LFT (or CMP, CBC)

   d. Antibiotics (doxycycline or chloramphenicol)

   e. Fluid bolus and antipyretics

O. Examiner instructions

   a. This is a case of Rocky Mountain spotted fever (RMSF). RMSF is a tick-borne illness that peaks in the summer months of June and July. The classic presentation includes a history of tick bite followed by progression of fever then rash with nausea, vomiting, and headache. Many cases do not specifically report a known tick bite, especially in pediatric populations; therefore, it is important to obtain a history of travel to an endemic area or participating in camping or other activities that would place the patient in closer contact with ticks. In this particular case, it is important to elicit a history that includes recent travel and activity as well as a thorough examination that will reveal a rash. Additional findings might include a headache, pedal edema, nausea, vomiting, conjunctival injection, and altered mental status. In order to best treat this patient, it is important to manage the acute clinical findings, including fever and tachycardia with fluids and antipyretics. After these interventions, the patient's status begins to improve while further investigation proceeds. Once the diagnosis is suspected, it is imperative to initiate appropriate antibiotic therapy. While the immediate laboratory findings are not diagnostic, they can often hint toward a diagnosis of RMSF where hyponatremia, thrombocytopenia, and transaminitis can be appreciated. More specific and definitive findings include antibody testing (elevation is usually not seen early on and the test results are not quickly available) and skin punch biopsy (specialized labs can expedite results, but they are not quickly obtained). Given the broad differential of a febrile and vomiting patient, other diagnostic imaging and laboratory tests might be considered, including chest and abdominal x-rays as well urine screening.

P. Pearls

   a. A travel history is central to developing the diagnosis of RMSF.

   b. The history of tick bite is not always provided, which is why it is important to determine the travel and activity history that places the patient in potential contact with ticks.

   c. The pathognomonic rash begins along the wrists and ankles, spreads to the hands and feet, then spreads centripetally to the trunk.

   d. Laboratory findings can help support the diagnosis and clinical suspicion where hyponatremia, transaminitis, and thrombocytopenia can be seen.

   e. Fever, rash, headache, and vomiting can be seen with a variety of illnesses; therefore, it is important to consider coexisting and additional diagnoses as well.

   f. RMSF can cause significant illness, including meningitis, renal failure, myocarditis, pneumonitis, pulmonary edema, and acute respiratory distress syndrome, as well as lethargy, confusion, and seizures.

Q. Figure legends

a. Figure 57.1 (Physical exam) Maculopapular rash to feet.

b. Figure 57.2 (CXR) Normal chest x-ray.

c. Figure 57.3 (Abdomen x-ray) Nonobstructive, normal abdomen x-ray.

R. References

a. *Tintinalli's Emergency Medicine: A Comprehensive Study Guide* (9th ed.): Chapters 161, Zoonotic Infections.

b. *Rosen's Emergency Medicine: Concepts and Clinical Practice* (10th ed.): Chapter 123, Tickborne Illnesses.

Sickle-Cell Disease

Oluwakemi Badaki-Makun, MD and Braden Hexom, MD

A. Chief complaint
a. 19-year-old male with a history of sickle-cell disease brought in by mother with the complaint of 3 days of back and now left-sided chest pain.

B. Vital signs
a. BP: 110/63, HR: 110, RR: 28, T: 37.9°C, Sat: 92% on RA, Wt: 65 kg

C. What does the patient look like?
a. Patient appears stated age, awake, and alert, responding to questions, but appears in severe pain and mildly tachypneic.

D. Primary survey
a. Airway: speaking in full sentences
b. Breathing: mild respiratory distress
c. Circulation: dry and cool skin, normal capillary refill

E. Action
a. Oxygen via NC or nonrebreather mask as needed to maintain >95% saturation
b. Large-bore peripheral IV line
c. Labs
    i. CBC, BMP, LFT, coagulation studies, blood type and crossmatch, ABG/VBG
    ii. Lactate, blood cultures, reticulocyte count, urinalysis, urine culture
d. CXR
e. EKG
f. Meds
    i. IV morphine and/or NSAID

F. History
a. HPI: A 19-year-old male college student with a history of sickle-cell disease (SS genotype) developed pain in the back and hips 3 days ago; pain has now become worse and is extending to the left chest. He took ibuprofen and hydrocodone at home without improvement. He is well known to the ED and is noted to have had multiple visits in the past year for pain crises. His last pain crisis was 2 weeks ago. He is admitted about twice a year. Today he notes cough and mild shortness of breath, but denies diarrhea, vomiting, headache, or neck pain. Chest pain is sharp, nonradiating, and worse with inspiration.
b. PMHx: History of sickle-cell disease with multiple ED visits and admissions. Baseline Hgb: 9. If asked about previous episodes, the patient will explain that most painful crises are in the

legs and arms and this is the first visit for chest pain. The mother states, "He has never had pain like this before." Normally pain responds to 2 mg Dilaudid or 16 mg morphine.

c. PSHx: none
d. Allergy: none
e. Meds: hydrocodone, ibuprofen
f. Social: sophomore in college, lives on campus; denies drugs/alcohol/smoking
g. FHx: mother and father with SS trait
h. PMD: Dr. Weber, pediatric hematologist

G. Nurse

a. EKG (Figure 58.1)
b. If oxygen and morphine given:
   i. BP: 108/62, HR: 90, RR: 22, T: 37.8°C, Sat: 97% on 2 L NC (or 100% on nonrebreather mask)
c. If no morphine or oxygen given:
   i. BP: 110/72, HR: 112, RR: 30, Sat: 89%
      1. Patient will develop worsening shortness of breath until oxygen is applied and will remain tachycardic until morphine is given for the severe pain.

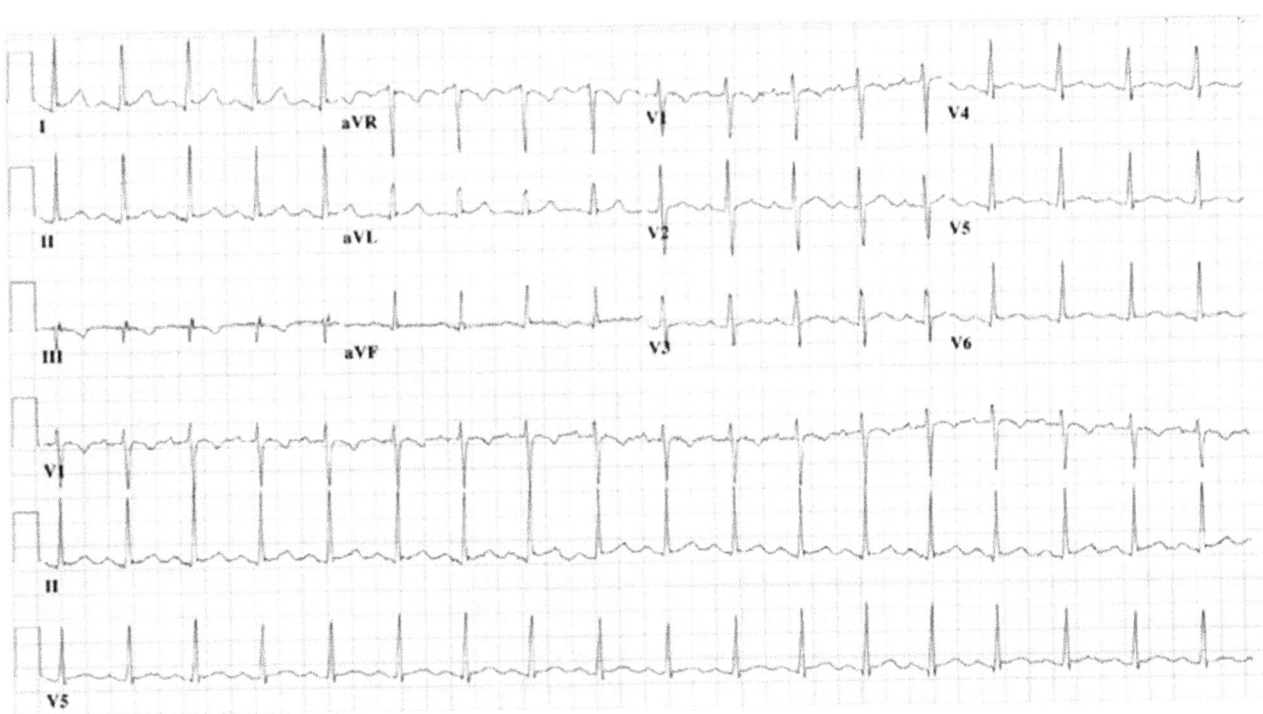

Figure 58.1

H. Secondary survey

a. General: alert, oriented × 3, in distress because of pain and mild shortness of breath
b. Head: normocephalic, atraumatic
c. Eyes: scleral icterus present, extraocular movements intact, pupils equal, reactive to light
d. Ears: normal tympanic membranes
e. Nose: no discharge
f. Neck: full range of motion, no jugular vein distension, no stridor
g. Pharynx: normal dentition, no lesions, no swelling
h. Chest: tender to palpation over sternum and ribs

i.   Lungs: (must ask) diminished breath sounds at left base, + crackles, dull to percussion, slightly diminished breath sounds at right lung base

j.   Heart: rate and rhythm regular, II/VI systolic flow murmur, no rubs or gallops

k.   Abdomen: normal bowel sounds, soft, nontender or distended, no hepatosplenomegaly

l.   Rectal: normal tone, brown stool, occult blood negative

m.   Extremities: no deformity, normal pulses, full range of motion

n.   Back: tender diffusely over spine and iliac crests

o.   Neuro: cranial nerves II to XII intact; normal sensation, strength; normal reflexes and gait

p.   Skin: pallor present, warm and dry

q.   Lymph: no lymphadenopathy

I. Action

a.   Meds
   i.   Morphine or Dilaudid

b.   Reassess
   i.   If less than a total of 10 mg morphine or 2 mg Dilaudid, pain continues
   ii. If total 10 mg morphine or 2 mg Dilaudid, pain improves

c.   Consultation
   i.   Hematology

d.   Imaging
   i.   CXR

J. Nurse

a.   CXR (Figure 58.2)

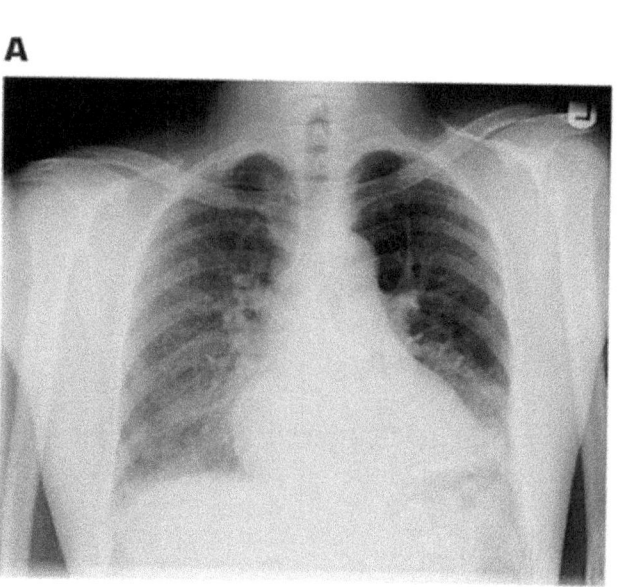
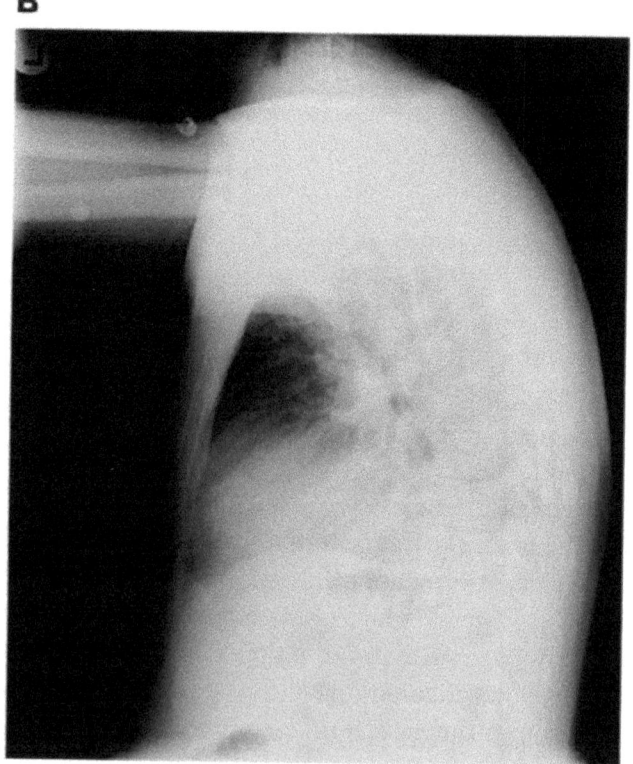

Figure 58.2

Case 58: Sickle-Cell Disease

K. Results

Table 58.1 Results table

Test	Result	Test	Result
Complete blood count:		T bili	2.8 mg/dL
WBC	18.9 × 10³/μL	D bili	0.1 mg/dL
Diff	93/6/1	Amylase	35 U/L
Hgb	7.9 g/dL	Lipase	23 U/L
Plt	325 × 10³/μL	Albumin	4.5 g/dL
		LDH	501 U/L
Basic metabolic panel:		**Urinalysis:**	
Na	134 mEq/L	SG	1.010–1.030
K	4.9 mEq/L	pH	5–8
Cl	108 mEq/L	Prot	Neg
CO$_2$	18.9 mEq/L	Gluc	Neg
BUN	23 mEq/dL	Ketones	Neg
Cr	0.7 mg/dL	Bili	Neg
Gluc	94 mg/dL	Blood	Neg
		LE	Neg
Coagulation panel:		Nitrite	Neg
PT	13 sec	Color	Yellow
PTT	25 sec		
INR	1.0	**Arterial blood gas:**	
		pH	7.35
Liver function panel:		pO$_2$	65 mmHg
AST	53 U/L	pCO$_2$	32 mmHg
ALT	40 U/L	HCO$_3$	19 mmol/L
Alk phos	106 U/L		

a. Reticulocyte count 10.6
b. Smear – occasional sickled cells, Howell–Jowell bodies, occasional target cells

L. Action
a. Meds
    i. Ceftriaxone (or cefotaxime) and azithromycin
    ii. Albuterol if patient has bronchospasm
b. Consult
    i. Hematology – recommends admission and consideration of simple packed red cell transfusion if patient severely anemic relative to baseline. Suggests discussing with ICU for admission if patient worsens in status.

M. Diagnosis

a.   Acute chest syndrome

N. Critical actions

a.   Oxygen (for hypoxia)
b.   Pain control with IV opiate and/or NSAIDs
c.   CXR and identification of a pulmonary infiltrate
d.   Antibiotics
e.   Albuterol if patient has bronchospasm
f.   IV fluids to maintain euvolemia
g.   Hematology consult for recommendations on transfusion (exchange vs. simple)
h.   Admission (may require medical ICU depending on severity of illness)

O. Examiner instructions

a.   This is a case of acute chest syndrome in a patient with sickle-cell disease. Acute chest syndrome is a severe complication of the disease that can rapidly progress to multisystem organ failure and death. The syndrome is defined by a new infiltrate on CXR plus one of the following: fever, cough, wheeze, tachypnea, or chest pain. Known etiologies include pulmonary fat embolism, pulmonary infarction, and infection with atypical organisms (*Mycoplasma pneumoniae*, *Chlamydia pneumoniae*) as well as viruses and other bacteria (e.g., *Streptococcus* and *Staphylococcus* species). Symptoms concerning for acute chest syndrome are chest pain, back pain, respiratory complaints, fever, and/or cough. Obtaining a CXR is key in this case; without it, the diagnosis cannot be made. Administration of oxygen, IV pain medications, and antibiotics are other critical actions for this case. If oxygen is not given, the patient's respiratory status will progressively worsen. If adequate IV pain medicine (10 mg of morphine or equivalent total) is not given, the patient will continue to have severe pain. Antibiotics should be given immediately after identification of an infiltrate on CXR. Albuterol should be given in patients with bronchospasm. A CBC and reticulocyte count should be obtained to evaluate the level of anemia and a type and hold should be sent as treatment often includes simple or exchange transfusions (based on the degree of anemia and the severity of illness). IV fluid boluses may be given if fluid resuscitation is necessary (e.g., if the patient is in shock), otherwise, a rate of 1.5× maintenance is recommended as excessive fluid resuscitation has been associated with worsening outcomes in acute chest syndrome.
b.   Curveball: The nurse approaches the candidate and states, "This guy is here all the time, and complains about pain until he gets his fix of narcotics." The nurse will be reluctant to give any narcotics until the MD reassures that the patient is experiencing pain common in sickle-cell crisis, and that his chronic use of narcotics (as part of his prescribed treatment) will raise his tolerance to this class of medicines significantly.

P. Pearls

a.   Painful crises that are not typical of the patient's usual symptoms should elicit a search for more serious complications of sickle-cell disease, including acute chest, aplastic crisis, splenic sequestration, hemolytic crisis, serious infection, stroke, or other end-organ infarct.
b.   Patients with sickle-cell disease who present with respiratory symptoms (with or without fever) should be evaluated for acute chest syndrome.
c.   IV pain medication, oxygen, antibiotics (IV cephalosporin + macrolide), bronchodilators, and/ or blood transfusion are mainstays of treatment for acute chest syndrome.
d.   In severe cases of acute chest, exchange transfusion is warranted.

Case 58: Sickle-Cell Disease

Q. Figure legends
a. Figure 58.1 (EKG) Sinus tachycardia.
b. Figure 58.2 (CXR) Retrocardiac infiltrate.

R. References
a. *Tintinalli's Emergency Medicine: A Comprehensive Study Guide* (9th ed.): Chapter 236, Sickle Cell Disease and Hereditary Hemolytic Anemias.
b. *Rosen's Emergency Medicine: Concepts and Clinical Practice* (10th ed.): Chapter 109, Anemia and Polycythemia.

Headache

Braden Hexom, MD, Jacob M. Stritch, MD, and James P. Gillen, MD

A. Chief complaint
a. 22-year-old male brought in by friends with the complaint of fever and headache

B. Vital signs
a. BP: 118/84, HR: 105, RR: 16, T: 38.9°C, Sat: 100% on RA, FS: 87 mg/dL

C. What does the patient look like?
a. Patient appears stated age, somewhat lethargic, appears ill, responding slowly to questions.

D. Primary survey
a. Airway: speaking in full sentences
b. Breathing: no respiratory distress, no cyanosis
c. Circulation: pale, clammy skin

E. Action
a. Large-bore peripheral IV line
   i. CBC, BMP, LFT, coagulation studies, blood type and crossmatch
   ii. Lactate, blood cultures, urinalysis, urine culture, alcohol level, acetaminophen level, salicylate level, urine toxicology screen
b. 1 L NS bolus
c. Monitor: BP: 118/84, HR: 105, RR: 16, T: 38.9°C, Sat: 100% on O_2

F. History
a. HPI: A 22-year-old male college student with no past medical history developed fever and headache this morning after attending an all-night drinking party. He denies any drug use but admits to drinking "a few drinks the night before." He woke up with a headache last night that he attributed to alcohol. He did not want to come to the hospital, but his roommate insisted when he developed a fever and was "not very awake." He describes a headache that does not go away and is bilaterally radiating down to the neck and shoulders. He has tried acetaminophen for the headache without improvement. Not the worst headache of his life, but significant pain, not sudden onset or thunderclap, no nausea, vomiting, blurry vision; + photophobia, + neck pain.
b. PMHx: none, immunizations reportedly up to date
c. PSHx: lives with roommate in college dormitory, does well in school, social drinking and smoking, no drugs
d. Allergy: none

e. Meds: none
f. FHx: no relevant history
g. PMD: school health services
h. Travel history (if asked): none

G. Nurse
a. With fluids
   i. BP: 112/88, HR: 87, RR: 16, Sat: 99%
b. No fluids
   i. BP: 90/70, HR: 110, RR: 16, Sat: 99%
c. Meds
   i. Ibuprofen or acetaminophen
      1. Does not improve headache or fever
   ii. Antiemetic
      1. Does not improve headache
d. Place patient into an isolation room, droplet precautions

H. Secondary survey
a. General: mildly lethargic but arousable, oriented × 3
b. Head: normocephalic, atraumatic, no sinus tenderness
c. Eyes: extraocular movement intact, pale conjunctivae, + photophobia, equal and reactive pupils, unable to visualize fundus
d. Ears: normal tympanic membranes
e. Nose: no discharge
f. Neck: pain and stiffness with flexion, no jugular vein distension, no stridor
g. Pharynx: normal dentition, no lesions, no swelling
h. Chest: nontender
i. Lungs: clear bilaterally
j. Heart: rate and rhythm regular, tachycardic, no murmurs, rubs, or gallops
k. Abdomen: normal bowel sounds, soft, nontender or distended
l. Rectal: normal tone, brown stool, occult blood negative
m. Urogenital: normal external genitalia
   i. Male: no discharge, normal testicular examination
n. Extremities: full range of motion, no deformity, normal pulses
o. Back: nontender
p. Neuro: cranial nerves II to XII intact; normal sensation, strength; normal reflexes and gait, hip and knee flexion with passive neck flexion, hamstring contraction with knee extension while hip flexed
q. Skin: warm and dry, diffuse petechial rash over complete trunk
r. Lymph: no lymphadenopathy

I. Action
a. Meds
   i. Dexamethasone 10 mg IV
   ii. Ceftriaxone or cefotaxime 2 g IV
   iii. Vancomycin 15–20 mg/kg IV loading dose

b. Imaging
   i.   CT head (will take 20 minutes to obtain if candidate does not order antibiotics)
   ii. CXR

J. Nurse

a. CT head (Figure 59.1)

K. Action

a. Lumbar puncture
   i.   Opening pressure
   ii. Send for Gram stain, culture, cell count, glucose, protein, PCR studies

L. Nurse

a. CXR (Figure 59.2)

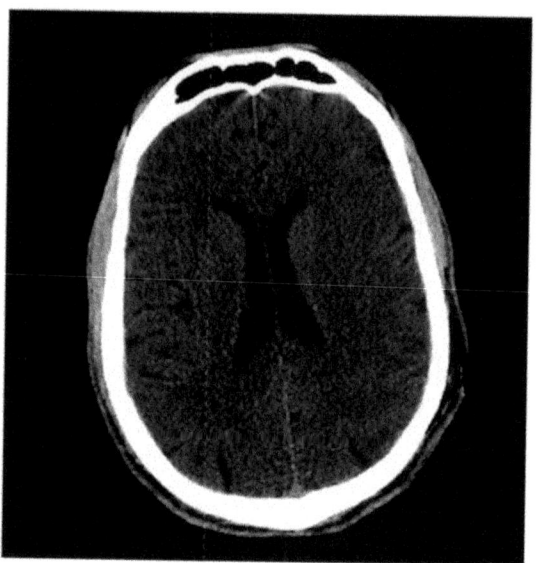

Figure 59.1

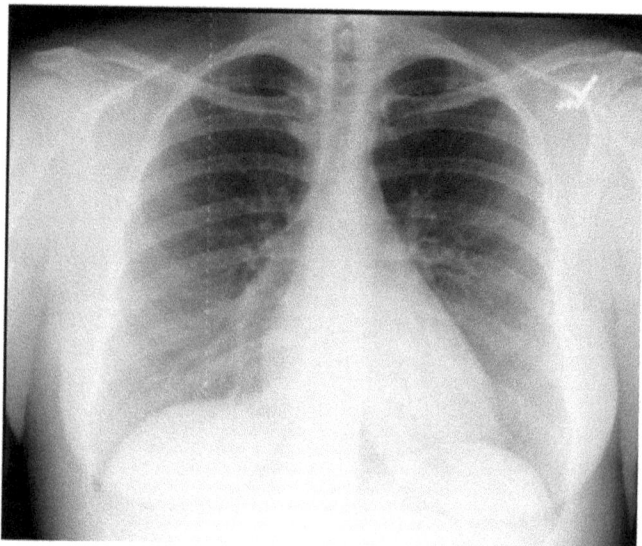
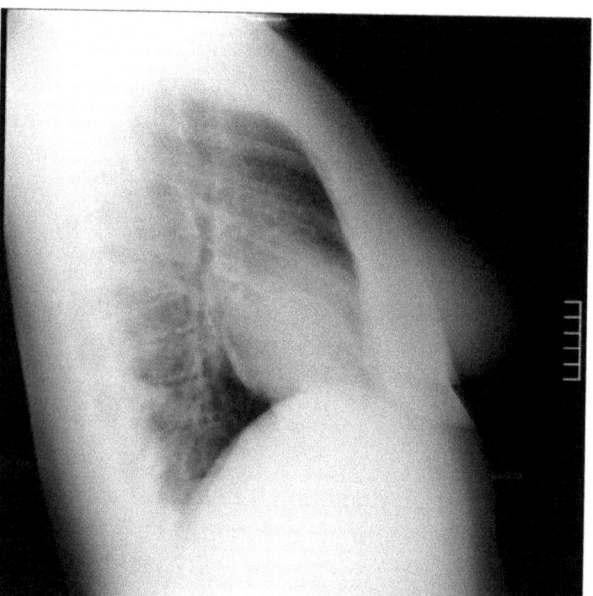

Figure 59.2

M. Results

Table 59.1 Results table

Test	Result	Test	Result
Complete blood count:		**Liver function panel:**	
WBC	$17.3 \times 10^3/\mu L$	AST	25 U/L
Diff	89.5/6.7/1.2	ALT	26 U/L
Hct	43%	Alk phos	220 U/L
Plt	$75 \times 10^3/\mu L$	T bili	0.6 mg/dL
		D bili	0.1 mg/dL
Basic metabolic panel:		Amylase	79 U/L
Na	121 mEq/L	Lipase	46 U/L
K	4.2 mEq/L	Albumin	3.9 g/dL
Cl	101 mEq/L		
CO_2	18.9 mEq/L	**Urinalysis:**	
BUN	23 mEq/dL	SG	1.010–1.030
Cr	0.7 mg/dL	pH	5–8
Gluc	94 mg/dL	Prot	Neg
		Gluc	Neg
		Ketones	Neg
Coagulation panel:		Bili	Neg
PT	13 sec	Blood	Neg
PTT	25 sec	LE	Neg
INR	1.0	Nitrite	Neg
		Color	Yellow

a. Serum and urine toxicology negative
b. Opening pressure 352 mmH$_2$O
c. Cerebral spinal fluid
   i. WBC: 1600
   ii. PMNs: 95%
   iii. RBC: 20
   iv. Glucose: 34
   v. Protein: 205
   vi. Gram stain: Gram-negative diplococci

N. Action

a. Admission to ICU setting, isolation bed
b. Public health
   i. Discussion with friends regarding prophylaxis
   ii. Call to dean or health services of college regarding possible campus health concern

iii. Prophylaxis to all exposed health providers

iv. Report case to Department of Public Health

O. Diagnosis

a. Bacterial meningitis

P. Critical actions

a. Appropriate antibiotic therapy before imaging or lumbar puncture

b. Lumbar puncture

c. Admission to isolation bed and ICU

d. Assessment of public health concerns

Q. Examiner instructions

a. This is a case of bacterial meningitis, a serious infection of the tissues surrounding the brain and usually fatal if not treated promptly. Classic symptoms are headache, fever, neck stiffness, and a petechial or purpuric rash. Seizure and altered mental status are common. Treatment must begin immediately with IV antibiotics as soon as the diagnosis is suspected. Antibiotics should be administered before CT and lumbar puncture if there will be an expected delay as these are diagnostic tests. If steroids are given, they should be administered before or with the antibiotics. The candidate should isolate the patient early in the course of the case and get in contact with college health services regarding prophylaxis of students and staff for meningitis.

R. Pearls

a. Empiric antibiotic therapy takes precedence over definitive diagnosis in patients with suspected meningitis (fever [95% of presentations], nuchal rigidity [88%], altered mental status [78%], headache [common]).

b. Antimicrobial therapy (vancomycin 15–20 mg/kg and ceftriaxone or cefotaxime 2 g IV) along with IV steroids (dexamethasone 10 mg IV) when indicated, should be administered as quickly as possible.

c. Consider adding acyclovir (10 mg/kg IV) if there is concern for HSV encephalitis; consider ampicillin (2 g IV) in patients >50 years of age to cover *L. monocytogenes*.

d. Indications for CT head prior to LP: focal neurologic deficit, new onset seizure, papilledema, immunocompromised state, malignancy, history of focal CNS disease, concern for mass CNS lesion, altered mental status or age > 60 years.

e. Kernig's (contraction of hamstrings in response to knee extension) or Brudzinski's (flexion of hips/knees in response to neck flexion) signs are insensitive but may aid in the diagnosis.

f. Immunocompromised patients require additional CSF testing and broader-spectrum antibiotics, as they are susceptible to a wider range of organisms, including *Tuberculosis*, *Cryptococcus*, *Staphylococcus*, and *Listeria*.

g. Chemoprophylaxis is recommended for close contacts of patients diagnosed with *N. meningitidis* and *H. influenzae* (rifampin 600 mg PO q 12 hr × 4 doses, ciprofloxacin 500 mg PO once, or ceftriaxone 250 mg IM once).

S. Figure legends

a. Figure 59.1 (Head CT) Normal head CT.

b. Figure 59.2 (CXR) Normal chest x-ray.

T. References

a. *Tintinalli's Emergency Medicine: A Comprehensive Study Guide* (9th ed.): Chapter 174, Central Nervous System and Spinal Infections.

b. *Rosen's Emergency Medicine: Concepts and Clinical Practice* (10th ed.): Chapter 95, Central Nervous System Infections.

Chest Pain

Monica Sethi, MD and Braden Hexom, MD

A. Chief complaint
a. 34-year-old male with chest pain

B. Vital signs
a. BP: 126/98, HR: 118, RR: 24, T: 37.9°C, Sat: 95% on RA, FS: 74 mg/dL

C. What does the patient look like?
a. Patient appears stated age, alert, oriented × 3, sitting up on stretcher, in no acute distress.

D. Primary survey
a. Airway: speaking full sentences
b. Breathing: mild tachypnea, but no apparent respiratory distress, no cyanosis
c. Circulation: dry and cool skin, normal capillary refill

E. Action
a. Oxygen via NC as needed to maintain >95% saturation
b. Large-bore peripheral IV lines
c. Labs
   i. CBC, BMP, LFT, coagulation studies, blood type and crossmatch
d. 1 L NS bolus
e. EKG

F. History
a. HPI: A 34-year-old male with no past medical history presenting with chest pain for the past 24 hours. He describes the pain as slow in onset, gradually worsening throughout the day. The pain is localized to the mid-chest, and is sharp, nonradiating, worse with inspiration. There is associated mild shortness of breath. If asked, the patient reports some new ankle swelling. If asked, he reports subjective fever, but no chills, diaphoresis, nausea, or vomiting. If asked, he reports the pain is made worse with lying down, better by sitting forward, and slightly worse when he is walking. If asked about recent illnesses, he states that he had "a bad cold" about two weeks ago that lasted one week and self-resolved; no recent travel; no leg pain, no recent immunizations.
b. PMHx: none
c. PSHx: lives with wife and young child, social drinking, no smoking or drugs
d. Allergies: none
e. Meds: none
f. FHx: no family history of heart disease, MI, or stroke
g. PMD: none

G. Nurse
a. EKG (Figure 60.1)
b. Medication
    i. Ibuprofen, indomethacin, or aspirin: pain improves
    ii. Codeine: no improvement

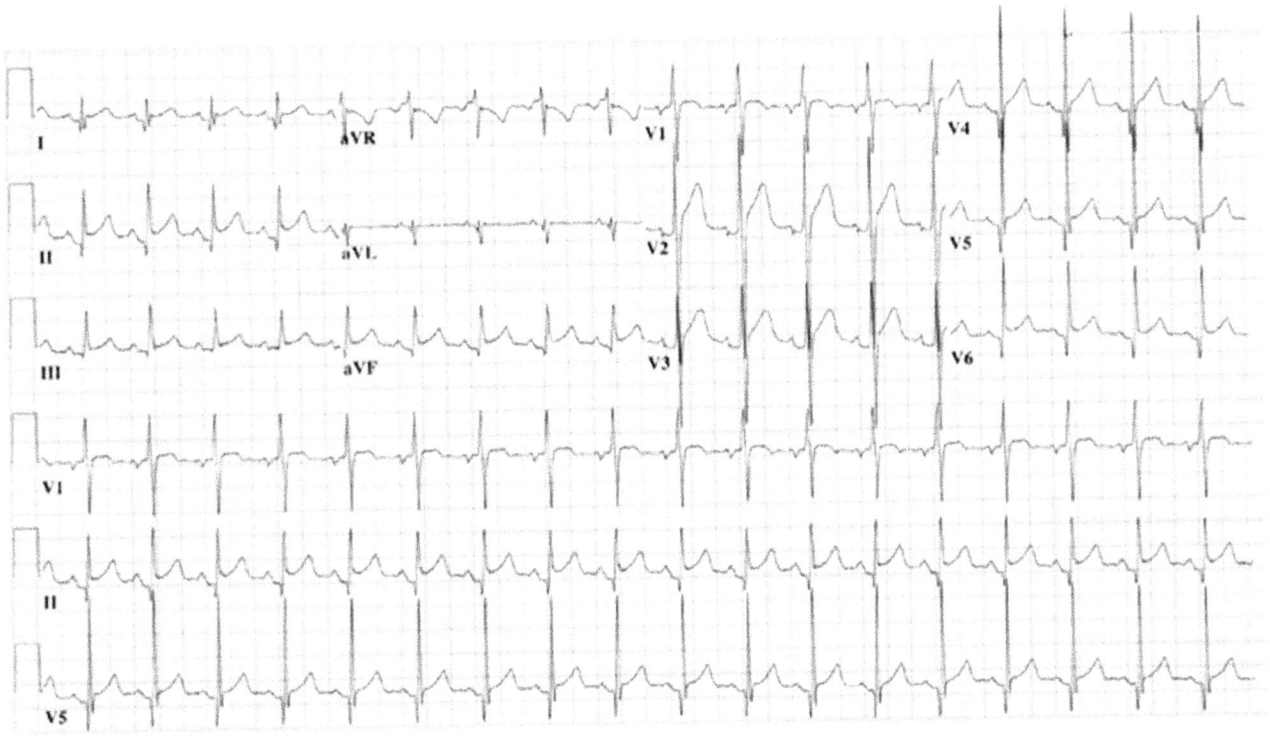

Figure 60.1

H. Secondary survey
a. General: alert, oriented × 3, sitting forward on stretcher, in no acute distress
b. Head: normocephalic, atraumatic
c. Eyes: extraocular movement intact, pupils equal, reactive to light
d. Ears: normal tympanic membranes
e. Nose: no discharge
f. Neck: full range of motion, no jugular vein distension, no stridor
g. Pharynx: normal dentition, no lesions, no swelling
h. Chest: nontender
i. Lungs: mild tachypnea, minimal crackles at the lung bases
j. Heart: friction rub is heard over the left apex (must ask), normal rate and rhythm
k. Abdomen: normal bowel sounds, soft, nontender or distended
l. Rectal: normal tone, brown stool, occult blood negative
m. Extremities: full range of motion, no deformity, normal pulses, trace edema in the feet and ankles bilaterally
n. Back: nontender
o. Neuro: cranial nerves II to XII intact; normal sensation, strength; normal reflexes and gait
p. Skin: warm and dry
q. Lymph: no lymphadenopathy

I. Action

a. Imaging

    i. Echocardiogram official (bedside ED US machine unavailable)

    ii. CXR

b. Labs

    i. Add on cardiac enzymes and D-dimer

c. Disposition

    i. Admit for serial echocardiography

J. Results

Table 60.1 Results table

Test	Result	Test	Result
Complete blood count:		**Liver function panel:**	
WBC	$10.3 \times 10^3/\mu L$	AST	45 U/L
Hct	43%	ALT	44 U/L
Plt	$75 \times 10^3/\mu L$	Alk phos	54 U/L
		T bili	0.5 mg/dL
Basic metabolic panel:		D bili	0.2 mg/dL
Na	133 mEq/L	Amylase	65 U/L
K	4.6 mEq/L	Lipase	23 U/L
Cl	105 mEq/L	Albumin	4.5 g/dL
CO_2	19 mEq/L		
BUN	24 mEq/dL	**Urinalysis:**	
Cr	0.9 mg/dL	SG	1.010–1.030
Gluc	77 mg/dL	pH	5–8
		Prot	Neg
Coagulation panel:		Gluc	Neg
PT	12.5 sec	Ketones	Neg
PTT	26.1 sec	Bili	Neg
INR	1.0	Blood	Neg
		LE	Neg
		Nitrite	Neg
		Color	Yellow

a. Cardiac enzymes

    i. Troponin 0.7 ng/mL

    ii. CK: 63 U/L

    iii. CK-MB: 4.8 U/L

b. D-dimer: negative

c. Echocardiogram: moderate amount of pericardial effusion, globally reduced EF of 35% with no specific wall motion abnormality, no evidence of cardiac tamponade

d. CXR (Figure 60.2)

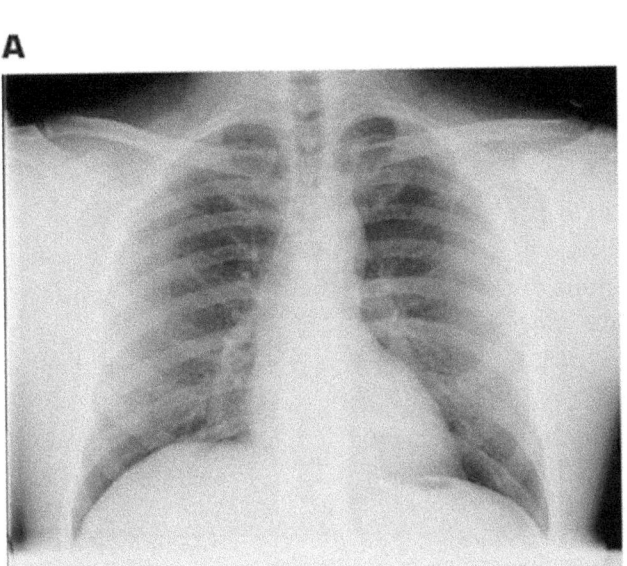
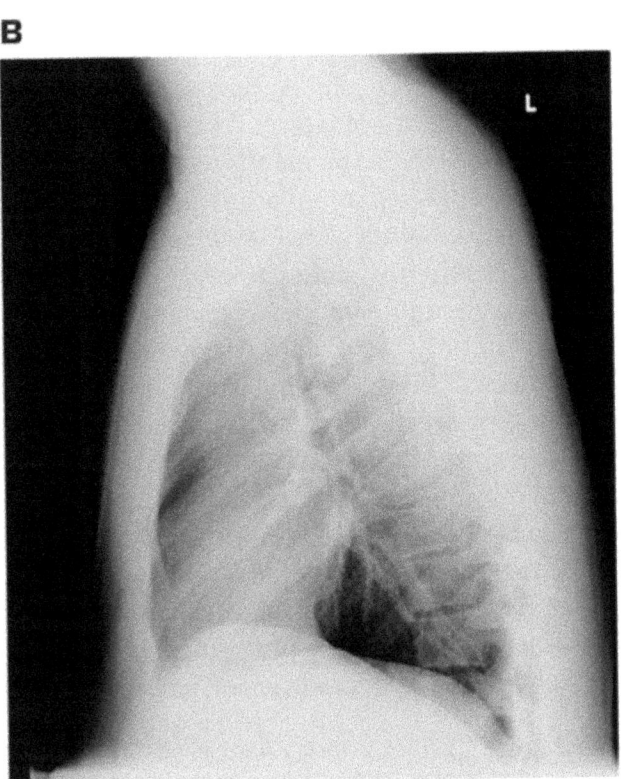

Figure 60.2

K. Diagnosis
a. Myopericarditis

L. Critical actions
a. EKG
b. Cardiac examination
c. Echocardiogram
d. NSAID
e. Cardiology consultation
f. Admission

M. Examiner instructions
a. This is a case of myopericarditis, an acute inflammation of the heart muscles and the lining of the heart. Often caused by viral illnesses (as in this case) or idiopathic, it is not an acute coronary syndrome, and can be the cause of chest pain in young people. Early actions include obtaining an EKG, NSAID, and echocardiogram. Upon diagnosing pericardial effusion and myocardial injury from myopericarditis, the patient should be admitted for observation and management. The patient should be monitored for worsening pericardial effusion, cardiac tamponade, and deteriorating cardiac function by echocardiography. The candidate should still

consider other diagnoses such as pulmonary embolism or myocardial infarction by reviewing risk factors such as family history of cardiac disease and recent travel history. Ultimately the patient has no risk factors for either pulmonary embolism or myocardial infarction and improves with NSAIDs.

N. Pearls

a. Myopericarditis may be caused by viral or bacterial illnesses, malignancy, radiation, or a variety of other causes.

b. Myopericarditis is a manifestation of an inflammatory syndrome spectrum, ranging from pure pericarditis to pure myocarditis. Symptoms include acute coronary-like chest pain, chest pain made worse with lying down and improved with sitting forward, dysphagia, dyspnea, and intermittent low-grade fevers. A friction rub is a frequently encountered physical finding.

c. Patients with myopericarditis may develop sinus tachycardia out of proportion to fever, and heart failure may develop in severe cases.

d. Diffuse ST elevation and T wave inversion are the most common EKG findings for myopericarditis, rarely corresponding to anatomical zones of infarction.

e. Laboratory testing (CBC, serial troponins, inflammatory markers), an EKG, a chest radiograph, and an echocardiogram establish the diagnosis, determine the presence of tamponade, grade disease severity, and help rule out alternative causes of chest pain.

f. Patients with viral myopericarditis with evidence of tamponade, myocardial injury, ventricular dysfunction, or arrhythmias should be admitted for cardiac monitoring and ongoing assessment of disease progression. Supportive care and NSAIDs are the mainstay of therapy.

g. Isolated viral pericarditis can be treated as an outpatient with 1–3 weeks of NSAID therapy.

O. Figure legends

a. Figure 60.1 (EKG) EKG showing sinus tachycardia; diffuse ST elevations/PR depressions suggestive of pericarditis.

b. Figure 60.2 (a) (CXR) Normal PA chest x-ray. (b) (CXR) Normal lateral chest x-ray.

P. References

a. *Tintinalli's Emergency Medicine: A Comprehensive Study Guide* (9th ed.): Chapter 55, Cardiomyopathies and Pericardial Disease.

b. *Rosen's Emergency Medicine: Concepts and Clinical Practice* (10th ed.): Chapter 68, Pericardial and Myocardial Disease.

Altered Mental Status

Braden Hexom, MD, David Orban, MD, and Matthew Beattie, MD

A. Chief complaint
a. 73-year-old female brought in by basic life support ambulance with complaint of confusion and facial droop; EMT call for a rule out stroke

B. Vital signs
a. BP: 153/104, HR: 105, RR: 16, T: 36.8°C, Sat: 100% on RA, FS: pending (if requested by candidate)

C. What does the patient look like?
a. Patient appears stated age, confused, garbled response to questions, with obvious facial droop on right side.

D. Primary survey
a. Airway: awake, garbled vocalizations
b. Breathing: no respiratory distress
c. Circulation: diaphoretic, pale, clammy skin

E. Action
a. Oxygen via NC or nonrebreather mask as needed to maintain >95% saturation
b. Two large-bore peripheral IV lines
c. Labs
    i.   CBC, BMP, LFT, coagulation studies, urinalysis, blood type and crossmatch
    ii. Finger stick glucose: (must ask) 22 mg/dL
d. 1 L NS bolus
e. EKG
f. Meds
    i.   D50 1–2 AMPS
    ii. Consider thiamine

F. History
a. HPI: A 73-year-old female is brought in after her husband found her on the sofa around 10 a.m. with confusion and slurred speech. She was brought immediately to the ED by ambulance (now 10:30 a.m.). Her husband states he last saw her around 7 a.m. when she was at her baseline. She has a history of hypertension, high cholesterol, diabetes, and hypothyroidism. The husband reports no recent illnesses or complaints. She suffers from mild dementia and forgetfulness, but is otherwise active, walks frequently, and is usually alert and conversational. Patient is confused and unable to answer questions.
b. EMS: no further history, only gave O_2 by mask
c. PMHx: hypertension, high cholesterol, diabetes (noninsulin dependent), hypothyroid

    d. PSHx: none

    e. Allergies: none

    f. Meds: lovastatin, metoprolol, aspirin, glyburide, metformin, levothyroxine

    g. Social: lives with husband, no smoking, alcohol, or drugs

    h. FHx: no relevant history

G. Nurse

    a. D50 push IV

        i. Patient's symptoms resolve completely. Patient is now awake, alert, and becomes oriented with supportive care. Upon questioning she states she took her regular medications but did not eat breakfast because she had a doctor's appointment at 1 p.m.

    b. If D50 is not given, patient will continue to be confused with focal neurological findings described below in secondary survey

    c. EKG (Figure 61.1)

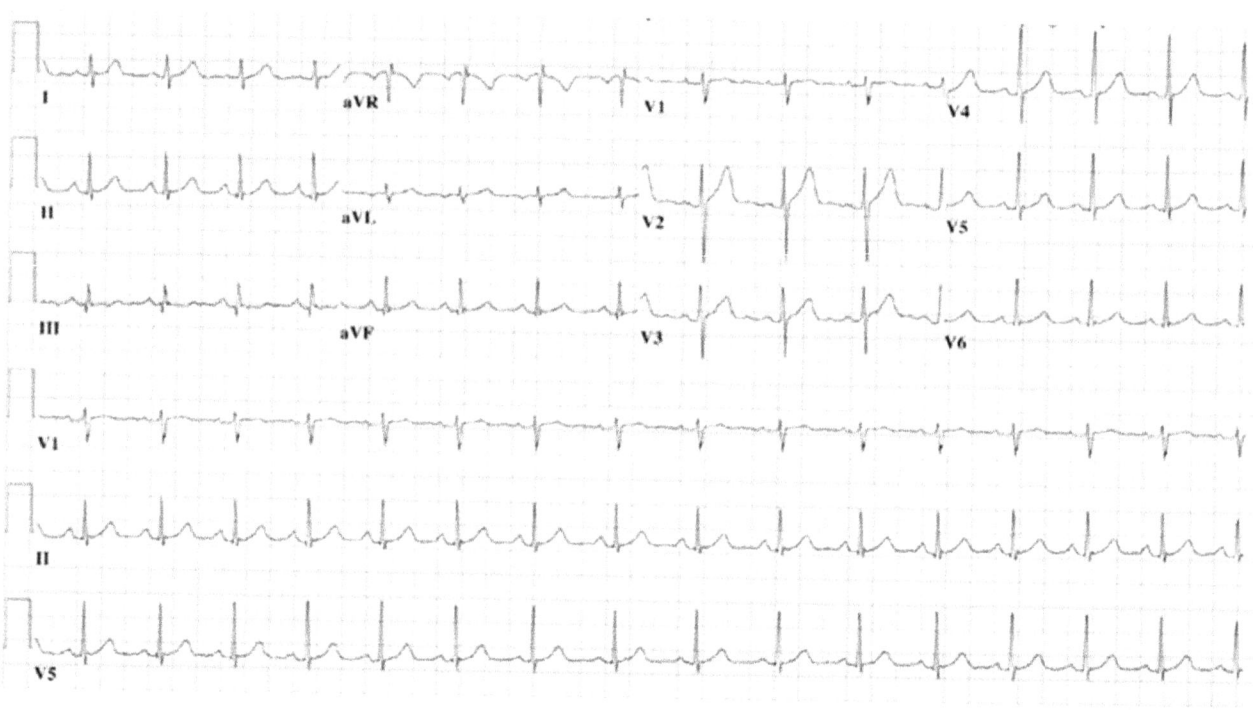

Figure 61.1

H. Secondary survey

    a. General

        i. Dextrose: alert and oriented × 3, in no acute distress

        ii. No dextrose: confused, not following commands

    b. Head: normocephalic, atraumatic

    c. Eyes: pale conjunctivae, extraocular movement intact, pupils equal, reactive to light

    d. Ears: normal tympanic membranes

    e. Nose: no discharge

    f. Neck: full range of motion, no jugular vein distension, no stridor

    g. Pharynx: normal dentition, no lesions, no swelling

    h. Chest: nontender

    i. Lungs: clear bilaterally

j. Heart: rate and rhythm regular, no murmurs, rubs, or gallops
k. Abdomen: normal bowel sounds, soft, nontender or distended
l. Rectal: normal tone, brown stool, occult blood negative
m. Urogenital: normal external genitalia
n. Extremities: full range of motion, no deformity, normal pulses
o. Back: nontender
p. Neuro:
    i. If dextrose given: cranial nerves II to XII intact; normal sensation, strength; normal reflexes and gait
    ii. If no dextrose: facial droop with garbled speech, does not cooperate with examination, reflexes normal, Babinski reflex normal, withdraws to pain
q. Skin: clammy
r. Lymph: no lymphadenopathy

I. Action
a. Further action required (candidate may opt for any combination, must do one)
    i.   Option 1: feed the patient
    ii. Option 2: D5 or D10 fluid administration at maintenance rate
    iii. Option 3: octreotide 50–150 mcg subcutaneously Q 6 h
    iv. If none of the above are given, patient's blood glucose will drop back down to 45 mg/dL and patient will once again become confused
b. Imaging
    i. CXR (Figure 61.2)
c. Admission

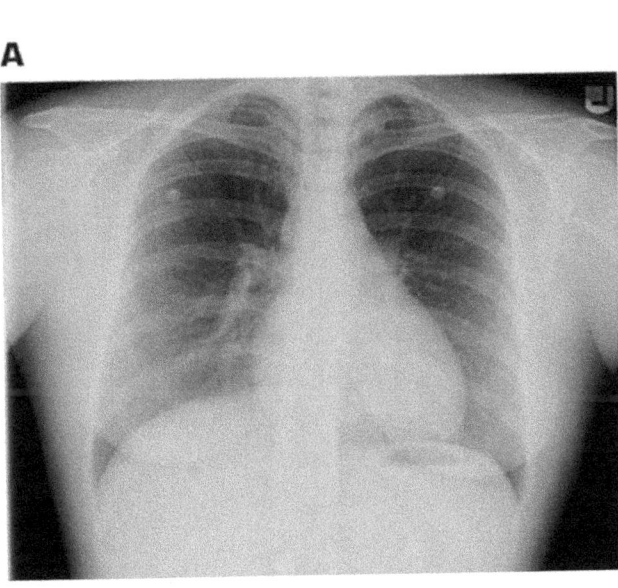
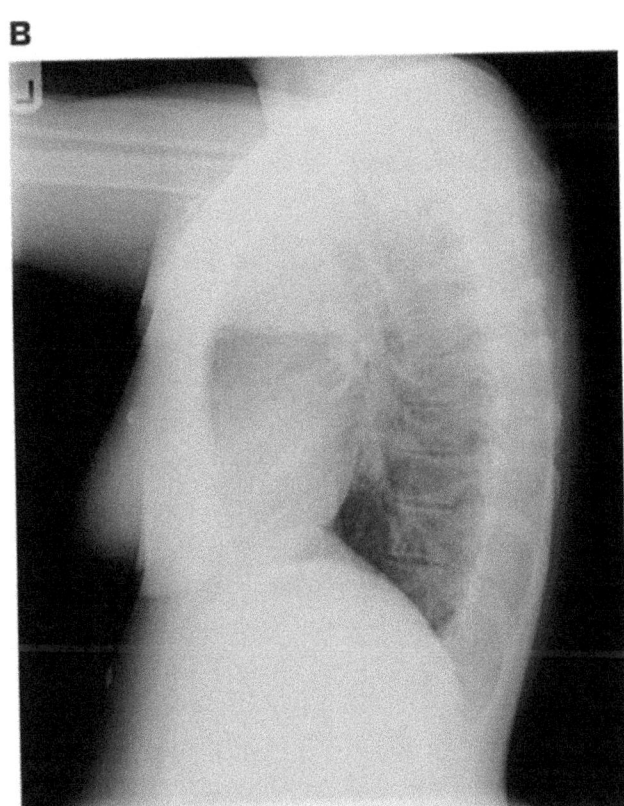

Figure 61.2

J. Nurse

a. CT head (Figure 61.3) if ordered – not necessary

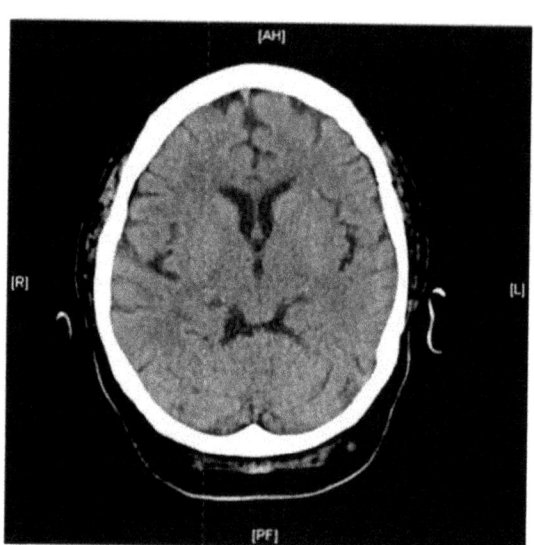

Figure 61.3

K. Results

Table 61.1 Results table

Test	Result	Test	Result
Complete blood count:		**Liver function panel:**	
WBC	$11.0 \times 10^3/\mu L$	AST	45 U/L
Hct	32%	ALT	44 U/L
Plt	$155 \times 10^3/\mu L$	Alk phos	54 U/L
		T bili	0.5 mg/dL
Basic metabolic panel:		D bili	0.2 mg/dL
Na	138 mEq/L	Amylase	65 U/L
K	4.3 mEq/L	Lipase	23 U/L
Cl	111 mEq/L	Albumin	4.5 g/dL
CO_2	21 mEq/L		
BUN	23 mEq/dL	**Urinalysis:**	
Cr	0.9 mg/dL	SG	1.010–1.030
Gluc	234 mg/dL	pH	5–8
		Prot	Neg
Coagulation panel:		Gluc	Neg
PT	13 sec	Ketones	Neg
PTT	25 sec	Bili	Neg
INR	1.0	Blood	Neg
		LE	Neg
		Nitrite	Neg
		Color	Yellow

L. Disposition
a. Admission for observation

M. Diagnosis
a. Hypoglycemia secondary to sulfonylurea

N. Critical actions
a. IV access
b. Finger stick glucose
c. IV dextrose
d. Further antihypoglycemic intervention (dextrose fluids, oral feeding, or octreotide)
e. Admission

O. Examiner instructions
a. This is a case of altered mental status with neurological deficits as a result of hypoglycemia. Hypoglycemia can mimic stroke, presenting with weakness and confusion, and can typically be reversed with the administration of dextrose. The hypoglycemia in this scenario is due to not eating breakfast after taking a diabetes medicine (glyburide, a sulfonylurea). Upon this patient's initial presentation, she exhibited signs of an acute stroke, which may lead the candidate to misdiagnose this patient and initiate a stroke protocol, including head CT, neurology consultation, intubation, or even thrombolysis. Obtaining an immediate blood glucose level is crucial to the diagnosis. With the ingestion in this case, further action is required beyond a rapid correction of blood glucose with dextrose. Blood sugar levels must be maintained because sulfonylurea drugs can cause delayed or rebound hypoglycemia for many hours. Feeding, fluids with dextrose, or octreotide are all adequate options, with two or all three sometimes required. Admission is mandatory.

P. Pearls
a. Symptoms of hypoglycemia are due to both the effects on the brain and a reflex sympathetic surge. Neurological effects include confusion, agitation, seizures, unresponsiveness, and focal neurological deficits. Autonomic effects include anxiety, irritability, vomiting, palpitations, tremor, and sweating.
b. If no clear cause of hypoglycemia is found, such as a missed meal or over-administration of medications, the patient should be evaluated for occult causes such as infection, renal dysfunction, or ischemia.
c. Rapid finger stick glucose is essential in all patients with altered mental status, especially with concern for stroke, as glucose <50 mg/dL is a contraindication to tPA.
d. An intervention beyond IV dextrose is usually required to maintain blood glucose levels. A carbohydrate-rich snack or juice is often sufficient, but D10 infusions may be required.
e. Hypoglycemia due to non-short-acting insulin or a sulfonylurea requires admission due to rebound hypoglycemia and long duration of action.
f. *Impaired awareness of hypoglycemia* is described as decreased ability to perceive the onset of hypoglycemia, placing the patient at risk for severe hypoglycemia. It is mainly seen in type 1 diabetics, the elderly, and the severely malnourished (e.g., patients with alcohol dependence).
g. Octreotide 50–150 mcg SQ inhibits release of insulin and is effective in the treatment of sulfonylurea-induced hypoglycemia. It is only recommended after initial glucose therapy has been initiated, as it primarily reduces the risk of recurrent hypoglycemia. If repeat episodes of

hypoglycemia are encountered, it can be repeated every 6 hours or started in a continuous IV infusion at 125 mcg/hr.

h. Glucagon 1 mg IM or SQ may be used when IV access is unattainable, but response is generally slower and is often not useful for patients with depleted glycogen stores, such as alcoholics.

Q. Figure legends
a. Figure 61.1 (EKG) Normal sinus rhythm.
b. Figure 61.2 (CXR) Normal chest x-ray.
c. Figure 61.3 (CT) Normal head CT.

R. References
a. *Tintinalli's Emergency Medicine: A Comprehensive Study Guide* (9th ed.): Chapter 168, Altered Mental Status and Coma. Chapter 223, Type 2 Diabetes Mellitus. Chapter 224, Type 2 Diabetes Mellitus.
b. *Rosen's Emergency Medicine: Concepts and Clinical Practice* (10th ed.): Chapter 12, Depressed Consciousness and Coma. Chapter 115, Diabetes Mellitus and Disorders of Glucose Homeostasis.

Headache

Hayley Neher, MD

A. Chief complaint
a. 32-year-old female presents with weakness, headache, and nausea for 1 day

B. Vital signs
a. BP: 140/90, HR: 105, RR: 20, T: 37.2°C, Sat: 99% on RA

C. What does the patient look like?
a. Patient appears stated age, uncomfortable, and well-nourished.

D. Primary survey
a. Airway: speaking in full sentences
b. Breathing: no respiratory distress, no cyanosis
c. Circulation: dry and cool skin, normal capillary refill

E. Action
a. Oxygen via 100% nonrebreather mask as needed to maintain >95% saturation
b. Large-bore peripheral IV line
c. Labs
   i. CBC, BMP, LFT, coagulation studies, blood type and crossmatch, urine pregnancy test
d. Monitor: BP: 140/90, HR: 100, RR: 22, Sat: 100%

F. History
a. HPI: A 32-year-old female with no past medical history presents to your community ED (located high in the mountains) with a 1 day history of "flu-like" illness with headache, generalized weakness, and nausea. Her friend brought her into the ED after she woke up this morning not feeling well. She arrived 2 days ago to go skiing and the symptoms started yesterday morning after waking up feeling "hung over" despite denying drinking more than one glass of wine the night before. This morning, they were planning to go skiing but the patient complained of worsening headache and unsteadiness; no chest pain, shortness of breath, palpitations, vomiting, diarrhea, fever, or blurry vision. No other contacts have similar symptoms. The friend states that others in the party had been in the area snowshoeing for the past week but the patient had an important work meeting and flew in late to join them.
b. PMHx: none
c. PSHx: none

d. Allergies: peanuts, no known drug allergies
e. Meds: daily multivitamin
f. Social: lives with roommate in a city apartment, denies tobacco and illicit drugs, reports 2–3 drinks of ETOH per week, is sexually active with IUD in place; works as a lawyer
g. FHx: no relevant history
h. PMD: Dr Miller
i. Travel history: arrived 2 days ago to the mountains by plane

G. Nurse
a. EKG (Figure 62.1)

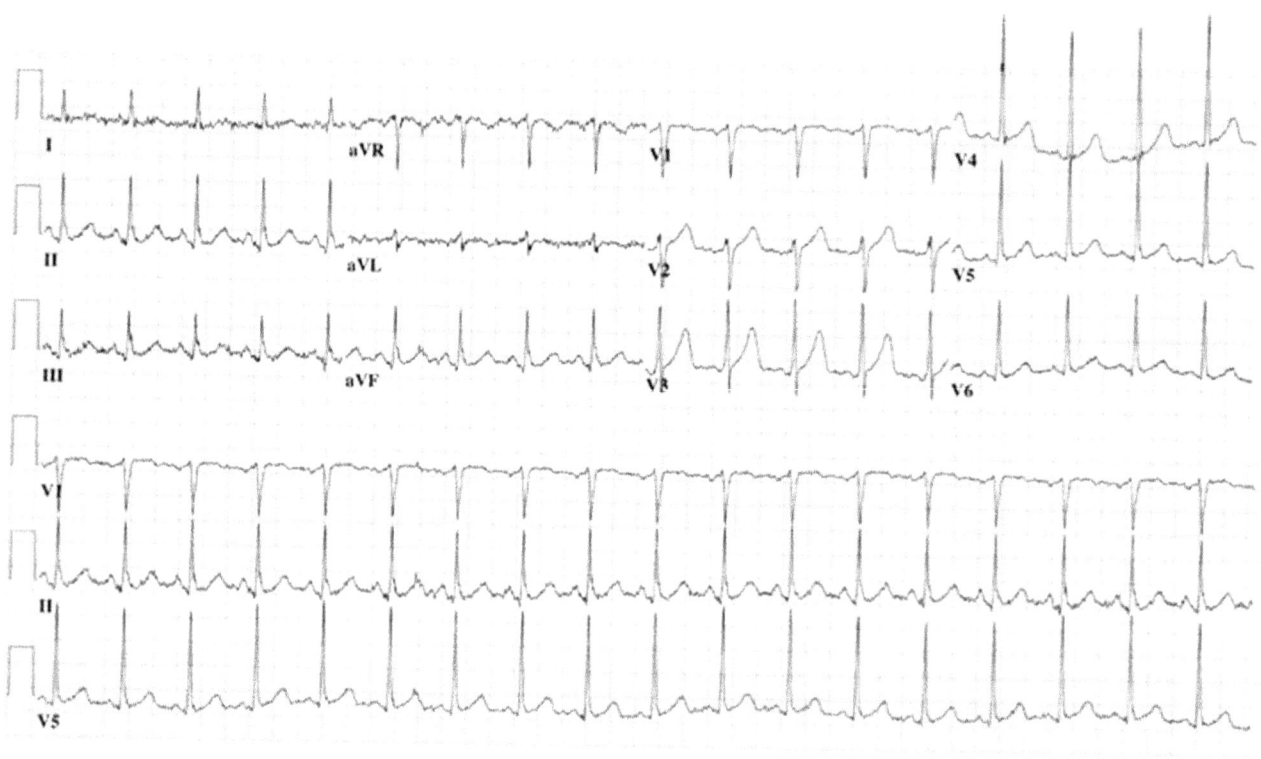

Figure 62.1

H. Secondary survey
a. General: appears sleepy but arousable, oriented × 3, uncomfortable
b. Head: normocephalic, atraumatic
c. Eyes: extraocular movement intact, pupils equal, reactive to light, no papilledema on fundoscopic examination
d. Ears: normal tympanic membranes
e. Nose: no discharge
f. Neck: full range of motion, no jugular vein distension, no stridor
g. Pharynx: normal dentition, no lesions, no swelling
h. Chest: nontender
i. Lungs: clear bilaterally
j. Heart: rate and rhythm regular, no murmurs, rubs, or gallops

k. Abdomen: normal bowel sounds, soft, nontender or distended
l. Pelvic: normal, no tenderness, discharge, bleeding or masses
m. Rectal: normal tone, brown stool, occult blood negative
n. Extremities: full range of motion, no deformity, normal pulses
o. Back: nontender
p. Neuro: intact reflexes throughout, ataxic on tandem gait, poor finger to nose, positive Romberg's test, no focal weakness, no sensory deficit
q. Skin: warm and dry
r. Lymph: no lymphadenopathy

I. Action
a. Meds
    i.   Acetazolamide
    ii. Dexamethasone
    iii. Ondansetron
b. Reassess
    i.   Patient still uncomfortable, now with worsening headache (HA), now vomited × 1.
c. Imaging
    i.   CT head without contrast
    ii. CXR

J. Nurse
a. BP: 130/90, HR: 90, RR: 16, Sat: 100% on nonrebreather mask
b. Patient: mildly confused, with continued HA
c. Imaging
    i.   CT head (Figure 62.2)
    ii. CXR (Figure 62.3)

Figure 62.2

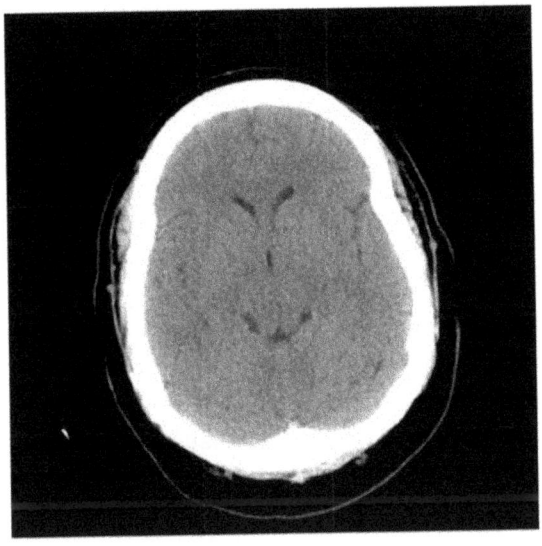

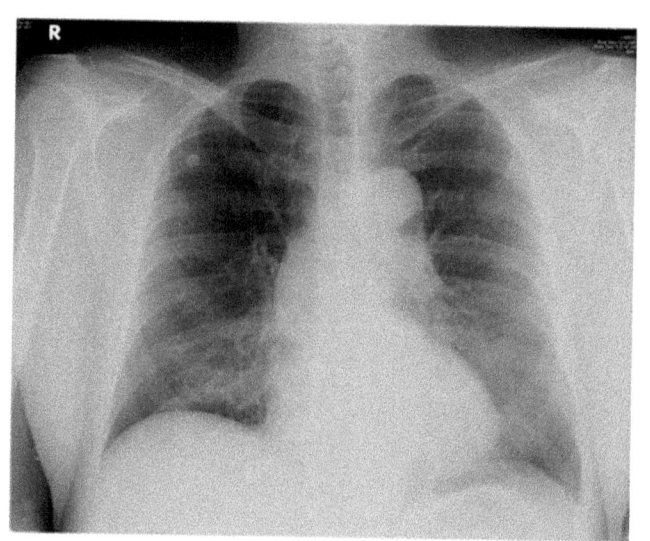

Figure 62.3

K. Results

Table 62.1 Results table

Test	Result	Test	Result
Complete blood count:		Alk phos	54 U/L
WBC	$9 \times 10^3/\mu L$	T bili	0.5 mg/dL
Hct	42%	D bili	0.2 mg/dL
Plt	$300 \times 10^3/\mu L$	Amylase	65 U/L
		Lipase	23 U/L
Basic metabolic panel:		Albumin	4.5 g/dL
Na	138 mEq/L		
K	4.9 mEq/L	**Urinalysis:**	
Cl	106 mEq/L	SG	1.010–1.030
CO_2	22 mEq/L	pH	5–8
BUN	18 mEq/dL	Prot	Neg
Cr	1.0 mg/dL	Gluc	Neg
Gluc	90 mg/dL	Ketones	Neg
		Bili	Neg
Coagulation panel:		Blood	Neg
PT	13 sec	LE	Neg
PTT	39 sec	Nitrite	Neg
INR	1.2	Color	Yellow
		Urine pregnancy	Negative
Liver function panel:			
AST	45 U/L		
ALT	44 U/L		

L. Action

a. Hyperbaric chamber

b. Arrange for transfer/descent to lower altitude

M. Diagnosis

a. High altitude cerebral edema (HACE)

N. Critical actions

a. Treatment with dexamethasone

b. Rapid descent

c. Oxygen

O. Examiner instructions

a. This is a case of acute mountain sickness that progresses to high altitude cerebral edema (HACE) without high altitude pulmonary edema (HAPE). HACE and HAPE are the most severe forms of high-altitude illnesses and are life-threatening. They can occur after a rapid ascent in altitude, progressing from acute mountain sickness. Our patient presents with flu-like symptoms 1 day after rapid ascent to the mountains by plane, which precipitates her illness. The history of being on a ski vacation can be given early in the case, but the candidate must ask specifically how she got to the resort to elicit the history of rapid ascent. Important early actions include recognition, oxygen, acetazolamide, steroids, and rapid descent. If the candidate does not recognize that the patient has HACE and initiate treatment, the patient will rapidly become more lethargic and confused, ultimately requiring intubation. With appropriate management, the patient will do well and will be stable for transfer to a low-altitude medical center.

P. Pearls

a. High-altitude illness typically occurs within the first 48 hours after rapid ascent above altitudes of 2000 m.

b. Acute mountain sickness (AMS) presents with flu-like or hangover-like symptoms, including nausea, vomiting, anorexia, headache, weakness, and decreased urination.

c. As symptoms of AMS worsen, it may progress to HACE with vomiting, altered mental status, and ataxia. Neurologic findings distinguish acute mountain sickness (absent) from HACE (present).

d. Treatment of HACE is rapid descent and steroids. Hyperbarics may be used as a temporizing measure, but may delay definitive descent (unless a portable hyperbaric bag is employed).

Q. Figure legends

a. Figure 62.1 EKG showing sinus tachycardia.

b. Figure 62.2 Normal noncontrast head CT.

c. Figure 62.3 Normal chest x-ray.

R. References

a. *Tintinalli's Emergency Medicine: A Comprehensive Study Guide* (9th ed.): Chapter 221, High Altitude Disorders.

b. *Rosen's Emergency Medicine: Concepts and Clinical Practice* (10th ed.): Chapter 132, High Altitude Medicine.

S. Acknowledgements

a. We would like to acknowledge Ravi Kapoor for their contribution to this chapter in the previous edition of this book, which has been updated by Hayley Neher.

Altered Mental Status

Bethany Johnston, MD and Tricia Swan, MD, MEd

A. Chief complaint
a. 65-year-old female brought in by EMS for altered mental status, vomiting and dizziness

B. Vital signs
a. BP: 93/50, HR: 42, RR: 18, T: 36.9°C, Sat: 99% on RA

C. What does the patient look like?
a. Patient appears stated age, appears fatigued and confused, groaning on stretcher. If asked, alert to self, states wrong president, date, and thinks location is a library.

D. Primary survey
a. Airway: speaking in full sentences
b. Breathing: no apparent respiratory distress, no cyanosis
c. Circulation: pale and cool skin, 4 second capillary refill

E. Action
a. Oxygen via peripheral NC or nonrebreather mask as needed to maintain >95% saturation
b. Two large-bore peripheral IVs
c. Monitor and/or place pads on patient: BP: 93/50, HR: 42, RR: 18, T: 36.9°C, Sat: 99% on RA
d. 1 L NS bolus
e. Labs
    i. CBC, BMP, LFT, magnesium, coagulation studies, urinalysis, fingerstick blood glucose
    ii. Lactate, blood cultures, urine culture, troponin
f. EKG

F. History
a. HPI: A 65-year-old female with a known history of congestive heart failure (CHF), hypertension (HTN), and diabetes presenting with progressive fatigue, confusion, dizziness, and nausea for the past 2 weeks. Her husband called the ambulance today because her symptoms became worse, she had one episode of nonbloody, nonbilious emesis, and was complaining of things "looking funny." If asked, husband will say she said things looked yellowish and hazy, but patient will not give this history herself.
b. PMHx: CHF, HTN, type 2 diabetes mellitus
c. PSHx: none
d. Allergies: none
e. Meds: metformin, atorvastatin, verapamil, digoxin, apixaban
f. Social: lives at home with husband, former smoker (quit 10 years ago), no alcohol or drug use

g. FHx: father passed away in his 70s from an acute myocardial infarction
h. PMD: her physician has recently been "going up" on one of her "heart medications" but husband is not sure which one

G. Nurse
a. EKG (Figure 63.1)
b. If 1 L NS given:
   i. BP: 95/65, HR: 45, RR: 18, Sat: 98% on O_2
c. If no fluids given:
   i. BP: 79/43, HR: 36, RR: 18, Sat 98% on O_2
d. Patient reports feeling dizzy and nauseated and appears diaphoretic
e. Fingerstick blood glucose: 155 mg/dL

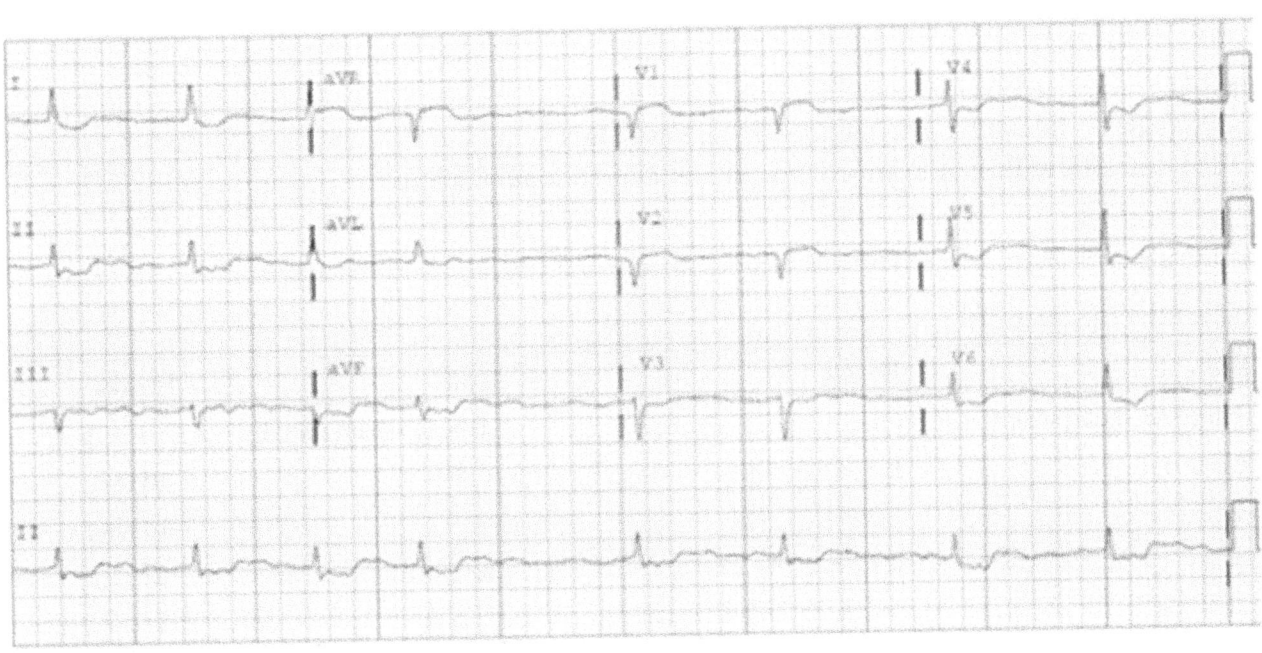

Figure 63.1

H. Secondary survey
a. General: alert, disoriented, groaning on exam table
b. HEENT: normocephalic, atraumatic, pupils equal, 3 mm and reactive bilaterally, extraocular movements intact, tympanic membranes normal, no nasal drainage, normal dentition, no oral lesions or swelling
c. Neck: full range of motion, no jugular vein distension, no stridor
d. Lungs: clear bilaterally
e. Heart: bradycardia, regular, no murmurs, rubs, or gallops
f. Abdomen: soft, nontender, nondistended, normal bowel sounds
g. Rectal: hemoccult negative brown stool, normal rectal tone
h. Urogenital: normal
i. Extremities: full range of motion, no deformity, pulses 1+ in extremities
j. Back: nontender
k. Neuro: unable to follow clear commands, strength appears normal, normal reflexes, unable to assess gait

l. Skin: pale, ashen, diaphoretic
m. Lymph: no lymphadenopathy

I. Action

a. Meds/fluids
    i. Atropine 0.5 mg IV
    ii. Ondansetron 4 mg IV
    iii. 1 L NS IV bolus
b. Imaging
    i. CXR
    ii. Repeat EKG
c. Lab: add digoxin level
d. Contact Poison Control
e. Place transcutaneous pacer pads on patient

J. Nurse

a. Vital signs: BP: 90/59, HR: 55, RR: 18, Sat: 98% on O_2
b. Patient: still with significant confusion and altered mental status

K. Results

Table 63.1 Results table

Test	Result	Test	Result
Complete blood count:		**Liver function panel:**	
WBC	$6.1 \times 10^3/\mu L$	AST	45 U/L
Hct	29.9%	ALT	44 U/L
Plt	$213 \times 10^3/\mu L$	Alk phos	54 U/L
		T bili	0.5 mg/dL
		D bili	0.2 mg/dL
Basic metabolic panel:		Amylase	65 U/L
Na	139 mEq/L	Lipase	23 U/L
K	6.1 mEq/L	Albumin	4.5 g/dL
Cl	104 mEq/L		
CO_2	21 mEq/L		
BUN	33 mEq/dL	**Urinalysis:**	
Cr	1.8 mg/dL	SG	1.020
Gluc	165 mg/dL	pH	6
Mg	1.0 mEq/L	Prot	Neg
		Gluc	Neg
Coagulation panel:		Ketones	Neg
PT	13.1 sec	Bili	Neg
PTT	25 sec	Blood	Neg

Table 63.1 (cont.)

Test	Result	Test	Result
INR	1.1	LE	Neg
		Nitrite	Neg
		Color	Yellow

a. No response to atropine
b. CXR (Figure 63.2)
c. Repeat EKG unchanged if no digoxin-specific Fab fragments and no pacing initiated
d. Lactate: 2.1 mmol/L
e. Digoxin level: 4.5 ng/mL
f. Troponin: 0.01 ng/mL

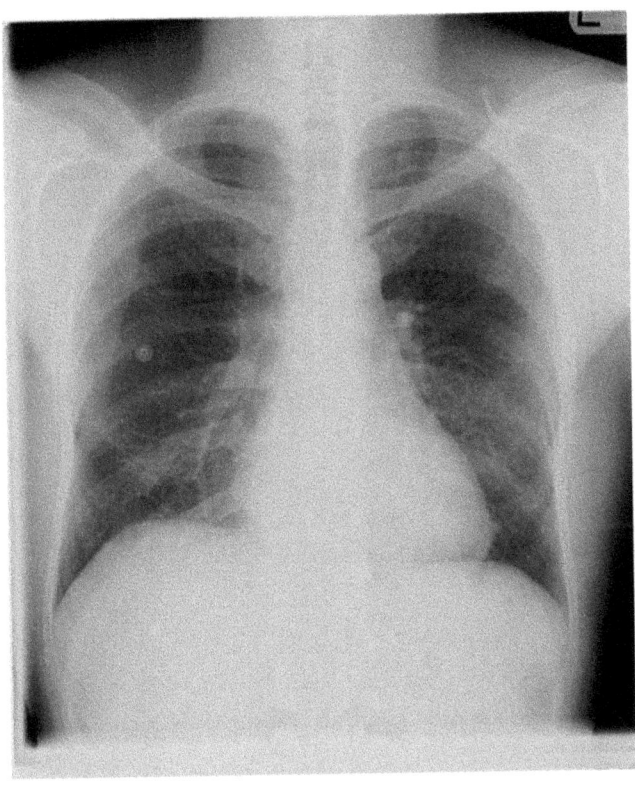

Figure 63.2

L. Action

a. Meds
   i. Digoxin-specific Fab fragments (Digibind™, DigiFab™) IV – 10 vials over 30 min
   ii. Magnesium sulfate 2 g IV
   iii. Dextrose 25 g (1 amp) + insulin 10 units IV
   iv. Bicarbonate 50 mEq (1 amp)
b. Repeat EKG after digoxin-specific FAB is given (Figure 63.3). Repeat EKG if *not* given is unchanged (Figure 63.1).
c. If transcutaneous pacing is initiated and no digoxin-specific Fab have been given, the pacer-defibrillator will not capture, the patient will become tachycardic, and a repeat EKG will show Figure 63.4. They will remain in this rhythm until digoxin-specific Fab is given.
d. MICU or cardiac ICU admission

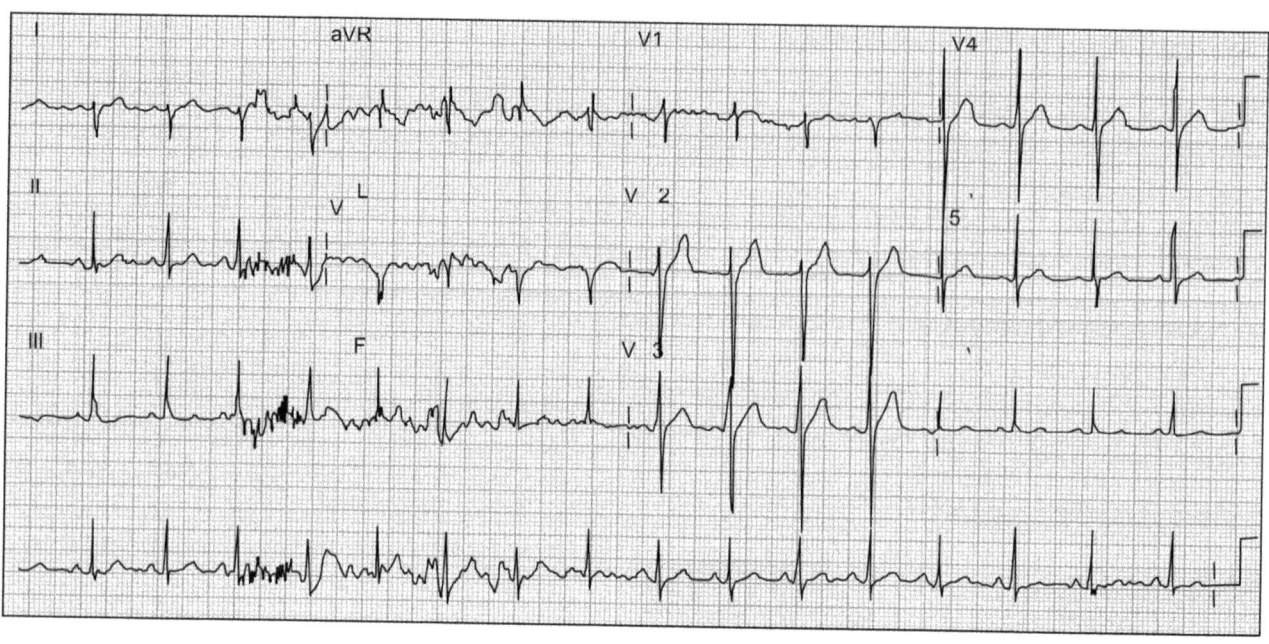

Figure 63.3

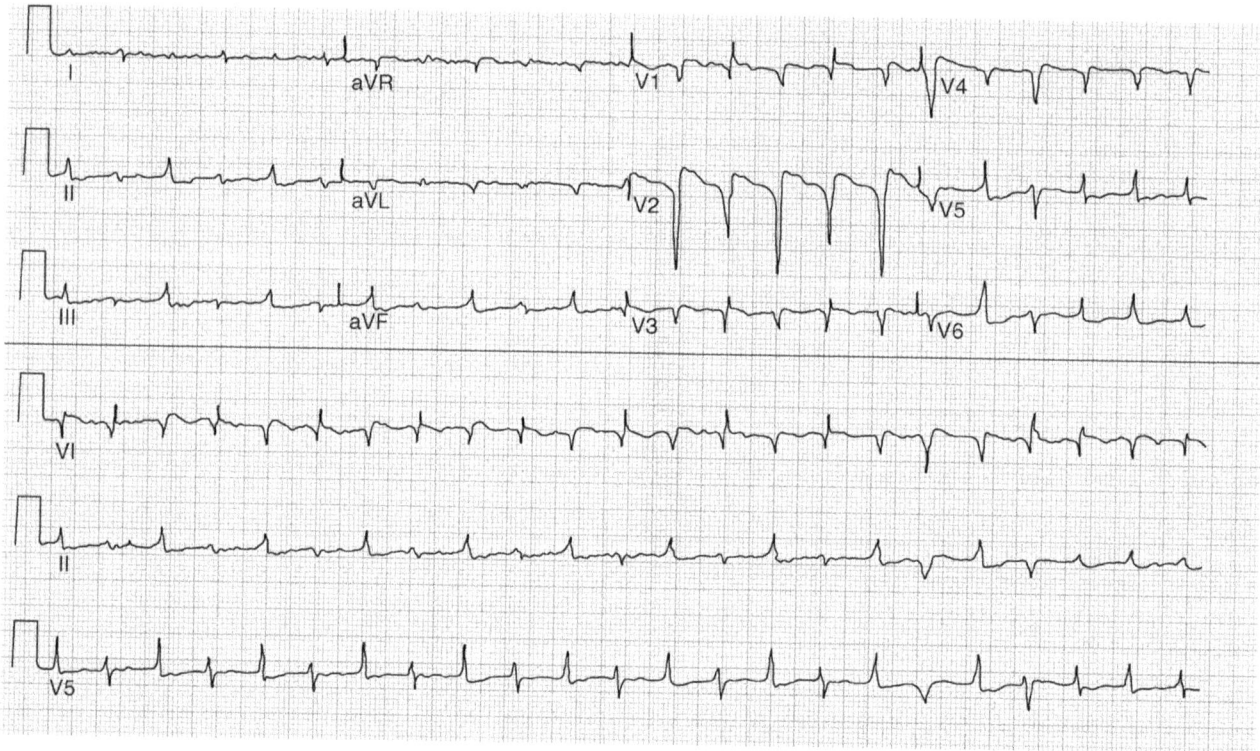

Figure 63.4

M. Diagnosis

a. Digitalis toxicity resulting in unstable bradycardia

N. Critical actions

a. Large-bore IV access and fluid bolus

b. Telemetry/EKG

c. Atropine

d. Digoxin-specific Fab antibody fragments

e. Treat electrolyte disturbances

f. ICU admission

O. Examiner instructions

a. This is a case of unstable bradycardia secondary to digoxin toxicity. Important early actions include administering IV fluids, IV atropine, treating for electrolyte abnormalities, obtaining serial EKGs and digoxin level, and treating with digoxin-specific antibody fragments. The candidate should not wait for digoxin level to treat with digoxin-specific Fab. Diagnosis should be made based off of clinical exam, history, and initial EKG. In this case, the digoxin toxicity was likely caused by the increased dose of her digoxin and the drug–drug interaction with verapamil. Digoxin toxicity can lead to life-threatening abnormalities in heart conduction. The patient presents with nonspecific symptoms of altered mental status, confusion, vomiting, and dizziness. The patient had also complained of visual disturbance prior to presentation. A classic visual complaint is xanthopsia, in which objects appear yellow/green. The candidate should initially cast a broad differential to exclude causes of altered mental status, such as hypoglycemia, hypoxia, stroke, myocardial infarction, electrolyte abnormalities, and infection. A thorough history should elicit her current medications, including digoxin, and a level should be ordered. As the case progresses, the patient becomes increasingly unstable, bradycardic, and hypotensive. The patient will not improve if digoxin-specific Fab is not administered despite attempting to correct hypovolemia and electrolyte disturbances and giving atropine and transcutaneous cardiac pacing. If the patient receives transcutaneous pacing, she will develop bidirectional ventricular tachycardia. At this time, the patient is clinically unstable and should be empirically treated with the antidote, digoxin-specific Fab.

P. Pearls

a. Digoxin toxicity can be acute or chronic (precipitated by a recent change in medication, medication interactions, change in renal function, etc.) and symptoms can be variable and vague, including gastrointestinal symptoms, visual changes, neurologic symptoms and cardiac arrhythmias.

b. The *critical* clinical manifestations of digoxin toxicity are those associated with cardiac arrhythmias. These include virtually all types of arrhythmias *except* for supraventricular tachycardias. Common EKG changes include bradycardia, ventricular bigeminy or trigeminy, ventricular tachycardia, AV nodal blockade, and bidirectional ventricular tachycardia.

c. Caution should be used when initiating transcutaneous pacing for bradycardia in digoxin toxicity, which can lead to potentially fatal arrhythmias.

d. In a patient taking digoxin, hyperkalemia (K > 5.5 mEq/L) is an indicator of acute digitalis toxicity, and an independent predictor of mortality.

e. Caution should be used if hyperkalemia is treated before being given the digoxin-specific Fab, as profound *hypo*kalemia may occur after the administration of the antidote.

f. Although traditional teaching is that calcium administration in digoxin-mediated hyperkalemia is dangerous, more recent evidence suggests that it is actually safe. However, the best therapy is still digoxin-specific antibody fragments.

g. For acute overdose, obtain a serum digoxin level on presentation and 6 hours post-ingestion (most accurate level is 6 hours post-ingestion). Levels are not as helpful in chronic toxicity and elevated serum digoxin levels alone should not be used for indication for treatment with digoxin-specific Fab.

h. Digoxin-specific antibody fragments are the treatment of choice in symptomatic digoxin toxicity. Indications for use include:
   i. Life-threatening hemodynamically unstable dysrhythmias
   ii. Hyperkalemia (K > 5 mEq/L)
   iii. Ingestion of massive quantities of digitalis (in children >0.1 mg/kg, in adults >10 mg)
   iv. Altered mental status attributed to digoxin toxicity
   v. Evidence of end-organ dysfunction due to hypoperfusion
i. Digoxin-specific Fab antibody fragments falsely elevate serum digoxin levels; therefore serial levels are of no utility. Resolution of toxicity is clinical.
j. Hemodialysis and hemoperfusion are ineffective to remove digoxin from the body.

Q. Figure legends
a. Figure 63.1 Junctional bradycardia with scooped ST segments or Salvador Dali moustache.
b. Figure 63.2 Normal chest x-ray.
c. Figure 63.3 Normal sinus rhythm.
d. Figure 63.4 Sinus tachycardia, bigeminy.

R. References
a. *Tintinalli's Emergency Medicine: A Comprehensive Study Guide* (9th ed.): Chapter 18, Cardiac Rhythm Disturbances. Chapter 193, Digitalis Glycosides.
b. *Rosen's Emergency Medicine: Concepts and Clinical Practice* (10th ed.): Chapter 65, Dysrhythmias. Chapter 142, Cardiovascular Drugs.

Shortness of Breath

Michael Marchick, MD and Garrett Snipes, MD

A. Chief complaint
a. 82-year-old female brought in by EMS for sudden onset of shortness of breath for 30 minutes

B. Vital signs
a. BP: 230/90, HR: 120, RR: 28, T: 37.2°C, Sat: 90% on 2 L NC

C. What does the patient look like?
a. Patient appears stated age, uncomfortable, sitting upright to breathe, cannot speak in full sentences, and diaphoretic.

D. Primary survey
a. Airway: unable to speak in full sentences but able to say her name
b. Breathing: tachypneic, very labored breathing with cyanosis and crackles
c. Circulation: diaphoretic, cool skin with intact pulses throughout

E. Action
a. Oxygen via increased NC O_2, VentiMask, or nonrebreather mask
b. Two large-bore peripheral IV lines
c. Labs
   i. CBC, BMP, troponin, brain natriuretic peptide (BNP), blood gas
   ii. Optional: coagulation studies, lactate, LFT, blood type and crossmatch
d. Monitor: BP: 230/90, HR: 120, RR: 34, Sat: 94% on nonrebreather mask, 87% if patient remains on 2 L NC
e. EKG
f. CXR

F. History
a. HPI: The patient is an 82-year-old female presenting via EMS for dyspnea. History is limited secondary to her labored breathing. Her husband, who accompanies the patient, states she has a history of hypertension, diabetes, and hypercholesterolemia and says that she has been feeling short of breath for the past 2 days. Patient has had difficulty sleeping at night, as she gets short of breath if she lies flat. She has not left the apartment recently, as they live on the third floor of a walk-up. She was fearful that she would not be able to make it back up the stairs if she left the building. The patient is able to deny cough, fever, or chest pain. This morning she woke up with acute worsening of her shortness of breath, prompting her presentation.
   i. EMS: bilateral crackles on chest examination. The patient was given 1 sublingual nitroglycerin and 2 L oxygen NC.

b. PMHx: hypertension, diabetes, and hypercholesterolemia, no prior cardiac work-up
c. PSHx: none
d. Allergies: none
e. Meds: does not know except a "water pill"
f. Social: lives with husband at home, leaving apartment less these days, denies alcohol, smoking, drugs, not sexually active
g. FHx: not relevant
h. PMD: Dr. Johnson

G. Nurse

a. BP: 220/90, HR: 120, RR: 35, Sat: 94% on 100% nonrebreather mask, 85% if patient remains on 2 L NC
b. EKG (Figure 64.1)
c. CXR (Figure 64.2)

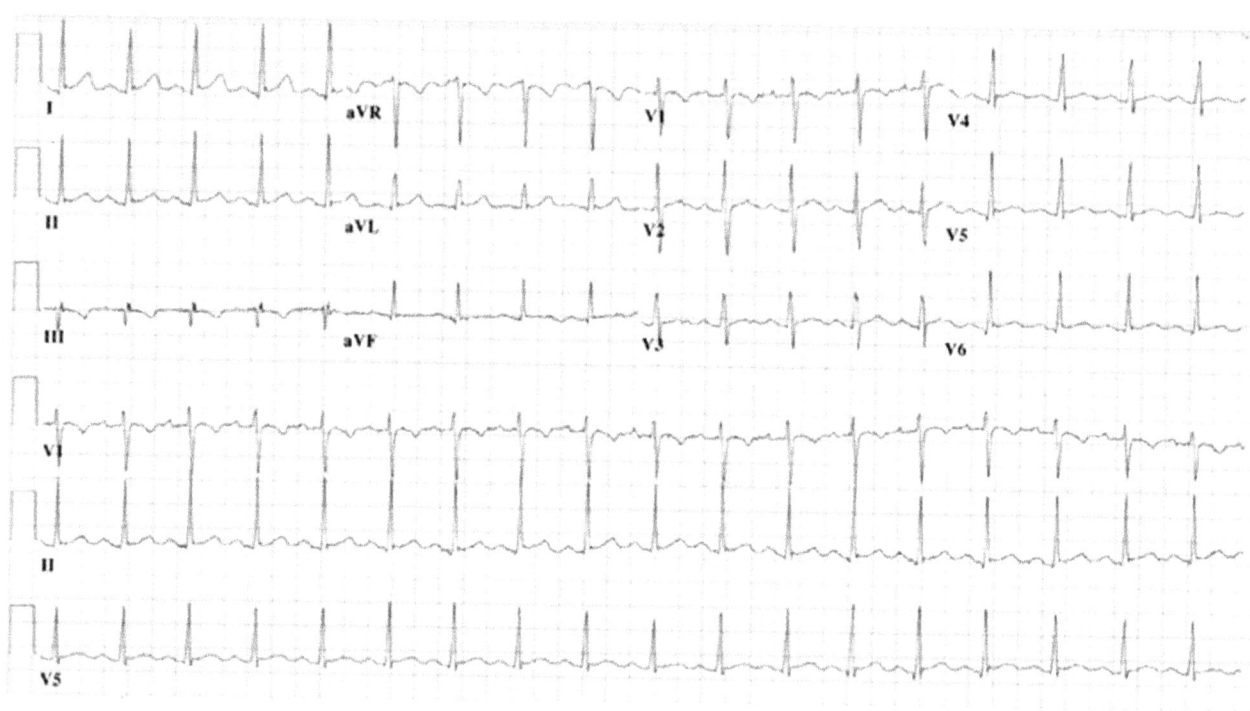

Figure 64.1

H. Action

a. Nitroglycerin 1 tablet sublingual
b. Furosemide IV

I. Secondary survey

a. General: severe respiratory distress, awake, unable to speak
b. Head: normocephalic, atraumatic
c. Eyes: extraocular movement intact, pupils equal, reactive to light
d. Ears: normal tympanic membranes
e. Nose: no discharge
f. Neck: full range of motion, + jugular vein distension, no stridor
g. Pharynx: normal dentition, no lesions, no swelling

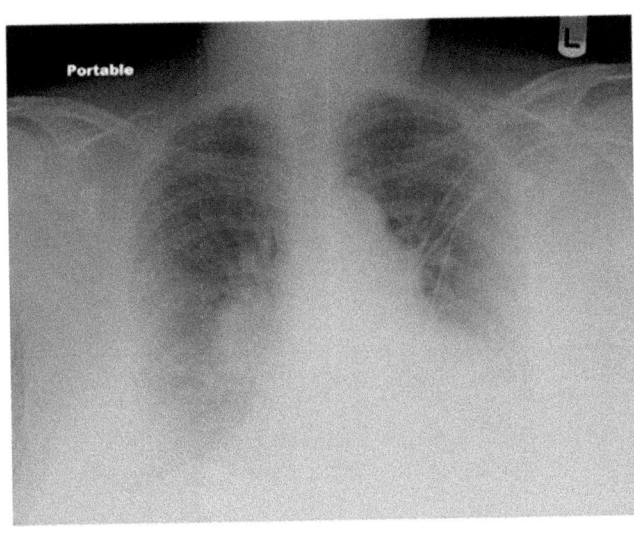

Figure 64.2

h. Chest: nontender
i. Lungs: diffuse crackles, minimal air movement
j. Heart: tachycardia, regular rhythm, no murmurs, rubs, or gallops
k. Abdomen: normal bowel sounds, soft, nontender or distended
l. Rectal: normal tone, brown stool, occult blood negative
m. Urogenital: deferred
n. Extremities: full range of motion, no deformity, normal pulses, 2+ pitting edema
o. Back: nontender
p. Neuro: cranial nerves II to XII intact; normal sensation, strength; normal reflexes and gait
q. Skin: cool, diaphoretic
r. Lymph: no lymphadenopathy

J. Action

a. Noninvasive ventilation
   i. CPAP/BiPAP: improvement of symptoms, vital signs
b. Meds
   i. Nitroglycerin high dose: mild improvement in shortness of breath
      1. Started at 50–100 mcg/min of IV nitroglycerin and titrated to relief of SOB, or
      2. Start sublingual nitroglycerin 0.4 mg SL every 5 minutes (at least two tablets, dosed sequentially)
   ii. If nitroglycerin is given in inappropriately low dose: worsening shortness of breath requiring intubation
      1. Less than 10 mcg/min of IV nitroglycerin
      2. Less than two tablets nitroglycerin 0.4 mg SL or not dosed sequentially
   iii. Diuretic (e.g. furosemide 1 mg/kg IV), if not previously administered
   iv. Aspirin 325 mg PO
c. Urinary output monitoring
d. Consider CCU consult

K. Nurse

Vitals depending on actions performed above:
   i. Optimal management (CPAP/BiPAP, with appropriate nitroglycerin and diuretic): BP: 150/70, HR: 105 RR: 20, Sat 97%

ii. Poor management (0 or only one of the three management options above): BP: 220/90, HR: 130, RR: 46, Sat: 90% on 100% FiO_2 (will decline further to respiratory arrest if not addressed)

iii. Intermediate-quality management (Two of three critical interventions above): BP: 170/80, HR: 110, RR: 24, Sat: 95%

L. Results

Table 64.1 Results table

Test	Result	Test	Result
Complete blood count:		T bili	0.9 mg/dL
WBC	$18 \times 10^3/\mu L$	D bili	0.3 mg/dL
Hct	27%	Amylase	60 U/L
Plt	$300 \times 10^3/\mu L$	Lipase	40 U/L
		Albumin	3.5 g/dL
Basic metabolic panel:			
Na	139 mEq/L	**Urinalysis:**	
K	4.9 mEq/L	pH	6
Cl	109 mEq/L	Prot	Neg
CO_2	20 mEq/L	Gluc	Neg
BUN	30 mEq/dL	Ketones	Neg
Cr	1.8 mg/dL	Bili	Neg
Gluc	90 mg/dL	Blood	Neg
		LE	Neg
Coagulation panel:		Nitrite	Neg
PT	13 sec	Color	Yellow
PTT	39 sec		
INR	1.0	**Arterial blood gas:**	
		pH	7.36
Liver function panel:		PO_2	60 mmHg
AST	25 U/L	PCO_2	35 mmHg
ALT	30 U/L	HCO_2	20 mmol/L
Alk phos	90 U/L		

a. Lactate: 1.6 mmol/L
b. Troponin: 0.20 ng/mL
c. BNP: 4000 pg/mL

M. Action

a. If intubated, continue management, with adequate sedation
b. Admit to CCU

N. Diagnosis
a. Congestive heart failure exacerbation

O. Critical actions
a. Oxygen
b. CPAP/BiPAP
c. High-dose nitroglycerin drip/sequential SL 0.4 mg nitroglycerin tablets
d. Diuretic (e.g. furosemide)
e. Aspirin
f. CCU consult

P. Examiner instructions
a. This is a patient presenting in extremis with pulmonary edema due to hypertensive acute decompensated heart failure. This results primarily from increased LV and pulmonary capillary hydrostatic pressures forcing a plasma ultrafiltrate across the pulmonary capillary membrane. This fluid then enters the pulmonary interstitium and alveoli, causing difficulty breathing. This patient presents with severe respiratory distress that must be managed aggressively to avoid intubation. If noninvasive positive pressure ventilation, appropriately dosed nitrates, and diuretics are started promptly, the patient will do well. If these interventions are not delivered promptly, the patient will continue to worsen and require intubation. Once the patient is improving, a search of the cause of CHF (e.g., myocardial infarction, medication noncompliance, dietary indiscretion, or infection) must begin.

Q. Pearls
a. Patients will often present with difficulty breathing on exertion.
b. The physical exam often outperforms diagnostic tests in this condition. Physical findings include pitting edema, crackles, wheezing ("not all that wheezes is asthma"), hypoxia, jugular venous distension, S3 or S4 on cardiac examination.
c. Five-year survival for patients with the diagnosis of CHF is 60% in men and 45% in women.
d. It is important to search for the root cause of exacerbation (e.g., MI, PNA, PE).
e. BNP is highly sensitive for CHF and can be sent in equivocal cases.
f. Treatment includes preload reduction with nitroglycerin, diuresis, and positive pressure ventilation (in severe exacerbations).
g. At low doses, nitrates act as venodilators, resulting in preload reduction. At higher doses, arterial dilation also occurs, resulting in reduced afterload as well.

R. Figure legends
a. Figure 64.1 (EKG) Sinus tachycardia; minimal voltage criteria for LVH.
b. Figure 64.2 (CXR) Cardiomegaly: pulmonary vascular congestion suggestive of CHF.

S. References
a. *Tintinalli's Emergency Medicine: A Comprehensive Study Guide* (9th ed.): Chapter 53, Acute Heart Failure.
b. *Rosen's Emergency Medicine: Concepts and Clinical Practice* (10th ed.): Chapter 67, Heart Failure.

T. Acknowledgements
a. We would like to acknowledge Ravi Kapoor for their contribution to this chapter in the previous edition of this book, which has been updated by Michael Marchick and Garrett Snipes.

Shortness of Breath

Christopher Strother, MD

A. Chief complaint
a. 10-day-old male with shortness of breath, "pulling," poor feeding

B. Vital signs
a. BP: 110/80, RUE HR: 175, RR: 90, T: 36.2°C, Sat: 95% on RA, FS: 70 mg/dL; Wt: 3 kg

C. What does the patient look like?
a. Patient appears stated age, lethargic, tachypneic, with intercostal and subcostal retractions.

D. Primary survey
a. Airway: patent, weak cry
b. Breathing: respiratory distress, diffuse mild crackles bilaterally
c. Circulation: capillary refill 2 seconds, diminished femoral pulses

E. Action
a. Oxygen supplementation (nonrebreather mask)
b. IV placement, place IO if any difficulty with IV access
c. Labs
   i. CBC, BMP, blood gas, blood culture, LFT, PT/PTT, blood type, urinalysis, urine culture
d. 20 mL/kg NS (60 mL) bolus, consider 10 mL/kg test if considering cardiac disease/failure clinically
e. Monitor: BP: 110/80, RUE HR: 175, RR: 85, Sat: 97% on O_2
   i. Unable to obtain LE blood pressure
f. EKG, CXR

F. History
a. HPI: A 10-day-old male, born full-term via normal spontaneous vaginal delivery at home. He is breastfed with some difficulty, often "tiring out" while feeding. He "sleeps a lot," and mother reports he "always breathes that fast." He was doing well until his tenth day of life (today), when he developed worsening shortness of breath, tachypnea, retractions, and refusing to breastfeed. He has exhibited worsening lethargy over the past few hours; denies fever, no vomiting or diarrhea, no cough, no rash, no sick contacts, and no medications given at home now or at birth.
b. PMHx: none
c. PSHx: none
d. Allergies: none
e. Social: lives with parents at home, no pets or siblings

   f. FHx: not relevant

   g. PMD: Dr. Chris

G. Nurse

   a. EKG (Figure 65.1)

   b. Lower extremity blood pressures

       i. BP: 50/palp

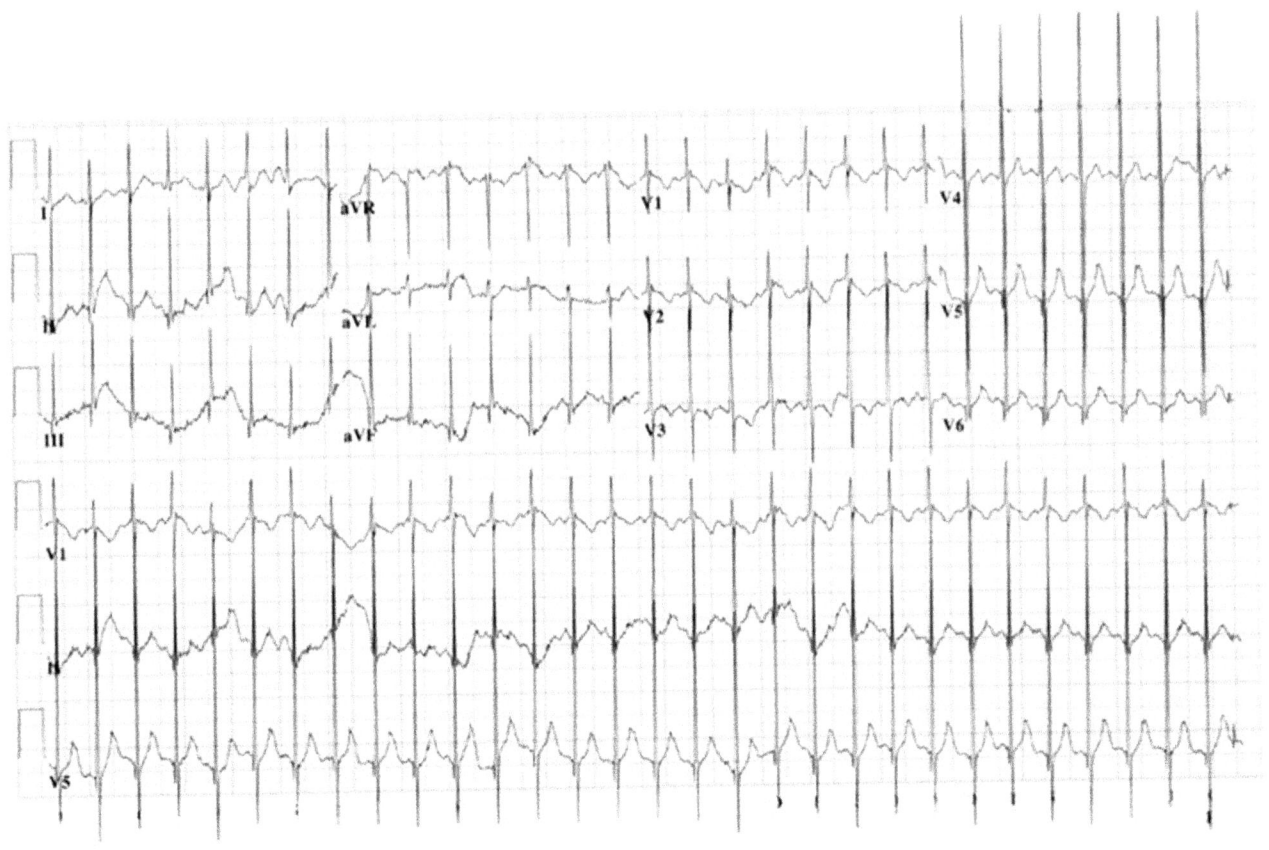

Figure 65.1

H. Secondary survey

   a. General: lethargic, moderate respiratory distress, severe tachypnea

   b. HEENT: normal

   c. Neck: normal

   d. Chest: mild diffuse rales, mild retractions, tachypnea

   e. Heart: S1S2, + systolic murmur at left sternal border and scapula

   f. Abdomen: liver palpable at 3 cm below costal margin, soft, nontender

   g. Rectal: normal

   h. Urogenital: normal

   i. Extremities: normal

   j. Back: normal

   k. Neuro: lethargic, nonfocal

   l. Skin: mottled, cyanotic

   m. Lymph: normal

I. Action

a. Procedures
  i. Endotracheal intubation via rapid sequence intubation
  ii. Ventilator settings: volume 10 mL/kg (30 mL) or with chest rise, O_2 100%, rate of 40
  iii. Consider central line placement
b. Meds
  i. Prostaglandin E1
c. Reassess
  i. Patient still with significant distress if not intubated, will begin to improve only after prostaglandin E1 administration
d. Consult
  i. Cardiology
e. Imaging
  i. CXR
f. Labs
  i. Urinalysis, urine culture

J. Nurse

a. Repeat vital signs
  i. If intubated: BP: 100/70, HR: 160, RR: 40 (vent), Sat: 100% (vent)
  ii. If not intubated: BP: 80/50, HR: 170, RR: 80, Sat: 92% on O_2
b. Patient: still in distress if not intubated

K. Results

Table 65.1 Results table

Test	Result	Test	Result
Complete blood count:		T bili	1.0 mg/dL
WBC	$9.5 \times 10^3/\mu L$	D bili	0.3 mg/dL
Hct	52.5%	Amylase	44 U/L
Plt	$150 \times 10^3/\mu L$	Lipase	18 U/L
		Albumin	3.4 g/dL
Basic metabolic panel:			
Na	139 mEq/L	**Urinalysis:**	
K	4.2 mEq/L	SG	1.010
Cl	110 mEq/L	pH	6
CO_2	20 mEq/L	Prot	Neg
BUN	9 mEq/dL	Gluc	Neg
Cr	0.6 mg/dL	Ketones	Neg
Gluc	90 mg/dL	Bili	Neg
		Blood	Neg
Coagulation panel:		LE	Neg
PT	11.1 sec	Nitrite	Neg

Table 65.1 (cont.)

Test	Result	Test	Result
PTT	28 sec	Color	Yellow
INR	1.0		
		Arterial blood gas:	
Liver function panel:		pH	7.45
AST	25 U/L	pO_2	140 mmHg
ALT	12 U/L	pCO_2	46 mmHg
Alk phos	115 U/L	HCO_3	28 mmol/L

a. Lactate: 1.2 mmol/L
b. Portable CXR (Figure 65.2)

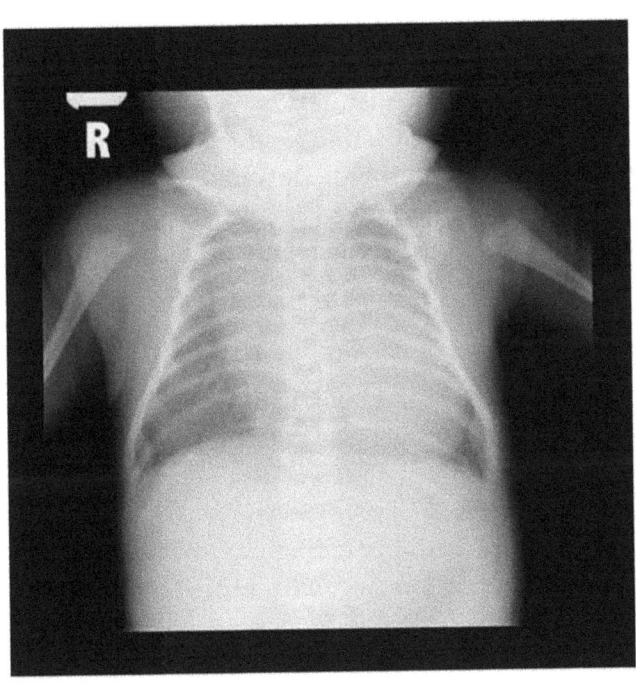

Figure 65.2

L. Action
a. Meds
   i. Antibiotics to cover sepsis (ampicillin and cefotaxime or gentamycin)
   ii. Prostaglandin drip
b. Cardiology consult
   i. For cardiac echo and admission: echo demonstrates critical aortic coarctation
   ii. Emergent operative repair needed
c. Discussion with family and PMD need for ICU admission and urgent repair of lesion

M. Diagnosis
a. Critical aortic coarctation

N. Critical actions

a. Recognition of respiratory distress
b. Oxygen administration, intubation
c. IV/IO access
d. EKG, CXR
e. Recognition of cardiomegaly and cardiac cause of respiratory distress
f. Cardiology consult
g. Prostaglandin E1 administration

O. Examiner instructions

a. This is a case of critical congenital heart disease that is dependent upon a patent ductus arteriosus to maintain blood flow to the body. A structural abnormality in the heart prevents blood from being oxygenated properly by the lungs. A fetal bypass pathway (the ductus arteriosus) allows some oxygenation to occur; when this closes, patients rapidly deteriorate. It is often clinically unrecognizable at birth, but patients develop obstructive heart failure which acutely worsens when the duct closes (normally at about 1 week). The newborn will have distress, and will have difficulty feeding due to the increased energy required to breathe. Infants often are described as "tired," "wears out," or "gets sweaty" when feeding. Important initial actions are oxygenation, IV access, CXR, and cardiology consultation. A congenital heart lesion must be considered in any newborn with shock or severe distress and prostaglandin should be given in case the lesion is duct-dependent. This patient will slowly improve with prostaglandin administration, but needs definitive intervention for true resolution of symptoms. Without prostaglandin the patient will develop steadily worsening heart failure and shock (blood pressure and oxygen level will fall, heart rate and respiratory rate will rise).

P. Pearls

a. Congenital heart disease should be considered in any newborn in shock or severe distress.
b. Early recognition of possible heart disease and initiation of prostaglandin and cardiology involvement is important.
c. Infants in extremis should also be treated for possible infection/sepsis. Sepsis work-up should be done with lumbar puncture performed only if the infant is stable enough to tolerate it.
d. Differential blood pressure and oxygen saturation from upper to lower extremities is a clue to congenital heart disease with a patent ductus arteriosus.

Q. Figure legends

a. Figure 65.1 (EKG) Sinus tachycardia, LVH, RVH.
b. Figure 65.2 (CXR) Cardiomegaly.

R. References

a. *Tintinalli's Emergency Medicine: A Comprehensive Study Guide* (9th ed.): Chapter 129, Congenital and Acquired Pediatric Heart Disease.
b. *Rosen's Emergency Medicine: Concepts and Clinical Practice* (10th ed.): Chapter 165, Pediatric Cardiac Disorders.

Flank Pain

Haley Godwin, MD and Megan Fix, MD

A. Chief complaint
a.   40-year-old male presents with flank pain for 2 days, worse today

B. Vital signs
a.   BP: 140/90, HR: 125, RR: 16, T: 37.4°C, Sat: O$_2$ 99% on RA 99

C. What does the patient look like?
a.   Patient appears stated age, speaking in full sentences, vomiting, uncomfortable, and writhing in bed.

D. Primary survey
a.   Airway: speaking in full sentences
b.   Breathing: no respiratory distress, no cyanosis
c.   Circulation: normal skin, warm

E. Action
a.   Obtain peripheral IV
b.   Labs
   i.   CBC, BMP, PT/PTT, urinalysis, type and screen
c.   1 L NS bolus IV
d.   Monitor: BP: 140/90, HR: 125, RR: 16, T: 37.4°C, Sat: 99% on RA
e.   Meds
   i.   Ketorolac IV or ibuprofen PO
   ii. Morphine IV
   iii. Metoclopramide, ondansetron, or equivalent antiemetic IV

F. History
a.   HPI: A 40-year-old male with a history of gout presents with left flank pain for 1 day. He has been on a long hiking trip and describes not drinking enough water. The pain is characterized as 10/10 in the left flank radiating to the groin. The patient states the pain began last night suddenly on the left side and was intermittent and associated with nausea. He took ibuprofen with mild relief but states that the pain returned this morning much worse than before, with three episodes of vomiting in the past 4 hours precipitating his visit. Patient states that he has never had this sensation before. Patient denies fever, chills, chest pain, shortness of breath, or headache; no hematemesis, no chest pain.
b.   PMHx: gout
c.   PSHx: none
d.   Allergies: none
e.   Meds: daily vitamins with calcium

f. Social: lives with wife at home; denies alcohol use, smoking, or illicit drug use, sexually active with one partner

g. FHx: not relevant

h. PMD: none

G. Nurse

a. If analgesia is given
   i.   BP: 130/80, HR: 105, RR: 16, T: 37.4°C, Sat: 99% on RA
   ii. Patient: feels significantly improved – mild dull pain to left flank

b. Without analgesia
   i.   BP: 160/100, HR: 120, RR: 16, T: 37.4°C, Sat: 99% on RA
   ii. Patient: still writhing in bed in significant pain

c. UA large blood, negative leukocyte esterase, negative nitrites

H. Secondary survey

a. General: alert, oriented
   i.   Analgesia – appears more comfortable
   ii. No analgesia – writhing in bed in pain

b. Head: normocephalic, atraumatic

c. Eyes: extraocular movement intact, pupils equal, reactive to light

d. Ears: normal tympanic membranes

e. Nose: no discharge

f. Neck: full range of motion, no jugular vein distension, no stridor

g. Pharynx: normal dentition, no lesions, no swelling

h. Chest: nontender

i. Lungs: clear bilaterally

j. Heart: rate and rhythm regular, no murmurs, rubs, or gallops

k. Abdomen: normal bowel sounds, soft, not tender or distended

l. Rectal: normal tone, brown stool, occult blood negative
   m. Urogenital: normal external genitalia, no hernia bilaterally
   i.   Male: no discharge, normal penile and testicular examination

n. Extremities: full range of motion, no deformity, normal pulses

o. Back: + costovertebral angle tenderness on the left

p. Neuro: cranial nerves II to XII intact; normal sensation, strength; normal reflexes and gait

q. Skin: warm and dry

r. Lymph: no lymphadenopathy

I. Action

a. Meds
   i.   IV analgesia as above if not given before

b. Imaging
   i.   CT abdomen and pelvis without contrast

J. Nurse

a. BP: 110/70, HR: 72, RR: 16, Sat: 98% on RA after pain medicine

b. Patient: no longer in pain, tachycardia resolved

c. Imaging
   i.   CT (Figure 66.1) – 3 mm stone in the left ureterovesicular junction (UVJ) with moderate hydronephrosis

Case 66: Flank Pain

K. Results

Table 66.1 Results table

Test	Result	Test	Result
Complete blood count:		**Coagulation panel:**	
WBC	$8 \times 10^3/\mu L$	PT	13.1 sec
Hct	41.5%	PTT	27 sec
Plt	$253 \times 10^3/\mu L$	INR	1.0
Basic metabolic panel:		**Urinalysis:**	
Na	139 mEq/L	SG	1.010–1.030
K	4.2 mEq/L	pH	5–8
Cl	101 mEq/L	Prot	Neg
CO_2	18.9 mEq/L	Gluc	Neg
BUN	20 mEq/dL	Ketones	Neg
Cr	1.0 mg/dL	Bili	Neg
Gluc	99 mg/dL	Blood	Large
		LE	Neg
		Nitrite	Neg
		Color	Yellow

A

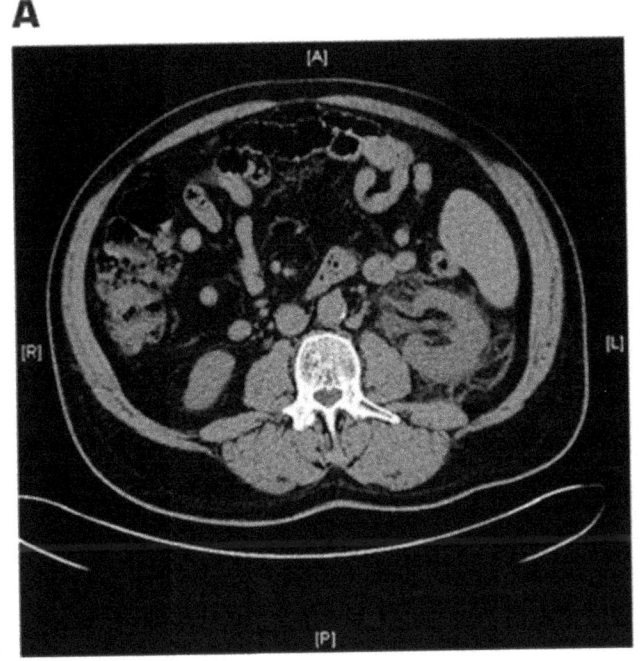

B

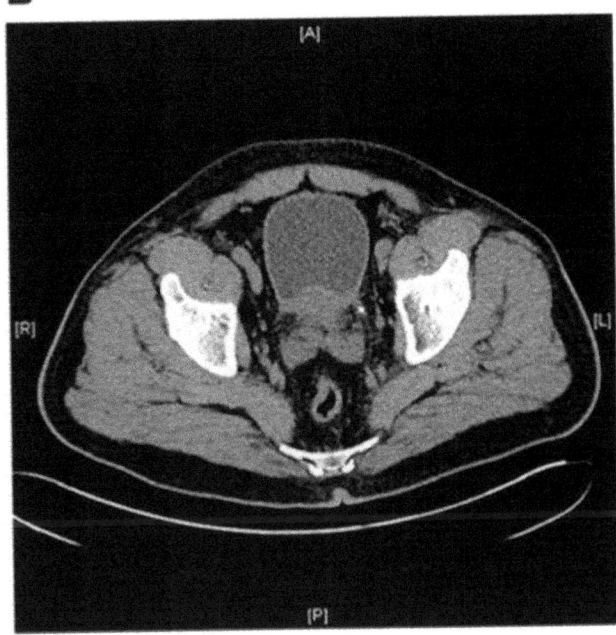

Figure 66.1

L. Action
a. Consult
   i.   Urology or PMD for follow-up
b. Discuss with patient the diagnosis of kidney stone, need for straining urine, and hydration with pain medications as needed
c. Disposition
   i.   Home
   ii. Pain medications
   iii. Consider alpha blockers (i.e. tamsulosin) for larger stones (<5 mm) or recurrent symptoms

M. Diagnosis
a. Renal colic

N. Critical actions
a. Large-bore IV access and hydration with at least 1 L NS
b. Early pain control
c. Confirmation of diagnosis of renal colic with CT abdomen and pelvis without contrast or renal ultrasound
d. Urinalysis
e. Temperature

O. Examiner instructions
a. This is a case of flank pain secondary to renal colic. This is an extremely painful condition caused by the passage of small stones from the kidney to the bladder. The patient has significant pain initially and appears extremely uncomfortable from the start. The candidate should address the patient's pain early in the encounter. No history is obtainable from the patient, except allergies, unless the pain is addressed. The key to diagnosing the patient's pain is in the history of symptoms and urinalysis. The history in this case is classic for renal colic. In addition, the patient has recently been dehydrated and has a history of gout, both of which are risk factors for nephrolithiasis. He takes a multivitamin with calcium, which may also be a risk factor. He also has physical findings suggesting the diagnosis with costovertebral angle tenderness in the absence of abdominal pain or tenderness.

P. Pearls
a. The ureterovesicular junction (UVJ) is the most common place to find stones on CT. At the time of diagnosis, up to 75% of stones are located in the distal one-third of the ureter.
b. Likelihood of the stone passing spontaneously is loosely related to the size of the stone. At 4 mm 90% pass, 4–6 mm 50% pass, and >6 mm 10% pass.
c. Flank pain in the absence of abdominal tenderness should suggest renal colic. However, aortic and iliac aneurysms or dissection may mimic the symptoms of renal colic. In addition, surgical emergencies such as appendicitis and cholecystitis should be considered in the differential.
d. Pain control should be initiated early.
e. Indications for admission for kidney stones include high-grade obstruction, intractable pain or vomiting, associated urinary tract infection, solitary or transplanted kidney.
f. Obtain urology consult for any stone over 6 mm, as they have an increased chance of requiring lithotripsy to pass.
g. Consider US as diagnostic tool instead of CT scan, especially in younger or pregnant patients.

Q. Figure legends

a. Figure 66.1 (a) (CT) Left perinephric stranding and hydronephrosis. (b) Figure 66.1 (CT) Left ureterovesicular junction calculus.

R. References

a. *Tintinalli's Emergency Medicine: A Comprehensive Study Guide* (9th ed.): Chapter 94, Urologic Stone Disease.

b. *Rosen's Emergency Medicine: Concepts and Clinical Practice* (10th ed.): Chapter 85, Urologic Disorders.

S. Acknowledgements

a. We would like to acknowledge Ravi Kapoor for their contribution to this chapter in the previous edition of this book, which has been updated by Haley Godwin and Megan Fix.

Seizure

Ellen Gilbertson, MD and Megan Fix, MD

A. Chief complaint

a. 45-year-old male brought in by EMS, seizing despite lorazepam IM

B. Vital signs

a. BP: 175/110, HR: 130, RR: 18, T: 37.6°C, Sat: 94% on RA, FS: 85 mg/dL (must ask)

C. What does the patient look like?

a. Patient in ED with tonic-clonic movements, bleeding from the mouth.

D. Primary survey

a. Airway: bleeding from the mouth but otherwise protecting airway
b. Breathing: no apparent respiratory distress, no cyanosis
c. Circulation: normal capillary refill

E. Action

a. Oxygen via NC or nonrebreather mask
b. Two large-bore peripheral IV lines
c. Labs
    i. CBC, BMP, LFT, coagulation studies, blood type and crossmatch
    ii. Lactate, alcohol level, acetaminophen level, salicylate level, urine toxicology screen, urinalysis, ABG.
d. 1 L NS bolus IV
e. Monitor: BP: 170/90, HR: 130, RR: 18, Sat: 98% on 2 L NC
f. EKG
g. Suction mouth
h. Meds
i. Lorazepam IM or IV
    1. Patient will continue to seize until a total of 8 mg lorazepam is given (multiple doses will likely need to be given to reach this threshold).
    2. Also acceptable to give midazolam (up to 10 mg IV/IM/intranasal) or diazepam 5–10mg IV, but patient won't stop seizing until given at least 10 mg of an IV benzodiazepine.

F. History

a. HPI: According to EMS, patient was walking outside with his girlfriend when he fell to the ground with rhythmic jerking movements. Per the girlfriend, he is a heavy alcohol user but had not been drinking for the last 3 days due to family visiting from out of state. She denies him having any prior seizures; denies that he has had fever, chills, vomiting, or abdominal pain; no sick contacts or recent travel.

b. PMHx: HTN, DM
c. Meds: none
d. PSHx: none
e. Allergies: no known drug allergies
f. Social: alcohol abuse in excess of 6 drinks/day; 1× weekly marijuana use; never tobacco user, currently unemployed
g. FHx: none
h. PMD: none

G. Nurse
a. EKG (Figure 67.1)
b. IF 1 L NS given
   i. BP: 170/90, HR: 110, RR: 18, Sat: 98% on 2 L NC

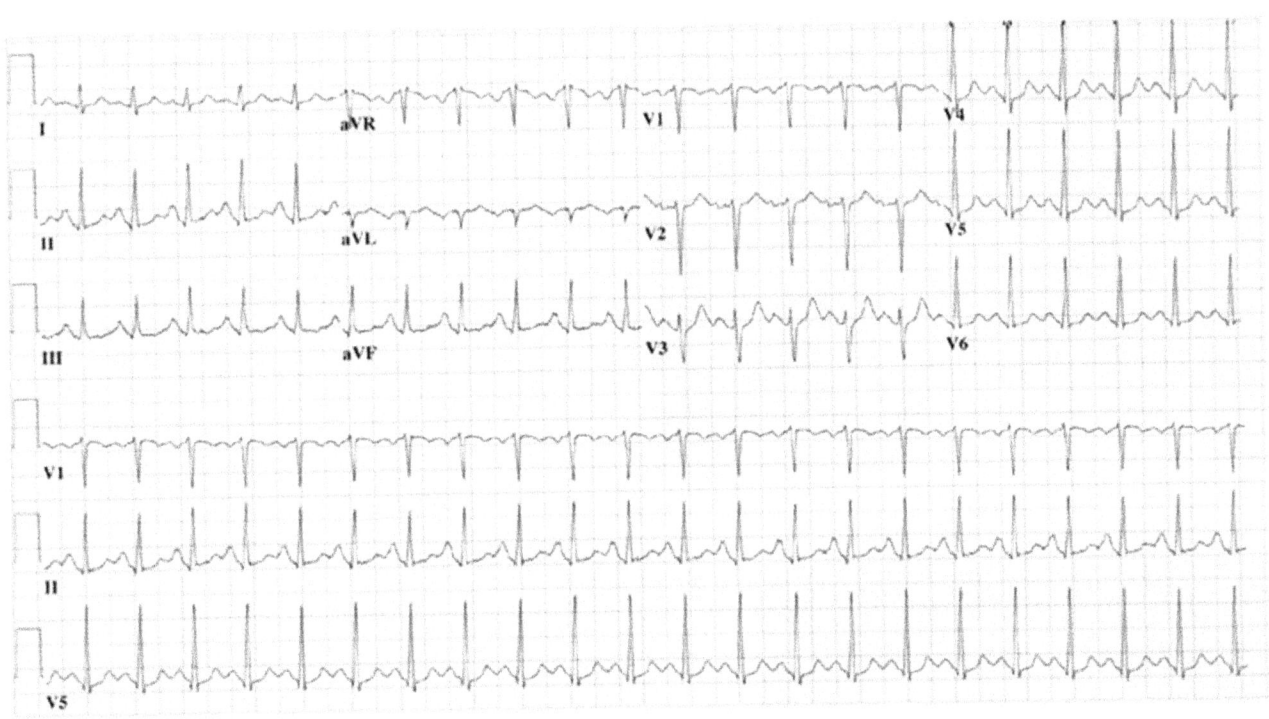

Figure 67.1

H. Secondary survey
a. General: somnolent, minimally responsive to painful stimuli only
b. HEENT: large contusion noted on occipital area with accompanying bloody laceration that has largely achieved hemostasis. Pupils equal round and reactive to light. Blood oozing from mouth; 1 cm lateral tongue laceration, minimally oozing.
c. Lungs: clear, fair air movement
d. Heart: tachycardic but regular

e. Abdomen: soft, nontender, nondistended; normoactive bowel sounds
f. Rectal: occult blood positive with brown stool
g. Urogenital: normal
h. Extremities: normal, voluntary movement difficult to assess due to AMS, bilateral AC lines in place
i. Back: normal, no stepoffs or deformities in vertebrae
j. Neuro: + gag reflex; GCS 9 (eye opening = 2, verbal = 3, motor = 4)
k. Skin: pale, no rashes, no edema, no cellulitis
l. Lymph: normal

I. Action

a. Imaging
    i.   CXR (Figure 67.2)
    ii. CT head (Figure 67.3)

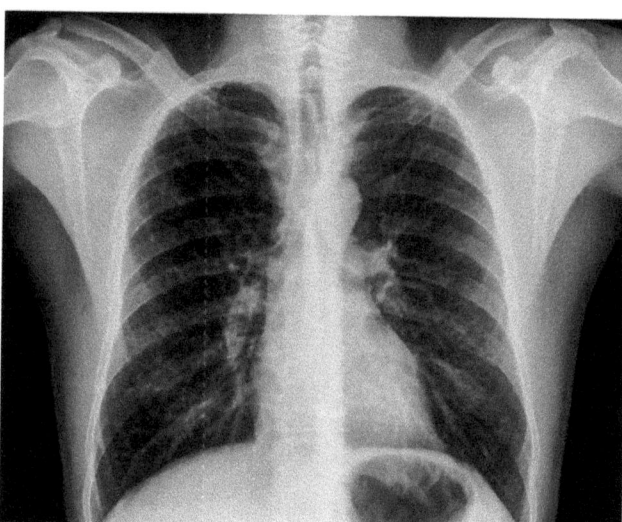

Figure 67.2

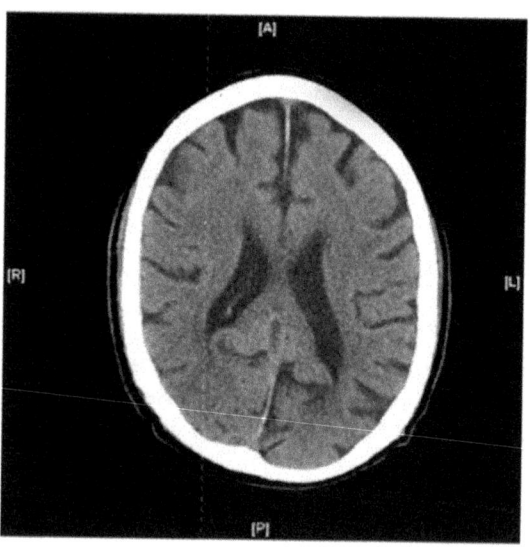

Figure 67.3

Case 67: Seizure

J. Results

Table 67.1 Results table

Test	Result	Test	Result
Complete blood count:		T bili	0.5 mg/dL
WBC	$15.1 \times 10^3/\mu L$	D bili	0.2 mg/dL
Hct	41.5%	Amylase	84 U/L
Plt	$253 \times 10^3/\mu L$	Lipase	50 U/L
		Albumin	4.5 g/dL
Basic metabolic panel:			
Na	128 mEq/L	**Urinalysis:**	
K	4.2 mEq/L	SG	1.020
Cl	101 mEq/L	pH	6
CO_2	18.9 mEq/L	Prot	Neg
BUN	35 mEq/dL	Gluc	Neg
Cr	1.6 mg/dL	Ketones	Neg
Gluc	202 mg/dL	Bili	Neg
		Blood	Neg
		LE	Neg
Coagulation panel:		Nitrite	Neg
PT	13.1 sec	Color	Yellow
PTT	26 sec		
INR	1.0	**Arterial blood gas:**	
		pH	7.35
Liver function panel:		pO_2	90 mmHg
AST	22 U/L	pCO_2	36 mmHg
ALT	20 U/L	HCO_3	22 mmol/L
Alk phos	100 U/L		

a. Lactate: 10 mmol/L
b. CT head (Figure 67.3)
c. CXR – normal
d. EtOH level <10 mg/dL, aspirin 0, acetaminophen 0
e. Patient starting to seize again, generalized tonic-clonic

K. Action

a. Consult
   i. Neurology for EEG
   ii. ICU
b. Discussion with family regarding status

    c. Meds

      i. Additional lorazepam 4 mg IVP (or other benzodiazepine) – seizure stops

      ii. Phenytoin or fosphenytoin 10 mg/kg load over 10 minutes

L. Diagnosis

a. Status epilepticus due to alcohol withdrawal

M. Critical actions

a. Finger stick blood glucose

b. IV access

c. IV benzodiazepine

d. Head CT to evaluate for intracranial pathology

e. Labs to exclude metabolic pathology

f. Serum toxicology

g. Neurology consult for new-onset seizure/status epilepticus

N. Examiner instruction

a. This is a case of status epilepticus likely due to alcohol withdrawal. The patient presents actively seizing with bleeding from a tongue laceration. Careful attention to ABCs is initially important, as is obtaining a blood glucose (normal) to determine if hypoglycemia is present. In this case, the seizure is not stopped with one dose of benzodiazepines as often occurs in alcohol withdrawal seizures. Here the definition of status can include seizures that persist despite benzodiazepines. The seizure must be treated, as seizure length is associated with damage to the brain and worsened prognosis. In this case, the history of alcohol abuse is not able to be obtained from the patient as he is actively seizing, and must be obtained from the girlfriend. She notes that he has not been drinking as family have been in town. Typically, alcohol withdrawal seizures occur 6–48 hours after the cessation of drinking. Of patients with seizures, 90% have 1–6 generalized tonic-clonic seizures; 60% experience multiple seizures within a 6-hour period. His seizures are therefore difficult to control and he will continue to seize until at least 8 mg of lorazepam (or other benzodiazepine) is given; if less than 8 mg lorazepam is given, the patient will continue to seize. Oxygen should be immediately provided once the airway has been suctioned and declared patent. The patient will be able to protect his own airway until the dosage of benzodiazepines surpasses 20 mg, at which point intubation will be required. If the patient is given phenobarbital before maxing out the dose of lorazepam, if he enters respiratory failure, or shows clinical signs of increased ICP, the patient will similarly require intubation via RSI. Additionally, the patient must be positioned in such a way as to avoid trauma from seizure recurrence. Examination of the patient's history, once airway and seizures have been controlled, is an integral step in determining the etiology of the seizures. The patient should be monitored continuously to ensure adequate cardiovascular (heart rate/blood pressure) and pulmonary function (respiratory rate/pulse oximetry).

O. Pearls

a. A rapid blood glucose level should be determined in all patients with seizure.

b. Status epilepticus is defined as a single seizure ≥5 minutes in length or two or more seizures without recovery of consciousness between seizures.

c. The most common causes of status epilepticus include subtherapeutic antiepileptic levels; preexisting neurologic conditions (prior CNS infection, trauma, hemorrhage, or stroke); anoxia or hypoxia; metabolic abnormalities; and alcohol or drug intoxication or withdrawal.

d. The main tenet of treatment of status epilepticus is to stop the seizure as quickly as possible and prevent recurrence.

e. Alcohol withdrawal should be considered in all patients presenting with seizure who have a history of alcohol abuse. Obtaining a thorough history from family or acquaintances is very helpful in this regard.

f. Anytime a patient presents with seizure, especially if the onset was unwitnessed, cranial imaging must be done to rule out trauma.

g. If the patient's airway is obstructed by the tongue, placement of an airway adjunct such as a nasopharyngeal or oropharyngeal airway will likely improve the patient's respiratory status.

h. The correct order of antiepileptic pharmacotherapy in status epilepticus is as follows: (1) benzodiazepines; (2) phenytoin; (3) barbiturates.

i. If seizures are unresponsive to treatment, consider INH overdose or tricyclic antidepressant overdose.

j. C spine precautions should be implemented if patient exhibits signs of trauma.

k. If patient is hyperthermic, treat with antipyretics and cooling blankets.

l. If the cause of the seizure is unknown, blood should be obtained in order to check serum electrolytes, glucose, sodium, calcium, magnesium, renal function, toxicology, antiepileptic drug levels (if indicated), and CBC.

m. If necessary, an intraosseous line can be used to administer all medications, including anticonvulsants.

P. Figure legends

a. Figure 67.1 (ECG) Sinus tachycardia.

b. Figure 67.2 (CXR) Normal chest radiograph.

c. Figure 67.3 (CT head) Normal head CT.

Q. References

a. *Rosen's Emergency Medicine: Concepts and Clinical Practice* (10th ed.): Chapter 14, Seizures. Chapter 88, Seizure.

b. *Tintinalli's Emergency Medicine: A Comprehensive Study Guide* (9th ed.): Chapter 171, Seizures and Status Epilepticus in Adults.

R. Acknowledgements

a. We would like to acknowledge Satjiv Kohli for their contribution to this chapter in the previous edition of this book, which has been updated by Ellen Gilbertson and Megan Fix.

Altered Mental Status

Tabitha Ford, MD and Robert Stephen, MD

A. Chief complaint

a. 56-year-old male presents by EMS after his family visited his home and found him to be confused

A. Vital signs

a. BP: 102/64, HR: 132, RR: 28, T: 39.6°C, Sat: 91% on RA

B. What does the patient look like?

a. Patient is somnolent, diaphoretic, moaning when he is awakened.

C. Primary survey

a. Airway: patent (GCS 12)
b. Breathing: tachypnea, but otherwise normal work of breathing
c. Circulation: slight mottling of extremities, palpable distal pulses

D. Action

a. Apply oxygen by nasal cannula or nonrebreather mask
b. Two large-bore peripheral IV lines
c. Labs
   i. CBC, CMP, VBG, troponin, lactate, blood cultures, urinalysis, urine culture, type and screen × 2
   ii. Glucose: 321 mg/dL
   iii. 1 L bolus IV (NS or LR)
   iv. Monitor: BP: 98/62, HR: 138, RR 28, Sat: 90% on RA or 98% on O_2
   v. EKG
   vi. CXR

E. History

a. HPI: A 56-year-old man with a history of poorly controlled diabetes, hypertension, hyperlipidemia, and alcoholism presents with concern for altered mental status. His family has not seen him in 3 days, but they visited his home and found him lying in a recliner moaning and answering questions inappropriately. Patient is not able to answer questions or provide further history.
b. PMHx: poorly controlled diabetes, hypertension, hyperlipidemia, alcoholism
c. PSHx: cholecystectomy 3 years ago
d. Allergies: none

e. Meds: insulin, metformin, atorvastatin, lisinopril
f. Social: frequent EtOH use, no drug use, lives alone
g. FHx: not available
h. PMD: Dr. Waters

F. Nurse
a. EKG: sinus tachycardia with no ischemic change
b. CXR: unremarkable
c. Fluids (post 1 L bolus)
    i.   BP 106/70, HR: 118, RR: 24, Sat: 99% on O_2
    ii. Mental status improving (GCS 14)
d. No fluids
    i.   BP 86/48, HR: 144, RR: 28, Sat: 99% on O_2

G. Secondary survey
a. General: more awake after fluids, disoriented speech, appears distressed
b. Head: normocephalic, atraumatic
c. Eyes: extraocular movement intact, pupils equal, reactive to light
d. Ears: external auditory canals without drainage, tympanic membranes clear and flat bilaterally
e. Nose: no rhinorrhea
f. Oropharynx: dry mucous membranes, no lesions or swelling
g. Neck: full range of motion without meningismus
h. Chest: nontender, no crepitus
i. Lungs: tachypnea with otherwise normal effort, clear bilaterally
j. Heart: tachycardic rate, rhythm regular, no murmurs
k. Abdomen: normal bowel sounds, soft, nontender, nondistended
l. Rectal: normal tone, brown stool, occult blood negative, no fluctuance
m. Urogenital (must ask): induration and erythema of left scrotum and perineum spreading to medial left thigh, significant tenderness to palpation, crepitus noted
n. Extremities: distal pulses intact, no joint swelling or erythema, moving all spontaneously
o. Back: nontender
p. Neuro: GCS 14 with confused speech, cranial nerves II through XII grossly intact, sensation to fine touch intact in all extremities, full strength in all extremities, no gross ataxia
q. Skin: hot and diaphoretic, perineal skin findings as noted above if asked
r. Lymph: no lymphadenopathy

H. Action
a. 1–2 L bolus (NS or LR)
b. Medication
    i.   Broad-spectrum antibiotics (e.g., vancomycin, ceftriaxone, plus clindamycin)
c. General surgery or urology consult
    i.   OR for debridement
d. CT head to assess for any intracranial injury given altered mental status and history of alcoholism
e. Consider CT pelvis to assess extent of infection if patient remains stable
f. Discussion with family regarding emergency surgical debridement

I. Nurse

a. CT resulted
   i. Head with no acute abnormality
   ii. Pelvis (Figure 68.1) showing subcutaneous air and stranding/infection tracking along fascial planes

b. Second liter fluids
   i. BP 110/74, HR: 104, RR: 24, Sat: 99% on O_2
   ii. Surgery ready to take patient to the OR

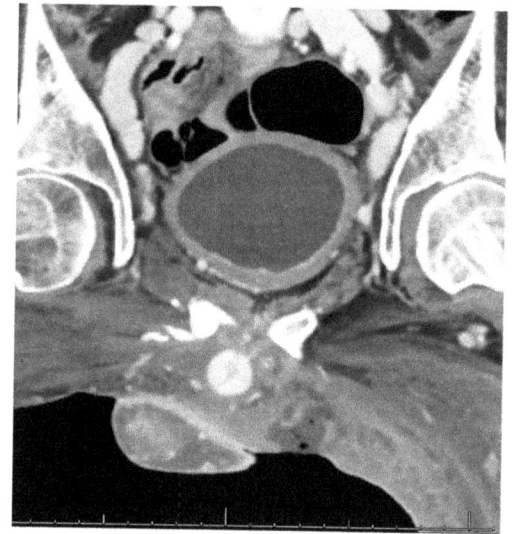
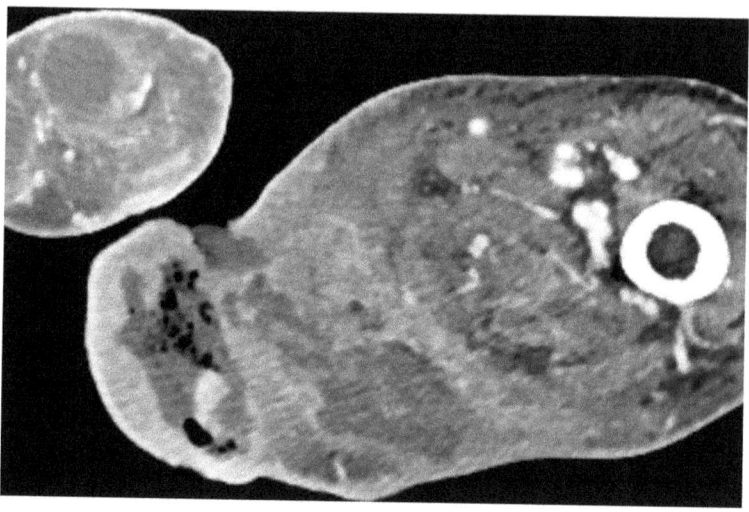

Figure 68.1

J. Results

Table 68.1 Results table

Test	Result	Test	Result
Complete blood count:		Alk phos	87 U/L
WBC	$28.6 \times 10^3/\mu L$	T bili	0.7 mg/dL
Hct	36.2%	Albumin	4.1 g/dL
Plt	$223 \times 10^3/\mu L$		
		Urinalysis:	
Basic metabolic panel:		SG	1.030
Na	126 mEq/L	pH	6
K	4.1 mEq/L	Prot	Neg
Cl	97 mEq/L	Gluc	+
CO_2	13 mEq/L	Ketones	Neg
BUN	46 mEq/dL	Blood	Neg
Cr	1.4 mg/dL	LE	Neg
Gluc	318 mg/dL	Nitrite	Neg
		Color	Yellow

Table 68.1 (cont.)

Test	Result	Test	Result
Coagulation panel:		**Venous blood gas:**	
PT	12.5 sec	pH	7.29
PTT	26 sec	PCO_2	30 mmHg
INR	1.0	HCO_3	14 mmol/L
Liver function panel:			
AST	118 U/L		
ALT	56 U/L		

a. Lactate: 7.6 mmol/L

K. Diagnosis
a. Fournier's gangrene

L. Critical actions
a. Bilateral large bore IV access and fluid bolus
b. Check blood glucose
c. Perform thorough exam (including genitalia) to localize source of infection
d. Early IV antibiotics
e. Surgery consult

M. Examiner instructions
a. This is a case of Fournier's gangrene, a necrotizing polymicrobial bacterial infection of the perineum. The infection may rapidly spread through fascial planes to the abdominal wall, and can be fatal, even if treated appropriately. Important actions in this case include early recognition of sepsis and appropriately aggressive treatment with intravenous fluids and prompt broad-spectrum antibiotics after obtaining cultures. Additionally, it is imperative to recognize that all patients with a fever and unknown source of infection should have a thorough skin exam, including the genitalia. This is especially true when the patient is unable to provide a clear history. If the provider does not perform a genital exam and recognize the soft tissue infection or manages the patient inappropriately without fluids, antibiotics, and surgical consult, the patient will continue to decompensate with increasing heart rate, decreasing blood pressure, and worsening altered mental status until the provider is forced to start vasopressor support and intubate the patient. At that time, the case will end. If the provider does make the diagnosis, it is essential to give broad-spectrum antibiotics and obtain immediate surgical consult for definitive treatment in the OR, at which time the case will end. The provider may order a CT scan if the patient has stabilized, but it is not absolutely necessary as the suspicion is high on clinical exam. If the surgeon requests a CT and the patient is stable, this may help solidify the diagnosis.

N. Pearls
a. Fournier's gangrene is a rapidly spreading, polymicrobial, necrotizing infection of the perineum or genitals.

b. Typically begins as a simple infection or abscess.
c. More common in diabetic patients or those with alcohol abuse.
d. Pain out of proportion to exam is a red flag for necrotizing infection.
e. Be sure to assess for crepitus on examination as subcutaneous air should significantly increase suspicion for necrotizing infection.
f. Microthrombus formation in small subcutaneous vessels causes local gangrene.
g. Treatment should include broad-spectrum antibiotics covering Gram-positive, Gram-negative, and anaerobic bacteria:
    i.   Piperacillin–tazobactam, imipenem, or meropenem **plus**
    ii. Vancomycin **plus**
    iii. Clindamycin (may decrease bacterial toxin formation)
h. Imaging cannot definitively rule out a necrotizing infection, although it may demonstrate signs such as subcutaneous air (Figure 68.1) or infection tracking along fascial planes.
i. This is ultimately a clinical diagnosis. When suspected, emergent surgical consultation is mandatory as these patients frequently require debridement.
j. These patients should be admitted to an intensive care unit as they have a very high mortality rate (20–40%).

O. Figure legends

a. Figure 68.1 (a) (CT) Left-coronal image of perineum. (b) (CT) Right-axial image of proximal left lower extremity and scrotum.

P. References

a. *Tintinalli's Emergency Medicine: A Comprehensive Study Guide* (9th ed.): Chapter 93, Male Genital Problems.
b. *Rosen's Emergency Medicine: Concepts and Clinical Practice* (10th ed.): Chapter 126, Skin and Soft Tissue Infections.

Vomiting

Amit Patel, MD

A. Chief complaint
a. 11-month-old male with fussiness and vomiting

B. Vital signs
a. BP: 90/60, HR: 150, RR: 30, T: 37.4°C, Sat: 98% on RA, FS: 85 mg/dL, Wt: 9.4 kg

C. What does the patient look like?
a. Patient being held by mom, lethargic appearing

D. Primary survey
a. Airway: patent
b. Breathing: no apparent respiratory distress, no cyanosis
c. Circulation: pale, clammy skin, 2+ distal pulses bilaterally; capillary refill 3 seconds

E. Action
a. Establish IV access
b. 20 mL/kg NS bolus (180–200 mL)
c. Labs
    i. CBC, BMP, urinalysis

F. History
a. HPI: As per mother, patient has "not been acting his usual happy self," interspersed with episodes of nonbilious, nonbloody vomiting for the past 4 days. During the episodes, the patient is not consolable. The episodes last 10–15 minutes. Patient is not drinking as much as normal and for the past 2 days is having fewer wet diapers. Mother states that the child had diarrhea about 1 week prior to this illness. No fever, chills, cough, diarrhea, hematemesis, rashes. No sick contacts or travel history.
b. PMHx: born at term, immunizations up to date
c. PSHx: none
d. Social: lives at home with parents and two older siblings
e. FHx: not relevant
f. PMD: Dr. Johnson

G. Nurse
a. If no fluids or inadequate fluids given
    i. BP: 80/50, HR: 165, RR: 30, Sat: 98% on RA
b. After adequate fluid bolus
    i. BP: 100/60, HR: 140, RR: 30, Sat: 98% on RA

H. Secondary survey

a. General: lethargic, sleeping in mother's arms; arousable to verbal stimuli
b. HEENT: mucous membranes dry; throat without exudates or erythema; tympanic membranes intact bilaterally
c. Neck: supple without lymphadenopathy
d. Lungs: clear to auscultation bilaterally
e. Heart: tachycardic but regular; no murmurs, rubs, or gallops
f. Abdomen: soft, moderately tender diffusely; nondistended; no rebound or guarding; hyperactive bowel sounds, no hepatosplenomegaly
g. Rectal: guaiac +; no gross blood
h. Extremities: normal
i. Back: normal
j. Neuro: lethargic, otherwise normal
k. Skin: pale, no rashes, no edema, no cellulitis
l. Lymph: normal

I. Action

a. Abdominal x-ray
b. Abdominal US
c. Reevaluate
   i. Monitor: BP: 100/60, HR: 140

J. Results

Table 69.1 Results table

Test	Result	Test	Result
Complete blood count:		**Liver function panel:**	
WBC	$10.3 \times 10^3/\mu L$	AST	10 U/L
Hct	39%	ALT	40 U/L
Plt	$312 \times 10^3/\mu L$	Alk phos	180 U/L
		T bili	0.5 mg/dL
Basic metabolic panel:		D bili	0.1 mg/dL
Na	138 mEq/L	Amylase	24 U/L
K	3.9 mEq/L	Lipase	18 U/L
Cl	100 mEq/L	Albumin	4.2 g/dL
CO_2	17.9 mEq/L		
BUN	9 mEq/dL	**Urinalysis:**	
Cr	0.2 mg/dL	SG	1.01
Gluc	80 mg/dL	pH	7.1
		Prot	Neg
Coagulation panel:		Gluc	Neg
PT	11.3 sec	Ketones	1+
PTT	32.1 sec	Bili	Neg

Table 69.1 (cont.)

Test	Result	Test	Result
INR	0.8	Blood	Neg
		LE	Neg
		Nitrite	Neg
		Color	Yellow

a. Abdominal x-ray (Figure 69.1)
b. Abdominal US (Figure 69.2)

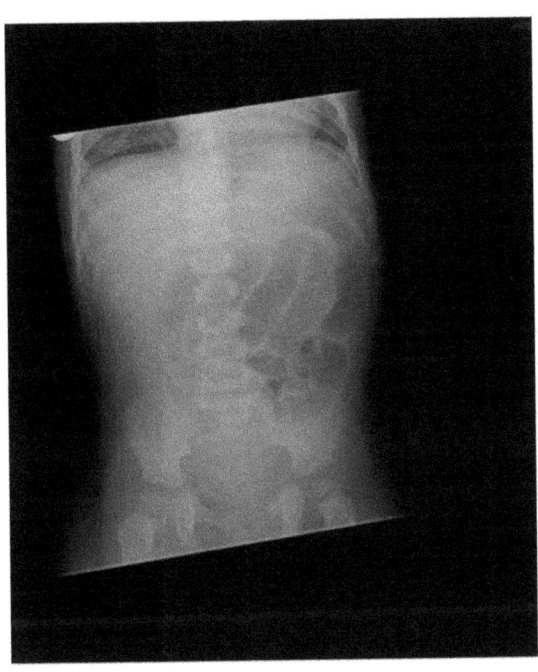

Figure 69.1

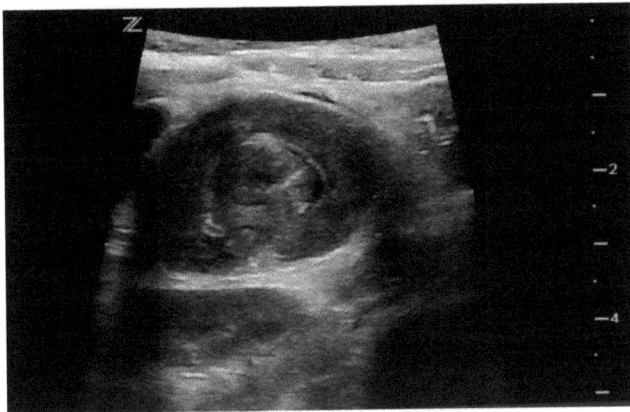

Figure 69.2

K. Action

a. Surgery consult
b. Discussion with family and PMD regarding possibility for emergent OR if no improvement with barium enema/air insufflation enema
c. Therapeutic study: contrast enema/air insufflation enema

L. Nurse

a. X-ray with barium (Figure 69.3)

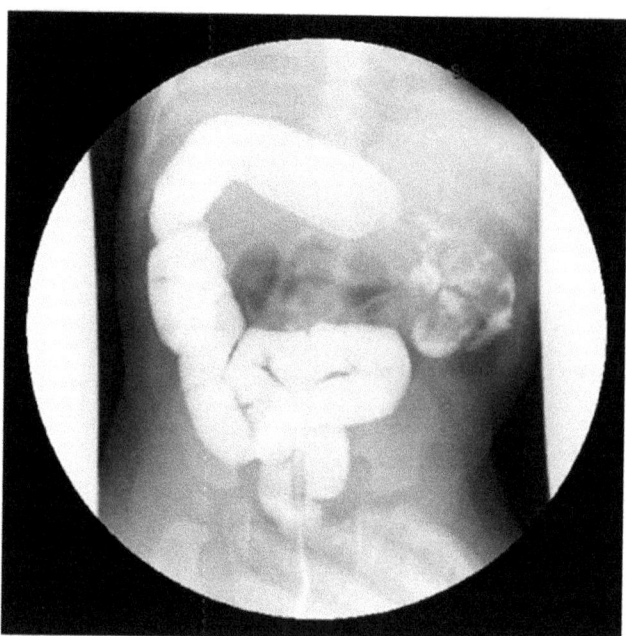

Figure 69.3

M. Diagnosis

a. Intussusception

N. Critical actions

a. NS bolus (20 mL/kg)
b. Complete physical examination
c. Barium enema/air insufflation enema
d. Pediatric surgical consult

O. Examiner instructions

a. This is a case of intussusception, a condition that results from the patient's intestine involuting into itself. The treatment is reduction of the telescoped bowel. If untreated, the patient can become obstructed or develop a perforation of the intestine. Early actions include IV access, fluid support, prompt surgical consultation, and either an initial US or barium enema. In this patient, the mother was concerned because the patient has been having intermittent episodes of inconsolable crying and vomiting which is consistent with intussusception in this age group. The infant should intermittently appear well but then have sudden episodes where he is inconsolable. Unless the diagnosis is established by US or enema, the patient's physical examination will progress to peritonitis requiring emergent surgical intervention. If the diagnosis is made with rapid reduction by enema, the patient will do well with observation.

P. Pearls

a. Intussusception is the most common cause of intestinal obstruction in children younger than 2 years old and occurs most commonly in infants 3–12 months old.
b. The exact etiology is unclear, but the most prevalent theory suggests a lead point that causes invagination of one segment of bowel into a more distal segment. The most common intussusception is ileocolic; other variations include ileoilieal and colocolic. As the process

continues and intensifies, edema develops, compressing the mesenteric veins and arteries resulting in ischemia of the bowel wall. As ischemia of the bowel wall continues, bleeding can lessen but the bowel may perforate leading to peritonitis.

c. A preceding viral illness can sometimes be seen a few days prior to the onset of the abdominal pain.

d. The classic triad of symptoms in intussusception is abdominal pain, vomiting, and bloody stools. All three symptoms occur in 20% of patients; however, three-quarters of patients with intussusception have two findings, and the remainder have either none or only one.

e. Diarrhea containing mucus and blood constitutes the classic "currant jelly" stool, but it is important to note that this is a late finding. However, 50–75% of cases have occult blood on rectal examination.

f. In a typical case, the child presents with cyclical episodes of severe abdominal pain. The pain typically lasts 10–15 minutes and has a periodicity of 15–30 minutes. During the painful episodes, the child is inconsolable, often described as drawing the legs up to the abdomen and screaming in pain.

g. Dance's sign: palpation of the abdomen may reveal a sausage-like mass in the right upper quadrant representing the actual intussusception and an empty space in the right lower quadrant representing the movement of the cecum out of its normal position. This finding is pathognomonic for intussusception.

h. Flat and upright films in the child with at least 6–12 hours of symptoms may show an obstructive pattern with distended bowel/air fluid levels. It may also show a soft tissue mass surrounded by a crescent of gas or a paucity of gas in the right lower quadrant.

i. Ultrasound has a 98–100% sensitivity for intussusception. A typical ileocolic intussusception has the appearance of a peripheral hypoechoic ring (target sign) with central echogenicity (the pseudo-kidney sign). It is also important to note that if there is a lack of Doppler blood flow within the intussusception there is a higher likelihood of bowel necrosis and the rate of successful reduction is lower.

j. Surgery should be consulted promptly and be present or immediately available for the enema in case of bowel perforation during the procedure.

k. Ill-appearing or febrile children require broad-spectrum, triple-antibiotic coverage with ampicillin, gentamycin, and either clindamycin or metronidazole.

Q. Figure legends
a. Figure 69.1 (Abdominal x-ray) Dilated loops of bowel.
b. Figure 69.2 (Abdominal ultrasound) Telescoping of intestines suggesting intussusception.
c. Figure 69.3 (X-ray with barium) Contrast filled loops of bowel up to the area of intussusception.

R. References
a. *Rosen's Emergency Medicine: Concepts and Clinical Practice* (10th ed.): Chapter 166, Pediatric Gastrointestinal Disorders.
b. *Tintinalli's Emergency Medicine: A Comprehensive Study Guide* (9th ed.): Chapter 133, Acute Abdominal Pain in Infants and Children.

S. Acknowledgements
a. We would like to acknowledge Satjiv Kohli for their contribution to this chapter in the previous edition of this book, which has been updated by Amit Patel.

Fever

Nicholas Levin, MD and Brendan Cummins, MD

A. Chief complaint
a. 45-year-old male arrives to the ED complaining of fever

B. Vital signs
a. BP: 105/50, HR: 110, RR: 24, T: 39.4°C, Sat 88% on RA

C. What does the patient look like?
a. Patient is warm to touch and diaphoretic.

D. Primary survey
a. Airway: speaking in full sentences
b. Breathing: no apparent respiratory distress, no cyanosis
c. Circulation: warm and wet skin, normal capillary refill

E. Action
a. Oxygen via nonrebreather mask
b. Two large-bore peripheral IV lines
c. Labs
    i. CBC, BMP, LFT, coagulation studies, LDH, ABG
    ii. Lactate, blood cultures, urinalysis, urine culture, LDH, stool culture, stool ova and parasites
d. Meds
    i. Acetaminophen
e. 1 L NS bolus
f. Monitor: BP: 95/60, HR: 115, RR: 24, Sat: 95% on NRB mask O_2
g. EKG
h. Imaging
i. CXR

F. History
a. HPI: A 45-year-old male with stage 3 HIV (last known CD4 count of 150), noncompliant with medical treatment, who states that he has been coughing with green sputum for the last 3 days. He is also complaining of fever, shortness of breath, pleuritic chest pain, and nonbloody diarrhea. He denies headache, hemoptysis, night chills, vomiting, abdominal pain, or melena; no recent travel, camping, or sick contacts.
b. PMHx: HIV
c. PSHx: none
d. Allergies: none

e. Meds: noncompliant, does not know
f. Social: lives in apartment alone; daily smoker and occasional EtOH use, but denies illicit drug use; not sexually active
g. FHx: not relevant
h. PMD: clinic

G. Nurse
a. EKG normal sinus tachycardia
b. CXR (Figure 70.1)

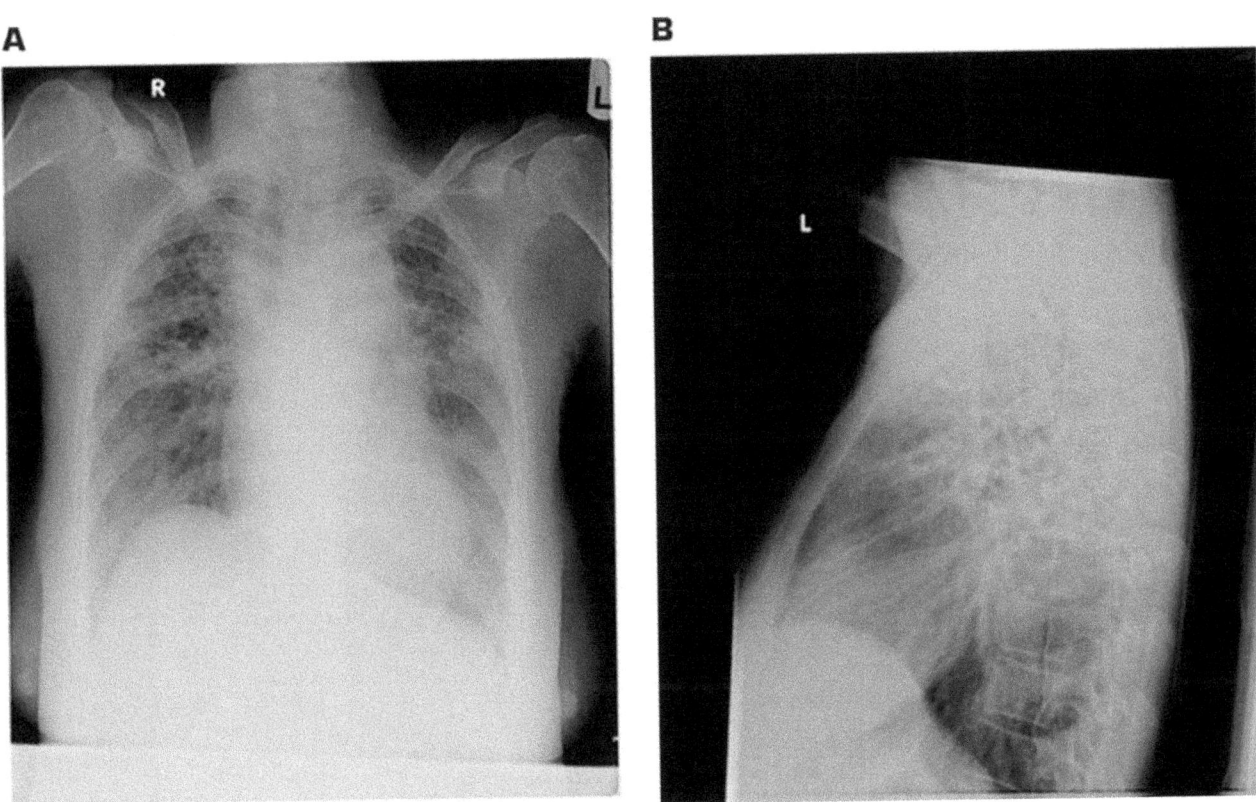

Figure 70.1

H. Secondary survey
a. General: alert, oriented × 3, mild respiratory distress
b. Head: cachectic, atraumatic
c. Eyes: extraocular movement intact, pupils equal, reactive to light
d. Ears: normal tympanic membranes
e. Nose: no discharge
f. Neck: full range of motion, no jugular vein distension, no stridor
g. Pharynx: poor dentition, throat without exudates, + thrush
h. Chest: nontender
i. Lungs: decreased breath sounds bilaterally with crackles
j. Heart: rate and rhythm regular, no murmurs, rubs, or gallops
k. Abdomen: normal bowel sounds, soft, nontender, or distended
l. Rectal: normal tone, brown stool, occult blood negative

m. Urogenital: normal external genitalia
   i.   Male: no discharge, normal testicular examination
n. Extremities: full range of motion, no deformity, normal pulses
o. Back: nontender
p. Neuro: cranial nerves II to XII intact; normal sensation, strength; normal reflexes and gait
q. Skin: warm and dry
r. Lymph: no lymphadenopathy

I. Action

a. Move patient to negative pressure isolation room (droplet precautions)
b. Meds
   i.   Prednisone
   ii. Ceftriaxone
   iii. Azithromycin
   iv. Sulfamethoxazole trimethoprim (Bactrim)
c. Reassess
   i.   Patient: continued shortness of breath, mildly improved

J. Nurse

a. 1 L NS
   i.   BP: 105/60, HR: 105, RR: 24, Sat: 95% on NRB mask O_2

K. Results

Table 70.1 Results table

Test	Result	Test	Result
Complete blood count:		Alk phos	45 U/L
WBC	$1.1 \times 10^3/\mu L$	T bili	0.8 mg/dL
Diff	88.6/8.4/1.8	D bili	0.2 mg/dL
Hct	41.50%	Amylase	55 U/L
Plt	$253 \times 10^3/\mu L$	Lipase	60 U/L
		Albumin	3.6 g/dL
Basic metabolic panel:		LDH	420
Na	139 mEq/L		
K	4.2 mEq/L	**Urinalysis:**	
Cl	101 mEq/L	SG	1.02
CO_2	18.9 mEq/L	pH	6
BUN	52 mEq/dL	Prot	Neg
Cr	1.6 mg/dL	Gluc	Neg
Gluc	202 mg/dL	Ketones	+
		Bili	Neg

Table 70.1 (cont.)

Test	Result	Test	Result
Coagulation panel:		Blood	Neg
PT	13.1 sec	LE	Neg
PTT	26.5 sec	Nitrite	Neg
INR	1.1	Color	Yellow
Liver function panel:		**Arterial blood gas:**	
AST	25 U/L	pH	7.3
ALT	28 U/L	pO_2	56 mmHg
		pCO_2	35 mmHg
		HCO_3	19 mmol/L

a. Lactate: 3.6 mmol/L

L. Actions

a. Admit to isolation with a monitored bed

M. Diagnosis

a. HIV pneumonia, likely *Pneumocystis jiroveci* pneumonia (previously known as *P. Carinii* or PCP)

N. Critical actions

a. Oxygen supplementation
b. IV fluids
c. CXR
d. Urinalysis
e. Antibiotics
f. Respiratory isolation
g. Prednisone

O. Examiner instructions

a. This is a case of fever in a HIV patient, likely caused by pneumonia. Important early actions included recognizing the fever, tachycardia, and hypoxia, and providing IV fluids, O_2 supplementation, and acetaminophen. The patient has significant shortness of breath secondary to his diffuse interstitial pneumonia and hypoxia. Supplemental oxygen improves his symptoms. With early antibiotics and steroids, the patient's symptoms and oxygen saturation will improve. If pneumonia is not recognized and the patient does not receive antibiotics early, the patient will continue to complain of worsening shortness of breath and cough and ultimately become septic, with increased heart rate and hypotension. Given the patient's risk for tuberculosis, he should be placed in a room with respiratory precautions to prevent spread to health care workers.

P. Pearls

a. Fever is a common presenting complaint for patients with uncontrolled HIV brought to the ED. Evidence of an infectious cause or other reason for fever should be sought by careful history and physical examination.

b. Tests ordered should include complete blood count, electrolytes, liver function tests, urinalysis and culture, blood cultures (aerobic, anaerobic, and fungal), and CXR. If the patient has diarrhea, stool culture and stool examination for ova and parasites should be sent. If PCP is suspected, LDH and ABG can be sent. Elevations in LDH are sensitive but not specific for PCP; however, in the setting of pulmonary infiltrates they should raise clinical concern for PCP infection.

c. The causative organism is a fungus (*Pneumocystis jiroveci*). It used to be classified as a protozoan (*Pneumocystis carinii*, or PCP). At the time of this writing, *Rosen's*, *Tintinalli's*, and the Centers for Disease Control all abbreviate the organism *Pneumocystis jiroveci* as "PCP."

d. If there are neurologic signs or symptoms or if no other source of fever is identified, lumbar puncture (LP) should be performed after a noncontrast head CT.

e. Development of pulmonary disorders is often related to CD4 counts. In patients with pulmonary involvement and CD4 counts >500, encapsulated bacteria, tuberculosis (TB), and malignancies are common. With lower CD4 counts, PCP, atypical mycobacteria, fungal infections, CMV, lymphoma, lymphoproliferative disorders, and Kaposi's sarcoma may also be seen.

f. A focal infiltrate on plain chest radiography often suggests bacterial pneumonia.

g. A diffuse interstitial or perihilar, granular pattern on chest radiography is associated with PCP. However, 20% of radiographs can be negative in cases of PCP.

h. Give steroids to patients with a partial pressure of arterial oxygen <70 mmHg or an alveolar–arterial gradient of >35 mmHg, typically oral prednisone 40 mg BID × 21 days.

Q. Figure legends

a. Figure 70.1 (CXR) Diffuse bilateral patchy infiltrates.

R. References

a. *Rosen's Emergency Medicine: Concepts and Clinical Practice* (10th ed.): Chapter 121, HIV.

b. *Tintinalli's Emergency Medicine: A Comprehensive Study Guide* (9th ed.): Chapter 155, Human Immunodeficiency Virus Infection.

S. Acknowledgements

a. We would like to acknowledge Satjiv Kohli for their contribution to this chapter in the previous edition of this book, which has been updated by Nicholas Levin and Brendan Cummins.

Palpitations

Shawn Zhong, MD

A. Chief complaint
a. 39-year-old female with history of hypertension brought in by EMS with the complaint of palpitations

B. Vital signs
a. BP: 161/112, HR: 160, RR: 22, T: 37.1°C, Sat: 99% on RA

C. What does the patient look like?
a. Patient appears stated age, slightly apprehensive, and sitting up on stretcher.

D. Primary survey
a. Airway: speaking in full sentences
b. Breathing: mildly increased respiratory rate, no respiratory distress, no cyanosis
c. Circulation: extremities warm and well perfused

E. Action
a. Oxygen via NC or nonrebreather mask to maintain saturation >95%
b. Two large-bore peripheral IV lines
c. Labs
    i. CBC, BMP, TSH
    ii. Urine pregnancy test
d. 1 L NS bolus
e. Monitor: BP: 152/65, HR: 162, RR: 22, Sat: 100% on O_2
f. EKG

F. History
a. HPI: A 39-year-old female with a history of hypertension states that she has had sudden onset of palpitations for the last hour; denies any chest pain; slightly short of breath and dizzy; denies any nausea, vomiting, fevers, chills, headache, neck pain, or pain in other parts of the body; no recent illnesses.
b. PMHx: hypertension
c. PSHx: none
d. Allergies: none
e. Meds: hydrochlorothiazide
f. Social: lives with husband and children at home; drinks alcohol socially; denies any smoking; denies any cocaine or other illicit drugs; is sexually active with husband only

g. FHx: mother had heart attack at age 68; father has diabetes
h. PMD: Dr. Fischer

G. Nurse
a. BP: 150/112, HR: 160, RR: 23, Sat: 99% on 2 L
b. Patient: complaints of mild shortness of breath and dizziness
c. EKG (Figure 71.1)

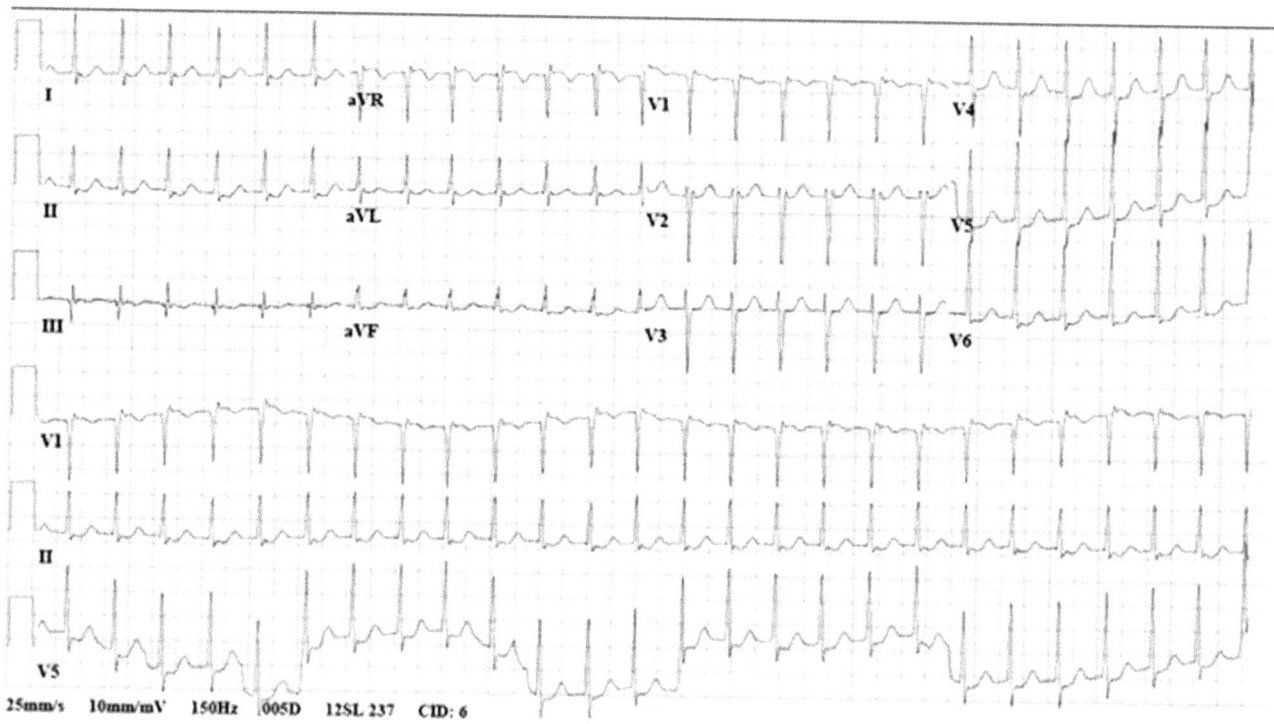

Figure 71.1

H. Secondary survey
a. General: alert, oriented × 3, mildly increased respiratory rate
b. Head: normocephalic, atraumatic
c. Eyes: extraocular movement intact, pupils equal, reactive to light
d. Ears: normal tympanic membranes
e. Nose: no discharge
f. Neck: full range of motion, no jugular vein distension, no stridor, no carotid bruit
g. Pharynx: normal dentition, no lesions, no swelling
h. Chest: nontender
i. Lungs: clear bilaterally
j. Heart: tachycardiac, rhythm regular, no murmurs, rubs, or gallops
k. Abdomen: normal bowel sounds, soft, nontender, or distended
l. Rectal: normal tone, brown stool, occult blood negative
m. Extremities: full range of motion, no deformity, normal pulses
n. Back: nontender
o. Neuro: cranial nerves II to XII intact; normal sensation, strength; normal reflexes, normal gait
p. Skin: warm and dry
q. Lymph: no lymphadenopathy

Case 71: Palpitations

I. Action

a. Maneuvers
    i. Vagal maneuvers (no response)
    ii. Carotid massage (should be discouraged in adult patients)
    iii. Ice packs on face
    iv. Valsalva maneuver
b. Meds
    i. Adenosine 6 mg rapid IVP (via three way stopcock or other method to ensure a rapid delivery)
    ii. Rhythm strip running; defibrillator at bedside
    iii. Warn patient of side effects

J. Nurse

a. BP: 152/98, HR: 150, RR: 20, Sat: 97% on 2 L
b. Patient felt nauseated during injection of adenosine, but now again feels mildly dizzy and with palpitations

K. Action

a. Meds
    i. Adenosine 12 mg rapid IVP
    ii. Rhythm strip running; defibrillator at bedside
    iii. Warn patient of side effects

L. Nurse

a. BP: 152/98, HR: 95, RR: 16, Sat: 98% on 2 L

M. Results

Table 71.1 Results table

Test	Result	Test	Result
Complete blood count:		T bili	1.0 mg/dL
WBC	$5.3 \times 10^3/\mu L$	D bili	0.3 mg/dL
Hct	42%	Amylase	50 U/L
Plt	$350 \times 10^3/\mu L$	Lipase	25 U/L
		Albumin	4.7 g/dL
Basic metabolic panel:			
Na	138 mEq/L	**Urinalysis:**	
K	4.3 mEq/L	SG	1.010–1.030
Cl	105 mEq/L	pH	5–8
CO_2	30 mEq/L	Prot	Neg
BUN	12 mEq/dL	Gluc	Neg
Cr	1.1 mg/dL	Ketones	Neg
Gluc	100 mg/dL	Bili	Neg

Table 71.1 (cont.)

Test	Result	Test	Result
Coagulation panel:		Blood	Neg
PT	12.6 sec	LE	Neg
PTT	26.0 sec	Nitrite	Neg
INR	1.0	Color	Yellow
Liver function panel:		**Arterial blood gas:**	
AST	23 U/L	pH	7.43
ALT	26 U/L	pO_2	95 mmHg
Alk phos	42 U/L	pCO_2	35 mmHg
		HCO_3	24 mmol/L

a. Urine pregnancy test: negative
b. Patient with significant improvement and resolution of symptoms
c. EKG (Figure 71.2)

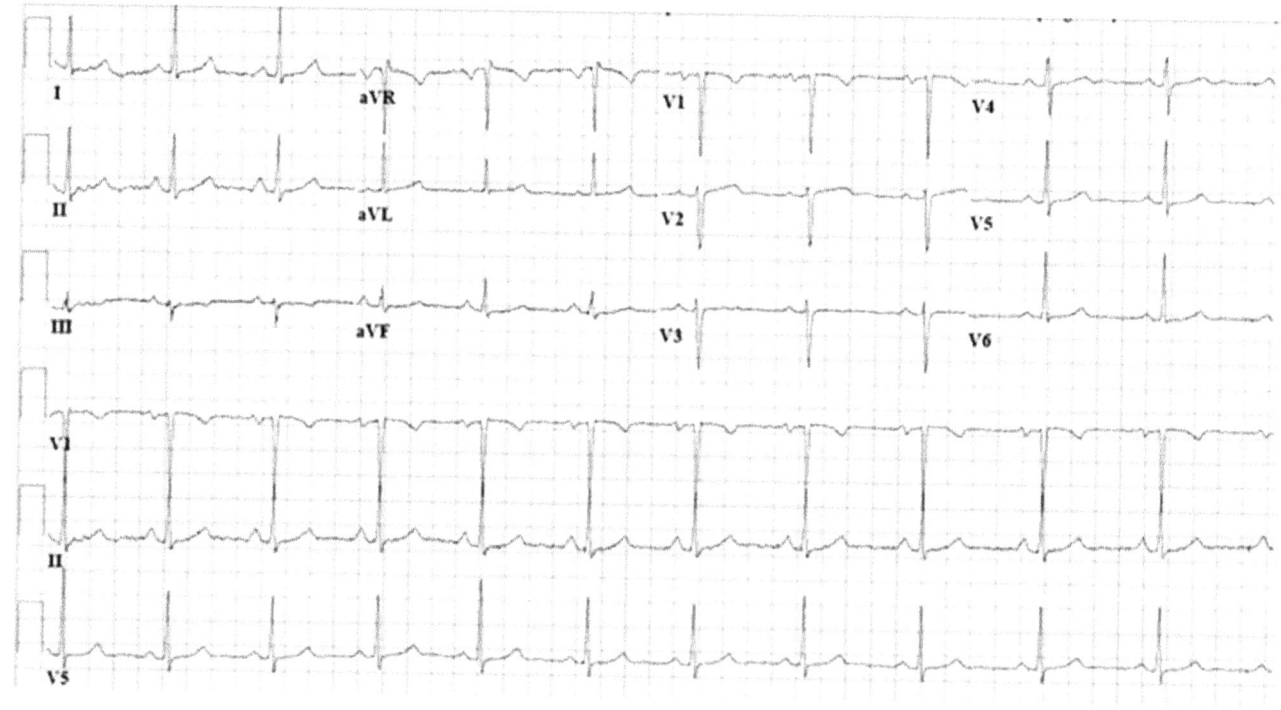

Figure 71.2

N. Action

a. Discussion with patient regarding diagnosis and instruction on vagal maneuvers
b. Follow-up with cardiology and PMD for further work-up

O. Diagnosis

a. Supraventricular tachycardia (SVT)

Case 71: Palpitations

P. Critical actions
a. Large-bore IV access
b. EKG
c. Discussion with patient regarding side effects of adenosine
d. Adenosine with rhythm strip – must specify a rapid push of adenosine
e. Repeat EKG and vitals after breaking rhythm

Q. Examiner instructions
a. This is a case of hemodynamically stable supraventricular tachycardia that responds to adenosine. This is a type of irregular rapid heart rate that is typically not dangerous and responds to treatment. The patient's main symptoms are palpitations and dizziness with stable vitals. Important early actions include large-bore IV access and EKG. After obtaining an EKG, the decision must be made to determine the rhythm. Upon conversion of the rhythm to a slow rate, the candidate must repeat the EKG and vital signs to ensure stability. The patient can be safely discharged once the rate is normal, and referred to a cardiologist for further assessment for the cause of the arrhythmia.

R. Pearls
a. Vagal maneuvers can be used before adenosine.
b. Adenosine must be given IV push rapidly in a large-gauge IV, as close to the heart as possible.
c. Should warn patient of adenosine side effects – flushing, sense of impending doom, dizziness.
d. Calcium channel blockers are another class of drugs that can be used.
    i. Diltiazem can be pushed.
    ii. Verapamil should be given at a slower rate (no IVP) and has more potential for blood pressure effects.
e. β-blockers is another class of drugs that can be used.
    i. Esmolol drip or propranolol
f. Cardioversion is required for unstable SVT.
g. If there is concern for myocardial ischemia as a cause for SVT, consider cardiac enzymes and admission or cardiology consult.

S. References
a. *Tintinalli's Emergency Medicine: A Comprehensive Study Guide* (9th ed.): Chapter 18, Cardiac Rhythm Disturbances.
b. *Rosen's Emergency Medicine: Concepts and Clinical Practice* (10th ed.): Chapter 65, Dysrhythmias.

Cough

Shawn Zhong, MD

A. Chief complaint

a. 45-year-old female brought in by friend, with shortness of breath, cough, and fever

B. Vital signs

a. BP: 78/32, HR: 125, RR: 30, T: 40.2°C, Sat: 90% on RA

C. What does the patient look like?

a. Patient appears stated age, tachypneic, moderate respiratory distress, somnolent, but awakens easily.

D. Primary survey

a. Airway: speaking in full sentences
b. Breathing: increased respiratory rate, moderate distress, no cyanosis
c. Circulation: warm, increased capillary refill

E. Action

a. Oxygen via NC or nonrebreather mask
b. Two large-bore peripheral IV lines
c. Labs
    i. CBC, BMP, LFT, coagulation studies, blood type and crossmatch
    ii. Lactate, blood cultures, urinalysis, urine culture
d. 2 L NS bolus
e. Monitor: BP: 77/40, HR: 112, RR: 26, Sat: 100% on nonrebreather mask
f. EKG
g. CXR

F. History

a. HPI: A 45-year-old female with no past medical history here with fever and shortness of breath for 3 days. Patient states symptoms started with a cough for 2 days but since yesterday with fevers of 40.2°C and chills. At times she feels like her entire body is shaking. Today she experienced increased shortness of breath, and had difficulty sleeping last night secondary to cough and shortness of breath. She denies any headache, nausea, vomiting, abdominal pain, or diarrhea. No recent travel. No hospitalizations within last 3 months (must ask).
b. PMHx: none
c. PSHx: none
d. Allergies: none
e. Meds: none

f. Social: denies alcohol use or illicit drug use; smokes one pack per day for 30 years; lives with boyfriend in apartment; sexually active without protection; tested negative for HIV 6 months ago

g. FHx: not relevant

h. PMD: none

G. Secondary survey

a. General: somnolent but arousable, oriented × 3, tachypneic, mild respiratory distress on oxygen

b. Head: normocephalic, atraumatic

c. Eyes: extraocular movement intact, pupils equal, reactive to light

d. Ears: normal tympanic membranes

e. Nose: no discharge

f. Neck: full range of motion, no jugular vein distension, no stridor

g. Pharynx: normal dentition, no lesions, no swelling

h. Chest: nontender

i. Lungs: crackles bilaterally, no wheezes/rhonchi

j. Heart: tachycardic, rhythm regular, no murmurs, rubs, or gallops

k. Abdomen: normal bowel sounds, soft, nontender or distended

l. Rectal: normal tone, brown stool, occult blood negative

m. Urogenital: normal external genitalia
   i. Female: no blood or discharge, cervical os closed, no cervical motion tenderness, no adnexal tenderness

n. Extremities: full range of motion, no deformity, normal pulses

o. Back: nontender

p. Neuro: cranial nerves II to XII intact; normal sensation, strength; normal reflexes and gait

q. Skin: warm and clammy

r. Lymph: no lymphadenopathy

H. Nurse

a. 2 L fluids
   i. BP: 110/78, HR: 110, RR: 20, Sat: 97% on NRM

b. 1 L fluids
   i. BP: 80/68, HR: 120, RR: 24, Sat: 97% on NRM

c. 1 L fluids with low dose norepinephrine (<3 mcg/kg/min) or neosynephrine (<30 mcg/min)
   i. BP: 108/64, HR: 110, RR: 22, Sat: 97% on NRM

d. No fluids
   i. BP: 62/48, HR: 130, RR: 28, Sat: 97% on NRM

I. Results

Table 72.1 Results table

Test	Result	Test	Result
Complete blood count:		T bili	1.0 mg/dL
WBC	$17.2 \times 10^3/\mu L$	D bili	0.3 mg/dL
Diff	92% N/6 bands	Amylase	50 U/L
Hct	39.50%	Lipase	25 U/L
Plt	$350 \times 10^3/\mu L$	Albumin	4.7 g/dL

Table 72.1 (cont.)

Test	Result	Test	Result
Basic metabolic panel:		**Urinalysis:**	
Na	138 mEq/L	SG	1.010–1.030
K	4.3 mEq/L	pH	5–8
Cl	105 mEq/L	Prot	Neg
CO_2	30 mEq/L	Gluc	Neg
BUN	32 mEq/dL	Ketones	Neg
Cr	1.1 mg/dL	Bili	Neg
Gluc	100 mg/dL	Blood	Neg
		LE	Neg
Coagulation panel:		Nitrite	Neg
PT	12.6 sec	Color	Yellow
PTT	26.0 sec		
INR	1.0	**Arterial blood gas:**	
		pH	7.35
Liver function panel:		pO_2	65 mmHg
AST	23 U/L	pCO_2	35 mmHg
ALT	26 U/L	HCO_3	20 mmol/L
Alk phos	42 U/L		

a. Lactate: 2 mmol/L
b. CXR
c. EKG sinus tachycardia

J. Action
a. Respiratory support: high-flow nasal cannula
b. Meds
    i. Levofloxacin or moxifloxacin, or
    ii. beta-lactam (ceftriaxone or cefotaxime or ceftaroline or ampicillin–sulbactam or ertapenem) *and* macrolide (azithromycin, clarithromycin, erythromycin) or doxycycline
c. Admit patient to ICU for IV antibiotics (patient's pneumonia severity index is 120, placing them in class IV. This is associated with a 8.2–9.3% mortality risk.)

K. Diagnosis
a. Community-acquired pneumonia

L. Critical actions
a. IV access
b. NS fluid bolus >2 L
c. CXR

d. Antibiotics

e. Admission

M. Examiner instructions

a. This is a case of community-acquired pneumonia in a healthy patient without medical problems. Pneumonia is most commonly a bacterial infection of the lungs that needs treatment with antibiotics. The seriousness of the infection relates to both the type of bacteria and the patient's ability to fight infection (medical history and age). Early actions with our patient include the recognition and treatment of abnormal vital signs, low blood pressure, high pulse, and low oxygen saturation despite supplemental oxygen and generous IV fluids. If the provider only gives 1 L of fluids, the BP should remain low and will only increase with more fluids or pressors. CXR should be taken, antibiotics should be given early, and the patient will need to be admitted to the ICU for antibiotics, given the severity of pneumonia represented by vital signs.

N. Pearls

a. Obtain CXR early.

b. Antibiotics should be given early.

c. If blood cultures are sent, antibiotics should be started ideally after the cultures are drawn.

d. In a patient who appears septic, use lactate to help guide treatment.

e. Risk classification guides such as the pneumonia severity index can be used to help identify patients at risk for mortality, but ultimately clinical judgment should be used.

O. References

a. *Tintinalli's Emergency Medicine: A Comprehensive Study Guide* (9th ed.): Chapter 65, Community-Acquired Pneumonia, Aspiration Pneumonia, and Noninfectious Pulmonary Infiltrates. Chapter 12, Approach to Nontraumatic Shock.

b. *Rosen's Emergency Medicine: Concepts and Clinical Practice* (10th ed.): Chapter 62, Pneumonia. Chapter 3, Shock.

Drowning

Shawn Zhong, MD

A. Chief complaint

a. 27-year-old male brought in by EMS after diving into the shallow end of a pool and losing consciousness, was immediately rescued by lifeguards, no CPR needed, unable to move arms and legs immediately after, complains of neck pain, immobilized with a C collar and backboard

B. Vital signs

a. BP: 90/40, HR: 65, RR: 15, T: 36.2°C, Sat: 98% on RA

C. What does the patient look like?

a. Patient appears stated age, lying on stretcher, wet from the pool, and not moving.

D. Primary survey

a. Airway: speaking in full sentences
b. Breathing: no apparent respiratory distress, no cyanosis
c. Circulation: warm and well perfused
d. Disability
    i. Opens eyes to commands, able to abduct arms and flex biceps but minimal extension of arms; no other movement in four extremities; CN grossly intact
    ii. Sensation intact in all extremities
e. Exposure: no other obvious injuries/deformities noted

E. Action

a. Oxygen via NC or nonrebreather mask
b. Two large-bore peripheral IV lines
c. Remove wet clothing
d. Labs
    i. CBC, BMP, LFT, coagulation studies, blood type and crossmatch
e. Fluids
    i. If no fluids given, BP: 72/32, HR: 55, RR: 26, Sat: 100% on 2 L
    ii. If 1 L fluids given, BP: 82/42, HR: 55, RR: 24, Sat: 100% on 2 L
    iii. If 1 L fluid and 1 unit pRBC given or vasopressors given, BP 92/52, HR 55, RR: 22, Sat: 100% on 2 L
f. FAST (Figure 73.1)
g. Imaging
    i. CT scan of head and C-spine
    ii. CT scan of neck, chest, abdomen, and pelvis with IV contrast

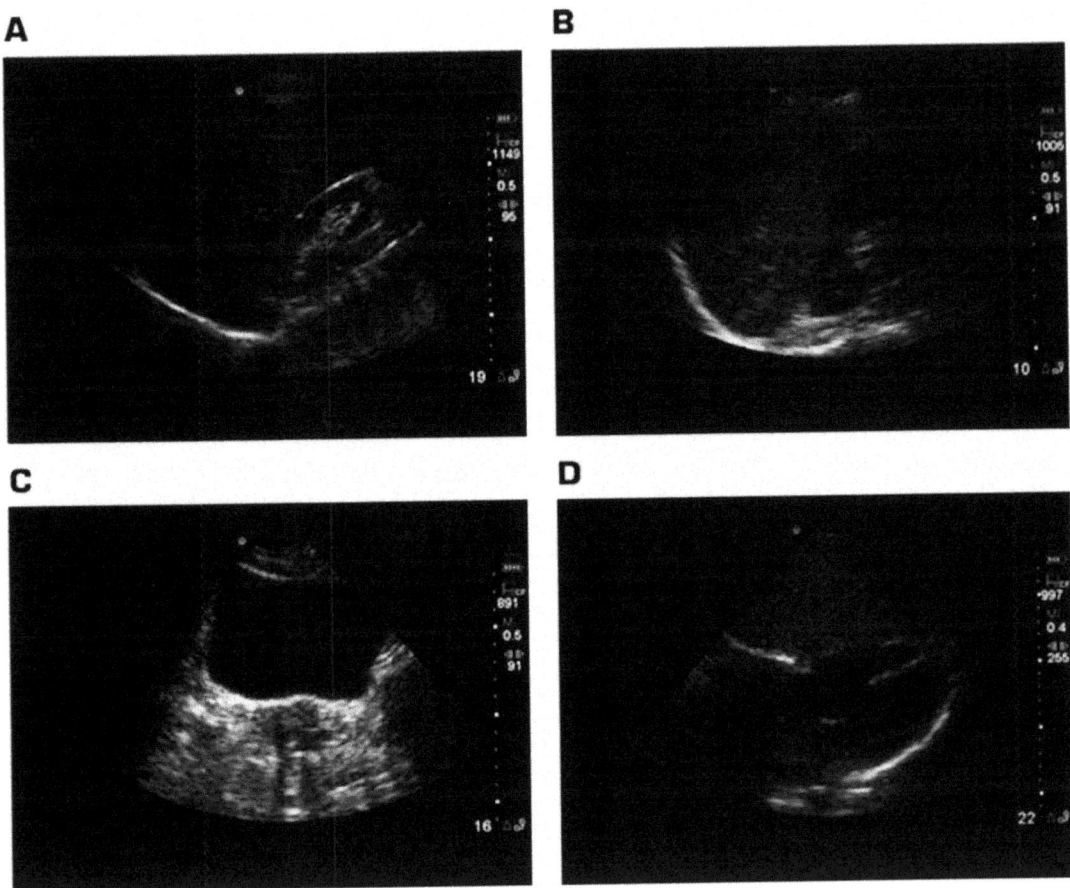

Figure 73.1

  iii. CXR

  iv. Pelvis x-ray

 h. Trauma surgery (trauma activation or consult)

F. History

a. HPI: A 27-year-old male with no past medical history. Patient was at local pool and dove into the shallow end. He lost consciousness, was rescued by lifeguard, and awoke unable to move. Bystanders called EMS; currently states that he cannot move his extremities below his shoulders; denies headache, nausea, vomiting, blurry vision, chest pain, or shortness of breath.

b. PMHx: none

c. PSHx: none

d. Allergies: no known drug allergies

e. Social: lives with wife, no children; denies smoking; drinks socially; denies illicit drug use

f. FHx: DM in father

G. Secondary survey

a. General: alert, oriented × 3, very anxious

b. Head: 4 cm contusion to forehead, no stepoffs

c. Eyes: extraocular movement intact, pupils equal, reactive to light

d. Ears: normal tympanic membranes

e. Nose: no discharge

f. Neck: no stridor, C collar in place

g. Pharynx: normal dentition, no lesions, no swelling
h. Chest: no evidence of trauma
i. Lungs: clear bilaterally
j. Heart: rate and rhythm regular, no murmurs, rubs, or gallops
k. Abdomen: normal bowel sounds, soft, nontender, distended suprapubically
l. Rectal: no tone, brown stool, occult blood negative, incontinent of stool
m. Urogenital: normal external genitalia
   i. Male: no discharge, normal testicular examination
n. Extremities: no deformity, normal pulses
o. Back: no evidence of trauma; unable to feel
p. Neuro: cranial nerves II to XII intact; opens eyes to commands, able to abduct arms and flex biceps but minimal extension of arms bilaterally; 0/5 motor strength of lower extremities, no sensation of lower extremities, decreased sensation below C5 dermatome, upgoing toes bilaterally
q. Skin: warm and dry (cover patient with blanket)
r. Lymph: no lymphadenopathy

H. Nurse
a. Vitals
   i. BP: 92/50, HR: 55, RR: 28, Sat: 98% on O_2; increase use of intercostals

I. Results

Table 73.1 Results table

Test	Result	Test	Result
Complete blood count:		**Liver function panel:**	
WBC	$5.3 \times 10^3/\mu L$	AST	23 U/L
Hct	41.5%	ALT	26 U/L
Plt	$350 \times 10^3/\mu L$	Alk phos	42 U/L
		T bili	1.0 mg/dL
Basic metabolic panel:		D bili	0.3 mg/dL
Na	138 mEq/L	Amylase	50 U/L
K	4.3 mEq/L	Lipase	25 U/L
Cl	105 mEq/L	Albumin	4.7 g/dL
CO_2	30 mEq/L		
BUN	12 mEq/dL	**Urinalysis:**	
Cr	1.1 mg/dL	SG	1.010–1.030
Gluc	100 mg/dL	pH	5–8
		Prot	Neg
Coagulation panel:		Gluc	Neg
PT	12.6 sec	Ketones	Neg
PTT	26.0 sec	Bili	Neg

Table 73.1 (cont.)

Test	Result	Test	Result
INR	1.0	Blood	Neg
		LE	Neg
		Nitrite	Neg
		Color	Yellow

a. CXR (Figure 73.2)
b. Pelvic x-ray (Figure 73.3)
c. CT C-spine (Figure 73.4)
   i. C4 burst fracture into canal
d. CT head, chest, abdomen, pelvis – negative
e. Repeat vitals
   i. BP: 90/48, HR: 70, RR: 32, Sat: 98% on O_2; shallow breaths; intercostal muscle use very visible

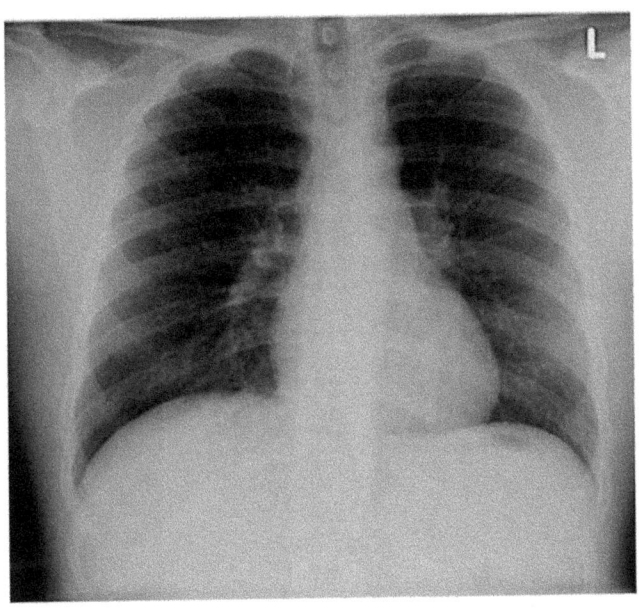

Figure 73.2

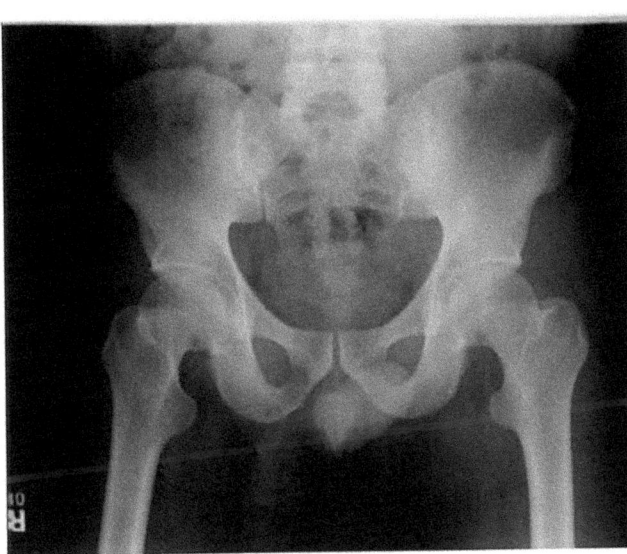

Figure 73.3

A   **B**

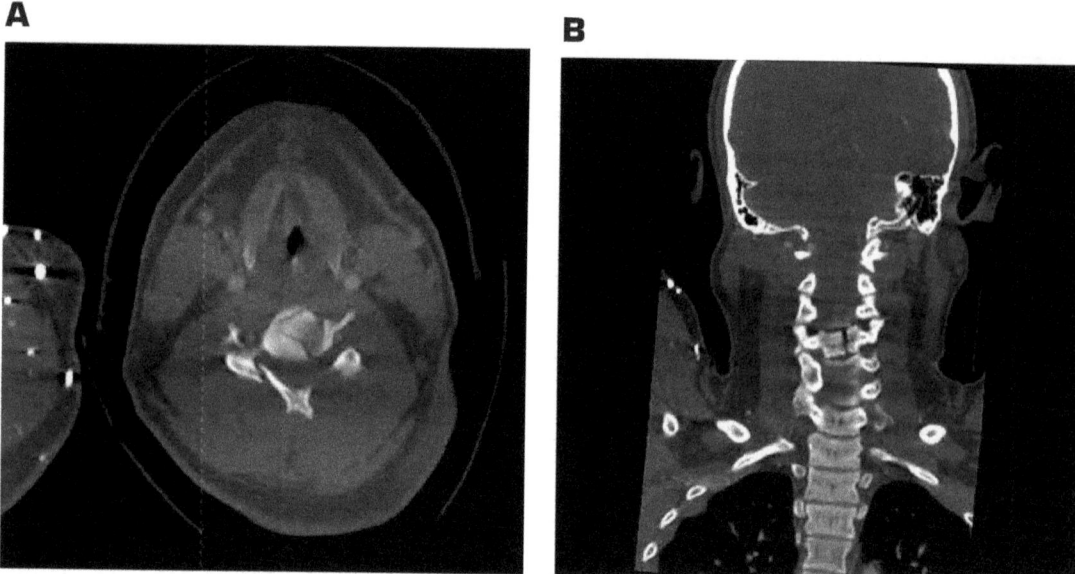

Figure 73.4

J. Action

a. Discussion with patient regarding results of CT and need for intubation given concern for inability of the diaphragm to sustain work of breathing

b. Consult
   i. Neurosurgery

c. Intubate
   i. Maintain C-spine immobilization
   ii. Intubation successful

K. Nurse

a. BP: 82/42, HR: 45, Sat: 100% on mechanical ventilation

L. Action

a. ICU consult

b. Start vasopressors (norepinephrine preferred) or increase if already started

M. Diagnosis

a. C-spine fracture

b. Spinal cord injury

c. Neurogenic shock

N. Critical actions

a. Large-bore IV access and fluid/blood administration. Shock in trauma must be treated as hemorrhagic shock until proven otherwise.

b. C-spine precautions

c. CT C-spine

d. Neurosurgery consult

e. Intubation

f. Recognition of neurogenic shock and treatment with vasopressors. Candidate should not identify as spinal shock as that is a separate entity.

O. Examiner instructions

a. This is a case of spinal cord injury and neurogenic shock after a cervical spine fracture. This is a devastating injury to the neck that leads to quadriplegia. In this patient, the injury to the spinal cord has led to damage of associated nerves that maintain blood pressure and breathing. Initial actions should be aimed at the trauma assessment of this injured patient, including fluid/blood administration for trauma shock, FAST, surgery consult, CT of the head, neck, chest, abdomen, and pelvis. Fluids should be limited and intravascular volume should be replaced by blood product administration as part of the initial trauma work-up. If the candidate makes the diagnosis of neurogenic shock early, they may give blood product or vasopressors, and the blood pressure will improve. It is important to note that neurogenic shock is an uncommon cause of hypotension in trauma patients and should be made after other etiologies such as hemorrhage or tension pneumothorax have been excluded. In this case, all work-up will be negative except for the cervical spine injury that should necessitate an emergent neurosurgery consultation. Steroids should not be administered. Once the candidate has established that this is a case of neurogenic shock, they must administer vasopressors (norepinephrine preferred). The patient is hypotensive secondary to neurogenic shock but should have fluids/blood transfusion initially as part of the trauma work-up and ultimately vasopressors to treat the neurogenic shock. If the patient is not started on vasopressors, he should become more hypotensive. The patient will also need intubation given increased work of breathing from lack of function of the diaphragm from his spinal cord injury. If the patient is not intubated, he will become more short of breath and hypoxic. The patient will need to be admitted to the ICU.

P. Pearls

a. In blunt trauma, spinal injuries should be presumed and should be treated as unstable until proven otherwise – maintain C-spine immobilization.
b. Hypotension in trauma should be treated with fluids and blood initially.
c. Neurogenic shock can occur in injuries above T6 – hypotension and bradycardia.
d. Neurogenic shock is manifested by hemodynamic changes (hypotension and bradycardia) due to loss of autonomic tone after a spinal cord injury. Severe neurogenic shock is more likely to occur in high cervical injuries and may not respond to fluid/blood challenge and requires vasopressors (norepinephrine preferred).
e. Diaphragm involvement (caused by phrenic nerve injury from lesions above C5) can occur and respiratory failure must be anticipated.
f. Steroids should not be used.

Q. Figure legends

a. Figure 73.1 FAST exam images (a) RUQ, (b) LUQ, (c) bladder, (d) cardiac.
b. Figure 73.2 Chest x-ray.
c. Figure 73.3 Normal Pelvis x-ray.
d. Figure 73.4 CT C-spine.

R. References

a. *Tintinalli's Emergency Medicine: A Comprehensive Study Guide* (9th ed.): Chapter 215, Drowning. Chapter 258, Spine Trauma.
b. *Rosen's Emergency Medicine: Concepts and Clinical Practice* (10th ed.): Chapter 133, Drowning. Chapter 35, Spinal Trauma.

Abdominal Pain

Javier Rosario, MD and Sheler Sadati, MD

A. Chief complaint
a. 61-year-old man brought in by EMS for severe epigastric pain for 1 day as well as 4 hours of nausea and vomiting

B. Vital signs
a. BP: 95/65, HR: 112, RR: 20, T: 38.3°C, Sat: 95% on RA

C. What does the patient look like?
a. Patient appears in moderate distress due to pain; refuses to lie down on the stretcher.

D. Primary survey
a. Airway: speaks full sentences
b. Breathing: no apparent respiratory distress; no cyanosis
c. Circulation: slightly diaphoretic; normal capillary refill

E. Action
a. Oxygen via NC or nonrebreather mask
b. Two large-bore peripheral IV lines
c. Labs
    i. CBC, BMP, LFT, coagulation studies, blood type and crossmatch
    ii. Lactate, blood cultures, urinalysis, urine culture, EtOH level
d. 1 L NS bolus
e. Monitor: BP: 95/65, HR: 112, RR: 20, T: 38.3°C, Sat: 99% on NC
f. EKG
g. Image
    i. Upright CXR

F. History
a. HPI: A 61-year-old man with past medical history of hypertension, high cholesterol, and hypertriglyceridemia presents with severe epigastric pain for the past day. The pain started yesterday after lunchtime. The patient reports that he was at a local fast-food restaurant with his wife right before the symptoms started. He reports feeling "fine" until about 3 hours after eating. Patient describes the pain as sharp and stabbing, radiating to his back associated with nausea. He reports history of frequent "heartburn" after eating, but never this severe. He reports four episodes of nonbilious, nonbloody vomiting since the pain started; no diarrhea; no blood per rectum; denies fever or chills; denies any urinary symptoms or flank pain; denies similar episodes of pain in the past; denies recent alcohol consumption; denies any insect or scorpion bites.

b. PMHx: hypertension, hypertriglyceridemia
c. PSHx: appendectomy 40 years ago
d. Allergies: none
e. Meds: noncompliant
f. Social: married 30 years; smoker (30 packs/year), drinks alcohol occasionally (once every 2–3 months); denies any drug abuse
g. FHx: mother with hypertension
h. PMD: Dr. Peterson

G. Nurse
a. Fluids
  i. BP: 106/67, HR: 110, RR: 20, Sat: 99% on NC
b. No fluids
  i. BP: 86/57, HR: 120, RR: 20, Sat: 99% on NC
c. EKG (Figure 74.1)
d. CXR (Figure 74.2) negative for free air under diaphragm

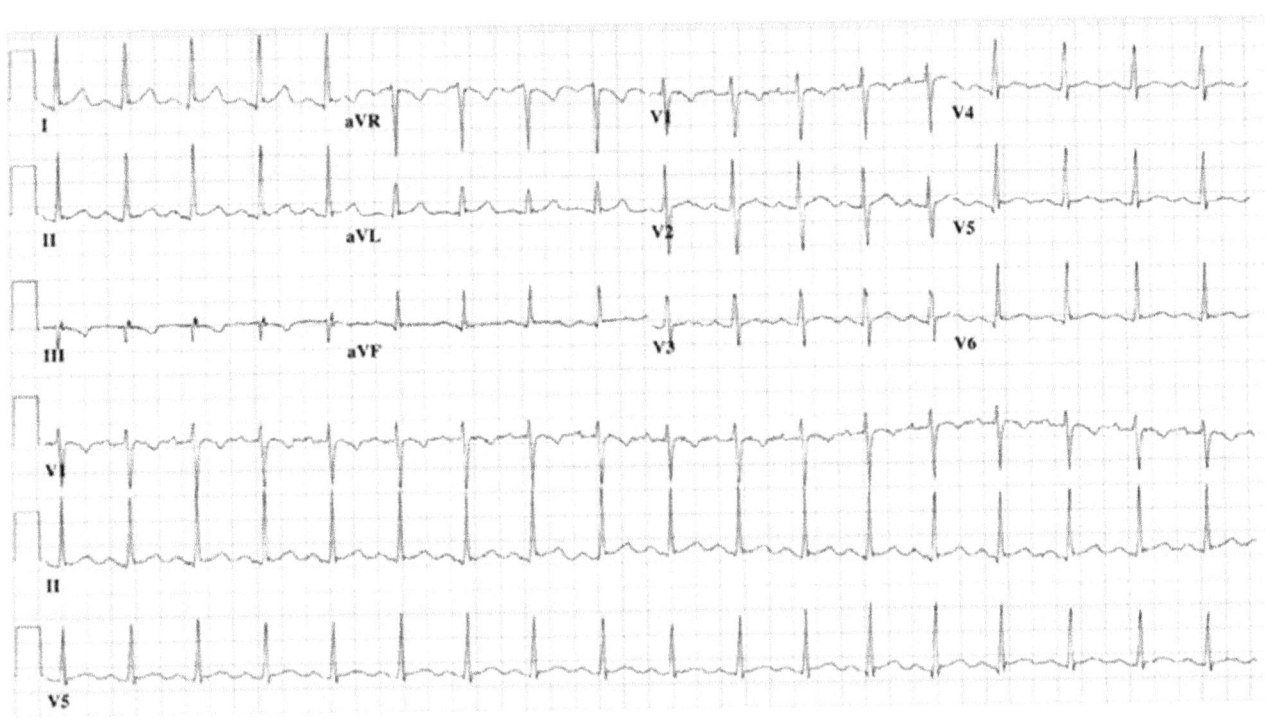

Figure 74.1

H. Secondary survey
a. General: alert, oriented × 3, appears in severe distress and uncomfortable due to pain
b. Head: normocephalic, atraumatic
c. Eyes: extraocular movement intact, pupils equal, reactive to light, mild icteric conjunctivae
d. Ears: normal tympanic membranes
e. Nose: no discharge
f. Neck: full range of motion, no jugular vein distension, no stridor
g. Pharynx: normal dentition, no lesions, no swelling
h. Chest: nontender
i. Lungs: clear bilaterally

B

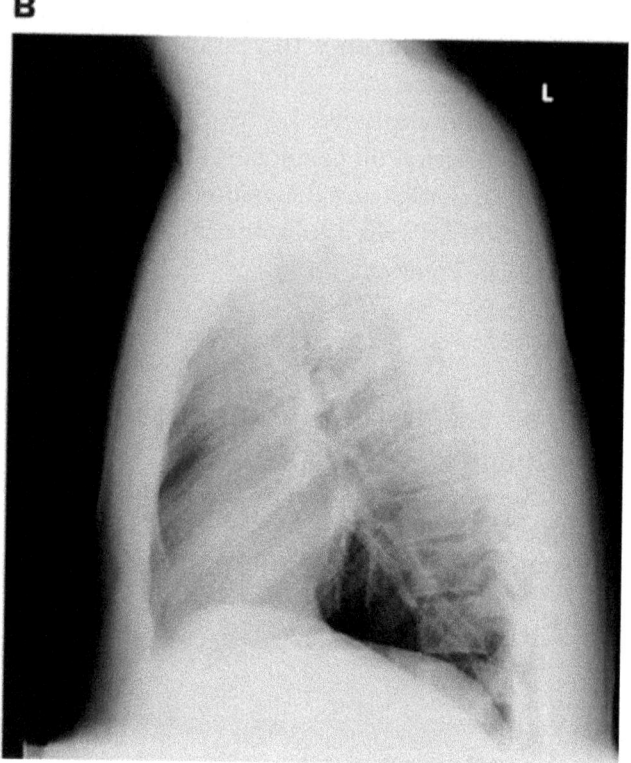

A

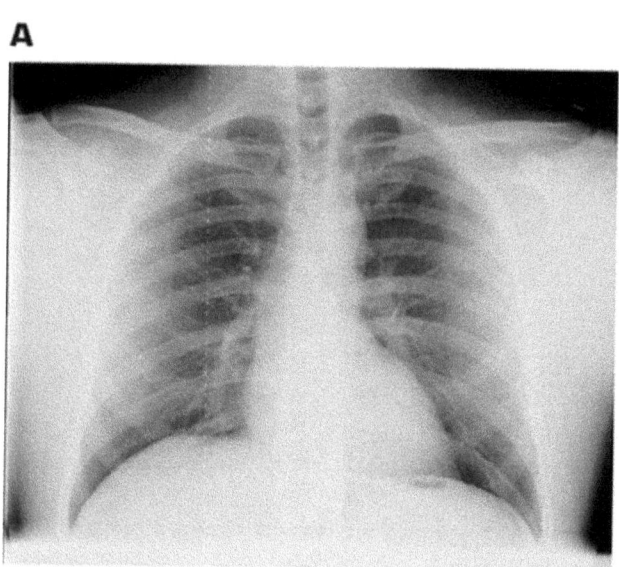

Figure 74.2

j. Heart: tachycardic rate, rhythm regular, no murmurs, rubs, or gallops
k. Abdomen: bowel sounds hypoactive, mildly distended, obese, tenderness in epigastric area and RUQ with guarding; no rebound; no rigidity; positive Murphy's sign
l. Rectal: normal tone, brown stool, occult blood negative
m. Urogenital: normal external genitalia
   i. Male: no discharge, normal testicular examination
n. Extremities: full range of motion, no deformity, normal pulses
o. Back: nontender
p. Neuro: cranial nerves II to XII intact; normal sensation, strength; normal reflexes and gait
q. Skin: warm and dry, slight jaundice
r. Lymph: no lymphadenopathy

I. Results

Table 74.1 Results table

Test	Result	Test	Result
Complete blood count:		**Liver function panel:**	
WBC	$17.4 \times 10^3/\mu L$	AST	93 U/L
Hct	38%	ALT	150 U/L
Plt	$350 \times 10^3/\mu L$	Alk phos	210 U/L
		T bili	4.3 mg/dL
Basic metabolic panel:		D bili	3.1 mg/dL
Na	138 mEq/L	Lipase	3120 U/L

Table 74.1 (cont.)

Test	Result	Test	Result
K	4.3 mEq/L	Albumin	4.7 g/dL
Cl	105 mEq/L		
CO_2	30 mEq/L	**Urinalysis:**	
BUN	34 mEq/dL	SG	1.010–1.030
Cr	1.1 mg/dL	pH	5–8
Gluc	256 mg/dL	Prot	Neg
		Gluc	Neg
Coagulation panel:		Ketones	Neg
PT	12.6 sec	Bili	+
PTT	26.0 sec	Blood	Neg
INR	1.4	LE	Neg
		Nitrite	Neg
		Color	Yellow

a. Calcium: 7.8 mg/dL
b. Lipid panel: triglycerides 210 mg/dL

J. Action
a. Meds
   i. IV morphine (or IV fentanyl if concerned about hypotension)
   ii. Acetaminophen
   iii. IV antiemetics
b. Imaging
   i. RUQ US: bedside or radiology department (Figure 74.3)
   ii. CT abdomen and pelvis with contrast (optional)
c. NPO
d. 2 L NS

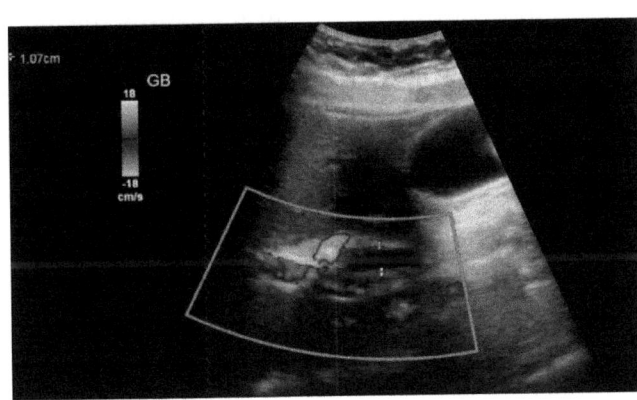 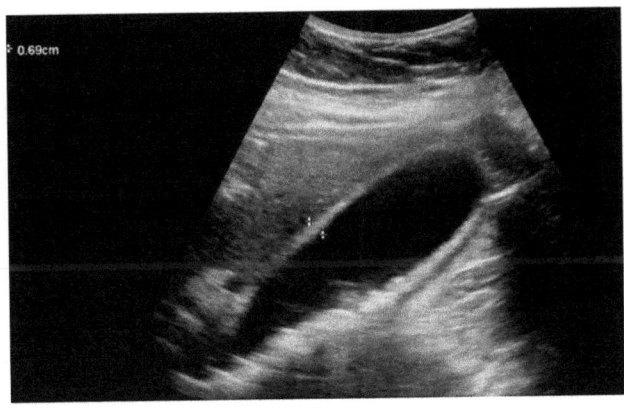

Figure 74.3

K. Nurse

a. BP: 100/67, HR: 90, RR: 20, Sat: 99% on NC
b. Patient: improvement of pain
c. RUQ US: bedside or radiology report: cholecystitis; dilated common bile duct
d. CT abdomen and pelvis with contrast (optional): peripancreatic inflammatory changes without necrosis or abscess; cholecystitis with common bile duct dilation and possible stone in biliary duct

L. Action

a. Consult surgery: admission for IV antibiotics, possible cholecystectomy after endoscopic retrograde cholangiopancreatography (ERCP)
b. Consult gastroenterology: will schedule patient for ERCP
c. IV antibiotics (piperacillin/tazobactam, ertapenem, or metronidazole + ceftriaxone)
d. Discussion with patient regarding diagnosis and surgery

M. Diagnosis

a. Pancreatitis due to gallstones (gallstone pancreatitis)

N. Critical actions

a. 2 L IV NS
b. Ultrasound
c. Pain medication: opiates
d. Surgical consultation
e. Intravenous antibiotics

O. Examiner instructions

a. This is a case of pancreatitis due to gallstones (gallstone pancreatitis) in a patient with a history of frequent "heartburn" after eating. These episodes of "heartburn" were likely episodes of biliary colic. Pancreatitis is an inflammation of the pancreas typically caused by heavy alcohol consumption, gallstones, or hypertriglyceridemia in the United States. As in our patient, the pain is typically sharp and constant in nature, radiating to the back, and associated with nausea and vomiting. If the patient does not receive opioid pain medications, he should start getting more upset and agitated. If the patient does not get at least 2 L of fluids, the blood pressure will decline and the patient will become more agitated. The patient should ultimately be admitted to the hospital, receive antibiotics covering GI pathogens (i.e., piperacillin/tazobactam, ertapenem, or metronidazole + ceftriaxone), while surgery and gastroenterology are consulted, and be kept NPO (no food or drink by mouth, to allow the pancreas to rest).

P. Pearls

a. The degree of elevation in amylase and lipase does not correlate with severity of the disease.
b. Ranson's criteria is just a tool for prognosis and does not change the emergency management of these patients.
c. These patients require aggressive fluid resuscitation due to sequestration of large volumes of fluid in the retroperitoneum.
d. Bluish discoloration in the left flank (Turner's sign) and around the umbilicus (Cullen's sign) are rarely seen, but indicate hemorrhagic pancreatitis.
e. Ultrasound is the imaging modality of choice for acute cholecystitis diagnosis.

f. In patients with acute pancreatitis where biliary disease has not been excluded, an ultrasound of the gallbladder should be strongly considered.

g. CT scan is not a sensitive test to diagnose pancreatitis. It is most useful to rule out complications such as pancreatic phlegmon or abscess.

h. Patients with chronic pancreatitis do not usually have elevation of pancreatic enzymes due to chronic damage to the organ.

i. The most common causes of acute pancreatitis are ethanol, gallstones, and hypertriglyceridemia.

j. Hypertriglyceridemia (generally >1000 mg/dL) can cause pancreatitis and would be treated with insulin.

k. Patients with gallstone pancreatitis need urgent surgical consultation for cholecystectomy and admission.

l. The most common electrolyte abnormality is hypocalcemia.

m. Causes of mortality include ARDS, hemorrhagic shock, sepsis, and DIC.

Q. Figure legends

a. Figure 74.1 (EKG) Sinus tachycardia.

b. Figure 74.2 (CXR) Normal chest X-ray; no air under diaphragm.

c. Figure 74.3 (Ultrasound) (a) Acute cholecystitis with thickening of the gallbladder wall, pericholecystic fluid, multiple gallstones. (b) Dilated common bile duct.

R. References

a. *Rosen's Emergency Medicine: Concepts and Clinical Practice* (9th ed.): Chapter 81, Pancreas.

b. *Tintinalli's Emergency Medicine: A Comprehensive Study Guide* (9th ed.): Chapter 77, Pancreas. Chapter 76, Liver and Biliary Tract Disorders.

Abdominal Pain

David H. Cisewski, MD

A. Chief complaint
a. 73-year-old female presents with the sudden onset of diffuse abdominal pain

B. Vital signs
a. BP: 116/91, HR: 121, RR: 16, T: 37.9°C, Sat: 97% on RA, FS: 129 mg/dL (must ask)

C. What does the patient look like?
a. Patient appears in pain, clutching stomach, laying in a lateral decubitus position, writhing in pain as she moves from side to side due to the discomfort.

D. Primary survey
a. Airway: speaking in full sentences, phonating well
b. Breathing: no apparent respiratory distress, noncyanotic
c. Circulation: pulses full in upper and lower extremities, skin warm and well perfused; normal capillary refill; if asked, pulses are irregular

E. Action
a. Oxygen: delivery via peripheral nasal canula or nonrebreather mask
b. Intravenous access: two large-bore peripheral IV lines placed
c. Cardiac monitor
    i. BP: 135/86, HR: 115, RR: 16, Sat: 100% on O_2
    ii. Irregular rhythm on monitor with narrow complexes
d. Labs
    i. CBC, BMP, LFT, lipase, coagulation studies (PT/INR, PTT), troponin, blood type and crossmatch
    ii. Venous blood gas, serum lactate
e. Intravenous fluid: 1 L intravenous fluid bolus (normal saline, Ringer's lactate, or Plasmalyte)
f. EKG

F. History
a. HPI: A 73-year-old female with a history of diabetes, hypertension, and hyperlipidemia presents with the sudden onset of cramping and diffuse abdominal pain that began 2 hours prior to arrival. The pain was sudden in onset in the setting of walking her dog, severity 10/10, maximal at onset, with one episode of diarrhea consisting of dark, watery stool 30 minutes prior to arrival. Patient currently has nausea without vomiting. Patient denies dysuria or hematuria. Patient has been compliant with her medications and was in her usual state of health prior to this episode.

b. PMHx: diabetes, hypertension, hyperlipidemia; history of palpitations 10 years ago without a formal diagnosis
c. PSHx: appendectomy, cholecystectomy
d. Allergies: seasonal allergies, no known drug allergies
e. Meds: metformin, atorvastatin, aspirin
f. Social: 1–2 drinks per week (socially); denies smoking or illicit drug use
g. FHx: father and mother had adult-onset hypertension and diabetes

G. Nurse
a. EKG (Figure 75.1)
b. Patient still with pain

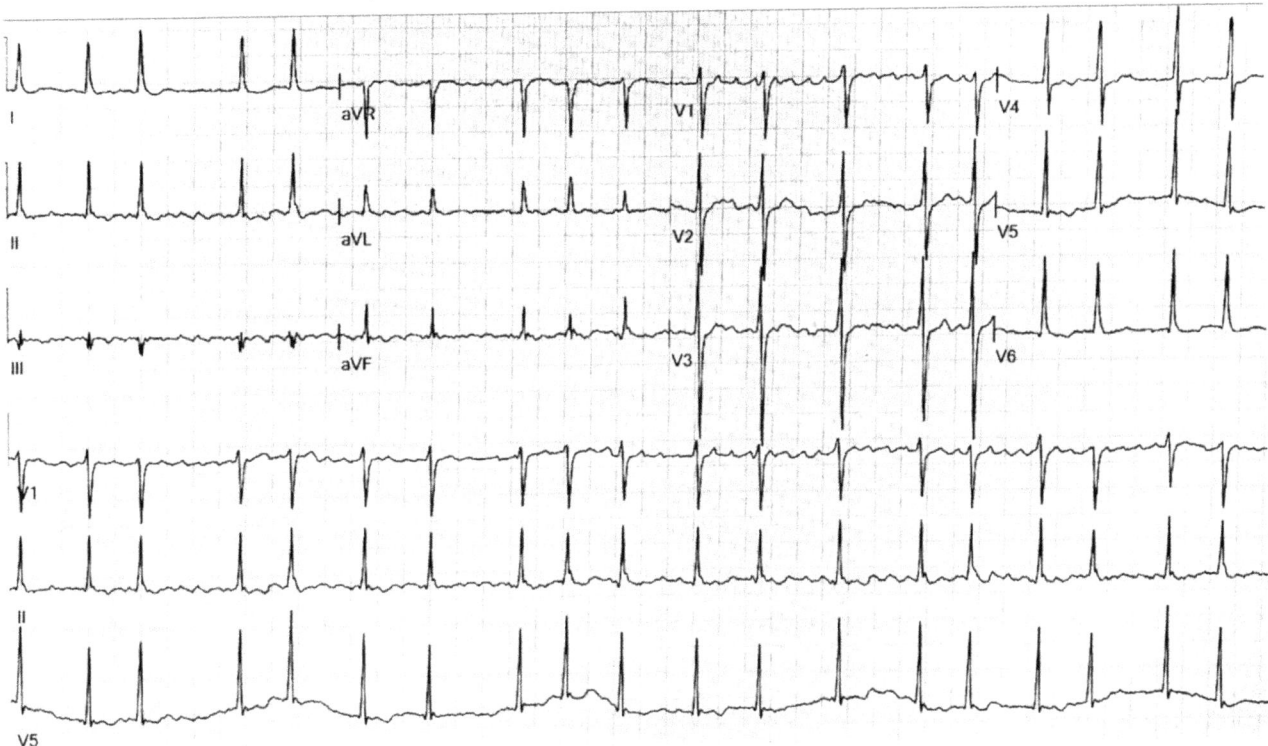

Figure 75.1

H. Secondary survey
a. General: alert, oriented × 3, appears in moderate distress due to abdominal pain
b. Head: normocephalic, atraumatic
c. Eyes: extraocular movement intact, pupils equal and reactive to light
d. Ears: tympanic membranes nonbulging, nonerythematous
e. Nose: clear; no rhinorrhea or discharge
f. Neck: full range of motion, no jugular vein distension, no stridor, no carotid bruit
g. Pharynx: normal dentition, no lesions, no swelling
h. Chest: nontender, no overlying rashes or erythema
i. Lungs: breath sounds equal bilaterally, clear to auscultation bilaterally
j. Heart: tachycardic, irregular rhythm, no rubs or gallops
k. Abdomen: soft, nondistended, bowel sounds normoactive, mild tenderness to palpation diffusely, no rebound or guarding, no costovertebral angle tenderness
l. Rectal: normal tone, brown stool, fecal occult blood positive

m. Urogenital: normal external genitalia
n. Vaginal: no bleeding or discharge
o. Extremities: full range of motion, no deformity, normal pulses
p. Back: no central spinal tenderness, no stepoffs
q. Neuro: cranial nerves II to XII intact; normal sensation, strength; normal reflexes and gait
r. Skin: warm, mildly diaphoretic, no rashes or erythema
s. Lymph: no lymphadenopathy

I. Action

a. Medication
    i. Fentanyl IV (or morphine IV)
    ii. Ceftriaxone IV (or ciprofloxacin)
    iii. Metronidazole IV
b. Imaging
    i. Upright chest radiograph (Figure 75.2) and abdominal series (Figure 75.3)
    ii. CT-angiography: abdomen

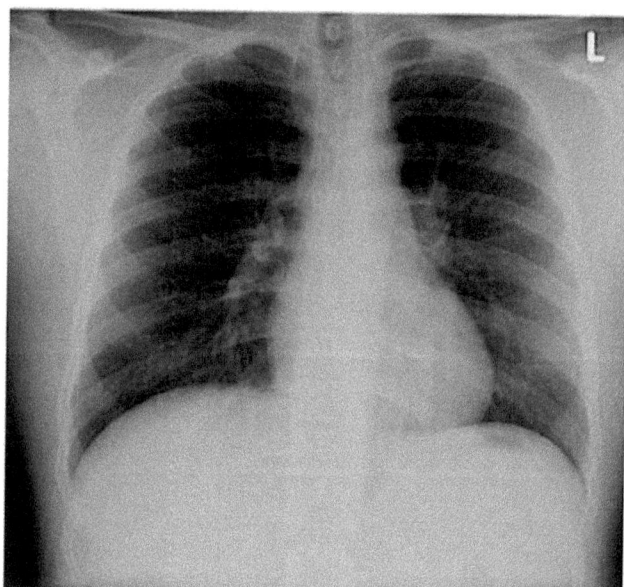

Figure 75.2

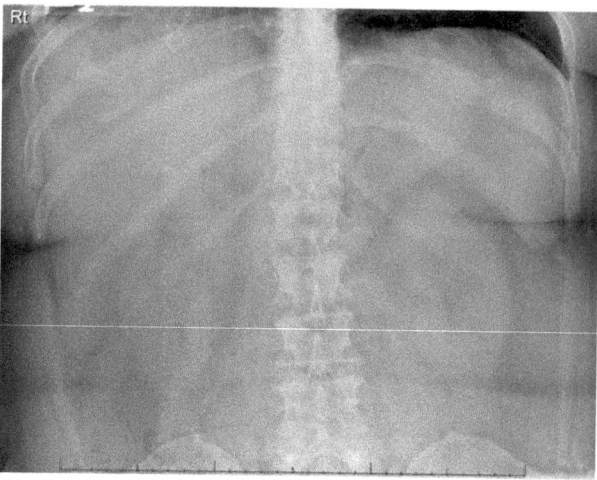
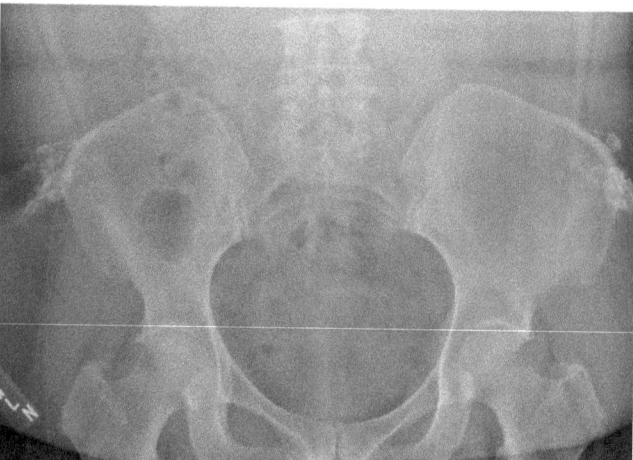

Figure 75.3

Case 75: Abdominal Pain

J. Nurse
a. Chest radiograph (Figure 75.2)
b. Abdominal series (Figure 75.3)
c. CT-angiography demonstrates superior mesenteric arterial thrombus located 3 cm distal to the abdominal aorta, pneumatosis intestinalis, and bowel wall thickening along the ascending colon with continuation midway through the transverse colon

K. Results

Table 75.1 Results table

Test	Result	Test	Result
Complete blood count:		D bili	0.3 mg/dL
WBC	$14.9 \times 10^3/\mu L$	Amylase	120 U/L
Hct	38%	Lipase	65 U/L
Plt	$350 \times 10^3/\mu L$	Albumin	4.7 g/dL
Basic metabolic panel:		**Urinalysis:**	
Na	138 mEq/L	SG	1.010–1.030
K	3.3 mEq/L	pH	5–8
Cl	105 mEq/L	Prot	Neg
CO_2	18 mEq/L	Gluc	Neg
BUN	32 mEq/dL	Ketones	Neg
Cr	1.2 mg/dL	Bili	Neg
Gluc	120 mg/dL	Blood	Neg
		LE	Neg
Coagulation panel:		Nitrite	Neg
PT	12.6 sec	Color	Yellow
PTT	26.0 sec		
INR	1.0	**Arterial blood gas:**	
		pH	7.4
Liver function panel:		pO_2	95 mmHg
AST	23 U/L	pCO_2	41 mmHg
ALT	26 U/L	HCO_3	24 mmol/L
Alk phos	42 U/L		
T bili	1.0 mg/dL		

a. Lactate: 6.2 mmol/L

L. Action
a. Consult requests
   i. General surgery (or vascular surgery) for possible embolectomy

  ii. Interventional radiology for possible catheter-directed intervention

  iii. ICU consult regarding plan for admission

 b. Discussion with patient regarding diagnosis and plan for admission and potential surgical intervention

 c. Intravenous unfractionated heparin (80 units/kg bolus followed by an infusion at 18 units/kg/hr)

 d. Analgesia – fentanyl (or morphine)

 e. NPO

 f. Intravenous fluid, continuous

M. Diagnosis

 a. Acute mesenteric ischemia secondary to embolism to superior mesenteric artery

N. Critical actions

 a. IV fluid: 1–2 L normal saline, Ringer's lactate, or Plasmalyte

 b. CT-angiography of abdomen and pelvis

 c. Antibiotics: ceftriaxone (or ciprofloxacin) and metronidazole

 d. IV unfractionated heparin (80 units/kg bolus followed by an infusion at 18 units/kg/hr)

 e. Surgery consult or interventional radiology consult

 f. Analgesic medication: IV fentanyl or morphine

O. Examiner instructions

 a. This is a case of acute mesenteric ischemia, presumably due to an embolic clot from the left atrium or left ventricle in the setting of atrial fibrillation. The patient's symptoms of pain out of proportion to exam – writhing pain and abdominal pain despite a soft abdomen – are secondary to a sudden onset of reduced blood flow to the intestinal mesentery. Atrial fibrillation, an irregular heart rhythm, has predisposed the patient to blood clot development within her atrium or ventricles. This case represents a classic presentation: female patient older than 50 years, history of palpitations, sudden onset of writhing pain, and abdominal pain despite a soft abdomen (pain out of proportion to exam). Early critical actions include pain control, recognition of diagnosis with initiation of work-up including CT-angiography, IV antibiotics, and surgery and/or interventional radiology consult once the diagnosis has been made. Surgery consult will recommend admission to the intensive care unit without immediate surgical intervention. If the patient is allowed to be admitted to the ICU without treatment (embolectomy, catheter-directed lysis, or papaverine infusion) the patient will become hypotensive, complain of worsening abdominal pain despite analgesic therapy, and develop peritoneal signs on abdominal examination – rebound, guarding, and rigidity.

P. Pearls

 a. The classic presentation of acute mesenteric ischemia includes an elderly patient with an acute-onset writhing pain despite a soft abdomen (or peritoneal signs if late presentation), bloody diarrhea or vomiting, history of palpitations, irregular heartbeat, known atrial fibrillation or recent myocardial infarction.

 b. Mesenteric arterial embolus is the most common cause (40–50%), typically cardiac in origin, arising from left atrial or ventricular mural thrombi or valvular lesions.

 c. The superior mesenteric artery is most frequently affected because of the large vessel caliber and narrow takeoff angle from the abdominal aorta (embolus typically lodges less than 10 cm distal to the origin of the superior mesenteric artery).

d. Acute mesenteric ischemia is a rapidly progressing disease pathology; structural damage occurs within 15 minutes, with complete transmural necrosis by 6 hours.
e. Serial serum lactate is the most useful blood test.
f. CT-angiography of the abdomen and pelvis is the gold standard imaging modality in the emergent setting.
g. Early treatment is essential and includes fluid resuscitation, antibiotic coverage, and prompt surgical consult.
h. Acute mesenteric ischemia carries a 60–80% mortality rate, even with diagnosis.

Q. Figure legends
a. Figure 75.1 ECG; atrial fibrillation (irregularly irregular).
b. Figure 75.2 Upright chest x-ray.
c. Figure 75.3 Abdominal series; non-specific bowl gas pattern.

R. References
a. *Rosen's Emergency Medicine: Concepts and Clinical Practice* (10th ed.): Chapter 78, Small Intestine.
b. *Tintinalli's Emergency Medicine: A Comprehensive Study Guide* (9th ed.): Chapter 71, Acute Abdominal Pain.

Shortness of Breath

Ryan McKenna, DO and Sheler Sadati, MD

A. Chief complaint

a. 59-year-old male with history of COPD brought in by EMS for severe respiratory distress

B. Vital signs

a. BP: 168/84, HR: 114, RR: 30, T: 37.8°C, Sat: 90% on 4 L NC O_2

C. What does the patient look like?

a. Patient alert and awake with anxious affect; moderate respiratory distress; using accessory muscle to breathe.

D. Primary survey

a. Airway: able to speak in one-word sentences only, secondary to shortness of breath
b. Breathing: moderate respiratory distress, cyanotic around lips and fingertips; diffuse wheezing
c. Circulation: does not appear pale; normal capillary refill

E. Action

a. Oxygen via increasing NC or nonrebreather mask or CPAP or bilevel positive air pressure
b. Two large-bore peripheral IV lines
c. Labs
    i. CBC, BMP, LFT, coagulation studies, blood type and crossmatch
    ii. VBG/ABG with lactate
d. 1 L NS bolus
e. Monitor: BP: 168/84, HR: 114, RR: 30, Sat: 90% on 4 L NC O_2
f. EKG
g. Meds
    i. Albuterol via nebulizer, continuous treatment
    ii. Ipratropium bromide via nebulizer, continuous treatment
    iii. Methylprednisolone or equivalent steroids, IV
    iv. Magnesium IV
h. Imaging
i. CXR

F. History

a. HPI: A 59-year-old male, morbidly obese with a history of hypertension and COPD with dry cough and runny nose over the past 3 days. The patient has been taking his albuterol treatment via nebulizer at home, but today despite multiple treatments developed severe shortness of breath and called EMS. The patient denies fever, chills, headache, nausea, vomiting, diarrhea, or chest pain.

b. PMHx: COPD, hypertension
c. PSHx: none
d. Allergies: none
e. Meds: hydrochlorothiazide, albuterol, aspirin
f. Social: heavy smoker (30 packs per year) recently decreased the number of cigarettes to 6–7 per day; denies alcohol or drug abuse; lives at home alone
g. FHx: unsure; patient is adopted

G. Nurse
a. Patient: mild improvement of symptoms but still in moderate respiratory distress, despite increase in O_2 by NC or NRB
b. BP: 168/84, HR: 114, RR: 25, Sat 90% on 4 L NC O_2 (if increase to 6 L NC O_2, then patient will be saturating 92%, if increase to NRB mask then saturating 95%)
c. EKG (Figure 76.1)
d. CXR (Figure 76.2)

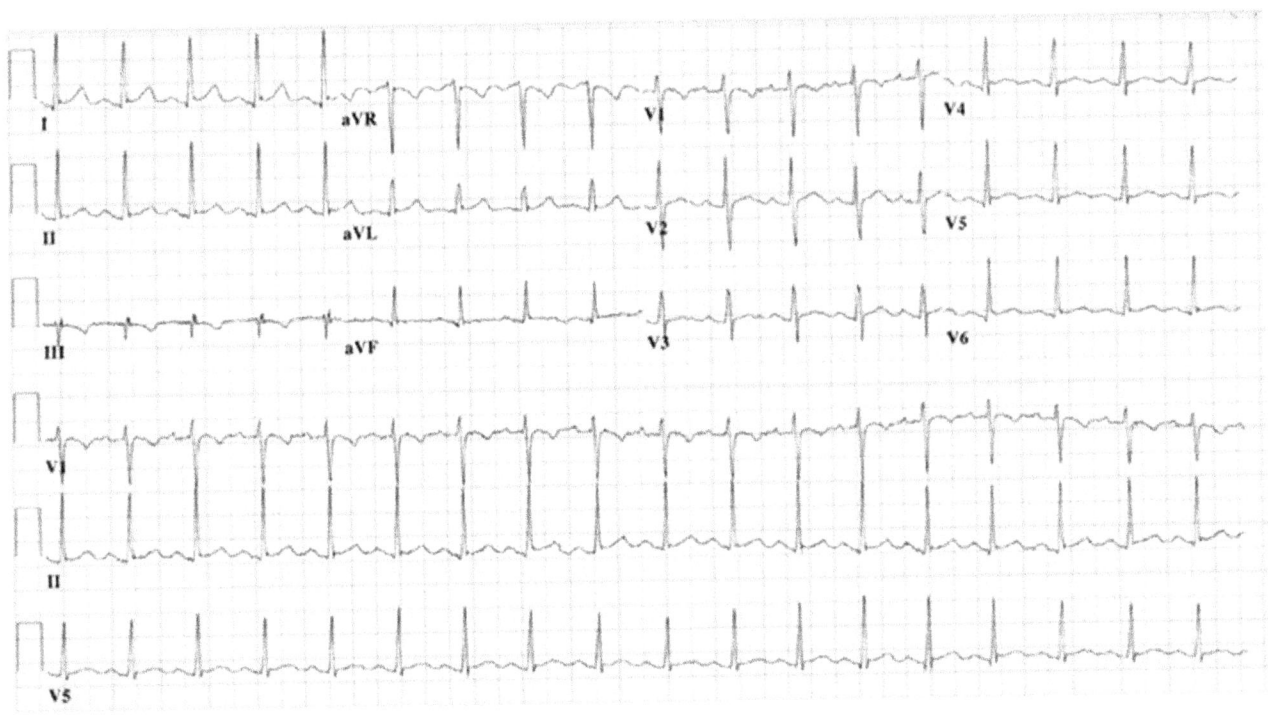

Figure 76.1

H. Secondary survey
a. General: moderate respiratory distress, diaphoretic and anxious
b. Head: normocephalic, atraumatic
c. Eyes: extraocular movement intact, pupils equal, reactive to light
d. Ears: normal tympanic membranes
e. Nose: no discharge
f. Neck: full range of motion, no jugular vein distension, no stridor
g. Pharynx: normal dentition, no lesions, no swelling
h. Chest: nontender
i. Lungs: tachypneic, using accessory muscles to breathe, diffuse wheezing bilaterally, scattered rhonchi

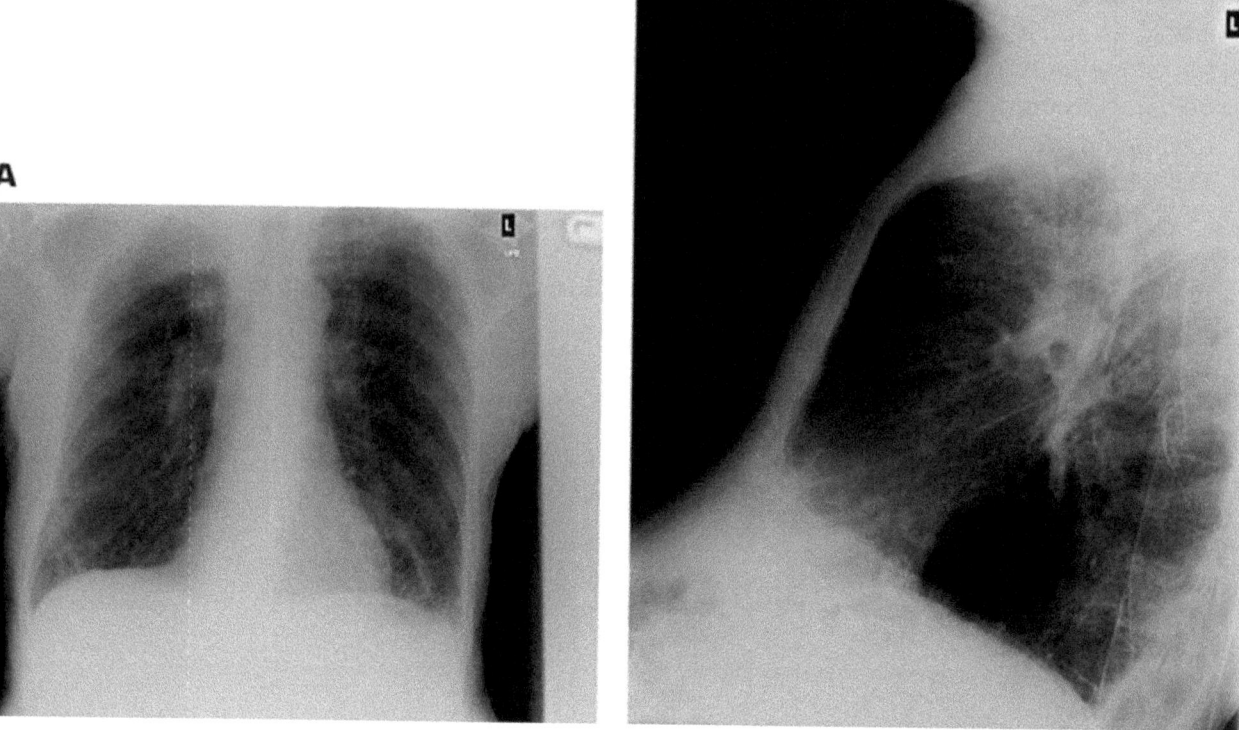

Figure 76.2

j. Heart: tachycardic rate, rhythm regular, no murmurs, rubs, or gallops
k. Abdomen: normal bowel sounds, soft, nontender or distended
l. Rectal: normal tone, brown stool, occult blood negative
m. Extremities: full range of motion, no deformity, normal pulses
n. Back: nontender
o. Neuro: cranial nerves II to XII intact; normal sensation, strength; normal reflexes
p. Skin: warm and dry
q. Lymph: no lymphadenopathy

I. Action

a. BiPAP or CPAP
b. Prepare for possible intubation
c. Meds
   i. Continuous albuterol and ipratropium bromide nebulizer treatment
   ii. Ceftriaxone and azithromycin or levofloxacin

J. Results

Table 76.1 Results table

Test	Result	Test	Result
Complete blood count:		T bili	1.0 mg/dL
WBC	$11.8 \times 10^3/\mu L$	D bili	0.3 mg/dL
Hct	41.5%	Amylase	50 U/L
Plt	$350 \times 10^3/\mu L$	Lipase	25 U/L
		Albumin	4.7 g/dL
Basic metabolic panel:			
Na	138 mEq/L	**Urinalysis:**	
K	4.3 mEq/L	SG	1.010–1.030
Cl	105 mEq/L	pH	5–8
CO_2	38 mEq/L	Prot	Neg
BUN	12 mEq/dL	Gluc	Neg
Cr	1.1 mg/dL	Ketones	Neg
Gluc	100 mg/dL	Bili	Neg
		Blood	Neg
Coagulation panel:		LE	Neg
PT	12.6 sec	Nitrite	Neg
PTT	26.0 sec	Color	Yellow
INR	1.0		
		Arterial blood gas:	
		pH	7.2
Liver function panel:		pO_2	65 mmHg
AST	23 U/L	pCO_2	65 mmHg
ALT	26 U/L	HCO_3	30 mmol/L
Alk phos	42 U/L		

K. Nurse

a. Patient's breathing improved significantly on BiPAP, O_2 Sat 98%; mental status improved. Patient appears more comfortable.

L. Action

a. Continue BiPAP or CPAP
b. Continuous albuterol treatment
c. Medical ICU consult

M. Diagnosis

a. Chronic obstructive pulmonary disease (COPD) exacerbation

N. Critical actions

a. O_2 supplementation
b. β-agonist and anticholinergic treatment via nebulizer
c. Steroids
d. CXR
e. BiPAP or CPAP or intubation

O. Examiner instructions

a. This is a case of COPD, likely secondary to viral infection versus pneumonia. COPD is a disease affecting the lungs, causing difficulty with air exchange. In severe exacerbations, patients can stop breathing. This patient's COPD was worsened because of a recent lung infection, and he comes into the ED in significant respiratory distress. Unless aggressive management is instituted with albuterol, ipratropium, steroids, and magnesium, the patient's shortness of breath will worsen. If noninvasive ventilatory support such as BiPAP or CPAP is given, the patient will not need to be intubated, but will still need ICU admission. If BiPAP or CPAP is not attempted, the patient will become more confused and lethargic, retain CO_2, and becoming unresponsive with low oxygenation. The patient will require intubation and admission to the medical ICU.

P. Pearls

a. Antibiotics should be administered to all COPD patients being admitted to the ICU or requiring BiPAP or CPAP.
b. Anticholinergic agents such as ipratropium bromide work on larger central airways as opposed to β-agonists agents, such as albuterol, which work on the small peripheral airways. Ipratropium bromide has a synergistic effect when used with albuterol, although it has slower onset of action.
c. Magnesium sulfate at a dose of 2 g has been shown to be effective in some cases of COPD exacerbation, although the mechanism of action is not well known and its use is still controversial.
d. Steroid use is less compelling compared to asthma exacerbation, but still should be given in all acute COPD exacerbations.
e. If the patient requires intubation, the ventilator setting should be adjusted, such as lower tidal volumes, lower RR (to allow the patient to exhale as COPD is an obstructive process), low or no PEEP, minimizing complications such as pneumothorax.
f. The risk of oxygen-induced apnea if the patient is tachypneic is less compared to when the patient is bradypneic. Regardless of whether the patient is in respiratory distress, oxygen should be given in high concentrations.

Q. Figure legends

a. Figure 76.1 (EKG) Sinus tachycardia; minimal voltage criteria for LVH.
b. Figure 76.2A (a) (CXR, PA) Bilateral increased interstitial markings. (b) (CXR, lateral) Bilateral increased interstitial markings.

R. References

a. *Tintinalli's Emergency Medicine: A Comprehensive Study Guide* (9th ed.): Chapter 70, Chronic Obstructive Pulmonary Disease.
b. *Rosen's Emergency Medicine: Concepts and Clinical Practice* (10th ed.): Chapter 60, Chronic Obstructive Pulmonary Disease.

Altered Mental Status

Megha George, MD and Sheler Sadati, MD

A. Chief complaint
a. 48-year-old male with altered mental status

B. Vital signs
a. BP: 183/105, HR: 136, RR: 20, T: 38.0°C, Sat: 97% on RA

C. What does the patient look like?
a. Patient appears unkempt and covered in urine, confused but awake, agitated, and uncooperative with staff.

D. Primary survey
a. Airway: speaking and maintaining his airway
b. Breathing: no apparent respiratory distress, no cyanosis
c. Circulation: diaphoretic, skin warm with normal capillary refill

E. Action
a. Ask EMS to stay
b. Obtain fingerstick: 254 mg/dL (must ask)
c. Oxygen via NC or nonrebreather mask
d. Two large-bore peripheral IV lines
   i. While trying to place an IV line, patient becomes verbally and physically abusive to nursing staff (the candidate will be unable to move on from this step until the patient is restrained and/or medication is given for sedation)
   ii. Attempts to verbally deescalate fail
e. Meds
   i. Haloperidol 5 mg IM and midazolam 2 mg IM (or lorazepam 2 mg IM)
   ii. Physical restraints

F. Nurse
a. Patient more cooperative after sedation

G. Action
a. EKG
b. Imaging
   i. CT head noncontrast

c. Labs
   i. CBC, BMP, LFT, coagulation studies, blood type and crossmatch
   ii. Alcohol level, acetaminophen level, salicylate level, urine toxicology screen
d. Monitor: BP: 183/105, HR: 136, RR: 20, Sat: 97% on RA (refusing O_2)

H. History

a. HPI: The patient was found sleeping on the sidewalk. Police tried to question him and EMS was called because the patient was unresponsive.
   i. EMS (must ask): As per EMS, this patient is well-known to them and is typically brought to various hospitals for intoxication. Today he looks much different because he is confused and minimally arousable. There are no signs of trauma and there was an empty vodka bottle at the scene. EMS was able to establish IV access and administered 1 amp of IV D50, 0.4 mg of IV naloxone, and 100 mg of IV thiamine with minimal improvement. Patient subsequently pulled the IV out.
b. PMHx: unknown
c. PSHx: unknown
d. Allergies: unknown
e. Meds: unknown
f. Social: unknown
g. FHx: unknown

I. Nurse

a. EKG (Figure 77.1)

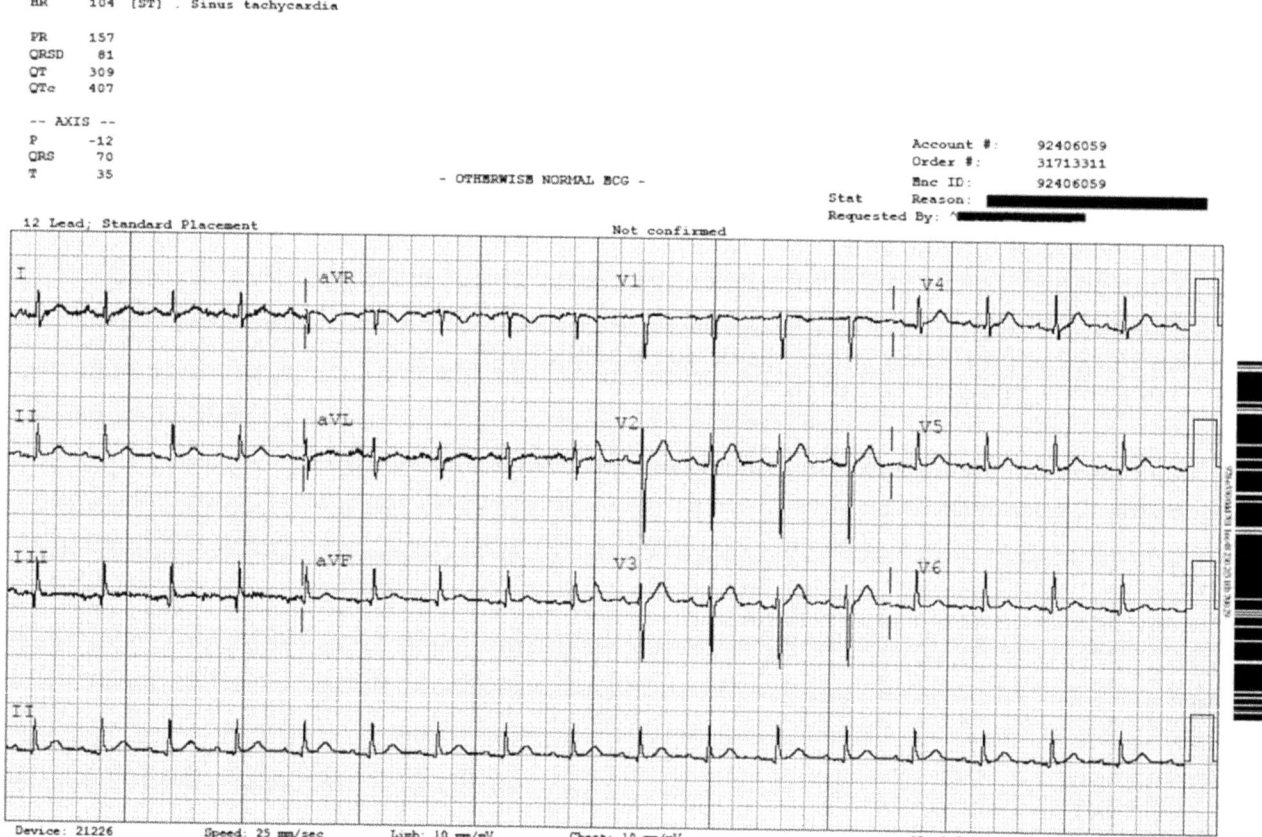

Figure 77.1

J. Secondary survey
a. General: sedated and sleeping, protecting airway
b. Head: normocephalic, atraumatic
c. Eyes: pupils equal, round, and reactive to light; no nystagmus
d. Ears: normal tympanic membranes
e. Nose: no bleeding, no septal hematoma
f. Neck: nontender
g. Pharynx: poor dentition, no acute bleeding
h. Chest: nontender
i. Lungs: clear bilaterally
j. Heart: regular rate and rhythm, no murmurs, rubs, or gallops
k. Abdomen: normal bowel sounds, soft, nontender, and nondistended
l. Rectal: deferred
m. Urogenital: deferred
n. Extremities: moving all extremities, no deformity, normal pulses
o. Back: nontender
p. Neuro: sedated, but when aroused is uncooperative with examination; patient is confused while awake; appears to be oriented to person; unsure of date or location; affect agitated; no focal deficits noted
q. Skin: diaphoretic and warm
r. Lymph: no lymphadenopathy

K. Nurse
a. Patient: develops a generalized tonic-clonic seizure

L. Action
a. Oxygen via NC or nonrebreather mask
b. Meds
   i. Lorazepam (will need a total of 8 mg for patient to stop seizing)
c. Place patient on monitor

M. Nurse
a. BP: 173/90, HR: 125, RR: 14, Sat: 97% on O_2

N. Results

Table 77.1 Results table

Test	Result	Test	Result
Complete blood count:		**Liver function panel:**	
WBC	$14.3 \times 10^3/\mu L$	AST	23 U/L
Hct	34%	ALT	26 U/L
Plt	$126 \times 10^3/\mu L$	Alk phos	42 U/L
		T bili	1.0 mg/dL
		D bili	0.3 mg/dL
Basic metabolic panel:		Amylase	50 U/L
Na	138 mEq/L		

Table 77.1 (cont.)

Test	Result	Test	Result
K	3.4 mEq/L	Lipase	25 U/L
Cl	105 mEq/L	Albumin	4.7 g/dL
CO$_2$	22 mEq/L		
BUN	21 mEq/dL	**Urinalysis:**	
Cr	1.1 mg/dL	SG	1.010–1.030
Gluc	241 mg/dL	pH	5–8
		Prot	Neg
Coagulation panel:		Gluc	Neg
PT	12.6 sec	Ketones	Neg
PTT	26.0 sec	Bili	Neg
INR	1.0	Blood	Neg
		LE	Neg
		Nitrite	Neg
		Color	Yellow

a. Lactate: 2.7 mmol/L
b. Urine toxicology screen negative, alcohol 56 mg/dL, acetaminophen 0, aspirin 0
c. CXR (Figure 77.2)
d. CT head noncontrast (Figure 77.3) is negative for hemorrhage or mass; mild atrophy reported

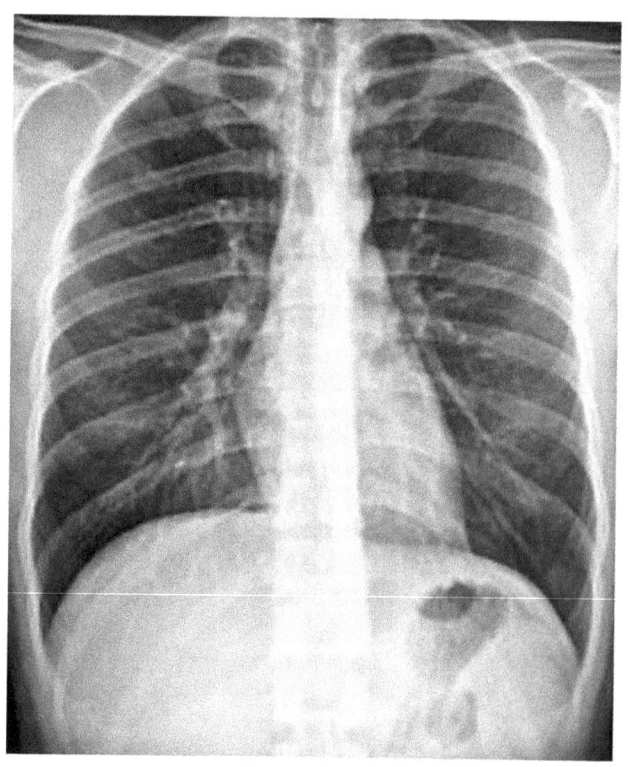
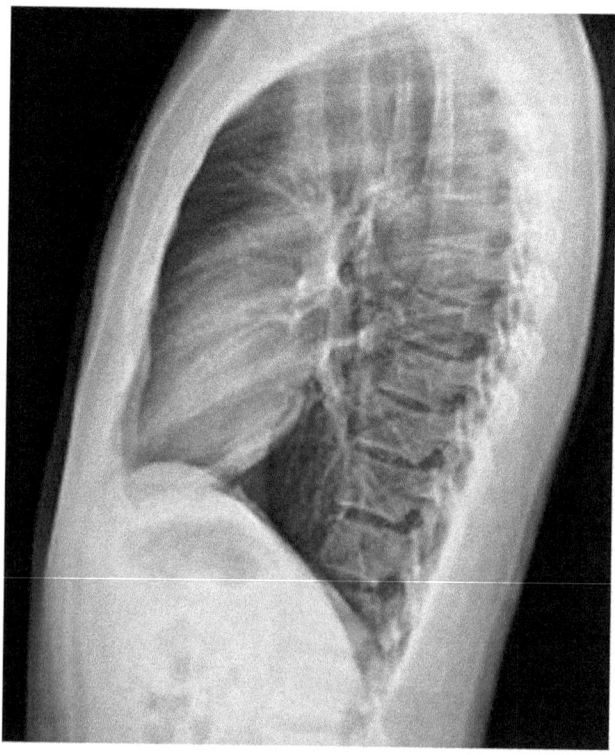

Figure 77.2

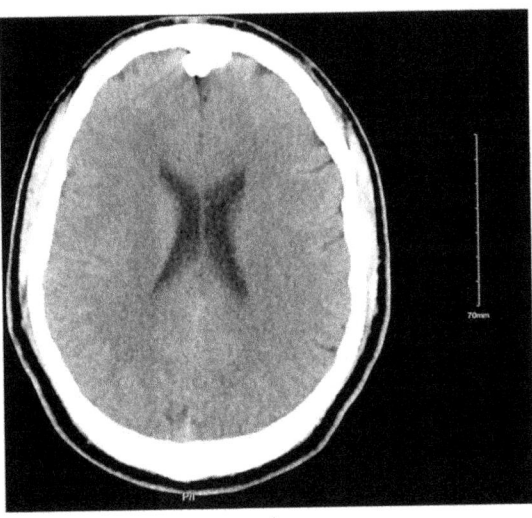

Figure 77.3

O. Actions
a. Admit to ICU for alcohol withdrawal seizures
b. Meds
   i. Multivitamins
   ii. Folic acid

P. Diagnosis
a. Alcohol withdrawal with seizure

Q. Critical actions
a. Management of the agitated patient
b. Fingerstick glucose
c. Benzodiazepine until seizure stops
d. Head CT

R. Examiner instructions
a. This is a case of a patient with alcohol withdrawal seizure. Seizure secondary to the cessation of alcohol in a chronic user can be a life-threatening condition if left untreated. The patient was found by EMS in the postictal period with minimal response to the "coma cocktail" of naloxone, thiamine, and dextrose. The candidate must get the history from EMS of alcohol use by the patient. The patient is confused and agitated because of a recent unwitnessed seizure in the field and will continue to become more agitated and abusive to staff until proper medication or restraints are applied. If haloperidol is given, the patient will initially calm down, but will seize a few minutes later. Early actions include finger stick glucose, IV access, CT head, and blood tests including toxicology screens. The patient will proceed to have a generalized tonic-clonic seizure that will only respond to lorazepam 8 mg, or equivalent. The patient should be admitted to a monitored bed and continued on benzodiazepines for withdrawal.

S. Pearls
a. "Coma cocktail" includes D50, naloxone, and thiamine.
b. Benzodiazepines are the medication of choice for alcohol withdrawal.
c. Any patient with seizure activity should be assessed for possible alcohol-related seizures.

d. Alcoholic patients are prone to hypoglycemia due to decreased reservoir of glycogen secondary to chronic liver damage; blood glucose should be assessed for all alcoholics with mental status changes and all seizure patients.

e. Glucose should not be given before thiamine in suspected alcoholics since it can precipitate Wernicke's encephalopathy or Korsakoff's syndrome with potentially irreversible brain damage.

f. Always assess intoxicated patients fully for trauma, infection, and metabolic abnormalities.

g. Alcohol withdrawal syndrome usually develops 6–24 hours after the reduction of alcohol intake and can last up to 7 days. Monitoring these patients closely in inpatient units is recommended until the signs and symptoms of withdrawal resolve completely.

T. Figure legends

a. Figure 77.1 (EKG) Sinus tachycardia.

b. Figure 77.2 (CXR) Normal AP and lateral chest X-ray.

c. Figure 77.3 (CT head noncontrast) Normal CT head.

U. References

a. *Rosen's Emergency Medicine: Concepts and Clinical Practice* (10th ed.): Chapter 12, Depressed Consciousness and Coma. Chapter 137, Alcohol-Related Disease.

b. *Tintinalli's Emergency Medicine: A Comprehensive Study Guide* (9th ed.): Chapter 168, Altered Mental Status and Coma. Chapter 185, Alcohols.

Weakness

Matthew Constantine, MD and Matthew Steimle, DO

A. Chief complaint
a. 66-year old male brought in by EMS with sudden-onset right-sided paralysis and slurred speech

B. Vital signs
a. BP: 192/109, HR: 85, RR: 18, T: 36.9°C, Sat: 95% on RA

C. What does the patient look like?
a. Patient appears stated age, comfortable and in no apparent distress, with a right facial droop.

D. Primary survey
a. Airway: speaking in full sentences, but speech is slurred
b. Breathing: no apparent respiratory distress, no cyanosis
c. Circulation: warm and dry skin, normal capillary refill
d. Neuro: alert and oriented to person, place, and time; right facial droop and slurred speech

E. Action
a. Monitors:
   i. Cardiac
   ii. Supplemental oxygen as needed to maintain O_2 saturation at or above 95%
b. Establish IV access
c. Finger stick blood glucose (89 mg/dL; must ask)
d. Brain imaging within 20 minutes of patient arrival
e. EKG
f. Labs
   i. CBC, BMP, LFT, coagulation studies, blood type and crossmatch
   ii. Troponin

F. History
a. HPI: This is a 66-year-old, right-handed male with a history of hypertension, who states that he awoke from sleep normally this morning; however, he was unable to get out of bed. He states that he felt paralyzed on his entire right side. His wife called EMS. EMS notes that they found the patient in bed and unable to move his right side. The patient also notes a right-sided facial droop. He feels as if his right arm and leg are numb; he could not feel EMS move them. He states that the last time he felt normal was when he went to sleep at 11:00 p.m. He awoke in his normal routine at 6:00 a.m. He presently denies any other symptoms, including headache, nausea, vomiting, vertigo, vision or hearing changes, left-sided symptoms, fevers, chills, chest

pain, or shortness of breath. He reports that he had one episode of similar symptoms 3 days ago. He states that he was watching TV when he felt weakness on the right arm greater than the leg; however, the symptoms only lasted for 10–15 minutes. He was about to call EMS when the symptoms resolved.

b. PMHx: hypertension
c. PSHx: none
d. Allergies: none
e. Meds: lisinopril, hydrochlorothiazide
f. Social: lives with wife at home, 28 pack per year smoking history, social EtOH use
g. FHx: father with CAD, mother with CVA at age 66
h. PMD: none, patient has not seen MD in 5+ years

G. Nurse
a. EKG (Figure 78.1)
b. No fluids
    i. BP: 205/110, HR: 64, RR: 20, Sat: 98%

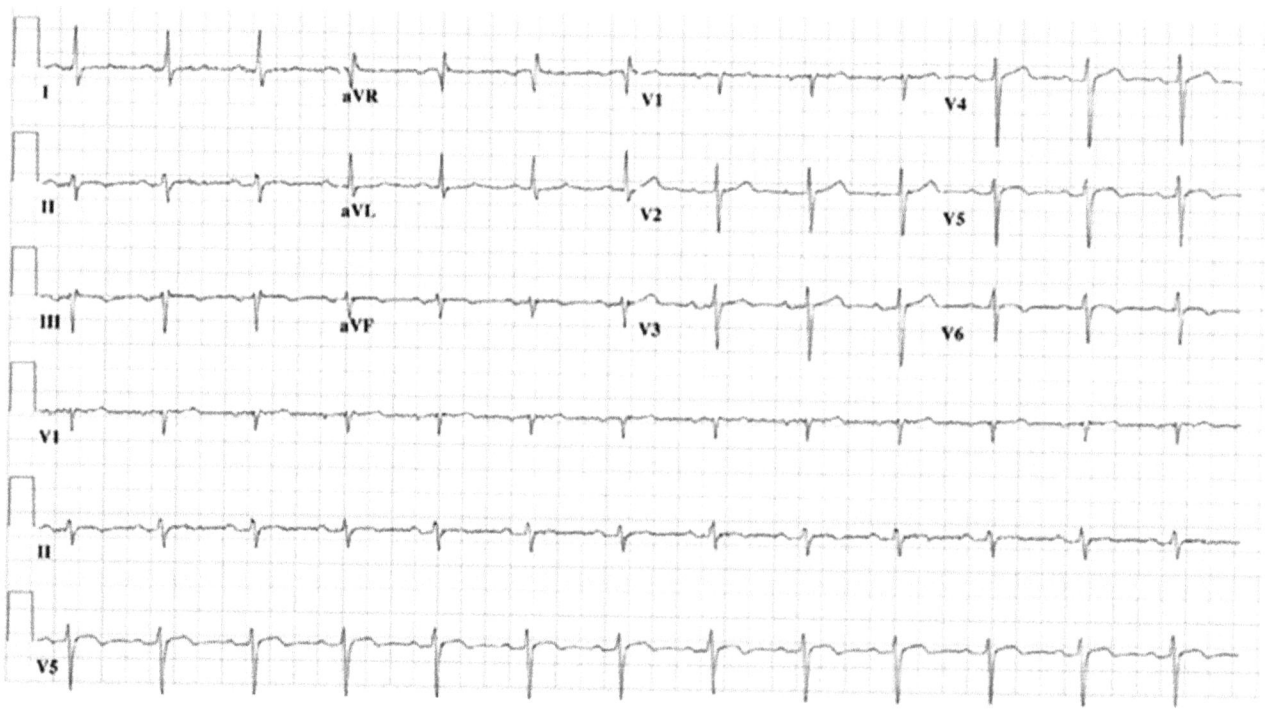

Figure 78.1

H. Secondary survey
a. General: alert and oriented to person, place, and time, right-sided facial droop and slurred speech obvious when talking to patient
b. HEENT: right facial droop, normocephalic, atraumatic; tympanic membranes normal bilaterally; extraocular movement intact; pupils equal, round, reactive; conjunctiva normal; no nasal discharge; palate normal, normal dentition, no lesions, no swelling

c. Neck: full range of motion, no jugular vein distension, no stridor
d. Chest: nontender
e. Lungs: clear bilaterally
f. Heart: rate and rhythm regular, no murmurs, rubs, or gallops
g. Abdomen: normal bowel sounds, soft, nontender or distended
h. Rectal: normal tone, brown stool, occult blood negative
    i. Male: no discharge, normal testicular examination
i. Urogenital: normal external genitalia
j. Extremities: no deformity, normal pulses
k. Back: nontender
l. Neuro:
    i. Alert and oriented to person, place, and time; cooperative
    ii. 0/5 motor strength in right upper and 2/5 in right lower extremity
    iii. Loss of fine touch and pain on right upper and lower extremities
    iv. Cranial nerves: right-sided facial droop with forehead sparing, otherwise cranial nerves intact
    v. Unable to cooperate with right-sided cerebellar examination or gait/Romberg testing
    v. Does not acknowledge MD's presence when on the patient's right side and does not voluntarily turn to look to right
    vi. When filling in clock face, he only writes numbers on the left side
    vii. Does not recognize common objects such as his watch or glasses
    viii. Memory is intact; however, he notes lack of ability to concentrate or maintain attention for longer than several minutes
m. Skin: warm and dry, capillary refill 1–2 seconds centrally and peripherally
n. Lymph: normal

I. Action
a. Meds
    i. Aspirin should not be given until after head CT or within 24 hours of receiving thrombolytics
    ii. blood pressure control is not recommended initially unless candidate for thrombolytics or reperfusion measures
b. Imaging
    i. Noncontrast head CT within 20 minutes of patient arrival
    ii. CT angiography of the head and neck is typically recommended concurrently with initial head CT, but do not delay thrombolytic treatment if initial head CT qualifies for thrombolytic therapy
    iii. Routine CXR not recommended unless symptomatic or thrombolytic management concerns
c. Consult
    i. Neurology stroke service
d. Additional testing for stroke mimic if applicable (urine, toxicologic, pregnancy)

J. Nurse
a. BP: 235/139, HR: 69, RR: 18, Sat: 98% on O_2
b. Patient: no change in neurological examination

K. Results

Table 78.1 Results table

Test	Result	Test	Result
Complete blood count:		T bili	1.0 mg/dL
WBC	$5.3 \times 10^3/\mu L$	D bili	0.3 mg/dL
Hct	41.5%	Amylase	50 U/L
Plt	$350 \times 10^3/\mu L$	Lipase	25 U/L
		Albumin	4.7 g/dL
Basic metabolic panel:			
Na	138 mEq/L	**Urinalysis:**	
K	4.3 mEq/L	SG	1.010–1.030
Cl	105 mEq/L	pH	5–8
CO_2	30 mEq/L	Prot	Neg
BUN	12 mEq/dL	Gluc	Neg
Cr	1.1 mg/dL	Ketones	Neg
Gluc	100 mg/dL	Bili	Neg
		Blood	Neg
Coagulation panel:		LE	Neg
PT	12.6 sec	Nitrite	Neg
PTT	26.0 sec	Color	Yellow
INR	1.0		
		Arterial blood gas:	
Liver function panel:		pH	7.4
AST	23 U/L	pO_2	95 mmHg
ALT	26 U/L	pCO_2	41 mmHg
Alk phos	42 U/L	HCO_3	24 mmol/L

a. Troponin: normal
b. Head CT (Figure 78.2) negative for acute hemorrhage, mass, or edema; ischemic changes in the left MCA distribution with hyperdense MCA sign

L. Action

a. Neurology consult
   i. Admission for further evaluation, observation, and further imaging
   ii. In some centers, this patient may be a candidate for mechanical thrombectomy
b. Discussion with family
c. Meds
   i. Aspirin 325 mg may be given as this is an ischemic stroke and since patient is not a candidate for rtPA since last normal >3–4.5 hours

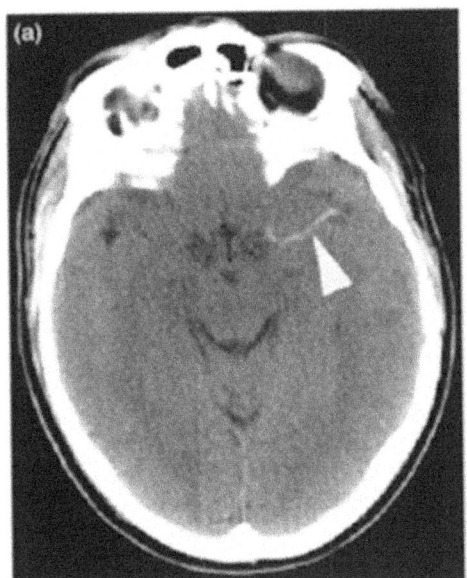
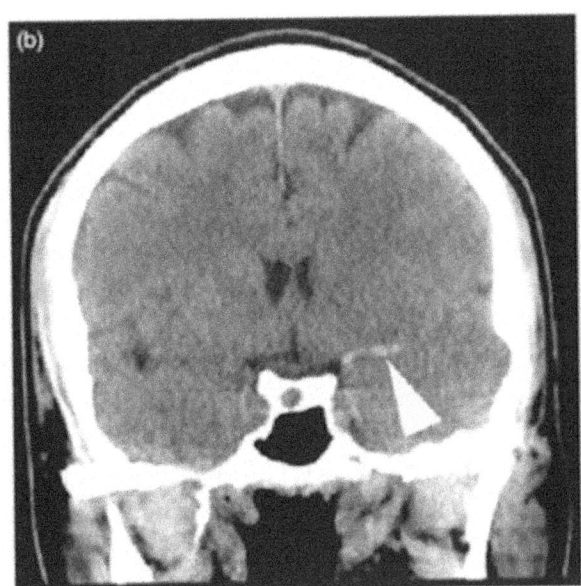

Fig. 4.1. (a) Axial and (b) coronal images demonstrating a hyperdense left MCA in keeping with acute intraluminal thrombus (arrowhead).

Figure 78.2

   ii. Antihypertensives at this point may be given, considering that SBP is >230 and or DBP is >130; options include but are not limited to
     1. β-blockers such as labetalol 10–20 mg IV push
     2. Calcium channel blockers such as nicardipine, starting at 5 mg/hr IV
     3. Sublingual nifedipine or nitroglycerin are not recommended
   iii. rtPA is not indicated at this time because time of onset cannot be established at less than 3–4.5 hours as the patient was last seen before sleep

M. Diagnosis
a. Stroke: left MCA

N. Critical actions
a. Finger stick glucose
b. Head CT (within 20 minutes "time is brain")
c. Neurology stroke team notification
d. Neurological examination
e. BP control with IV agents

O. Examiner instructions
a. This is a case of left–middle cerebral artery stroke, a condition caused by a cessation of flow to one of the arteries supplying the brain, resulting in death of the tissue. The patient's symptoms include neurological deficits that are consistent with the left motor and sensory centers in the brain (dominant hemisphere), which are fed by this artery. Early critical actions include establishing the time of onset (or time last known to be without deficit), IV access, glucose check, monitoring, immediate head CT and neurology consult. Because the CT is negative for signs of intracranial hemorrhaging, the symptoms are assumed to be the result of either a thrombotic, embolic, or hypoperfusion-related process. Subsequently, antiplatelet,

anticoagulation, and thrombolytic therapies are considered. Blood pressure monitoring and management is important throughout the case.

P. Pearls

a. Approximately 87% of strokes are ischemic as opposed to hemorrhagic. Ischemic strokes can be subdivided into three categories: thrombotic, embolic, or hypoperfusion-related.

b. Time of symptom onset is key to treatment consideration as rtPA protocols call for administration within 3 hours (with extended window parameters 3–4.5 hours) of symptoms onset. Longer extended window parameters are available with endovascular therapies (up to 6 hours). Mechanical thrombectomy should be considered in parallel with rtPA for select patients. In select patients, this intervention can be considered up to 24 hours from when last known well.

c. Patient must have an immediate CT of the head to rule out intracranial hemorrhage.

d. Early consultation with an experienced stroke physician is critical for management.

e. No antiplatelet agent should be given within 24 hours of rtPA.

f. Thrombotic, hypoperfusion-related, and embolic strokes may be preceded by TIAs with a stuttering or waxing and waning deficit.

g. Patients with atrial fibrillation have a fivefold increased risk for development of stroke.

h. ACEP recommends not using the $ABCD^2$ score to identify patients who can be safely discharged home.

i. For patients who are not candidates for thrombolytics or reperfusion measures, the guidelines call for permissive hypertension, with no active attempts to lower blood pressure unless the systolic or diastolic blood pressure is >220/120 mmHg, or the mean arterial pressure is >130 mmHg, or if the patient has another medical condition that would benefit from lowering blood pressure. If BP management is initiated, suggested target is 15% reduction in SBP over 24 hours.

j. Blood pressure control is essential prior to, during, and after thrombolytic therapy. A systolic or diastolic blood pressure >185/110 mmHg is a contraindication to the use of rtPA. The patient must meet these entry parameters to use rtPA to avoid hemorrhagic transformation.

k. It is extremely helpful to calculate an NIH stroke scale when making management decisions with the stroke specialist.

l. It is critical to review the inclusion and exclusion criteria of rtPA before administration.

m. Optimize general supportive care measures to minimize neuronal injury, including temperature control, glucose control, and hydration, and maintain adequate cerebral perfusion. Too much or too little of any of these can be harmful (Goldilocks principle).

n. It is critical to get stroke patients to a stroke facility quickly: "drip and ship."

o. Mechanical thrombectomy.

Q. Figure legends

a. Figure 78.1 (EKG) Normal sinus rhythm; biphasic T waves V5–6.

b. Figure 78.2 (a) Axial and (b) coronal images demonstrating a hyperdense left MCA in keeping with acute intraluminal thrombus (arrowhead).

R. References

a. *Tintinalli's Emergency Medicine: A Comprehensive Study Guide* (9th ed.): Chapter 167, Stroke Syndromes.

b. *Rosen's Emergency Medicine: Concepts and Clinical Practice* (10th ed.): Chapter 87, Stroke.

Pedestrian Struck

Rachel Semmons, MD and Matthew Constantine, MD

A. Chief complaint
a. 57-year-old female brought in by EMS after being struck by an automobile. Patient complains of right leg pain and lower back pain. She is immobilized with a backboard and collar.

B. Vital signs
a. BP: 145/77, HR: 105, RR: 25 T: 36.2°C, Sat: 98% on RA, FS: 131 mg/dL

C. What does the patient look like?
a. Patient appears stated age, uncomfortable-appearing, and in moderate distress, lying supine on the backboard and in a cervical collar.

D. Primary survey
a. Airway: speaking in full sentences
b. Breathing: mildly tachypneic, no cyanosis
c. Circulation: warm and dry, normal capillary refill
d. Disability: GCS 15
e. Exposure
   i. Open right ankle fracture noted; multiple ecchymoses on right leg, thigh, and hip

E. Action
a. Two large-bore peripheral IV lines
b. Labs
   i. CBC, BMP, LFT, coagulation studies, blood type and crossmatch two units
   ii. Point of care hematocrit
c. 1 L NS bolus
d. Antibiotics for open fracture
e. Monitor: BP: 139/91, HR: 120, RR: 20, Sat: 98% on RA, 100% if on O_2
f. EKG (Figure 79.1)
g. FAST (Figure 79.2)
h. Imaging
   i. CXR (Figure 79.3)
   ii. Pelvic x-ray (Figure 79.4)
   iii. C-spine x-ray (Figure 79.5)
i. Consults
   i. Surgery/trauma
   ii. Orthopedics

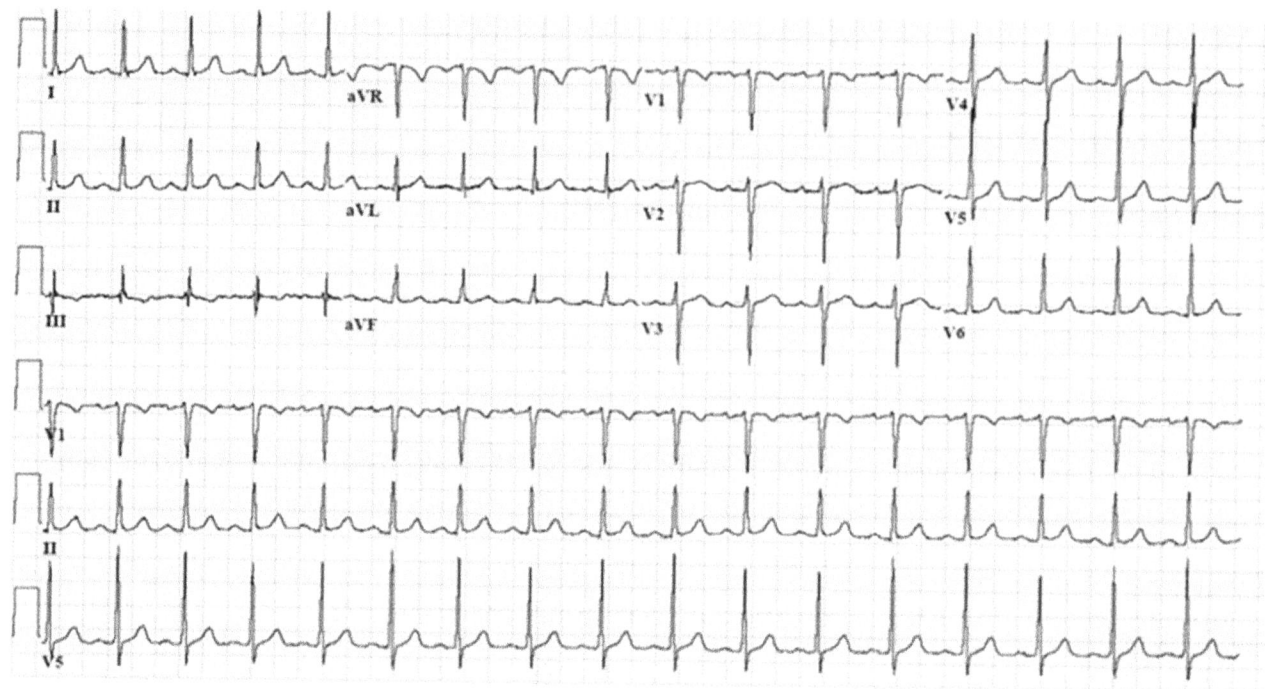

Figure 79.1

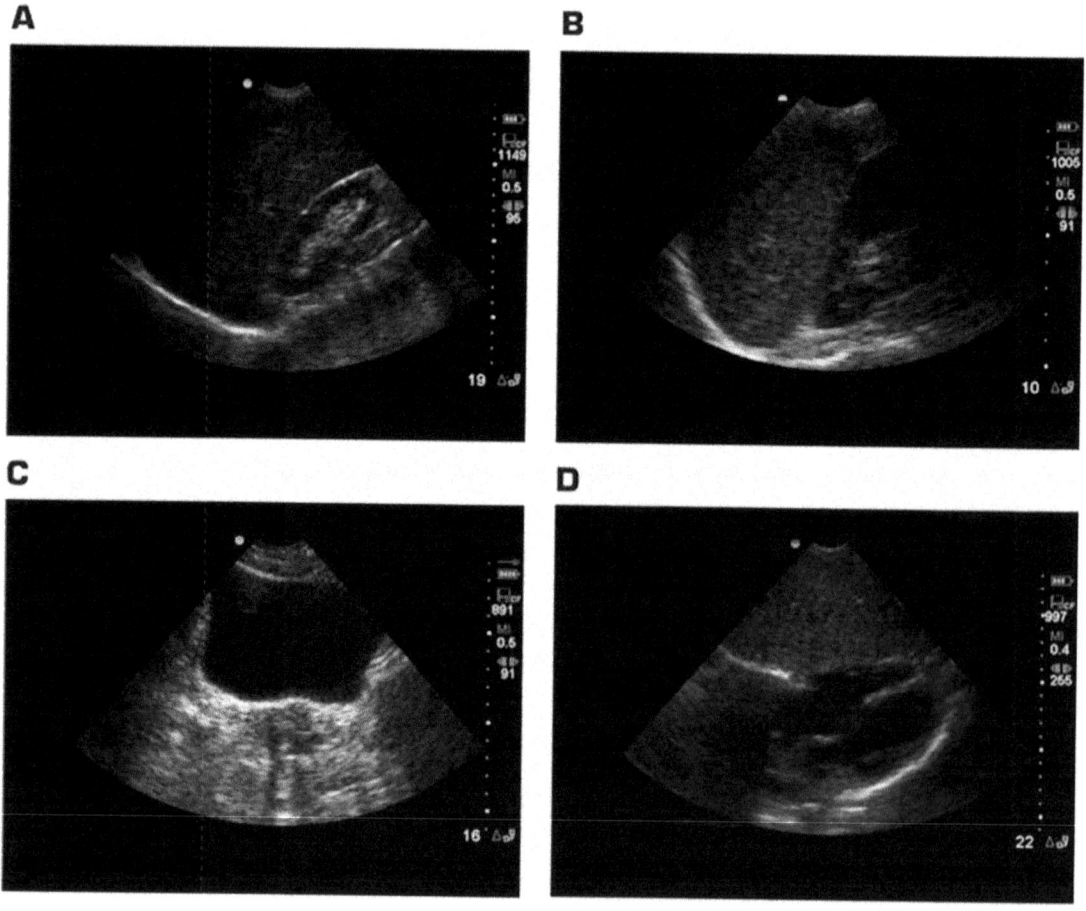

Figure 79.2

Figure 79.3

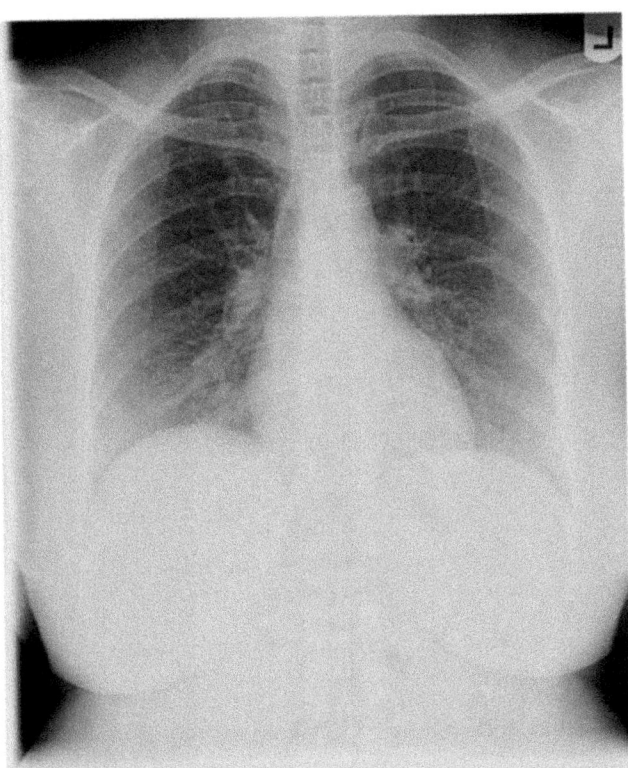

Figure 79.4

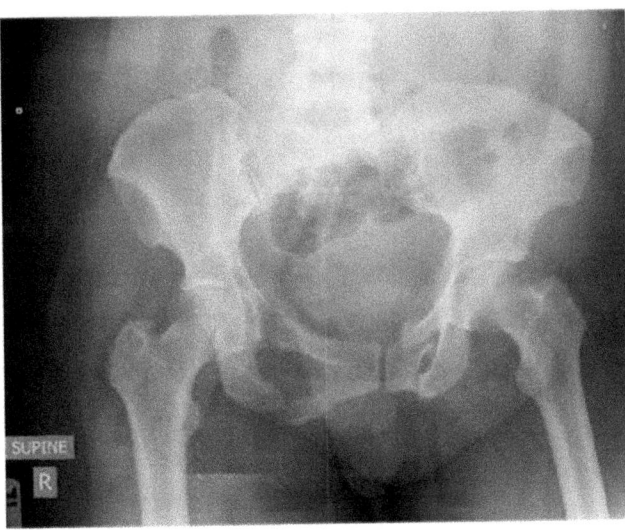

F. History

a. HPI: This is a 57-year-old female struck by a car at low speed (~10 mph) while crossing an intersection. The patient was struck on the right side, knocked onto the hood and then landed ~4 feet in front of the vehicle. She presently complains of pain in her right lower extremity at the ankle as well as at the right hip and lower back. She denies LOC, vision or hearing changes, vertigo, neck pain, chest pain, shortness of breath, nausea, vomiting, or abdominal pain. She denies recent alcohol or drug use. Her last tetanus is unknown.

b. PMHx: hypertension

c. PSHx: none

d. Allergies: none

e. Meds: amlodipine

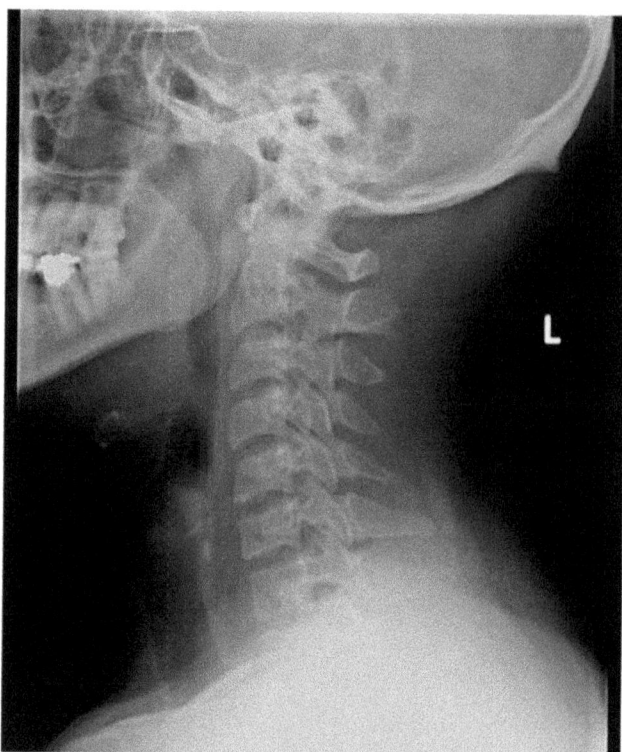

Figure 79.5

f.   Social: lives alone, social EtOH, denies smoking or drug use
g.   FHx: not relevant
h.   PMD: Dr. Pine

G. Nurse

a.   EKG (Figure 79.1)
b.   Hematocrit: 32%
c.   2 L NS
     i.   BP: 100/66, HR: 120, RR: 22, Sat: 98% on O_2
d.   If no fluids given then
     i.   BP: 80/45, HR: 125, RR: 22, Sat: 98% on O_2

H. Secondary survey

a.   General: alert, oriented × 3, moderate distress secondary to pain
b.   Head: contusion to left forehead, no scalp lacerations or bony deformities noted
c.   Eyes: no periorbital ecchymoses, extraocular movement intact, pupils equal, reactive to light
d.   Ears: normal tympanic membranes, no blood in external auditory canals
e.   Nose: no deformity, no nasal septal hematoma or epistaxis
f.   Neck: cervical collar in place, trachea midline, no stridor, no midline cervical tenderness noted to palpation
g.   Pharynx: normal dentition, no lesions, no swelling
h.   Chest: nontender, no contusions/abrasions, no crepitus
i.   Lungs: tachypnea, no accessory muscle movement or retractions, clear bilaterally
j.   Heart: tachycardic rate, rhythm regular, no murmurs, rubs, or gallops
k.   Abdomen: normal bowel sounds, soft, nontender, nondistended, no ecchymosis
l.   Pelvis: inward pressure to both femoral heads causes significant tenderness and 4 cm movement
m.   Rectal: normal tone, brown stool, occult blood negative

n. Urogenital: normal external genitalia
   i. Female: no vaginal bleeding
o. Extremities: open, nonangulated fracture of the medial right ankle with swelling and ecchymosis with minimal bleeding. Right knee and femur are nontender to palpation. Palpation of right hip reproduces same right-sided pelvic and back pain that was elicited on pelvic examination. ROM at ankle, knee, and hip are limited due to patient discomfort. 2+ dorsalis pedis and posterior tibial pulses, good capillary refill and sensation intact to light touch.
p. Back: no midline tenderness, no ecchymosis noted; patient complains of right paraspinal tenderness
q. Neuro: GCS – eyes open spontaneously, moves upper and left lower extremities on command and without discomfort, responds appropriately to questions, GCS = 15; no sensory deficits noted; CNs II–XII intact; finger-to-nose testing is normal.
r. Skin: pale and cool now (different from primary survey), other lesions as noted elsewhere on examination
s. Lymph: no lymphadenopathy

I. Nurse

a. BP: 72/25 HR: 140 RR: 25 Sat 98% on O_2
b. C-spine x-ray (Figure 79.5)
c. CXR (Figure 79.3)
d. AP pelvis (Figure 79.4)

J. Action

a. IV access: two 16-gauge IVs are acceptable; if central access obtained, the best choice is 8 Fr introducer in the subclavian vein
   i. Avoid femoral access as patient with obvious RLE injury and suspected pelvic fracture
   ii. Internal jugular difficult to access secondary to C collar
b. Orthopedics reductions
   i. The pelvis requires stabilization with a sheet wrapped/tied around pelvis or a commercial pelvic binder. Avoid further testing of the pelvis. With pelvic laxity and dropping BP in the setting of a negative FAST and CXR, pelvic hemorrhage is high on the differential
c. Blood products
   i. Two units packed red blood cells (no type-specific available, must ask for O+ or O− blood)
d. Meds
   i. Tetanus toxoid
   ii. Cefazolin 1 g IV and gentamicin 6 mg/kg IV
   iii. Fentanyl and/or ketamine (at sub-dissociative dose)
e. Consult
   i. Interventional radiology for emergent pelvic angiography
f. Imaging
   i. Patient will require CT head and cervical spine, and CT of chest, abdomen, and pelvis (currently unavailable given hemodynamic instability of patient)
   ii. Right lower extremity films (these are not critical at this point and can wait until the patient is stable)

K. Nurse

a. Reassess
   i. Patient: still with pain

ii. Vitals
   1. Two units blood
      a. BP: 100/61, HR: 110, RR: 25, Sat: 98% on 100% NRB O_2
   2. No blood
      a. BP: 70/25, HR: 150, RR: 30, Sat: 98% on O_2

L. Results

Table 79.1 Results table

Test	Result	Test	Result
Complete blood count:		**Liver function panel:**	
WBC	$10 \times 10^3/\mu L$	AST	23 U/L
Hct	30.5%	ALT	26 U/L
Plt	$251 \times 10^3/\mu L$	Alk phos	42 U/L
		T bili	1.0 mg/dL
Basic metabolic panel:		D bili	0.3 mg/dL
Na	138 mEq/L	Amylase	50 U/L
K	4.3 mEq/L	Lipase	25 U/L
Cl	100 mEq/L	Albumin	4.7 g/dL
CO_2	18 mEq/L		
BUN	12 mEq/dL	**Urinalysis:**	
Cr	1.1 mg/dL	SG	1.010–1.030
Gluc	100 mg/dL	pH	5–8
		Prot	Neg
Coagulation panel:		Gluc	Neg
PT	12.6 sec	Ketones	Neg
PTT	26.0 sec	Bili	Neg
INR	1.0	Blood	Neg
		LE	Neg
		Nitrite	Neg
		Color	Yellow

a. Lactate: 4 mmol/L

M. Action
a. Discussion with patient (and family, if available) about the need for emergent embolization for presumed pelvic fracture with bleeding
b. Meds
   i. Fentanyl and/or ketamine (analgesic dose)
c. Interventional radiology for emergent embolization
d. Surgery to continue management with further imaging and admission to SICU

N. Diagnosis
a. Unstable pelvic fracture with hemorrhage
b. Open right ankle fracture

O. Critical actions
a. IV access with at least two large-bore catheters
b. Maintain C-spine protection due to distracting injuries
c. Blood transfusion
d. Immediate activation of surgery/trauma service
e. FAST examination
f. X-ray: chest and pelvis
g. Reduction and fixation of pelvis
h. Consulting IR for angiographic intervention

P. Examiner instructions
a. This is a case of a pelvic fracture secondary to trauma, a serious condition due to the proximity of many large blood vessels that can be injured as a result of the fracture. Initially our patient had outward signs of significant lower extremity trauma and a mechanism severe enough to cause such an injury. The patient, although injured, appears stable initially in terms of mental status, GCS, and vital signs. However, over the course of the case the patient becomes more hypotensive and tachycardic. Immediate actions after ensuring adequate airway, breathing, and circulation are to establish adequate IV access with large-bore catheters, fluid boluses, and to activate any trauma service available or consult surgery. The secondary survey shows that the patient has no evidence of significant injuries other than the right lower extremity and the pelvis. The candidate will need to address the likely source of bleeding in the pelvis with definitive treatment: embolization by interventional radiology. If the candidate attempts to wait for CT of the head, chest, abdomen, and pelvis, the patient should become more hypotensive and the surgery consult should indicate that the patient appears too unstable to go to the scanner.

Q. Pearls
a. Mechanism of injury is a key historical factor in predicting clinical course.
b. Pelvic injury carries a significant mortality and evaluation is a key part of the trauma work-up.
c. Pelvic fractures associated with instability require immediate intervention.
d. Early consultation of trauma services, orthopedics, and possibly interventional radiology should be obtained as pelvic fractures may decompensate quickly.
e. Resuscitative endovascular balloon occlusion of the aorta (REBOA) may be used as a possible temporizing intervention in patients with pelvic fractures with significant hemodynamic instability, but CT angiography or operative fixation is the mainstay of therapy.

R. Figure legends
a. Figure 79.1 (EKG) Sinus tachycardia.
b. Figure 79.2 (a) (US) No free fluid in Morison's pouch. (b) (US) No free fluid in splenorenal recess. (c) (US) No free fluid in pelvis. (d) (US) No pericardial effusion.
c. Figure 79.3 (X-ray) Normal chest x-ray.
d. Figure 79.4 (X-ray) Bilateral pelvic rami fractures.
e. Figure 79.5 (X-ray) Normal cervical spine x-ray.

S. References

a. *Tintinalli's Emergency Medicine: A Comprehensive Study Guide* (9th ed.): Chapter 272, Pelvis Injuries.
b. *Rosen's Emergency Medicine: Concepts and Clinical Practice* (10th ed.): Chapter 41, General Principles of Orthopedic Injuries. Chapter 46, Pelvic Trauma.

Back Pain

Chanteil D. Ulatowski, MD and Nicholas G. Maldonado, MD, FACEP

A. Chief complaint
a. 30-year-old female presents to the emergency department with complaints of back pain

B. Vital signs
a. BP: 95/65, HR: 115, RR: 22, T: 38.1°C (oral), Sat: 98% on RA, FS: 105 mg/dL

C. What does the patient look like?
a. Patient appears her stated age; however, she appears ill and in moderate distress. She is sitting up in bed with her hand on her right flank.

D. Primary survey
a. Airway: speaking in full sentences
b. Breathing: no apparent respiratory distress or cyanosis
c. Circulation: skin is warm and dry with <3 second capillary refill

E. Action
a. Peripheral IV lines
b. Place patient on cardiac monitor
c. Obtain a weight (kg)
d. Labs:
    i. CBC, BMP, LFT, lipase, lactic acid, urinalysis, urine culture, urine pregnancy test
e. 30 mL/kg NS or LR bolus
f. Rectal temperature: 39°C
g. Meds:
    i. Acetaminophen
h. Vitals: BP: 115/68, HR 112, RR: 17, Sat: 99%

F. History
a. HPI: This is a 30-year-old female with a history of ovarian cysts who presents to the emergency department with complaints of right-sided back pain. She states the pain started 2 days ago and has gotten progressively worse. The pain is a 7/10 in severity and located in the right mid-back with radiation to the flank. She notes that she had subjective fevers for the last 24 hours and has been suffering from nausea and vomiting. She also notes that for the last week she has been experiencing urinary frequency which she has attributed to increased thirst and drinking more water. She also states that she has been sexually active with her fiancé where they occasionally use condoms. She denies hematuria or any vaginal discharge, rash, or itching to her genital area. She has a history of irregular menses, thus her LMP is unable to be determined.
b. PMHx: ovarian cysts

c. Obstetric/gynecologic history: nulliparous, irregular menses, ovarian cysts
d. PSHx: none
e. Allergies: penicillin (rash)
f. Meds: none
g. Social: lives at home with her fiancé, social EtOH, denies any tobacco or illicit drug use
h. FHx: diabetes, HTN
i. PCP: Dr. Smith

G. Nurse
a. Vitals
    i. After 30 mL/kg NS: BP: 110/68, HR: 96, RR: 16, Sat: 99%
    ii. If no fluids: BP: 87/65, HR: 122, RR: 24, Sat: 99%
b. Patient
    i. Patient still appears in mild distress and is shivering with chills.
    ii. If no antiemetic given, patient continues complaining of nausea and vomits
c. Urine pregnancy: positive

H. Secondary survey
a. General: alert and oriented × 3, increasing distress secondary to pain
b. Head: normocephalic, atraumatic
c. Eyes: extraocular movement intact, pupils equal, round, reactive to light and 3 mm in diameter
d. Ears: bilateral tympanic membranes without erythema or bulging
e. Nose: no nasal discharge
f. Neck: supple, full ROM, no jugular vein distension or stridor
g. Pharynx: normal dentition, no swelling or lesions
h. Chest: atraumatic with no tenderness to palpation
i. Lungs: clear to auscultation bilaterally
j. Heart:
    i. If fluids given: normal rate and rhythm, no murmur, rubs, or gallops, intact distal pulses
    ii. If no fluids given: tachycardic, with normal rhythm, no murmur, rubs, or gallops, intact distal pulses
k. Abdomen: normal bowel sounds, soft, nondistended, mild tenderness to suprapubic region
l. Urogenital: normal external genitalia
    i. Female: no blood or discharge from cervical os; cervical os is closed; no cervical motion tenderness, adnexal tenderness, or masses noted
m. Extremities: full ROM, no deformity
n. Back: right-sided CVA tenderness; no left-sided CVA tenderness
o. Neuro: cranial nerves II–XII intact, normal sensation, 5/5 strength in bilateral upper and lower extremities, normal reflexes and gait
p. Skin: warm and dry without rashes
q. Lymph: no lymphadenopathy

I. Actions:
a. Labs: HCG quantitative
b. Meds:
    i. Pain: morphine
    ii. Fever: acetaminophen (avoid NSAIDs)
    iii. N/V: ondansetron (Zofran) or metoclopramide (Reglan) or promethazine (Phenergan)

c. Reassess
  i. Patient appears in less distress and is no longer tachycardic after IV fluids. She is no longer vomiting after the use of antiemetics and no longer febrile after antipyretic. She states her pain is now a 2/10 after the pain medication.
d. Imaging possibilities
  i. CXR
  ii. Pelvic ultrasound
  iii. Renal ultrasound
  iv. A noncontrast CT may have been ordered prior to hCG results being known, but should not be done given pregnancy status and alternative options

J. Nurse
a. Vitals: BP: 100/50, HR: 92, RR: 17, Sat 98% on RA

K. Results

Table 80.1 Results table

Test	Result	Test	Result
Complete blood count:		Alk phos	55 U/L
WBC	$16.2 \times 10^3/\mu L$	T bili	1.0 mg/dL
PMN	94%	D bili	0.3 mg/dL
Hct	39.20%	Lipase	27 IU/L
Plt	$246 \times 10^3/\mu L$	Albumin	3.8 g/dL
Basic metabolic panel:		**Urinalysis:**	
Na	139 mEq/L	SG	1.012
K	4.0 mEq/L	pH	7.0
Cl	105 mEq/L	Prot	100
CO_2	26 mEq/L	Gluc	Neg
BUN	27 mEq/dL	Ketones	Trace
Cr	1.2 mg/dL	Bili	Neg
Gluc	104 mg/dL	Blood	Moderate
		LE	+
Coagulation panel:		Nitrite	+
PT	12.8 sec	Color	Yellow
PTT	25.3 sec	Clarity	Turbid
INR	1.1	RBC	58
		WBC	244
		WBC clumps	Many
Liver function panel:		POCT pregnancy	+
AST	27 U/L		
ALT	20 U/L		

a. Urine culture: pending
b. CXR (Figure 80.1)
c. HCG quantitative: 198,000 mIU/mL
d. Lactic acid: 2.1 mmol/L

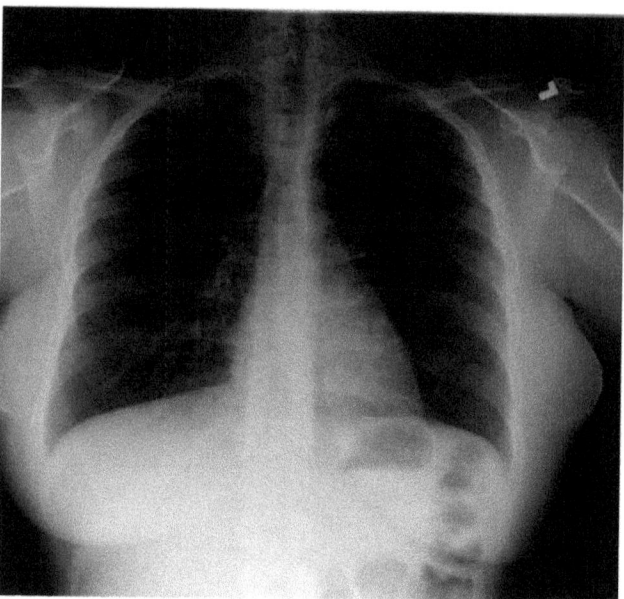

Figure 80.1

L. Action

a. Meds:
    i. Known pregnancy and allergy to penicillin: IV third- or fourth-generation cephalosporin (i.e., ceftriaxone or cefepime given low likelihood of cross-reactivity)
b. Optional:
    i. Transabdominal point-of-care obstetric US (Figure 80.2)
    ii. Renal US to rule out hydronephrosis from nephrolithiasis (Figure 80.3)

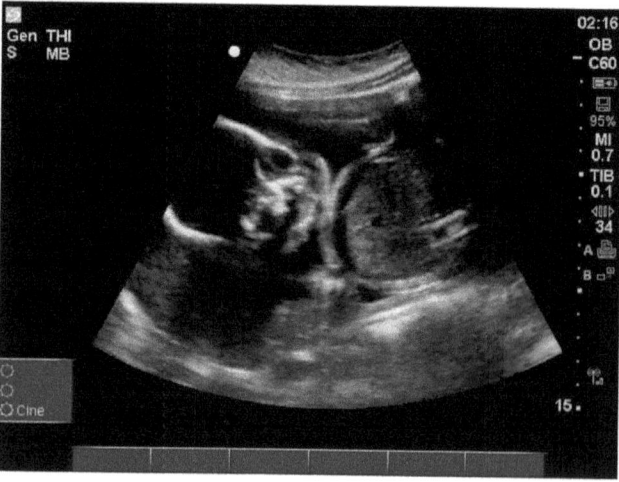

Figure 80.2

c. Disposition:
    i. Admission for IV antibiotics and IV fluid hydration due to acute pyelonephritis in pregnancy

M. Diagnosis

a. Acute pyelonephritis in pregnancy

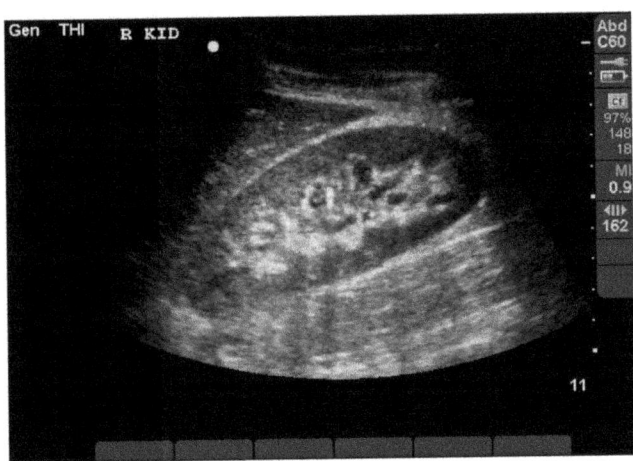

Figure 80.3

N. Critical actions

a. IV fluids: 30 mL/kg bolus of isotonic crystalloid
b. Pain control (avoid NSAIDs)
c. Symptomatic treatments (antipyretic/antiemetic)
d. Identifies penicillin allergy
e. Urine pregnancy test
f. Antibiotics (avoid penicillins and fluoroquinolones)
g. Avoid CT given pregnant status
h. Admission for IV antibiotics and fluid resuscitation

O. Examiner instructions

a. This is a case of acute pyelonephritis in pregnancy. Acute pyelonephritis is a bacterial infection of the urinary system affecting the kidneys. It can present with or without preceding lower urinary tract symptoms (dysuria, frequency, urgency, or hematuria), and with or without signs of sepsis. It complicates 1–2% of pregnancies, resulting in bacteremia in about 20% of cases, and is one of the most common reasons for hospitalization in this patient population. This patient presents with systemic inflammatory response syndrome (febrile, tachycardic, and tachypneic), as well as initial hypotension. Sepsis evaluation should be triggered, and given the patient's chief complaint of back pain, a urinary source should be suspected. Early actions for this patient include IV fluid resuscitation, parenteral antibiotics, and symptomatic treatments. The candidate should obtain a thorough history to establish medication allergy and possibility of pregnancy affecting pharmacotherapy. In addition, a thorough physical exam should be obtained to evaluate for other causes of fever, nausea, vomiting, and flank pain. Pregnancy status should be identified, altering pharmacologic management and image acquisition. Overall, actions harmful to the fetus should be avoided – NSAID use, fetotoxic antibiotics, ionizing radiation. Given the high incidence of complications in pregnant patients with acute pyelonephritis, admission for parenteral antibiotics, IV fluids, and observation is indicated.

P. Pearls

a. Acute pyelonephritis is a clinical diagnosis classically presenting with systemic symptoms, flank pain, and lower urinary tract symptoms, as well as signs of infection and costovertebral angle tenderness. One or more of these classic findings may be absent.
b. A negative urinalysis is insufficient to exclude the diagnosis. Imaging is rarely indicated to establish the diagnosis, but is helpful when complications are suspected (i.e., perinephric abscess, emphysematous pyelonephritis, obstructing ureterolithiasis, etc.).

c. Modifying factors that increase the likelihood of complications include: pregnancy, age >65 years, immunocompromised states, obstructive uropathy, renal transplantation, recent urologic procedure or instrumentation (i.e., stents, nephrostomy tubes), and a history of multidrug resistant organisms, among others.

d. Acute pyelonephritis complicates 1–2% of pregnancies, resulting in bacteremia in about 20% of cases, and is one of the most common reasons for hospitalization in this patient population. Women of child-bearing age with suspected pyelonephritis should be assessed for pregnancy, as this modifying factor alters pharmacologic management, image acquisition, and disposition.

e. Although ciprofloxacin and trimethoprim-sulfamethoxazole are appropriate first-line therapies for most cases of acute uncomplicated pyelonephritis in the setting of favorable local resistance data, they should be avoided in pregnancy. For pregnant patients, an extended-spectrum cephalosporin, extended-spectrum penicillin, or a carbapenem carry less risk to the developing fetus.

f. In patients with mild penicillin allergies, the risk of cross-reactivity with late-generation cephalosporins is low.

g. Given the high incidence of complications in pregnant patients with acute pyelonephritis, admission for parenteral antibiotics, IV fluids, and observation is indicated.

Q. Figure legends

a. Figure 80.1 (CXR) Normal chest x-ray (photo credit: Matthew Constantine, MD).

b. Figure 80.2 (Ultrasound) Ultrasound image showing normal intrauterine pregnancy (photo credit: Connor Nickels, MD, RDMS).

c. Figure 80.3 (Ultrasound) Ultrasound showing normal renal ultrasound (photo credit: Connor Nickels, MD, RDMS).

R. References

a. *Tintinalli's Emergency Medicine: A Comprehensive Study Guide* (9th ed.): Chapter 91, Urinary Tract Infections and Hematuria. Chapter 99, Comorbid Disorders in Pregnancy.

b. *Rosen's Emergency Medicine: Concepts and Clinical Practice* (10th ed.): Chapter 85, Urologic Disorders. Chapter 86, Gynecologic Disorders.

Altered Mental Status

Gail Knight, MD and Terri Davis MD

A. Chief complaint
a. 52 year-old male brought in by EMS with altered mental status

B. Vital signs
a. BP: 150/80, HR: 160, RR: 24, T: 38.6°C, Sat: 97% on RA
b. Point of care glucose (must ask): 150 mg/dL

C. What does the patient look like?
a. Patient appears older than stated age, restless-appearing, fiddling with sheet and telemetry wires, and with frequent cough

D. Primary survey
a. Airway: speaking in full sentences
b. Breathing: tachypneic, no cyanosis
c. Circulation: warm, mildly diaphoretic, capillary refill normal

E. Action
a. Two large-bore peripheral IV lines
b. 1 L NS bolus
c. Acetaminophen 975 mg orally
d. EKG
e. CXR
f. Labs
   i. CBC, BMP, LFT, PT/PTT, urinalysis
   ii. EtOH level, salicylate and APAP levels, TSH, free T4
   iii. Lactic acid, blood cultures, urine culture
g. Monitor: BP: 160/74, HR: 150, RR: 24, Sat: 97%

F. History
a. HPI: A 52-year-old male with a history of hypertension, diabetes, and tobacco use brought in by EMS at the behest of his wife for altered mental status. Wife reports that he has had a cough for the last 3 days getting progressively worse, but that she has never seen him like this before. Two days ago, he complained of throat pain, muscle pain, and a racing heart. She thought he had a cold, so she gave him acetaminophen. However, he has gradually become more confused and restless. She called EMS this morning because she found him in bed, mumbling, talking "out of his head." To her knowledge, he has experienced no falls or trauma. He is usually very active and mentally sharp. There were no pill or alcohol bottles on

scene, per wife. She volunteers that he "eats all the time" lately but seems to have been losing weight over the last 2 months.

ROS: Unable to provide. If specifically asked of wife: + diarrhea, + hair loss. Wife will also say he "looks different in his eyes" if asked about any changes in his appearance.

b. PMHx: hypertension, diabetes
c. PSHx: remote appendectomy (>10 years ago)
d. Allergies: none
e. Meds: hydrochlorothiazide, metformin
f. Social: lives with wife at home, smokes one pack a day for the last 10 years, nondrinker, denies drug use, monogamous with wife, works as an accountant
g. FHx: not relevant
h. PMD: switched doctors, hasn't seen one in about 8 months

G. Nurse

a. EKG (Figure 81.1)
b. If 1 L NS given:
    i. BP: 145/65, HR: 150, RR: 22, Sat: 100% on O_2
c. If no fluids given:
    i. BP: 106/60, HR: 160, RR: 24, Sat 100% on O_2
d. CXR (Figure 81.2)
e. If acetaminophen given: 37.9°C
f. If no acetaminophen given: 39.0°C

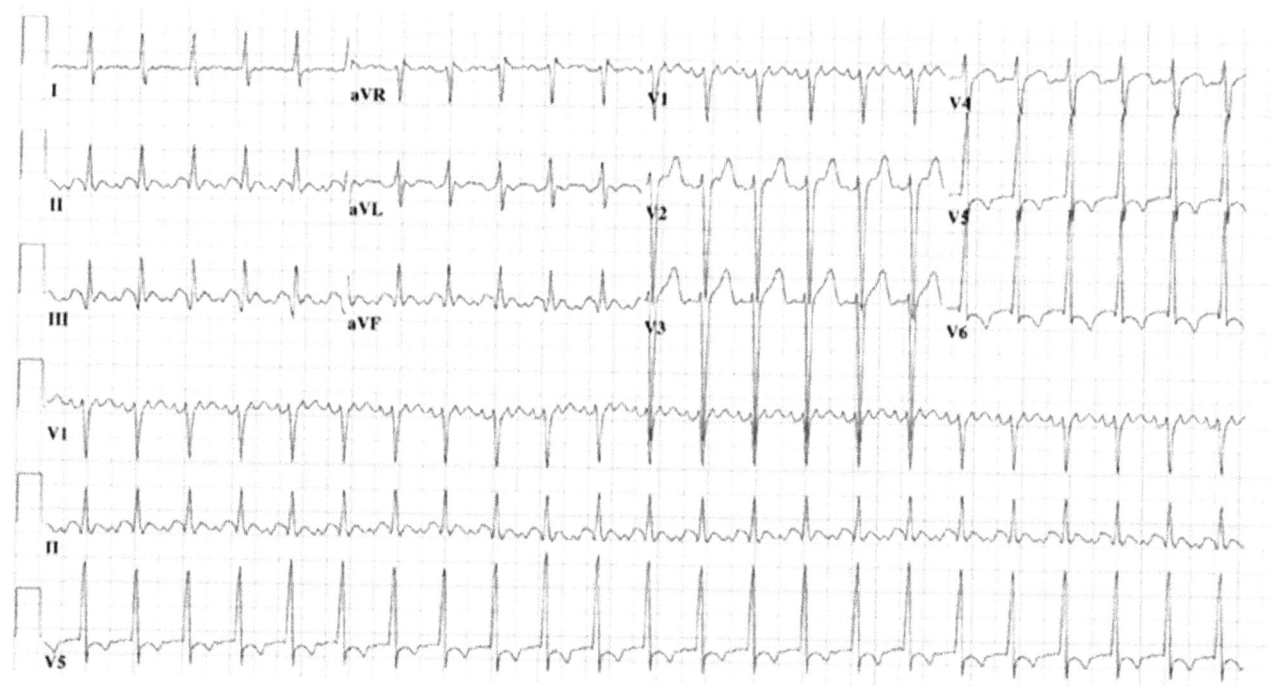

Figure 81.1

H. Secondary survey

a. General: alert, disoriented to place and time, muttering but often incomprehensible, is able to answer yes or no to simple questions like, "Do you have pain?"
b. Head: normal
c. Eyes: exophthalmos, but examiner should ask what the candidate is looking for (Figure 81.3)

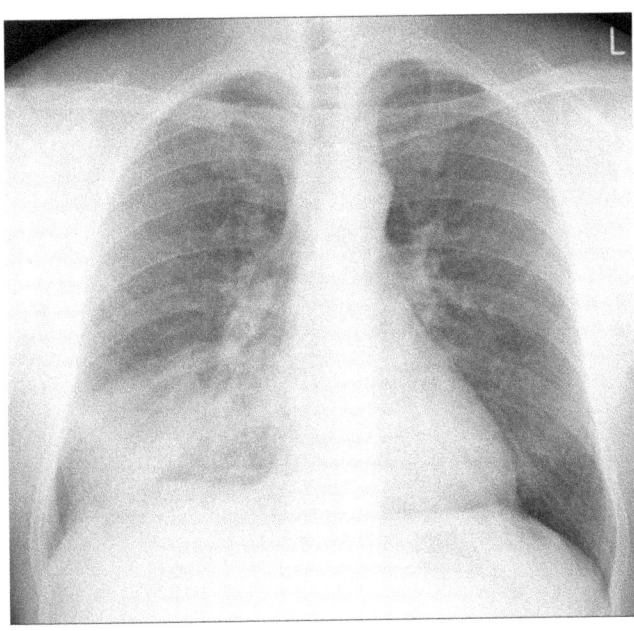

Figure 81.2

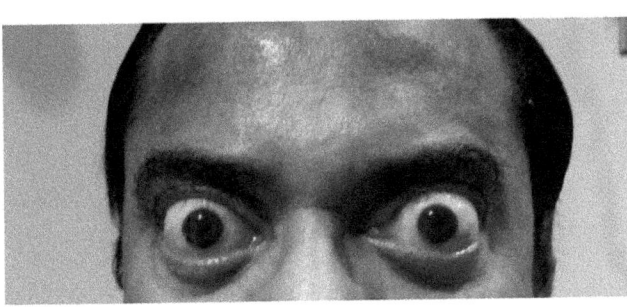

Figure 81.3

d. ENT: dry mucous membranes, otherwise normal
e. Neck: supple, nonnuchal, + thyromegaly, + tenderness to palpation, no jugular vein distension
f. Chest: tachypneic, expiratory wheeze bilaterally, diminished over right middle lung field
g. Heart: tachycardic to 150s
h. Abdomen: normal
i. Urogenital: normal
j. Extremities: no gross deformities, full range of motion
k. Back: normal
l. Neuro: alert, oriented × 1 (self), intermittently follows simple commands, mumbling incomprehensibly, moving all four extremities with good bulk tone, fine tremor, no gross deficits, brisk patellar reflexes bilaterally, no clonus, bilateral down-going Babinski, gait not tested
m. Skin: warm, diaphoretic
n. Lymph: normal

I. Action
a. Meds:
    i. 1 L IVF bolus (if not given already)
    ii. Appropriate antibiotics to treat pneumonia

b. Reassess
  i. Patient still altered
c. Imaging
  i. CT head, noncontrast

J. Nurse

a. Vital signs: same as prior
b. Patient: still restless, tremulous and tachycardic

K. Results

Table 81.1 Results table

Test	Result	Test	Result
Complete blood count:		**Liver function panel:**	
WBC	$18.0 \times 10^3/\mu L$	AST	23 U/L
Hct	41.5%	ALT	26 U/L
Plt	$421 \times 10^3/\mu L$	Alk phos	42 U/L
		T bili	1.0 mg/dL
Basic metabolic panel:		D bili	0.3 mg/dL
Na	138 mEq/L	Amylase	50 U/L
K	3.5 mEq/L	Lipase	25 U/L
Cl	105 mEq/L	Albumin	4.7 g/dL
CO_2	30 mEq/L		
BUN	21 mEq/dL	**Urinalysis:**	
Cr	1.1 mg/dL	SG	1.010–1.030
Gluc	105 mg/dL	pH	5–8
		Prot	Neg
Coagulation panel:		Gluc	Neg
PT	12.6 sec	Ketones	Neg
PTT	26.0 sec	Bili	Neg
INR	1.0	Blood	Neg
		LE	Neg
		Nitrite	Neg
		Color	Yellow

a. CT head (Figure 81.4)
b. Pending: TSH, free T4, T3, any other labs

L. Action

a. Lumbar puncture
b. Discussion with wife to perform lumbar puncture, obtain informed consent

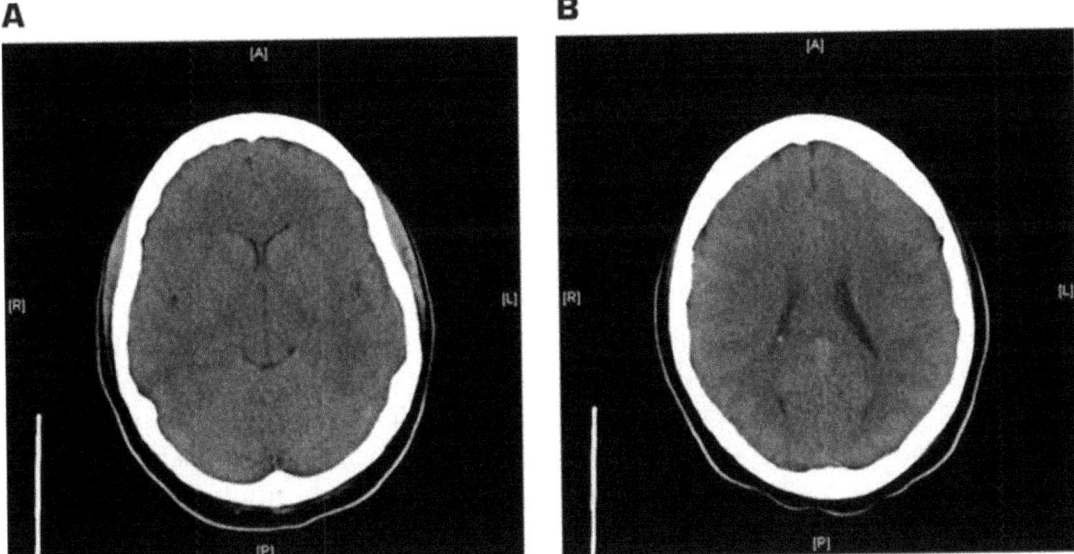

Figure 81.4

c. Meds:
   i. Propranolol (0.5–1 mg IV over 10 minutes; repeat doses of 1–2 mg IV over 10 minutes every 2 hours)
   ii. Methimazole 40 mg PO/NGT loading dose then 20 mg PO/NGT every 4 hours (Propylthiouracil (PTU) 600–1000 mg PO/NGT loading dose then 200 mg PO/NGT every 4 hours is an acceptable response, however it is less preferred due to an FDA boxed warning.)
   iii. After 1 hour, 10 drops of potassium iodide–iodine solution.
   iv. Steroids
   v. Antibiotics

M. Reassess
a. Appears calmer, tremor improved
b. BP: 130/70, HR: 100, RR: 20, Sat: 100% on O_2

N. Nurse:
a. Results: TSH, free T4

O. Action
a. Consult ICU for admission

P. Diagnosis
a. Thyrotoxicosis
b. Community-acquired pneumonia

Q. Critical actions
a. Large-bore IV access
b. IVF resuscitation 1–2 L
c. CXR
d. CT head

    e. Antibiotics

    f. Propranolol, methimazole (or PTU)

    g. Disposition to ICU

R. Examiner instructions

a. This is a case of an infectious process (community-acquired pneumonia [CAP]) triggering thyrotoxicosis, leading to altered mental status (AMS). Thyrotoxicosis is a clinical diagnosis and should be based upon a thorough history and a rigorous physical exam. It is important that the candidate is specific when enquiring about the eye and ENT portions of the physical exam. The examiner should probe, "What do you want to know?" which clues the examinee in, but also forces them to be specific. Thyrotoxicosis (or thyroid storm) can occur in untreated or incompletely treated Graves' disease followed by a provocative illness such as infection, trauma, diabetic crisis, myocardial infarction, childbirth, use of iodinated contrast studies, emotional stress, etc. Important early actions include administering IV fluids, appropriate antibiotics to treat CAP, and proper treatment of thyrotoxicosis with a β-blocker (preferably propranolol) and antithyroidal agents (PTU or methimazole). The CT head should be pursued in the setting of a patient with altered mental status, but is negative for acute process. Lumbar puncture is not a critical action if the examinee identifies the pneumonia early.

S. Pearls

a. Thyrotoxicosis is a clinical diagnosis, not a lab diagnosis. Do not wait for test results before starting treatment.

b. The Burch–Wartofsky point scale predicts the likelihood that thyrotoxicosis is thyroid storm. It utilizes a point scale based on the patient's temperature, CNS effects, gastrointestinal–hepatic dysfunction, heart rate, CHF, and atrial fibrillation.

c. When treating thyrotoxicosis, always give medications in the following order: propranolol, thionamides, then iodine.

    i. Propranolol blunts the sympathomimetic drive and symptoms of thyrotoxicosis. (Esmolol is preferred if the patient has congestive heart failure. Consider cardio-selective β-blockers [atenolol, metoprolol, or calcium channel blockers] in patients with reactive airway disease).

    ii. Methimazole is preferred over propylthiouracil for severe-but-not-life-threatening hyperthyroidism (except during pregnancy due to teratogenicity of methimazole). Propylthiouracil blocks the peripheral conversion of T4 to T3 (unlike methimazole), but has an FDA box warning for liver injury. PTU is the preferred medication for life-threatening thyroid storm.

    iii. Iodine is administered 1 hour after thionamide administration. It blocks the release of thyroid hormone, but if it is given earlier it will have the opposite effect.

d. Stressors such as infection, surgery, trauma, acute iodine load, myocardial infarction, and childbirth increase the risk of developing thyrotoxicosis in patients with an underlying thyroid disorder.

T. Figure legends

a. Figure 81.1 (EKG) EKG showing sinus tachycardia.

b. Figure 81.2 (CXR) Chest x-ray showing right lower lobe pneumonia (case courtesy of Dr. Sajoscha Sorrentino, Radiopaedia.org, rID: 14979).

c. Figure 81.3 (Photo) Exophthalmos (image reproduced with permission from Adam J Cohen, MD, published by Medscape Drugs & Diseases (https://emedicine.medscape.com/), Exophthalmos (Proptosis), 2020, available at https://emedicine.medscape.com/article/1218575-overview).

d. Figure 81.4 (CT) Normal noncontrast CT of the head.

U. References

a. *Tintinalli's Emergency Medicine: A Comprehensive Study Guide* (9th ed.): Chapter 229, Hyperthyroidism and Thyroid Storm.

b. *Rosen's Emergency Medicine: Concepts and Clinical Practice* (10th ed.): Chapter 117, Thyroid and Adrenal Disorders.

Abdominal Pain

Christopher Strother, MD

A. Chief complaint
a. 3-year-old male brought in by his mother with the complaint of abdominal pain and vomiting after falling off a stool at home

B. Vital signs
a. BP: 115/73, HR: 155, RR: 32 (crying), T: 36.8°C, Sat: 100% on RA

C. What does the patient look like?
a. Patient appears stated age, uncomfortable-appearing, and holding his abdomen.

D. Primary survey
a. Airway: patent, speaking normally, crying
b. Breathing: no apparent respiratory distress, no cyanosis
c. Circulation: pink, warm skin, normal capillary refill

E. Action
a. No immediate actions indicated

F. History
a. HPI: This is a 3-year-old male who presents with moderate to severe diffuse abdominal pain. His mother states that the child fell off a stool in the kitchen onto a marble floor, or possibly onto another chair, cried initially, calmed down, then fell asleep for a couple of hours. The incident was not witnessed by his mother as she was not home at the time. He awoke crying and has been crying about stomach pain for the past 30 minutes. He is refusing to eat or drink and has vomited (nonbloody, nonbilious). There has been no diarrhea. He denies pain anywhere else.
b. PMHx: none
c. PSHx: none
d. Allergies: none
e. Social: lives with mother and mother's boyfriend; no smoking or pets in the house
f. FHx: not relevant
g. PMD: Dr. Sanders

G. Secondary survey
a. General: alert but very fussy, moderate distress secondary to pain
b. HEENT: normal
c. Neck: normal, supple

d. Chest: normal
e. Heart: normal
f. Abdomen: diffuse tenderness and guarding, nondistended, no masses, no hernias, bowel sounds present, limited examination – patient uncooperative due to pain
g. Rectal: brown stool, hemoccult negative
h. Urogenital: normal
i. Extremities: normal except scattered bruises on forearms, upper arms, and thighs
j. Back: normal, no tenderness
k. Neuro: normal
l. Skin: normal except minor bruising as above
m. Lymph: normal

H. Action

a. Meds
  i. Pain control
  ii. NS 20 mL/kg
b. Consult
  i. Surgery
  ii. Social work
c. Imaging
  i. CT abdomen
  ii. Focused assessment with sonography in trauma (FAST): negative for free fluid
d. Monitor
e. One large-bore peripheral IV line
f. Labs
  i. CBC, BMP, LFT, blood type, PT/PTT, urinalysis

I. Nurse

a. BP: 98/75, HR: 125, RR: 26, Sat: 100% on RA
b. Patient: still with significant pain unless opioid given

J. Results

Table 82.1 Results table

Test	Result	Test	Result
Complete blood count:		**Liver function panel:**	
WBC	$20.1 \times 10^3/\mu L$	AST	14 U/L
Hct	34.5%	ALT	28 U/L
Plt	$553 \times 10^3/\mu L$	Alk phos	220 U/L
		T bili	0.4 mg/dL
		D bili	0.2 mg/dL
Basic metabolic panel:		Amylase	68 U/L
Na	142 mEq/L	Lipase	35 U/L
K	4.0 mEq/L	Albumin	3.5 g/dL
Cl	110 mEq/L		

Table 82.1 (cont.)

Test	Result	Test	Result
CO_2	21 mEq/L	Urinalysis:	
BUN	8 mEq/dL	SG	1.025
Cr	0.6 mg/dL	pH	7
Gluc	120 mg/dL	Prot	Neg
		Gluc	Neg
Coagulation panel:		Ketones	Neg
PT	13.1 sec	Bili	Neg
PTT	26 sec	Blood	Neg
INR	1.0	LE	Neg
		Nitrite	Neg
		Color	Yellow

a. CT abdomen (Figure 82.1) demonstrates splenic laceration

K. Action
a. Surgery consult
   i. Admit for serial examinations, observation
b. Social work consult
   i. The patient has an injury due to child abuse. The police and child protective services need to be contacted; they will likely temporarily remove the child from his home. The mother seems appropriate currently and is also a victim of domestic abuse by her boyfriend.
c. Ophthalmology consult
   i. No retinal hemorrhages
d. Discussion with family regarding need for admission, social work, child services due to severity of injury with inconsistent story (discussed sensitively with mother)
e. Meds
   i. Morphine or fentanyl
f. Radiology
   i. Skeletal survey for occult fractures

L. Diagnosis
a. Nonaccidental abdominal trauma
b. Splenic laceration

M. Critical actions
a. Recognition of potentially serious abdominal injury
b. CT abdomen
c. Recognition of inconsistent story, pattern of bruises, possible child abuse
d. Surgery consult
e. Social work/child services consult

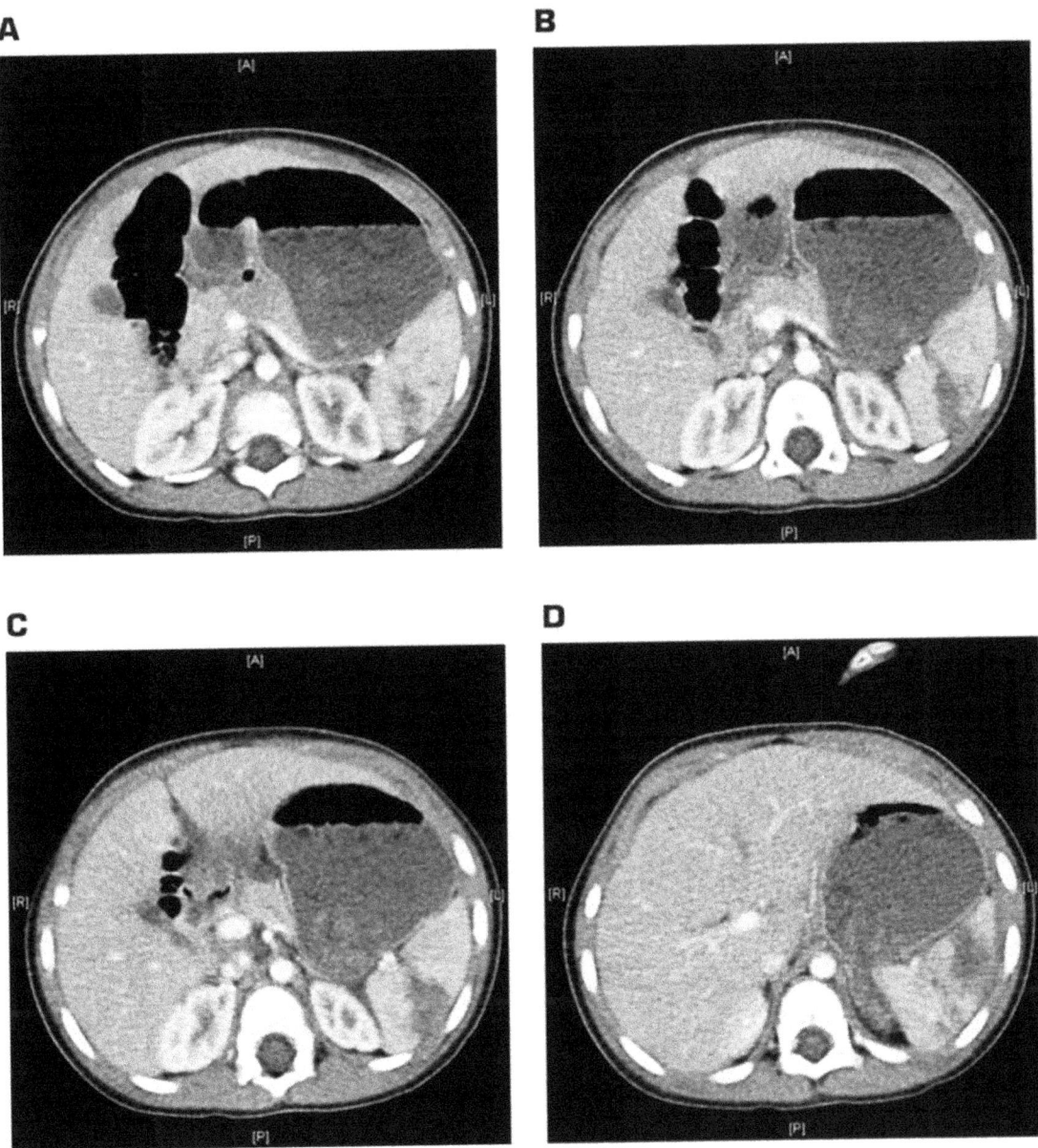

Figure 82.1

N. Examiner instructions

a. This is a case of nonaccidental trauma, or child abuse. The key to the case is that the story of falling off a chair is inconsistent with a serious abdominal injury. Also, the physical examination reveals bruising that is inconsistent with a typical 3-year-old's rough- housing. Knee and elbow scrapes and findings that are expected at this age, but soft tissue bruising of the upper arms and thighs is concerning. A 3-year-old is easily influenced and will likely agree with whatever story the mother gives initially. The real history is that the mother's abusive boyfriend kicked him when he dropped and broke a dish in the kitchen. The mother will only admit this if a social worker is called to speak with her, or if directly asked about the possibility of the boyfriend causing the injury.

b. The severe tenderness of the abdomen should prompt CT evaluation. Social work or child services should be notified in any case of suspected child abuse. If highly suspicious or confirmed nonaccidental trauma, ophthalmology should be consulted to evaluate for retinal hemorrhage as a sign of shaken baby syndrome. Particularly in younger children and infants, a full skeletal survey should be done to rule out occult injury and identify old injury patterns. Head CT should also be considered if findings of physical abuse are present.

O. Pearls

a. Physicians are mandated reporters – if child abuse is suspected, authorities must be notified.
b. The story should corroborate the injury.
c. Mothers who are abused often have children at risk and vice versa.
d. CT scan is the gold standard for diagnosis of blunt abdominal injury in children.
e. Splenic lacerations in stable children often do well with minimal intervention, observation, and supportive care; immediate laparotomy is *not* indicated. However, surgery should always be consulted.

P. Figure legends

a. Figure 82.1 (CT abdomen) Splenic laceration and hematoma

Q. References

a. *Tintinalli's Emergency Medicine: A Comprehensive Study Guide* (9th ed.): Chapter 110, Pediatric Trauma. Chapter 150, Child Abuse and Neglect.
b. *Rosen's Emergency Medicine: Concepts and Clinical Practice* (10th ed.): Chapter 160, Pediatric Trauma. Chapter 170, Child Abuse.

Abdominal Pain

Lisa Jacobson, MD

A. Chief complaint
a. 5-year-old boy presents with mild abdominal pain, cola-colored urine, and diarrhea

B. Vital signs
a. BP: 115/70, HR: 90, RR: 18, T: 38.0°C

C. What does the patient look like?
a. A well-developed, interactive child with a pale complexion, in mild distress.

D. Primary survey
a. Airway: speaking in full sentences
b. Breathing: regular rate
c. Circulation: distal pulses bounding

E. Action
a. Labs
    i. CBC, BMP, LFT, coagulation studies, blood type and crossmatch
b. IV access
c. Acknowledge hypertension by repeating blood pressure

F. History
a. HPI: This is a 5-year-old boy with 10 days of watery diarrhea and occasional nonbilious, nonbloody vomiting. His mother has noticed that he feels warm on occasion and has given him acetaminophen. He has consistently complained of lower abdominal pain that she thought was related to the diarrhea and she thought he just had a "stomach flu." When he started complaining that his urine looked funny, she brought him to the ER. The child endorses red material in his diarrhea at times over the past few days.
b. PMHx: none
c. PSHx: none
d. Allergies: penicillin
e. Social: lives with mom and dad, has one younger sister; attends kindergarten
f. FHx: maternal grandmother has diabetes; father has high blood pressure
g. PMD: Dr. Kline

G. Nurse
a. Repeat BP: 117/75

H. Secondary survey

a. General: pale, normally developed boy in mild distress
b. HEENT: pupils equal and reactive, mucous membranes moist, tympanic membranes clear
c. Neck: normal
d. Chest: CTA bilaterally, no wheeze/rhonchi/rales
e. Heart: regular rate and rhythm, no murmurs
f. Abdomen: soft, nondistended, mild tenderness in lower abdomen
g. Rectal: occult blood positive
h. Urogenital: circumcised, no lesions, bilateral descended testes, no hernias
i. Extremities: full range, no edema
j. Back: normal
k. Neuro: normal
l. Skin: occasional petechiae and ecchymoses on shins
m. Lymph: normal

I. Action

a. Labs
    i.   stool culture
b. IV hydration

J. Nurse

a. Vitals remain the same
b. Patient: still with abdominal discomfort; has had diarrhea during the visit

K. Results

Table 83.1 Results table

Test	Result	Test	Result
Complete blood count:		**Liver function panel:**	
WBC	$13.1 \times 10^3/\mu L$	AST	23 U/L
Hct	21.5%	ALT	26 U/L
Plt	$35 \times 10^3/\mu L$	Alk phos	42 U/L
		T bili	1.6 mg/dL
Basic metabolic panel:		D bili	0.3 mg/dL
Na	139 mEq/L	Amylase	50 U/L
K	4.8 mEq/L	Lipase	25 U/L
Cl	101 mEq/L	Albumin	4.7 g/dL
CO_2	18.9 mEq/L		
BUN	18 mEq/L	**Urinalysis:**	
Cr	1.1 mg/dL	SG	1.010–1.030
Gluc	89 mg/dL	pH	5–8
		Prot	+

Table 83.1 (cont.)

Test	Result	Test	Result
Coagulation panel:		Gluc	Neg
PT	12.6 sec	Ketones	Neg
PTT	26.0 sec	Bili	+
INR	1.0	Blood	+
		LE	Neg
		Nitrite	Neg
		Color	Yellow

a. Helmet and burr cells seen on CBC

L. Action

a. Consult
   i. Hematology, possible plasmapheresis if symptoms worsen
   ii. Nephrology
b. Admit
c. Discuss diagnosis with family
d. Meds
   i. IV hydration
e. EKG (Figure 83.1)
f. NPO
g. May type and cross for platelets, although this is unnecessary

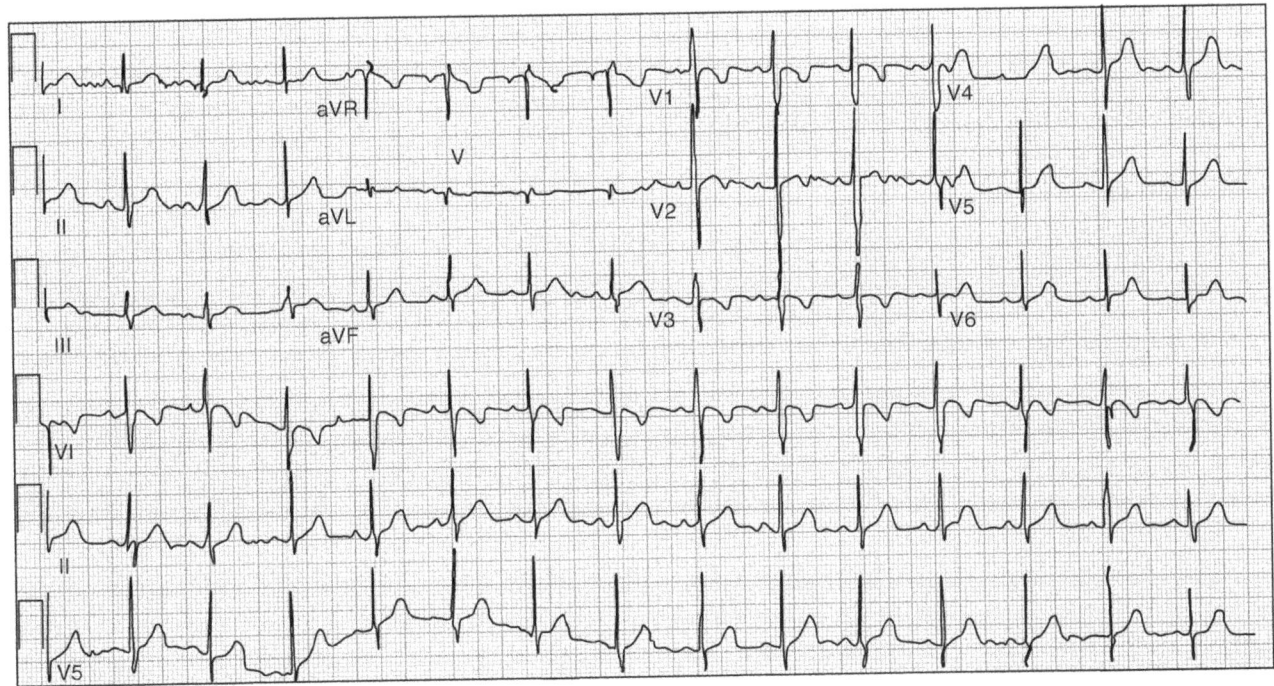

Figure 83.1

M. Diagnosis

a. Hemolytic uremic syndrome (HUS)

N. Critical actions

a. Large-bore IV access and fluid bolus
b. Discussion with family
c. Admission
d. Pediatric hematology consult

O. Examiner instructions

a. This is a case of hemolytic uremic syndrome (HUS) in a child following an episode of *Escherichia coli* O157:H7-mediated diarrheal illness. This condition is typically caused by ingesting bacteria from sources such as uncooked meats, and causes severe low red blood cell and platelet count and kidney problems. Early actions include IV access, CBC, and fluids. The use of antimotility agents is contraindicated in patients with *E. coli* infectious diarrhea. In children, advanced measures such as plasma exchange or infusion are rarely used as mortality is so low. Antibiotics are not indicated. The patient should be admitted for observation and hydration.

P. Pearls

a. Treatment with antimotility agents may lead to toxic megacolon.
b. Treatment with antibiotics may enhance toxin release.
c. Treat hyperkalemia.
d. Consider plasmapheresis if symptoms are severe.
e. Ninety percent recover with supportive treatment alone.
f. Up to 40% of patients may develop seizures from CNS involvement.
g. Consider thrombocytopenic purpura and disseminated intravascular coagulation in your differential.

Q. Figure legends

a. Figure 83.1 (EKG) Normal sinus rhythm.

R. References

a. *Tintinalli's Emergency Medicine: A Comprehensive Study Guide* (9th ed.): Chapter 237, Acquired Hemolytic Anemia.
b. *Rosen's Emergency Medicine: Concepts and Clinical Practice* (10th ed.): Chapter 168, Pediatric Genitourinary and Renal Tract Disorders.

Respiratory Distress

Lisa Jacobson, MD

A. Chief complaint
a. 2-year-old female with respiratory distress

B. Vital signs
a. BP: 90/60, HR: 125, RR: 40, T: 37.1°C, Sat: 90% on RA

C. What does the patient look like?
a. A well-developed, interactive child with pale complexion in moderate respiratory distress.

D. Primary survey
a. Airway: crying
b. Breathing: labored, fast
c. Circulation: distal pulses bounding

E. Action
a. Oxygen supplementation (blow-by O_2)
b. Airway management preparation
   i. Bag-valve mask and intubation tray
c. Peripheral IV access
d. Monitor: BP: 90/60, HR: 125, RR: 40, Sat: 93% on blow-by O_2

F. History
a. HPI: This is a 2-year-old girl brought in by her anxious mother who states that her daughter suddenly started to cry while she was playing in her room unattended for 5 minutes. The girl has appeared agitated and short of breath since. The mother states she only went to the other room to answer the phone. She thinks her daughter's lips look a little blue. The episode occurred 30 minutes ago, and the daughter has been inconsolable since, which is not like her.
b. PMHx: none, normal delivery full term, immunizations up to date
c. PSHx: none
d. Allergies: none
e. Meds: none
f. Social: lives with her parents, has one older sister; attends daycare
g. FHx: maternal grandmother has diabetes; father has high blood pressure
h. PMD: Dr. Stern

G. Nurse
a. BP: 90/69, Sat: 92% on blow-by O_2

H. Examination

a. General: alert, interactive, mild respiratory distress, drooling
b. Head: normocephalic, atraumatic
c. Eyes: extraocular movements intact, pupils equal, reactive to light
d. Ears: normal tympanic membranes
e. Nose: no discharge
f. Pharynx: no obvious foreign body in posterior pharynx (must ask), no exudates or injection of tonsils, cyanotic lips
g. Neck: full range of motion, no jugular vein distension, no stridor
h. Chest: nontender
i. Lungs: increased work of breathing with significant respiratory effort, breath sounds clear and equal bilaterally, retractions, grunting, air exchange fair
j. Heart: tachycardic, pulses 2+, equal bilaterally, no murmurs
k. Abdomen: soft, nontender, bowel sounds normal
l. Genital examination: Tanner I girl
m. Extremities: full range of motion, no deformity, normal pulses
n. Back: normal inspection
o. Neuro: awake, alert appropriate for age
p. Skin: warm and dry, no rash
q. Lymph: no lymphadenopathy

I. Action

a. Portable CXR
b. Foreign body extraction or ENT consult (ENT initially says they will be down in 1 hour – candidate must be persistent)
c. Conversation with mother to explain concern for foreign body

J. Nurse

a. CXR (Figure 84.1): upper airway foreign body visualized

K. Action

a. ENT is able to remove the foreign body (candidate must have visualized the foreign body on x-ray – ENT should ask what they saw on x-ray) *or* examinee is able to remove the foreign body with direct or video laryngoscopy
b. Repeat vital signs: BP: 90/60, HR: 115, RR: 22, Sat: 100%
c. Admit for observation or observe in ED and discharge with precautions

L. Diagnosis

a. Foreign body aspiration

M. Critical actions

a. Airway management preparation
b. Oxygen supplementation
c. CXR
d. ENT consult or foreign body removal

Figure 84.1

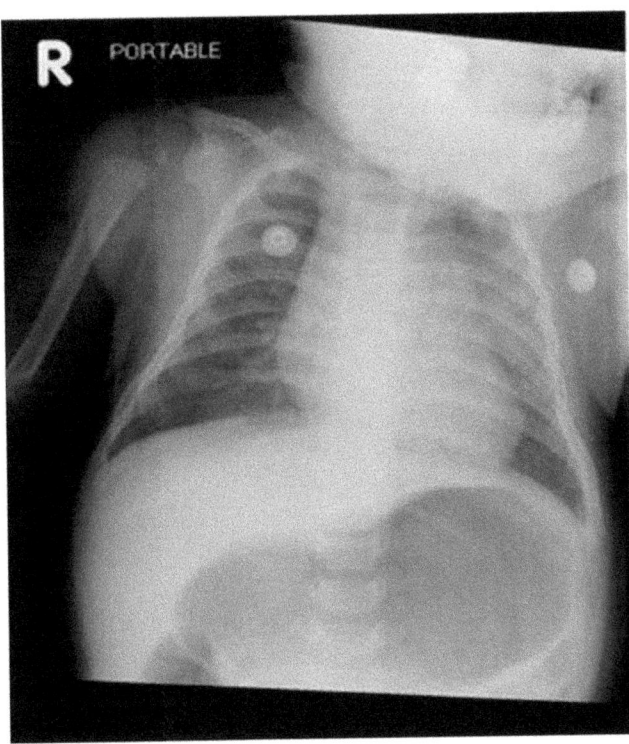

N. Examiner instructions

a. This is a case of aspiration of a foreign body found in the posterior pharynx. The child was left alone by her mother and swallowed something that has partially obstructed the airway. The candidate should prepare to manage the airway but should not intubate. A foreign body is visualized on x-ray and ENT consult can come immediately to remove the object, but initially the ENT consult will be resistant. In this case there is only one x-ray, but the candidate could ask for inspiratory and expiratory films and/or a neck x-ray. Foreign body management may also consist of abdominal thrusts in the upright or supine position, as the child is older than 1 year.

b. It is reasonable for the examinee to opt to treat on their own with BLS, direct laryngoscopy, and/or video laryngoscopy as well.

O. Figure legends

a. Figure 84.1 Chest x-ray.

P. References

a. *Rosen's Emergency Medicine: Concepts and Clinical Practice* (10th ed.): Chapter 162, Pediatric Upper Airway Obstruction and Infections.

b. *Tintinalli's Emergency Medicine: A Comprehensive Study Guide* (9th ed.): Chapter 126, Stridor and Drooling in Children.

Overdose

Lisa Jacobson, MD

A. Chief complaint

a. 45-year-old female with foot pain and depression

B. Vital signs

a. BP: 115/70, HR: 90, RR: 16, T: 37.0°C, Sat: 100% on RA, Wt: 50 kg

C. What does the patient look like?

a. Patient is a thin Caucasian woman with a flat affect.

D. Primary survey

a. Airway: speaking in full sentences
b. Breathing: no apparent respiratory distress, no cyanosis
c. Circulation: dry and cool skin, normal capillary refill

E. History

a. HPI: This is a 45-year-old female who sustained an ankle fracture 7 days ago and has been feeling frustrated by her current immobility. Eight hours ago, she was at home drinking wine and feeling sad and frustrated when she decided to take the remaining 29 of her 50 oxycodone/APAP tablets with the intention to commit suicide. She then went to bed. When she awoke this morning, she felt guilty and scared. Not wanting to die, she told her husband what had happened and was brought to the ER. She denies headache, nausea, vomiting, abdominal pain, chest pain, shortness of breath, numbness, tingling, or weakness. She has had no recent illness and denies co-ingestions or previous suicide attempts. She was in the ED 1 week ago for placement of a cast for her left ankle fracture.
b. PMHx: none
c. PSHx: none
d. Allergies: none
e. Meds: received Rx for 50 oxycodone/acetaminophen (5/325 mg) 7 days ago
f. Social: denies tobacco, drinks wine daily, denies illicit drug use
g. FHx: none

F. Action

a. Oxygen supplementation as needed
b. Two large-bore peripheral IV lines

c. Labs
  i. CBC, BMP, LFT, coagulation studies, blood type and crossmatch
  ii. Urine pregnancy test, alcohol level, acetaminophen level, salicylate level, urine toxicology screen
d. Monitor: BP: 115/70, HR: 90, RR: 16, Sat: 100% on O_2
e. EKG
f. CXR
g. Meds
  i. Charcoal can be given, though unlikely to provide benefit 8 hours post-ingestion
  ii. Empiric initiation of N-acetylcysteine
h. Psychiatric hold

G. Secondary survey
a. General: alert, oriented × 3, comfortable, gaze evading
b. Head: normocephalic, atraumatic
c. Eyes: extraocular movements intact, pupils pinpoint bilaterally
d. Ears: normal tympanic membranes
e. Nose: no discharge
f. Neck: full range of motion, no jugular vein distension, no stridor
g. Pharynx: normal dentition, no lesions, no swelling
h. Chest: nontender
i. Lungs: clear bilaterally
j. Heart: rate and rhythm regular, no murmurs, rubs, or gallops
k. Abdomen: normal bowel sounds, soft, nontender, nondistended
l. Rectal: normal tone, brown stool, occult blood negative
m. Extremities: normal pulses, full range, no edema, left lower extremity casted to mid-calf
n. Back: nontender
o. Neuro: cranial nerves II to XII intact; normal sensation, strength; normal reflexes and gait
p. Skin: warm and dry
q. Lymph: no lymphadenopathy

H. Action
a. Call Poison Control Center
b. Start N-acetylcysteine (NAC)
c. Psychiatry consult
d. Admit

I. Nurse
a. EKG (Figure 85.1)
b. CXR (Figure 85.2)

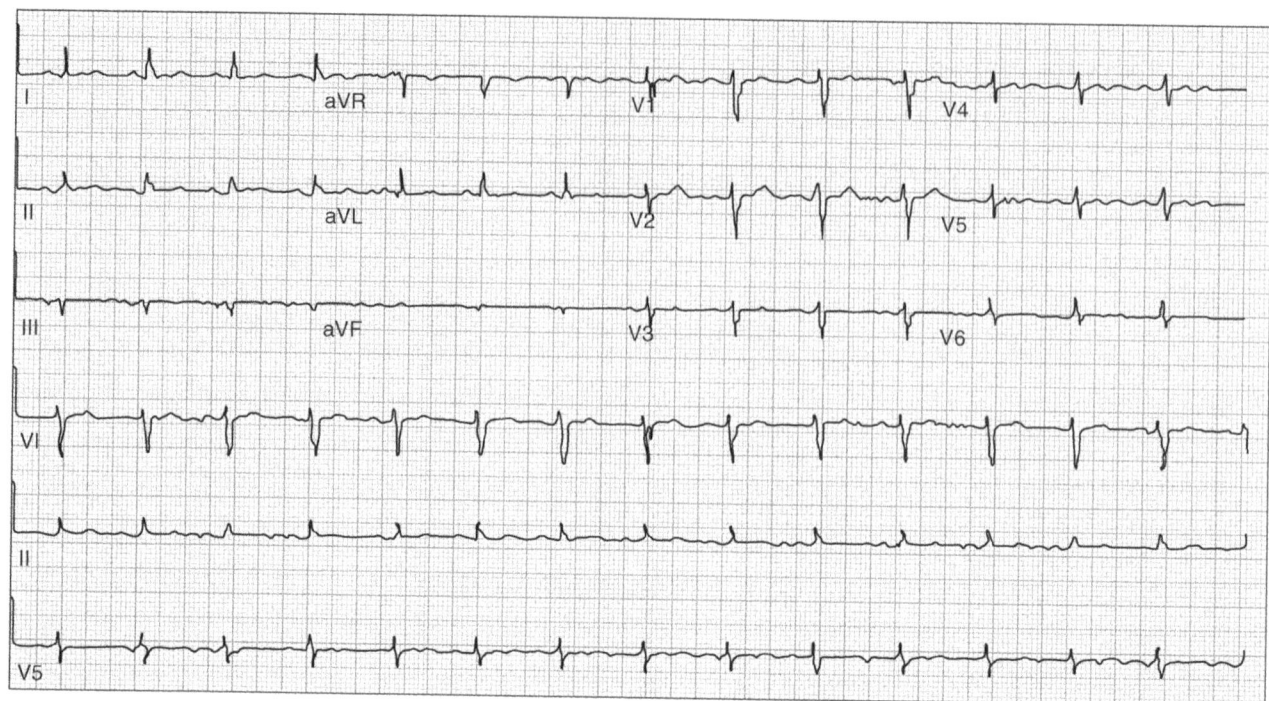

Figure 85.1

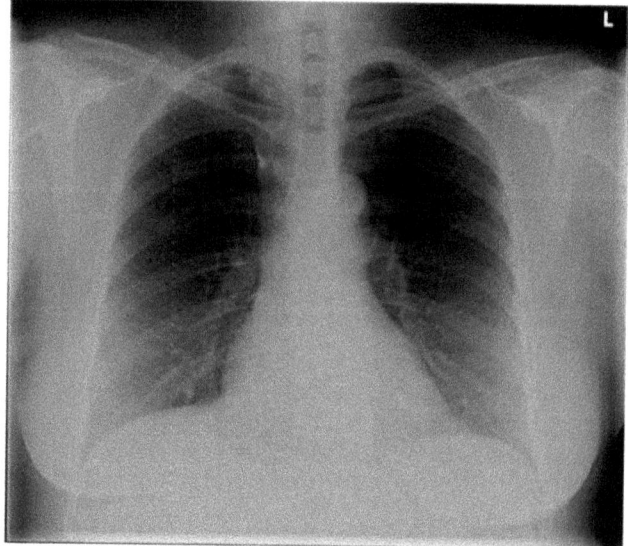

Figure 85.2

J. Results

Table 85.1 Results table

Test	Result	Test	Result
Complete blood count:		T bili	1.0 mg/dL
WBC	$5.3 \times 10^3/\mu L$	D bili	0.3 mg/dL
Hct	41.5%	Amylase	50 U/L
Plt	$350 \times 10^3/\mu L$	Lipase	25 U/L
		Albumin	4.7 g/dL
Basic metabolic panel:			
Na	138 mEq/L	**Urinalysis:**	
K	4.3 mEq/L	SG	1.010–1.030
Cl	105 mEq/L	pH	5–8
CO_2	30 mEq/L	Prot	Neg
BUN	12 mEq/dL	Gluc	Neg
Cr	1.1 mg/dL	Ketones	Neg
Gluc	100 mg/dL	Bili	Neg
		Blood	Neg
Coagulation panel:		LE	Neg
PT	12.6 sec	Nitrite	Neg
PTT	26.0 sec	Color	Yellow
INR	1.0		
		Arterial blood gas:	
Liver function panel:		pH	7.4
AST	23 U/L	PO_2	95 mmHg
ALT	26 U/L	PCO_2	41 mmHg
Alk phos	42 U/L	HCO_3	24 mmol/L

a. Urine pregnancy test: negative
b. Urine toxicology: negative
c. Alcohol level: 252 mg/dL
d. Salicylate level: <5 mg/dL
e. Acetaminophen: 167 mcg/dL

K. Diagnosis
a. Acetaminophen overdose

L. Critical actions

a. Determine timing of ingestion
b. Check acetaminophen level and potentially co-ingested substance levels
c. Start NAC immediately based on calculated dose greater than 140 mg/kg
d. Check EKG
e. Place patient on suicide watch

M. Examiner instructions

a. This is a case of acetaminophen overdose that presents at approximately 8 hours post-ingestion. This is a serious overdose given the amount of medication ingested and has a high risk for liver failure and death. Thus, the candidate needs to assess either for quantity of ingestion or check an immediate level and begin NAC, the antidote. As in any overdose or ingestion case, the candidate must also evaluate for co-ingestants and toxidromes. GI decontamination is not necessary so many hours post-ingestion.

N. Pearls

a. Toxic exposure to acetaminophen is likely with greater than 140 mg/kg ingestion in a single dose or when greater than 7.5 g is ingested within a 24-hour period.
b. Acetaminophen is typically metabolized mainly via glucuronidation and sulfation, but following overdose these mechanisms are easily saturated. A larger proportion of acetaminophen instead cycles through cytochrome P450 to NAPQI, which depletes glutathione stores. If stores are sufficiently depleted, NAPQI binds to other hepatic macromolecules, causing necrosis.
c. There are four stages of toxicity:
   i. First 24 hours – minimal signs and symptoms
   ii. 24–48 hours – RUQ pain, abnormal LFT
   iii. 72–96 hours – fulminant hepatic failure for some patients, causing metabolic acidosis, renal failure, encephalopathy
   iv. End of first week – recovery in survivors to full hepatic function
d. Children have increased hepatic sulfation and may be at decreased risk of hepatotoxicity compared to adults.
e. NAC is administered as:
   i. A 150 mg/kg loading dose over 15 minutes to 1 hour
   ii. Followed by an initial maintenance dose of 50 mg/kg over 4 hours
   iii. Followed by a second maintenance dose of 100 mg/kg over 16 hours.

O. Figure legends

a. Figure 85.1 (EKG) Normal sinus rhythm.
b. Figure 85.2 (CXR) Normal chest x-ray.

P. References

a. *Rosen's Emergency Medicine: Concepts and Clinical Practice* (10th ed.): Chapter 138, Acetaminophen.
b. *Tintinalli's Emergency Medicine: A Comprehensive Study Guide* (9th ed.): Chapter 190, Acetaminophen.

Chest Pain

Lisa Jacobson, MD

A. Chief complaint
a. 59-year-old male with chest pain

B. Vital signs
a. BP: 115/70, HR: 90, RR: 16, T: 37°C, Sat: 94% on RA

C. What does the patient look like?
a. Patient is an obese man, diaphoretic and clutching his chest.

D. Primary survey
a. Airway: speaking in full sentences
b. Breathing: no apparent respiratory distress, no cyanosis
c. Circulation: dry and cool skin, normal capillary refill

E. Action
a. Supplemental oxygen as needed to maintain O_2 above 95%
b. Peripheral IV line
c. Labs
   i. CBC, BMP, LFT, coagulation studies, blood type and crossmatch
   ii. Troponin
d. Monitor: BP: 115/70, HR: 90, RR: 16, T: 37°C
e. EKG

F. History
a. HPI: This is a 59-year-old who presents with sudden-onset chest pressure (8/10) radiating down his left arm for the past 2 hours. He has associated nausea and diaphoresis. He denies shortness of breath, vomiting, back pain, fever, chills, or cough. He has no history of cardiac disease. He reports decreased exercise tolerance for the past 2 weeks.
b. PMHx: hypercholesterolemia
c. PSHx: none
d. Allergies: none
e. Meds: atorvastatin
f. Social: denies drug or alcohol use, smokes one pack per day for 30 years, no cocaine
g. FHx: father with MI at 53
h. PMD: Dr. Silverstein

G. Nurse
a. EKG (Figure 86.1)

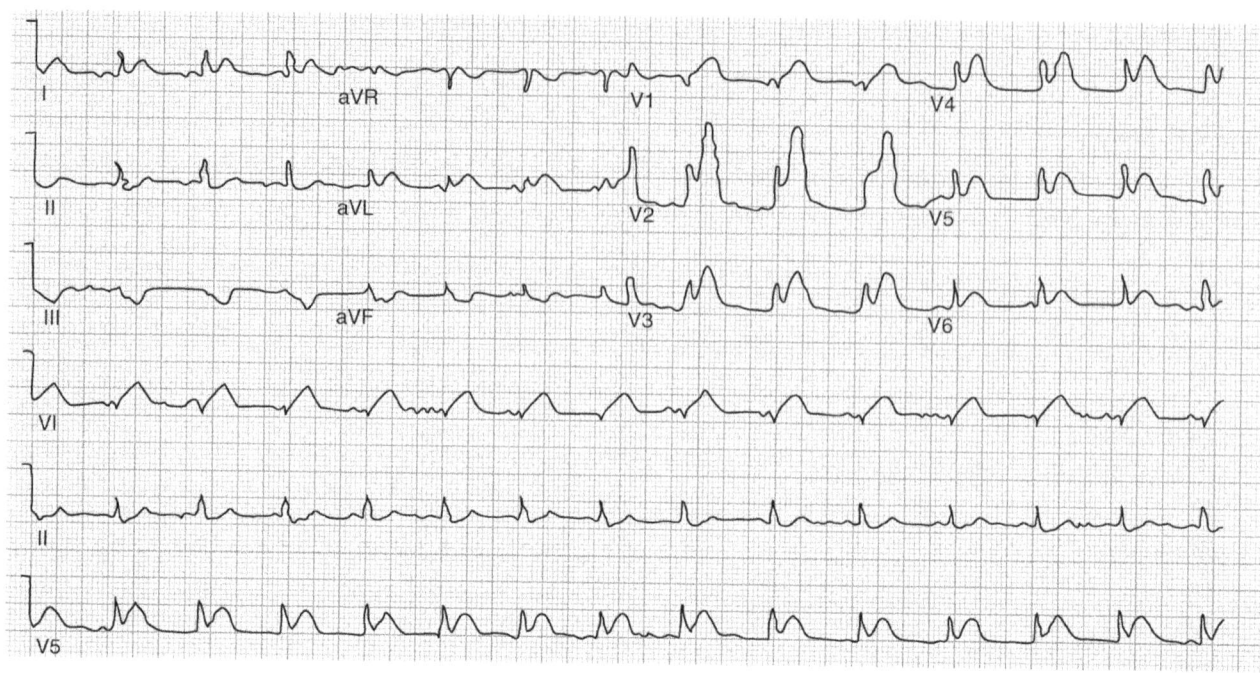

Figure 86.1

H. Secondary survey

a. General: alert, oriented × 3, uncomfortable, diaphoretic
b. Head: normocephalic, atraumatic
c. Eyes: extraocular movements intact, pupils equal, reactive to light
d. Ears: normal tympanic membranes
e. Nose: no discharge
f. Neck: full range of motion, no jugular vein distension, no stridor
g. Pharynx: normal dentition, no lesions, no swelling
h. Chest: nontender
i. Lungs: clear bilaterally
j. Heart: rate and rhythm regular, no murmurs, rubs, or gallops
k. Abdomen: normal bowel sounds, soft, nontender, nondistended
l. Rectal: normal tone, brown stool, occult blood negative
m. Extremities: full range of motion, no deformity, normal pulses
n. Back: nontender
o. Neuro: cranial nerves II to XII intact; normal sensation, strength; normal reflexes and gait
p. Skin: warm and diaphoretic
q. Lymph: no lymphadenopathy

I. Action

a. Consult
   i. Cardiology for catheterization
b. Discussion with patient regarding EKG results
c. Meds
   i. Aspirin chewable
   ii. Sublingual nitroglycerin and/or morphine IV for pain control
   iii. Antiplatelet such as clopidogrel
   iv. Heparin drip

d. Imaging
   i. Chest x-ray

J. Nurse

a. Nitroglycerin or morphine
   i. Vitals unchanged, pain improved 4/10
b. No nitroglycerin
   i. Vitals unchanged, pain worsens to 10/10

K. Results

Table 86.1 Results table

Test	Result	Test	Result
Complete blood count:		**Liver function panel:**	
WBC	$7.3 \times 10^3/\mu L$	AST	23 U/L
Hct	41.5%	ALT	26 U/L
Plt	$330 \times 10^3/\mu L$	Alk phos	42 U/L
		T bili	1.0 mg/dL
Basic metabolic panel:		D bili	0.3 mg/dL
Na	146 mEq/L	Amylase	50 U/L
K	4.0 mEq/L	Lipase	25 U/L
Cl	105 mEq/L	Albumin	4.7 g/dL
CO_2	27 mEq/L		
BUN	12 mEq/dL	**Urinalysis:**	
Cr	1.1 mg/dL	SG	1.010–1.030
Gluc	89 mg/dL	pH	5–8
		Prot	Neg
		Gluc	Neg
Coagulation panel:		Ketones	Neg
PT	12.6 sec	Bili	Neg
PTT	26.0 sec	Blood	Neg
INR	1.0	LE	Neg
		Nitrite	Neg
		Color	Yellow

a. Troponin: normal
b. Cardiac catheterization lab is ready for patient

L. Diagnosis

a. Anterolateral myocardial infarction

M. Critical actions

a. Cardiac monitoring
b. EKG within 10 minutes of arrival
c. Cardiology catheterization
d. Aspirin
e. Pain control with morphine or nitroglycerin

N. Examiner instructions

a. This is a case of anterolateral wall myocardial infarction (heart attack), in which there is a clot in the coronary artery preventing oxygen delivery to the heart muscle, causing cell death. The candidate should recognize this immediately upon seeing the EKG and should activate the cardiac catheterization lab to open the blocked artery as rapidly as possible. Treatment in the ED should include aspirin, nitroglycerin, and oxygen. There is no need to wait for laboratory results, and the candidate may successfully complete the case without asking for those results.

O. Pearls

a. Patients with myocardial infarction may present anywhere on the spectrum from well-appearing to extremely distressed and toxic.
b. Cardiac catheterization is currently the management of choice but in hospitals without ready access to coronary angioplasty, thrombolytic therapy should be administered.
c. The circumflex artery is most likely responsible for lateral wall ischemia as it wraps around the sulcus toward the right coronary territory. The left anterior descending artery is most often the source of anterior and septal blood supply to the heart.

O. Figure legends

a. Figure 86.1 (EKG) Anterior and lateral ST elevations with inferior depressions, likely acute anterolateral MI.

P. References

a. *Tintinalli's Emergency Medicine: A Comprehensive Study Guide* (9th ed.): Chapter 48, Chest Pain. Chapter 49, Acute Coronary Syndromes.
b. *Rosen's Emergency Medicine: Concepts and Clinical Practice* (10th ed.): Chapter 22, Chest Pain. Chapter 64, Acute Coronary Syndromes.

Fever

Edward R. Melnick, MD, MHS, Danielle Roberts, MD, and Marie-Carmelle Elie, MD, RDMS

A. Chief complaint
a. 89-year-old female brought in by EMS from a nursing home for evaluation of fever and altered mental status

B. Vital signs
a. BP: 141/87, HR: 98, RR: 24, T: 38.7°C, Sat: 93% on RA, FS: 209 (must ask), MAP: 67

C. What does the patient look like?
a. Patient appears stated age, pale, drowsy, and incoherent.

D. Primary survey
a. Airway: speaking several words at a time
b. Breathing: increased respiratory rate and work of breathing, but no apparent respiratory distress and no cyanosis
c. Circulation: pale and very warm skin, normal capillary refill

E. Action
a. Oxygen via NC or nonrebreather mask
b. Two large-bore peripheral IV lines
c. Labs
   i. CBC, BMP, LFT, coagulation studies, blood type and crossmatch
   ii. VBG/ABG, lactate, troponin, blood cultures, urinalysis, urine culture
d. 30 cc/kg of IV bolus only in the presence of hypotension or LA >4 mmol/L
e. Monitor: BP: 128/91, HR: 98, RR: 24, Sat: 97%, on 4 L NC
f. EKG
g. Imaging
   i. CXR

F. History
a. HPI: This is an 89-year-old female brought in by EMS from a nursing home for evaluation of fever and altered mental status. The patient cannot give a history due to her dementia and mental status changes. The nursing home transfer summary states that the patient has a history of diabetes, hypertension, and dementia. Yesterday, she was at her baseline, alert and conversant, but was noted today to be less coherent, drowsy, and febrile to 39°C.
b. PMHx: diabetes, hypertension, and dementia

c. PSHx: none

d. Allergies: none

e. Meds: insulin, diltiazem, aspirin

f.   Social: lives in nursing home, no family contact information listed in nursing home transfer summary

g. FHx: not relevant

h. PMD: nursing home staff physician

i.   Weight: 60 kg

G. Nurse

a. EKG (Figure 87.1)

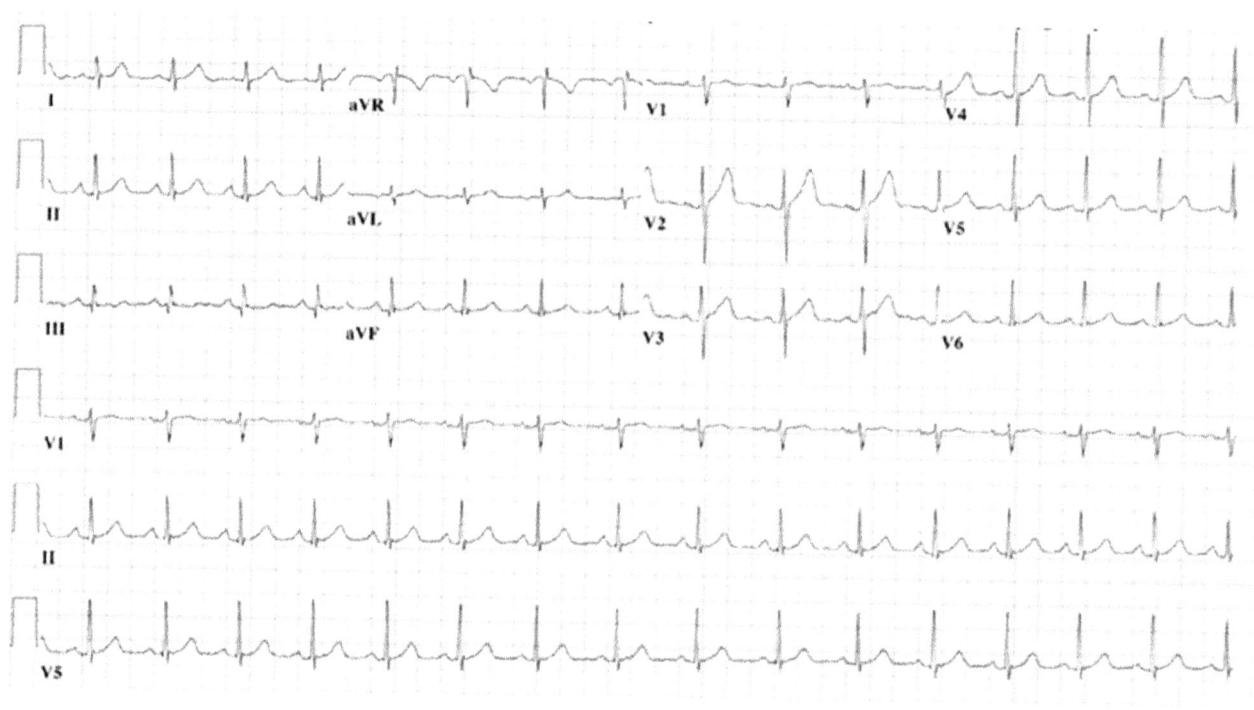

Figure 87.1

H. Secondary survey

a. General: pale, warm skin, drowsy, incoherent, not oriented to person, place, or time, increased work of breathing

b. Head: normocephalic, atraumatic

c. Eyes: extraocular movements intact, pupils equal, reactive to light

d. Mouth: pale dry mucous membranes

e. Ears: normal tympanic membranes

f.   Nose: no discharge

g. Neck: full range of motion, no jugular vein distension, no stridor

h. Pharynx: normal dentition, no lesions, no swelling

i. Chest: nontender
j. Lungs: increased respiratory rate and work of breathing, no respiratory distress, focal rhonchi at the right base, otherwise clear lungs
k. Cardiovascular: tachycardic rate, rhythm regular, no murmurs, rubs, or gallops; intact distal pulses
l. Abdomen: normal bowel sounds, soft, nontender, nondistended
m. Rectal: normal tone, brown stool, occult blood negative
n. Urogenital: normal external genitalia
   i. Female: no blood or discharge, cervical os closed, no cervical motion tenderness, no adnexal tenderness
o. Extremities: full range of motion, no deformity
p. Back: nontender
q. Neuro: cranial nerves II to XII intact; normal sensation, strength; normal reflexes and gait
r. Skin: warm and dry, poor turgor
s. Lymph: no lymphadenopathy

I. Nurse
a. BP: 101/67, HR: 105, RR: 24, Sat: 96% on 4 L NC, MAP 63
b. Labs sent but radiology is delayed because of technical problems – both portable and PA/lateral chest x-rays are unavailable

J. Action
a. Consider both possible infectious and noninfectious etiologies. Tailor antibiotic choice to the probable infectious causes such as respiratory.
   i. Broad-spectrum antibiotics to cover probable respiratory infection (e.g., cefepime and vancomycin)
   ii. consider anaerobic coverage for possible aspiration pneumonia
   iii. Additional 1 L IV bolus for persistent hypotension and MAP >65
b. Reassess
   i. Patient appears unchanged from prior examination

K. Nurse
a. With antibiotics
   i. BP: 128/75, HR: 90, RR: 18, Sat: 99% on 4 L NC
b. Without antibiotics
   i. BP: 89/57, HR: 117, RR: 26, Sat: 95% on 4 L NC
c. Administer fluid bolus 30 mL/kg for hypotension
d. Follow-up vitals post-fluid resuscitation
   i. BP: 110/73, HR: 100, RR: 24, Sat: 96% on 4 L NC
   ii. If no fluid bolus no change
e. CXR (Figure 87.2)

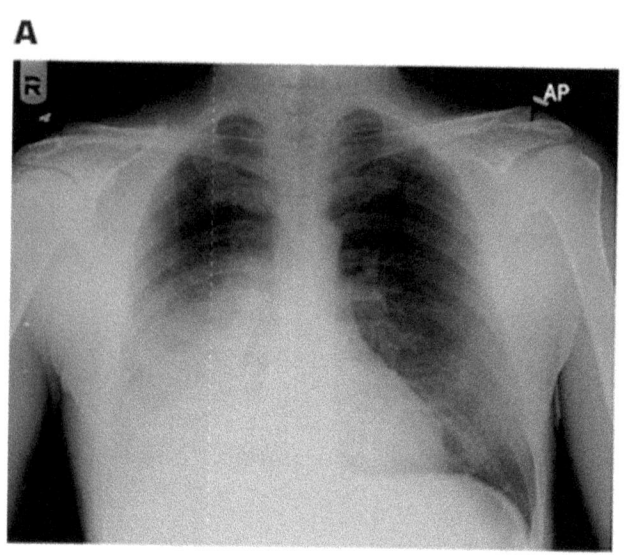

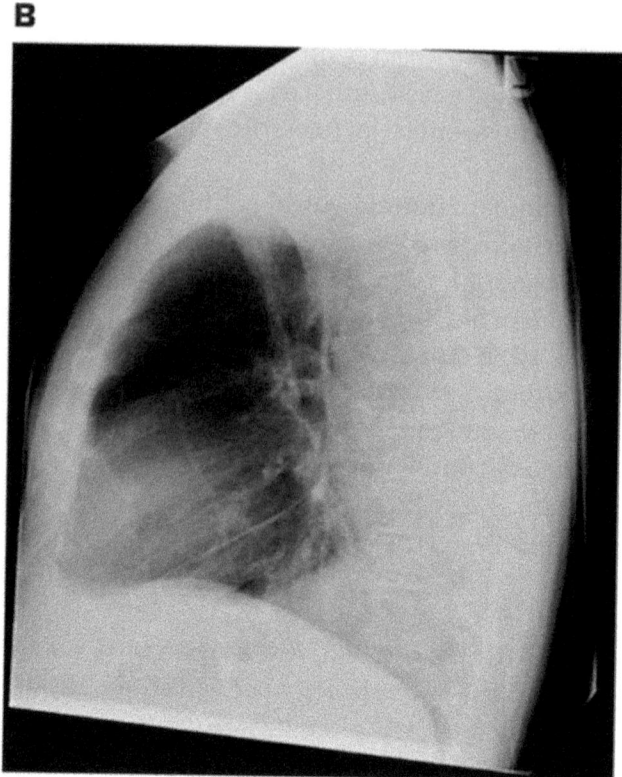

Figure 87.2

L. Results

Table 87.1 Results table

Test	Result	Test	Result
Complete blood count:		**Liver function panel:**	
WBC	$16.7 \times 10^3/\mu L$	AST	23 U/L
Hct	41.5%	ALT	26 U/L
Plt	$250 \times 10^3/\mu L$	Alk phos	42 U/L
		T bili	1.0 mg/dL
Basic metabolic panel:		D bili	0.3 mg/dL
Na	148 mEq/L	Amylase	50 U/L
K	4.3 mEq/L	Lipase	25 U/L
Cl	115 mEq/L	Albumin	4.7 g/dL
CO_2	21 mEq/L		
BUN	49 mEq/dL	**Urinalysis:**	
Cr	2.1 mg/dL	SG	1.020
Gluc	100 mg/dL	pH	7
		Prot	Neg

Table 87.1 (cont.)

Test	Result	Test	Result
Coagulation panel:		Gluc	Neg
PT	12.6 sec	Ketones	Neg
PTT	26.0 sec	Bili	Neg
INR	1.0	Blood	Neg
		LE	Neg
		Nitrite	Neg
		Color	Yellow

a. Lactate: 1.2 mmol/L with antibiotics (5.1 if no antibiotics given empirically)

M. Action

a. Medicine contact for admission.
b. If no antibiotics were given empirically already, initiate early goal-directed therapy (EGDT) with repeat assessments of hemodynamics and lactate.

N. Diagnosis

a. Sepsis due to pneumonia

O. Critical actions

a. IV access and fluid bolus 30 cc/kg for hypotension in the setting of sepsis
b. CBC
c. Blood and urine culture prior to antibiotic administration
d. CXR
e. Evaluate for sources of fever including cellulitis, decubitus ulcers, urinalysis
f. Early appropriate antibiotics (this should include beta-lactam antibiotic *or* third-/fourth-generation cephalosporin *plus* macrolide *or* fluroquinolone; may include vancomycin or linezolid) – alternatively, aggressively resuscitate if not given early and patient decompensates

P. Examiner instructions

a. This is a case of sepsis in a patient presenting with vital sign and clinical derangements consistent with systemic inflammatory response syndrome (SIRS), an inflammatory state that is commonly displayed with infection, due to nosocomial pneumonia. In this case, the patient's temperature, heart rate, respiratory rate, and WBC count fulfill SIRS criteria. Important early actions include obtaining appropriate IV access, prompt administration of broad-spectrum antibiotics tailored to the patient's suspected source of infection, IV fluid resuscitation with 30 cc/kg for hypotension or lactate >4.0 mmol/L, followed by diagnostics, including assessing lactate level, urinalysis, CBC, cultures, and CXR. Since the CXR is not immediately available, the candidate must decide to give antibiotics early based on the clinical suspicion of pneumonia in the presence of SIRS criteria. If antibiotics are not given, the patient begins to manifest signs of septic shock. At this point, in addition to giving broad-spectrum antibiotics, the candidate should perform one of the following:
    i.   Bedside ultrasound to assess volume status
    ii. Arterial line placement to assess pulse pressure variation

iii. Serial lactate measurement

iv. Global exam for assessment for perfusion (i.e., pulses, mottling, etc.)

Q. Pearls

a. Sepsis is defined as life-threatening organ dysfunction caused by a dysregulated host response to infection. This definition emphasizes the presence of both infection and organ dysfunction. Sepsis represents a continuum of severity ranging from sepsis to severe sepsis and septic shock. The latest sepsis guidelines aim to provide a clinical framework for identifying and managing patients with suspected infection and organ dysfunction, facilitating early recognition and intervention to improve patient outcomes.

b. Systemic inflammatory response syndrome is a clinical syndrome characterized by a dysregulated systemic inflammatory response to various insults, including infection, trauma, burns, pancreatitis, and others. Patients who meet two or more of these criteria are diagnosed with SIRS. It is important to recognize that SIRS is a nonspecific syndrome that can occur in response to a variety of insults, not just infection. Therefore, further evaluation is needed to determine the underlying cause of SIRS and guide appropriate management.

c. The criteria for diagnosing SIRS include the presence of two or more of the following clinical manifestations:

i. Fever (core body temperature >38°C) or hypothermia (core body temperature <36°C)

ii. Tachycardia (heart rate >90 bpm)

iii. Tachypnea (respiratory rate >20 breaths per minute) or hyperventilation ($PaCO_2$ < 32 mmHg)

iv. Leukocytosis (WBC count >12,000/μL), leukopenia (WBC count <4000/μL), or bandemia (band forms >10% of total WBC count)

d. A patient with two or more SIRS criteria with a suspected or confirmed infection can be categorized as follows:

i. Sepsis: Two SIRS criteria with a proven or suspected infection. Of note, the term formally known as severe sepsis describes sepsis plus the presence of end-organ dysfunction, such as hypotension, elevated lactate, renal dysfunction, hypoxia, thrombocytopenia, hyperbilirubinemia, or coagulopathies.

ii. Septic shock: sepsis as defined above with refractory hypotension despite isotonic crystalloid volume repletion of 30 cc/kg. The progression to this state typically coincides with reduced peripheral perfusion and one or more organ dysfunctions, associated with increased morbidity and mortality.

e. Sepsis or infection should always be considered in a patient who presents with SIRS criteria. Be vigilant in recognizing sepsis in high-risk populations such as elderly patients, immunocompromised individuals, those with chronic illnesses, and patients with recent surgeries or invasive procedures.

Figure legends

a. Figure 87.1 (EKG) Sinus tachycardia.

b. Figure 87.2 (AP and lateral CXR) Right lower lobe consolidation.

References

a. *Tintinalli's Emergency Medicine: A Comprehensive Study Guide* (9th ed.): Chapter 65, Community Acquired Pneumonia, Aspiration Pneumonia, and Non-Infectious Pulmonary Infiltrates. Chapter 151, Sepsis.

b. *Rosen's Emergency Medicine: Concepts and Clinical Practice* (10th ed.): Chapter 62, Pneumonia. Chapter 127, Sepsis Syndrome.

Altered Mental Status

Chelsea Allen, DO and David A. Caro, MD

A. Chief complaint
a. 81-year-old male brought in by EMS from home with the complaint of altered mental status

B. Vital signs
a. BP: 150/56, HR: 130, RR: 22, T: 43°C, Sat: 95% on RA, FS: 176 mg/dL (must ask)

C. What does the patient look like?
a. Patient is a disheveled, elderly male on stretcher mumbling incoherently, accompanied by his daughter.

D. Primary survey
a. Airway: maintaining airway
b. Breathing: no apparent respiratory distress, lungs CTA, no cyanosis
c. Circulation: warm and dry skin, normal capillary refill
d. Disability: altered mental status; no focal deficits, normal pupils
e. Exposure: undress the patient completely

E. Action
a. Oxygen via NC or nonrebreather mask as needed to maintain saturation >95%
b. Two large-bore peripheral IV lines
c. Labs
   i. BMP, LFT, CK, troponin, lactate
   ii. CBC, coagulation studies, blood type and screen
   iii. Urinalysis
   iv. Blood cultures, urine culture
d. 500 mL cooled NS bolus
e. Monitor: BP: 155/61, HR: 132, RR: 22, Sat: 100% on O_2
f. EKG (Figure 88.1)

F. History
a. HPI: An 81-year-old male with a history of hypertension, diabetes, and hypercholesterolemia brought in by EMS from home for altered mental status. EMS found the patient lying on the ground next to the bed in a very warm apartment. The daughter states that patient lives alone and is able to take care of himself at baseline. The patient mentioned to her a few days prior that his air conditioning had broken down. He had hoped that the landlord would fix it

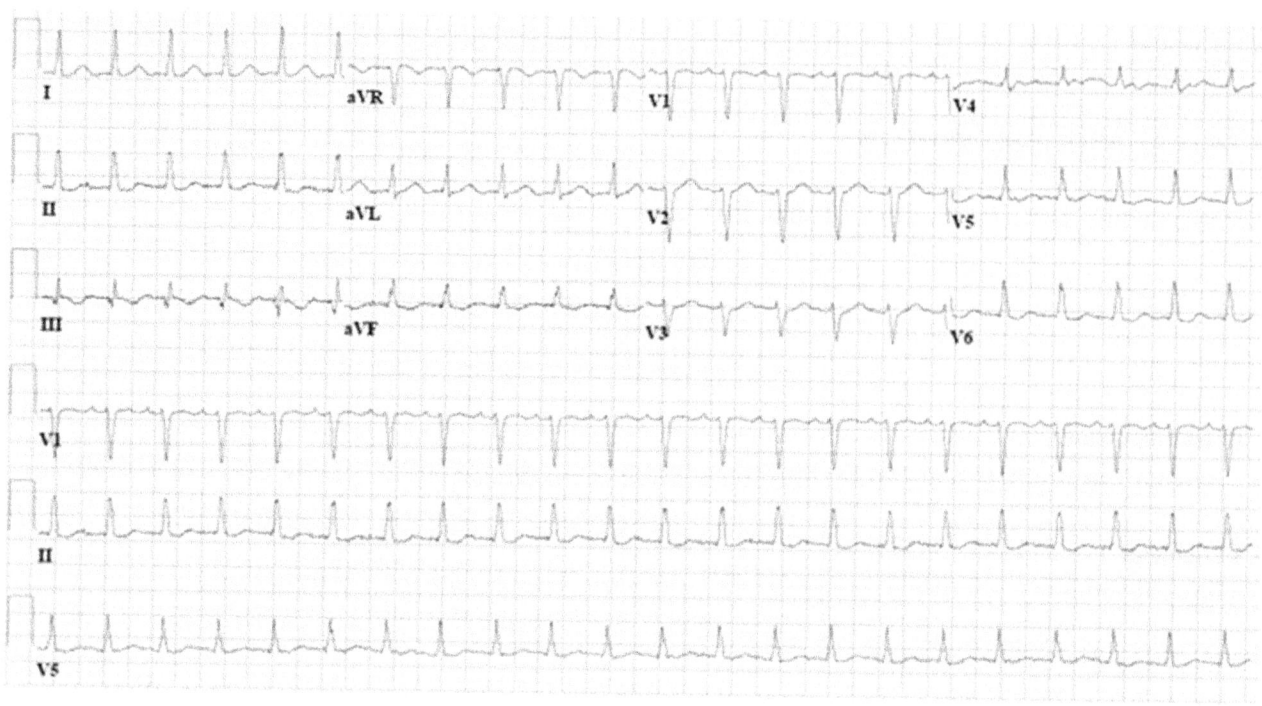

Figure 88.1

quickly as the summer temperature was rising outside. She has not seen him for 4 days and became concerned when he did not answer his phone the last few times she had called. This prompted her to call EMS.

b. PMHx: hypertension, diabetes, and hypercholesterolemia
c. PSHx: appendectomy over 30 years ago
d. Allergies: none
e. Meds: unknown
f. Social: lives alone, ex-smoker (quit 20 years ago), no drugs, not sexually active; does not drink alcohol
g. FHx: not relevant
h. PMD: Dr. Jagoda

G. Nurse
a. If IVF bolus given:
   i. BP: 140/66, HR: 125, RR: 20, T: 42.0°C, Sat: 98% on 2 L NC O_2
b. If no fluids given:
   i. BP: 155/61, HR: 132, RR: 22, Sat: 100% on O_2

H. Secondary survey
a. General: alert and oriented × 0, cachectic elderly male, muttering incoherently, very warm to touch, not following commands, no apparent distress
b. Head: normocephalic, atraumatic
c. Eyes: mildly pale conjunctiva, extraocular movement intact, pupils equal, reactive to light
d. Ears: normal tympanic membranes
e. Nose: no discharge

f.   Neck: full range of motion, no jugular vein distension, no stridor
g.   Pharynx: dry mucous membranes, normal dentition, no lesions, no swelling
h.   Chest: nontender
i.   Lungs: clear bilaterally
j.   Heart: tachycardic rate, rhythm regular, no murmurs, rubs, or gallops
k.   Abdomen: normal bowel sounds, soft, nontender, nondistended
l.   Rectal: normal tone, brown stool, occult blood negative
m.   Urogenital: normal external genitalia
n.   Male: no discharge, normal testicular examination
o.   Extremities: full range of motion, no deformity, normal pulses
p.   Back: nontender
q.   Neuro: moves extremities equally spontaneously and withdraws to painful stimuli,
     uncooperative with rest of examination
r.   Skin: hot to touch, dry, pale, no rashes, no edema, stage 1 ulcer on buttock, covered with stool
     and urine
s.   Lymph: no lymphadenopathy

I. Action
a.   Clean patient
b.   Hydration
     i.   IVF boluses: NS IVF 250 mL/hr
     ii. Evaluate current and ongoing hydration status
          1.   If available, evaluate IVC volume with POCUS. IVC collapsible on POCUS exam.
          2.   Monitor urine output – insert Foley catheter. Initial urine output minimal (50 cc), with
               dark yellow urine.
c.   Cooling (evaporative or immersion)
     i.   Evaporative cooling: position fans close to completely undressed patient and then spray
          tepid water on the patient
     ii. Immersion cooling: place undressed patient into a tub of ice water to cover trunk and
          extremities
          iii. Adjuncts: ice pack to neck, axillae, and groin
               1.   Continuous core temperature monitor (rectal or Foley probe thermometer)
d.   Discontinue cooling efforts if rectal temperature reaches 39–40°C to avoid overshoot
     hypothermia
e.   Additional labs and imaging
     i.   Consider myoglobin, TSH, toxicology screen, aspirin and acetaminophen levels
     ii. CT head (Figure 88.2)
     iii. CXR (Figure 88.3)
f.   Meds
     i.   Ceftriaxone IV (2 g)
     ii. Vancomycin IV (1 g)
     iii. Lorazepam prn IV (0.03–0.05 mg/kg IV to treat shivering)
g.   Reassess
     i.   BP: 140/76, HR: 120, RR: 18, T: 41°C, Sat: 98% on 2 L O_2 (after 1 L NS)
h.   Lumbar puncture (after CT head)

A

B

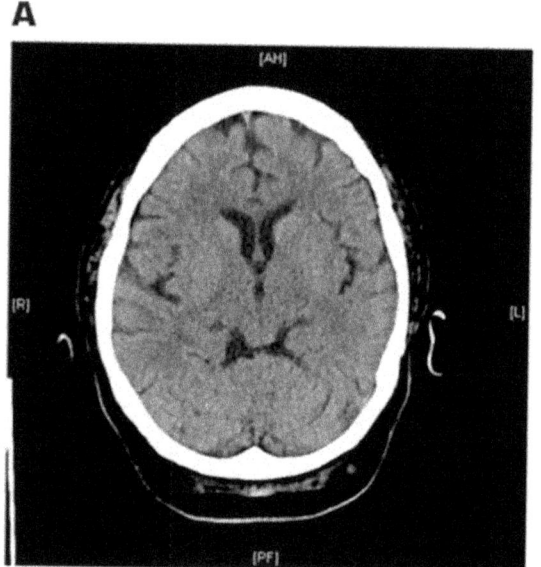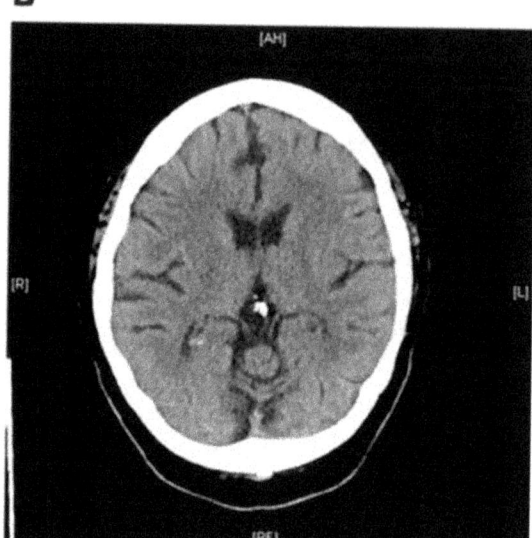

Figure 88.2

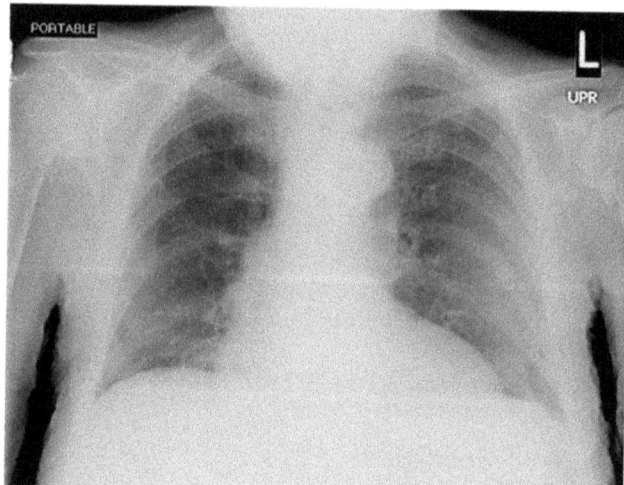

Figure 88.3

J. Results

Table 88.1 Results table

Test	Result	Test	Result
Complete blood count:		**Urinalysis:**	
WBC	$12.0 \times 10^3/\mu L$	SG	1.030
Diff	56.6/8.4/1.8	pH	7
Hct	36.5%	Prot	Neg
Plt	$91 \times 10^3/\mu L$	Gluc	Neg
		Ketones	Neg
Basic metabolic panel:		Bili	Neg
Na	155 mEq/L	Blood	Neg

Table 88.1 (cont.)

Test	Result	Test	Result
K	3.3 mEq/L	LE	Neg
Cl	121 mEq/L	Nitrite	Neg
CO_2	19 mEq/L	Color	Yellow
BUN	80 mEq/dL		
Cr	2.1 mg/dL	**Arterial blood gas:**	
Gluc	202 mg/dL	pH	7.4
Lactate	1.8 mmol/L	pO_2	95 mmHg
		pCO_2	41 mmHg
Coagulation panel:		HCO_3	24 mmol/L
PT	13.6 sec		
PTT	26.0 sec	**Toxicology screen negative:**	
INR	1.2	Troponin	<0.05
		CK	1580 U/L
		TSH	1.0 mIU/L
Liver function panel:		Myoglobin	45 mcg/L
AST	330 U/L		
ALT	230 U/L		
Alk phos	100 U/L	**Lumbar puncture:**	
T bili	1.0 mg/dL	Color	Clear
D bili	0.3 mg/dL	RBC	5
Amylase	50 U/L	WBC	2 (lymphocytes)
Lipase	25 U/L	Glucose	66
Albumin	4.7 g/dL	Protein	30
		Smear	Negative for organisms

K. Action

a. ICU consult
   i. Discuss with family regarding advanced directives
b. Hydration: continue volume resuscitation with isotonic solution

L. Diagnosis

a. Heatstroke

M. Critical actions

a. Remove clothing on primary survey
b. Check blood glucose
c. Large-bore IV access and fluid bolus
d. Add additional cooling measures

e. Place core temperature monitor
f. CT head
g. ICU admission

N. Examiner instructions

a. This is a case of classic heatstroke in an elderly patient who lives a sedentary lifestyle on medications for chronic illness. Heatstroke is a life-threatening condition in which the body loses its ability to regulate its temperature, causing dysfunction of multiple organ systems. It is caused by environmental heat exposure. The patient has been in a heated apartment with a broken air conditioner for days and presents with extremely high temperature. Important early actions include checking blood glucose, administering IV fluids, immediate cooling, continuous temperature monitor, and placement of Foley catheter to monitor urine output. In any patient presenting with altered mental status, it is paramount to rule out stroke and central nervous system infection; consider head CT head and lumbar puncture if warranted. It is also important to check for signs of end-organ and systemic injury (cardiac ischemia, pulmonary edema, elevated liver enzymes, renal failure, rhabdomyolysis, and coagulation disorders, for example). Patients who are intubated and hemodynamically labile require continued cooling and should be admitted to the ICU.

O. Pearls

a. The "classic" signs of heatstroke are CNS dysfunction, elevated temperature (usually above 40°C), and anhidrosis. This is a true medical emergency.

b. Anhidrosis (lack of sweating) may not be present for a variety of reasons, and is *not* considered an absolute diagnostic criterion.

c. Immediate, aggressive, rapid cooling down to 40°C is the mainstay of therapy. Morbidity is directly related to severity and duration of hyperthermia.

d. Supportive measures are critical – rehydration, cooling, and confirmation of no other causes of hyperpyrexia.

e. Administer oxygen as necessary.

f. Those with classic heatstroke need IV fluids but take care with rehydration (fluid requirements may not be large); ongoing rate of 250–300 mL/hr might be required.

g. Consider CVP monitoring to guide fluid therapy in the elderly or those with cerebral vascular disease.

h. Meds
   i. Use:
      1. Benzodiazepine or chlorpromazine: control shivering with as needed.
   ii. Do not use:
      1. Antipyretics (e.g., acetaminophen, aspirin, ibuprofen) are *not* useful because antipyretics interrupt the change in the hypothalamic set point caused by pyrogens.
      2. Dantrolene has *not* been demonstrated to be effective.
      3. Anticholinergic drugs are the most frequent cause of impaired sweating in classic heatstroke, so are *contraindicated*.
      4. Antiarrhythmics: tachydysrhythmias are common and respond to cooling. Do *not* cardiovert.

i. Management of encephalopathy is supportive, directed at minimizing cerebral edema by avoiding fluid overreplacement and assuring hemodynamic, thermal, and metabolic stability.

P. Figure legends
a. Figure 88.1 (EKG) Sinus tachycardia.
b. Figure 88.2 (Head CT) Normal head CT.
c. Figure 88.3 (CXR) Bilateral increased interstitial markings.

Q. References
a. *Tintinalli's Emergency Medicine: A Comprehensive Study Guide* (9th ed.): Chapter 168, Altered Mental Status and Coma. Chapter 210, Heat Emergencies.
b. *Rosen's Emergency Medicine: Concepts and Clinical Practice* (10th ed.): Chapter 12, Depressed Consciousness and Coma. Chapter 129, Heat Illness.

R. Acknowledgments
a. We would like to acknowledge Tiffany Truong for their contribution to this chapter in the previous edition of this book, which has been updated by Chelsea Allen and David A. Caro.

Shortness of Breath

Andrew Thomas, MD

A. Chief complaint
a. 59-year-old male presents for fatigue and shortness of breath for 4 days

B. Vital signs
a. BP: 96/50, HR: 130, RR: 22, T: 36.8°C, Sat: 97% on RA

C. What does the patient look like?
a. Cachectic male appears mildly short of breath, speaking in full sentences, and tachypneic.

D. Primary survey
a. Airway: speaking in full sentences
b. Breathing: rapid breathing; no apparent respiratory distress, no cyanosis
c. Circulation: cool, diaphoretic on the forehead, normal capillary refill

E. Action/nurse
a. Oxygen via NC or nonrebreather mask as needed to maintain saturation >95%
b. Two large-bore peripheral IV lines
c. 1 L NS bolus
d. Monitor: BP: 92/50, HR: 124, RR: 26, Sat: 98% on 2 L O_2
e. EKG or rhythm strip

F. History
a. HPI: A 59-year-old male with a history of deep vein thrombosis and pulmonary embolus on oral anticoagulation, and lung cancer diagnosed 2 months ago undergoing chemotherapy, presents for gradual-onset fatigue and dyspnea for 4 days. He has been compliant with all medications and chemotherapy sessions. Today he felt increasingly short of breath and presents for evaluation on the advice of his oncologist. He denies cough, fever, chills, nausea, vomiting, headache, chest pain, hemoptysis, calf pain, abdominal pain, urinary symptoms, lower extremity edema, or medication noncompliance.
b. PMHx: DVT, PE, lung cancer
c. PSHx: port placement in right chest
d. Allergies: iodinated contrast media (anaphylaxis)
e. Meds: apixaban and several infused chemotherapy medications
f. Social: lives at home, 40-pack-year tobacco use history with ongoing use and efforts to quit
g. FHx: not relevant
h. PMD: Dr. Beck

G. Nurse

a. EKG (Figure 89.1)

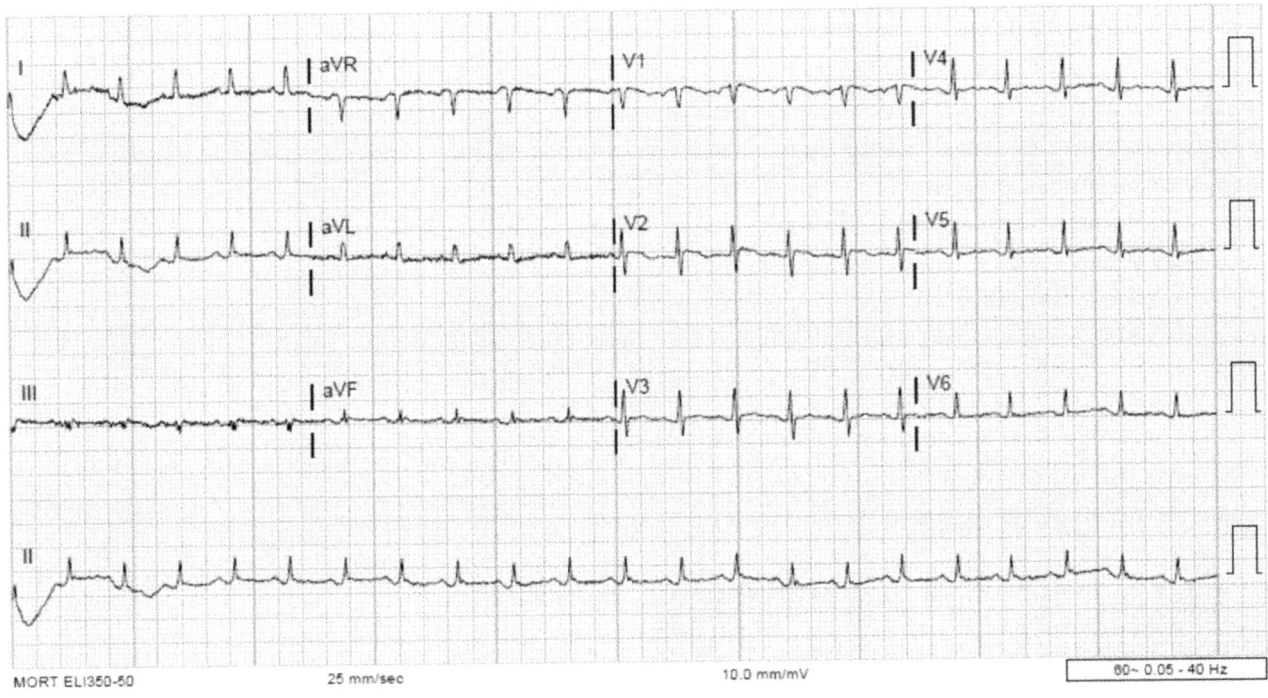

Figure 89.1

b. 1 L NS
   i. BP: 110/76, HR: 110, RR: 22, Sat: 96% on 2 L O_2
c. No fluids
   i. BP: 74/50, HR: 130, RR: 28, Sat: 92% on 2 L O_2

H. Secondary survey

a. General: alert and oriented × 3, cachectic male, speaking in full sentences, rapid breathing, mildly dyspneic, pulsus paradoxus (if asked)
b. Head: normocephalic, atraumatic
c. Eyes: extraocular movement intact, pupils equal, reactive to light
d. Ears: normal tympanic membranes
e. Nose: no discharge
f. Neck: full range of motion, trachea midline, + jugular vein distension, no stridor
g. Pharynx: normal dentition, no lesions, no swelling
h. Chest: nontender, with symmetric chest rise
i. Lungs: tachypnea, good air entry, no crackles, wheezes, or rhonchi; right chest port in place with no surrounding erythema or drainage
j. Heart: diminished heart sounds, tachycardic rate, regular rhythm, no gallops or rubs, + pulsus paradoxus (must ask about this and explain how to assess it)
k. Abdomen: normal bowel sounds, soft, nontender, nondistended
l. Rectal: normal tone, brown stool, occult blood negative
m. Urogenital: deferred
n. Extremities: full range of motion, no deformity, normal pulses, no edema, negative Homan's sign (if asked)

o. Back: nontender
p. Neuro: cranial nerves II to XII intact; normal sensation, strength; normal reflexes and gait
q. Skin: no rashes or lesions, no jaundice, no erythema
r. Lymph: no lymphadenopathy

I. Action

a. Place patient on nonrebreather mask
b. Reassessment of patient
    i. Consider additional fluid bolus
c. Imaging
    i. CXR (Figure 89.2)
    ii. Point of care ultrasound (POCUS) cardiac view (Figure 89.3)
    iii. If the candidate requests CT angiography of the chest, the patient reports anaphylactic allergy to iodinated contrast media
d. Consultation
    i. Cardiology
    ii. Cardiothoracic surgery

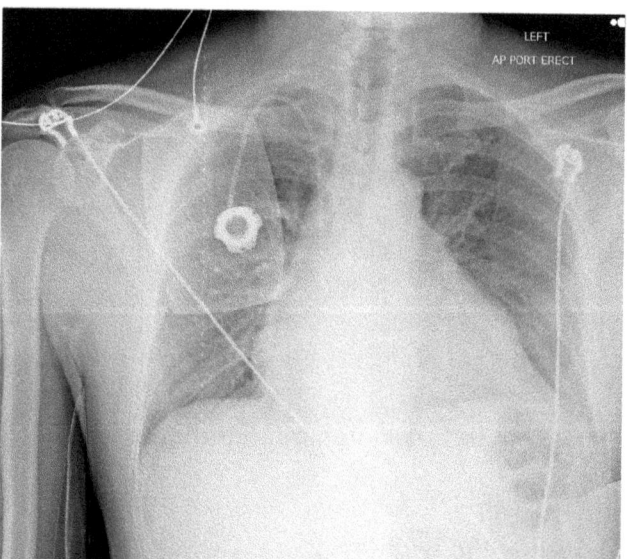

Figure 89.2

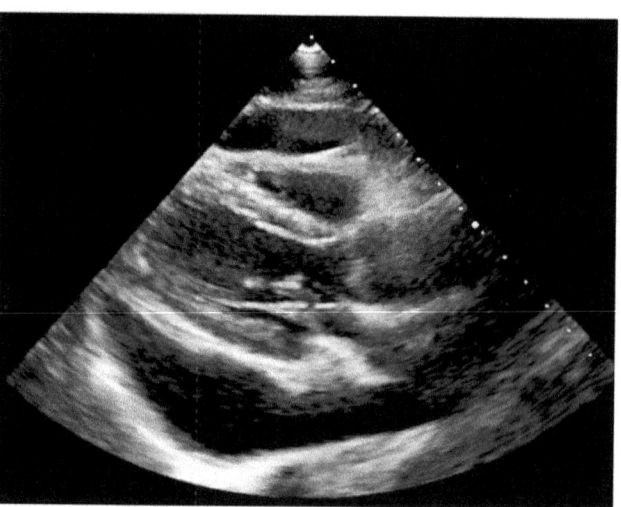

Figure 89.3

J. Nurse

a. CXR (Figure 89.2)

K. Results

Table 89.1 Results table

Test	Result	Test	Result
Complete blood count:		**Liver function panel:**	
WBC	$9.1 \times 10^3/\mu L$	AST	33 U/L
Hct	32.7%	ALT	36 U/L
Plt	$154 \times 10^3/\mu L$	Alk phos	92 U/L
		T bili	1.2 mg/dL
		D bili	0.4 mg/dL
Basic metabolic panel:		Lipase	30 U/L
Na	134 mEq/L	Albumin	3.4 g/dL
K	4.1 mEq/L		
Cl	101 mEq/L		
CO_2	22 mEq/L	**Urinalysis:**	
BUN	28 mEq/dL	SG	1.010–1.030
Cr	1.7 mg/dL	pH	5–8
Gluc	94 mg/dL	Prot	Neg
		Gluc	Neg
		Ketones	Neg
Coagulation panel:		Bili	Neg
PT	12.6 sec	Blood	Neg
PTT	26.0 sec	LE	Neg
INR	1.1	Nitrite	Neg
		Color	Yellow

a. Lactate: 1.9 mmol/L
b. Troponin: normal
c. B-natriuretic peptide: normal

L. Action

a. Consult
    i.   Cardiothoracic surgery for emergent pericardial window
b. Cardiology
    i.   Emergent echocardiography demonstrates presence of cardiac tamponade. This should be performed in the ED. If the patient is sent out of the ED for echo, he should collapse and be brought back to ED emergently with pulseless electrical activity.
    ii. Recommends emergent cardiothoracic surgery consult for pericardial window
c. Admission to OR

M. Diagnosis

a. Pericardial tamponade

N. Critical actions

a. Large-bore IV access and fluid bolus
b. CXR
c. EKG
d. Bedside cardiac ultrasound
e. Cardiothoracic surgery consult

O. Examiner instructions

a. This is a case of nontraumatic pericardial effusion with tamponade physiology. Tamponade is life-threatening because it impairs filling of the right ventricle and can lead to obstructive shock. This patient's initial vitals demonstrated hypotension, tachycardia, tachypnea, and shortness of breath concerning for shock. Additionally, his diaphoresis and medical comorbidities raise concern for several dangerous causes of his symptoms. The physical exam findings of Beck's triad were present on exam: hypotension, jugular venous distension, and diminished heart sounds. The diagnosis is further supported by low voltages on his EKG, though there is not obvious electrical alternans. Another clue is the enlarged cardiac silhouette on CXR. Finally, the diagnosis of pericardial effusion should be recognized on point-of-care cardiac ultrasound. A trained clinician may recognize features of impaired right ventricular filling consistent with tamponade; however, this could also be confirmed and quantified with comprehensive echocardiography. The physiologic changes of tamponade establish the diagnosis. Early administration of IV fluids and consultation to cardiothoracic surgery for pericardial window are necessary. It is important to be prepared to perform an emergent pericardiocentesis in the ED if this patient were to further decompensate.

P. Pearls

a. Atraumatic pericardial effusion can occur idiopathically, or can be seen in disease processes such as malignancy, following percutaneous procedures, as a complication of myocardial infarction, or in association with uremia, aortic dissection, or tuberculosis.
b. Classic clinical findings: Beck's triad (hypotension, jugular venous distension, and distant heart sounds), narrow pulse pressure, dyspnea, tachycardia, pulsus paradoxus (exaggerated drop in systolic pressure with inspiration).
c. EKG: diminished amplitude, low voltage QRS, may exhibit electrical alternans in a larger effusion.
d. Kussmaul's sign: rise in central venous pressure with spontaneous inspiration.
e. CXR: a large cardiac silhouette without pulmonary congestion, especially with a left-sided pleural effusion, may be seen in large pericardial effusions. A normal CXR cannot exclude pericardial effusion or tamponade because small volumes of pericardial effusion can induce tamponade physiology if the accumulation is rapid, as in the case of active bleeding.
f. Echocardiography: the gold standard for diagnosing pericardial effusion, and should be performed emergently if tamponade physiology is present. The imaging features that would suggest tamponade are diastolic collapse of right ventricle and right atrium, anechoic space behind left ventricle and in front of right ventricle, and paradoxical septal motion.
g. Fluid bolus can supply preload to the right ventricle and improve perfusion.

h. In the settings of hemodynamic collapse, pericardiocentesis should be performed emergently in the ED. Consider ultrasound guidance for this procedure.

i. Definitive therapy: pericardial window by cardiothoracic surgery.

Q. Figure legends

a. Figure 89.1 (EKG) Sinus tachycardia with low voltage.

b. Figure 89.2 (CXR) Mildly enlarged cardiac silhouette, right chest port.

c. Figure 89.3 (US) Significant pericardial effusion.

R. References

Tintinalli's Emergency Medicine: A Comprehensive Study Guide (9th ed.): Chapter 55, Cardiomyopathies and Pericardial Disease. Chapter 240, Emergency Complications of Malignancy.

Rosen's Emergency Medicine: Concepts and Clinical Practice (10th ed.): Chapter 68, Pericardial and Myocardial Disease.

S. Acknowledgments

a. We would like to acknowledge Tiffany Truong for their contribution to this chapter in the previous edition of this book, which has been updated by Andrew Thomas.

Stab to Chest

Qiaohua Zhang, MD

A. Chief complaint
a. 53-year-old female brought in by EMS for stab wound to chest and dyspnea

B. Vital signs
a. BP: 95/34, HR: 110, RR: 24, T: 37°C, Sat: 95% on RA

C. What does the patient look like?
a. Anxious-appearing, obese, middle-aged female with hemostatic stab wound to right anterior chest, alert and oriented × 3, but distracted by pain.
b. Patient is more tachypneic than initial triage vitals. Using abdominal muscles to aid in respiration.

D. Primary survey
a. Airway: speaking in one-word sentences
b. Breathing: severe respiratory distress. Not cyanotic. Breath sounds diminished in right upper chest; right side jugular venous distension; unable to assess if there is tracheal deviation due to obesity
c. Circulation: pink and warm skin, normal capillary refill, heart sounds present

E. Action
a. Oxygen via nonrebreather mask
b. Decompression of pneumothorax using finger or needle thoracostomy (describe site to examiner)
  i. If CXR or ultrasound is asked for before decompression, the patient immediate deteriorates, forcing an action
  ii. Decompression of pneumothorax
    1. BP: 110/56, HR: 84, RR: 18, Sat: 100% on O_2
    2. Patient: breathing more comfortably, states she feels less short of breath
  iii. No decompression
    1. BP: 70/50, HR: 140, RR: 36, Sat: 92% on O_2
    2. Patient: agitated, in severe respiratory distress.
  iv. If case persists with no decompression, patient codes

F. Nurse
a. Two large-bore peripheral IV lines
b. Labs
  i. CBC, chem 7, troponin, PT/PTT, type and crossmatch two units

c. 1 L NS bolus and/or activation of massive transfusion protocol (MTP) and/or uncrossed blood
d. Consults
    i. Thoracic surgery, trauma surgery, or general surgery

G. History

a. HPI: A 53-year-old female with a history of breast cancer presents to the ED with the complaint of shortness of breath and stab to chest. Patient stated that while standing outside a bar with her boyfriend she was stabbed once to the right anterior chest by an intoxicated male who ran away with her purse. She thought it looked like a small pocketknife. EMS stated that they found her sitting on the ground outside the bar complaining of difficulty in breathing. Patient denies any other injuries; no loss of consciousness.
b. PMHx: breast malignancy bilateral (ductal carcinoma in situ)
c. PSHx: hysterectomy 10 years ago, bilateral simple mastectomy with reconstruction with tissue expanders followed by bilateral insertion of permanent saline breast implants
d. Allergies: none
e. Meds: none
f. Social: divorced, lives alone, 1 pack per day smoker since age 18, no drugs
g. FHx: noncontributory
h. PMD: Dr. Deleon

H. Nurse

a. 1 L NS
    i. BP: 122/64, HR: 78, RR: 16, Sat: 100% on 2 L NC

I. Secondary survey

a. General: alert and oriented × 3, comfortable
b. Head: normocephalic, atraumatic
c. Eyes: extraocular movement intact, pupils equal, reactive to light
d. Ears: normal tympanic membranes
e. Nose: no discharge
f. Neck: full range of motion, no jugular vein distension (if chest tube in place), no stridor
g. Pharynx: normal dentition, no lesions, no swelling
h. Chest/lungs:
    i. Needle decompression: breath sounds slightly diminished on right side, good air entry to left side, no wheezing or crackles, no ecchymosis, no crepitus, no bony tenderness
    ii. Chest tube: chest tube in right fourth intercostal space, midaxillary line, good air entry bilaterally, no wheezing or crackles, 2 cm linear wound to right 3–4 intercostal space in the midaxillary line above chest tube, no ecchymosis, crepitus, and bony tenderness
i. Heart: rate and rhythm regular, no murmurs, rubs, or gallops
j. Abdomen: normal bowel sounds, soft, nontender or distended
k. Rectal: normal tone, brown stool, occult blood negative
l. Urogenital: deferred
m. Extremities: full range of motion, no deformity, normal pulses
n. Back: nontender
o. Neuro: cranial nerves II to XII intact; normal sensation, strength; normal reflexes and gait
p. Skin: warm and dry, no other injuries noted except as described above
q. Lymph: no lymphadenopathy

J. Action

a. Bedside FAST examination showing RUQ, LUQ, suprapubic, and subxiphoid views (Figure 90.1)
b. Meds
    i. IV opioid including morphine or fentanyl
    ii. IM tetanus
c. Follow-up CXR (Figure 90.2) to assess tube positioning and lung re-expansion

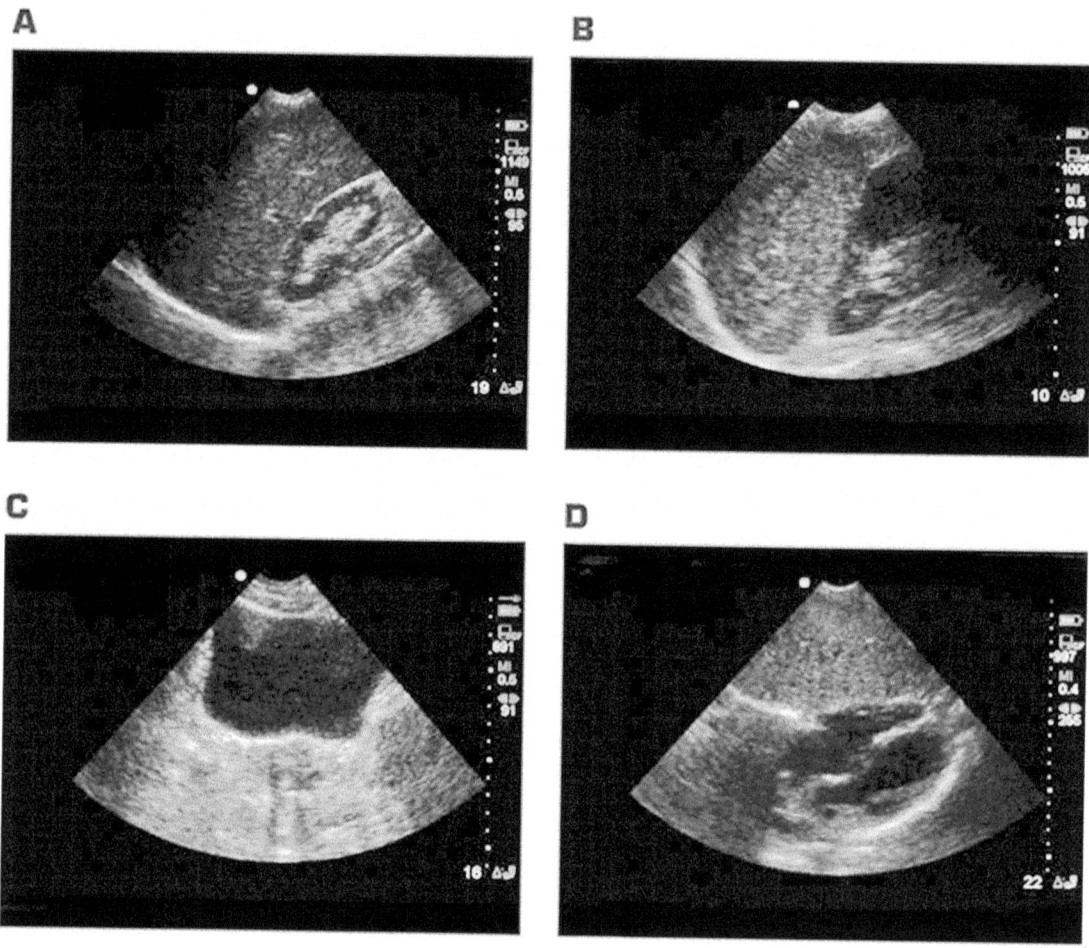

Figure 90.1

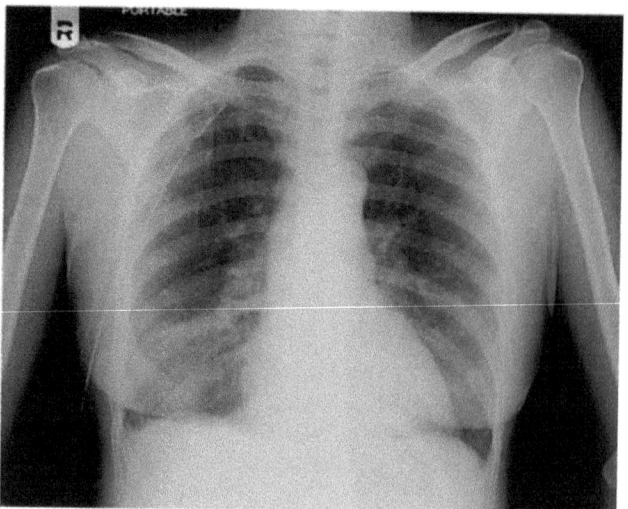

Figure 90.2

K. Nurse

a. BP: 125/79, HR: 88, RR: 16, Sat: 100% on 2 L O_2 (after 1 L)

b. Patient: feeling comfortable

L. Results

Table 90.1 Results table

Test	Result	Test	Result
Complete blood count:		T bili	1.0 mg/dL
WBC	$10.3 \times 10^3/\mu L$	D bili	0.3 mg/dL
Hct	39.1%	Amylase	50 U/L
Plt	$142 \times 10^3/\mu L$	Lipase	25 U/L
		Albumin	4.7 g/dL
Basic metabolic panel:			
Na	134 mEq/L	**Urinalysis:**	
K	4.3 mEq/L	SG	1.010–1.030
Cl	105 mEq/L	pH	5–8
CO_2	25 mEq/L	Prot	Neg
BUN	12 mEq/dL	Gluc	Neg
Cr	1.1 mg/dL	Ketones	Neg
Gluc	100 mg/dL	Bili	Neg
		Blood	Neg
		LE	Neg
Coagulation panel:		Nitrite	Neg
PT	12.6 sec	Color	Yellow
PTT	26.0 sec		
INR	1.0	**Arterial blood gas:**	
		pH	7.4
Liver function panel:		pO_2	95 mmHg
AST	23 U/L	pCO_2	41 mmHg
ALT	26 U/L	HCO_3	24 mmol/L
Alk phos	42 U/L		

M. Action

a. Consult

    i. Admitted to surgery

N. Diagnosis

a. Tension pneumothorax

O. Critical actions

a. Emergent decompression of tension pneumothorax via finger thoracostomy or needle decompression followed by immediate tube thoracostomy
b. FAST examination (eFAST looking for lung sliding and lung point sign can be performed to support diagnosis of pneumothorax when in question)
c. Pain management
d. CXR to confirm chest tube placement
e. Consult trauma team for admission

P. Examiner instructions

a. This is a case of a tension pneumothorax in a patient who suffered a stab wound to the chest. The condition is caused by a one-way air leak into the pleural space secondary to a punctured parietal pleura. This creates a one-way valve in which air accumulates in the space during inspiration, but is unable to exit during expiration. Expansion of this space causes anatomical compression and shift of mediastinal structures, causing decreased venous return and leading to hemodynamic instability. The patient presented with unstable vitals (hypotension, tachycardia, mild hypoxia, and tachypnea), moderate respiratory distress, and decreased breath sounds on the right side. Diagnosis of tension pneumothorax often requires a high level of suspicion in the presence of decreased or absent breath sounds on the affected side. The correct treatment is finger thoracostomy or emergent needle decompression followed by thoracostomy tube. If the candidate asks for a CXR before needle decompression or chest tube, the patient will become more short of breath and the oxygen saturation will drop to 88%. If the patient's pneumothorax is still not decompressed, the patient will go into cardiac arrest.

Q. Pearls

a. Tension pneumothorax is a life-threatening condition that requires prompt management.
b. Tension pneumothorax is primarily a clinical diagnosis based on patient presentation. Do not delay delivery of treatment modalities while waiting for imaging or lab studies.
c. After finger thoracostomy or needle decompression, immediately begin preparation to insert a thoracostomy tube. Then reassess the patient, as hemothorax is common with pneumothorax, especially in trauma. It may be necessary to place an additional thoracostomy tube.
d. Most common etiologies are trauma (blunt or penetrating) or iatrogenic, but pneumothorax has been seen in barotrauma secondary to positive-pressure ventilation, CPR, central venous catheter placement, or surgery.
e. Obtain a follow-up CXR to assess for lung re-expansion, thoracostomy tube positioning, and to correct any mediastinum deviation.
f. All patients with tension pneumothorax should be admitted to a surgical service.

R. Figure legends

a. Figure 90.1 (a) (US) No free fluid in Morison's pouch. (b) (US) No free fluid in splenorenal recess. (c) (US) No free fluid in pelvis. (d) (US) No pericardial effusion.
b. Figure 90.2 (CXR) Right chest tube in place; no pneumothorax.

S. References

a. *Tintinalli's Emergency Medicine: A Comprehensive Study Guide* (9th ed.): Chapter 261, Pulmonary Trauma.

b. *Rosen's Emergency Medicine: Concepts and Clinical Practice* (10th ed.): Chapter 37, Thoracic Trauma.

T. Acknowledgments
a. We would like to acknowledge Tiffany Truong for their contribution to this chapter in the previous edition of this book, which has been updated by Qiaohua Zhang.

Abdominal Pain

David Wein, MD and Edward Melnick, MD

A. Chief complaint
a. 50-year-old female brought in by EMS with the complaint of lower abdominal pain

B. Vital signs
a. BP: 135/83, HR: 115, RR: 18, T: 38.8°C, Sat: 99% on RA, FS: 94 mg/dL

C. What does the patient look like?
a. Patient appears stated age, in moderate distress due to pain.

D. Primary survey
a. Airway: speaking in full sentences
b. Breathing: no apparent respiratory distress, no cyanosis
c. Circulation: warm skin with mild diaphoresis, normal capillary refill

E. Action
a. Oxygen via NC or nonrebreather mask as needed to maintain saturations >95%
b. IV access
c. Labs
   i. CBC, BMP, LFT, coagulation studies, blood type and crossmatch, lactic acid
   ii. urinalysis, urine pregnancy test
d. 1 L NS bolus

F. History
a. HPI: A 45-year-old female with no past medical history was brought in by EMS with the complaint of lower abdominal pain. She describes the pain as sharp, constant, and progressively worsening for the last 36 hours, with nausea, vomiting, and subjective fevers and chills. The pain does not radiate and has not migrated. She denies back pain, urinary symptoms, and vaginal bleeding/discharge. She reports chronic constipation and denies diarrhea. Her last menstrual period was 3 weeks ago. ROS is otherwise not contributory.
b. PMHx: hypertension and hypercholesterolemia
c. PSHx: none
d. Allergies: none
e. Meds: none
f. Social: denies alcohol use, smoking, or illicit drug use; lives with husband at home, sexually active and monogamous
g. FHx: not relevant
h. PMD: Dr. Nelson

G. Secondary survey

a. General: alert, oriented × 3, moderate distress secondary to pain
b. Head: normocephalic, atraumatic
c. Eyes: extraocular movement intact, pupils equal, reactive to light
d. Ears: normal tympanic membranes
e. Nose: no discharge
f. Neck: full range of motion, no jugular vein distension, no stridor
g. Pharynx: normal dentition, no lesions, no swelling
h. Chest: nontender
i. Lungs: clear bilaterally
j. Heart: rate and rhythm regular, no murmurs, rubs, or gallops
k. Abdomen: normal active bowel sounds, soft with focal tenderness and voluntary guarding at LLQ, no masses, no hernias, nontender at McBurney's point, negative Murphy's sign, no rebound
l. Rectal: normal tone, brown stool, occult blood positive, nontender
m. Urogenital: normal female external genitalia; no blood or discharge, cervical os closed, no cervical motion tenderness, no adnexal tenderness
n. Extremities: full range of motion, no deformity, normal pulses
o. Back: nontender, no CVA tenderness
p. Neuro: cranial nerves II to XII intact; normal sensation, strength; normal reflexes and gait
q. Skin: warm and dry
r. Lymph: no lymphadenopathy

H. Nurse

a. Patient: still with significant pain
b. Urine pregnancy test negative

I. Action

a. Meds
  i. Morphine
  ii. Zofran
  iii. Acetaminophen
b. Reassess
  i. Patient still with significant discomfort, worsening until pain meds given, but doesn't fully resolve, also patient continues to have nausea and remains unable to tolerate POs despite antiemetic
c. Consult
d. Imaging
  i. CT abdomen/pelvis with IV contrast
e. Diet
  i. NPO

J. Nurse

a. Vital signs
  i. With IV fluid
    1. BP: 135/83, HR: 105, RR: 18, Sat: 99% on RA
  ii. Without IV fluid
    1. BP: 95/63, HR: 138, RR: 18, Sat: 99% on RA
b. Patient: still with significant pain until pain meds given, then pain improved

K. Results

Table 91.1 Results table

Test	Result	Test	Result
Complete blood count:		**Liver function panel:**	
WBC	$16 \times 10^3/\mu L$	AST	23 U/L
Diff	88.6/8.4/1.8	ALT	26 U/L
Hct	35.0%	Alk phos	42 U/L
Plt	$327 \times 10^3/\mu L$	T bili	1.0 mg/dL
		D bili	0.3 mg/dL
Basic metabolic panel:		Amylase	50 U/L
Na	138 mEq/L	Lipase	25 U/L
K	4.3 mEq/L	Albumin	4.7 g/dL
Cl	105 mEq/L		
CO_2	15 mEq/L	**Urinalysis:**	
BUN	20 mEq/dL	SG	1.020
Cr	0.7 mg/dL	pH	7
Gluc	100 mg/dL	Prot	Neg
		Gluc	Neg
Coagulation panel:		Ketones	Neg
PT	12.6 sec	Bili	Neg
PTT	26.0 sec	Blood	Neg
INR	1.0	LE	Neg
		Nitrite	Neg
Lactic acid	4.0 mEq/L	Color	Yellow

a. CT abdomen/pelvis without contrast (Figure 91.1)

L. Action

a. Surgery consult
b. Discussion with family and PMD regarding need for admission, IV antibiotics, and bowel rest
c. Meds
   i. Gentamycin (or tobramycin) and metronidazole (or clindamycin), or ciprofloxacin and metronidazole *or*
   ii. Ticarcillin–clavulanic acid, or imipenem, or piperacillin/tazobactam
   iii. If no antibiotics given, patient decompensates with worsening pain, low blood pressure, and high fever (sepsis)
d. NPO
e. Maintenance IV fluids

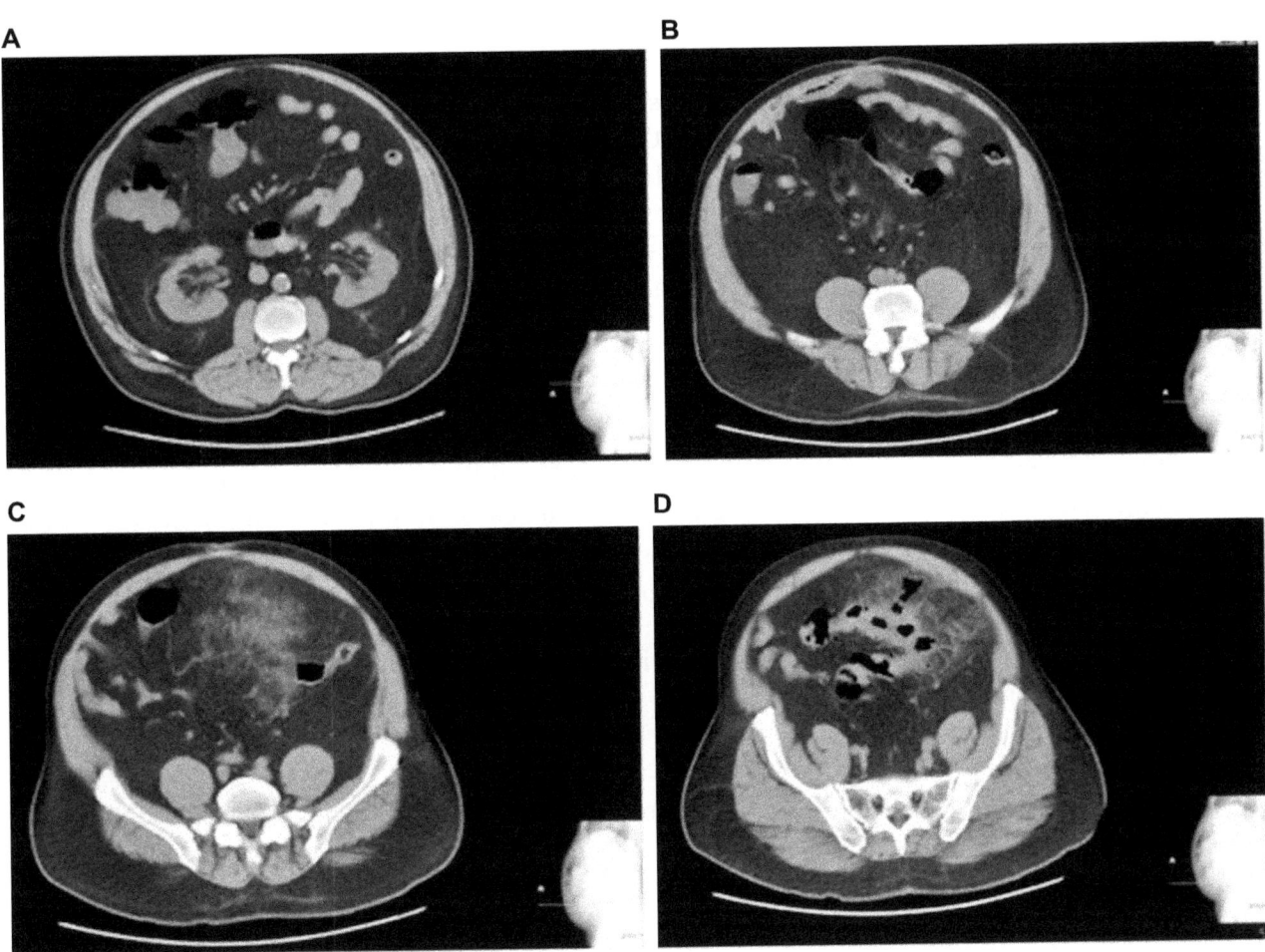

Figure 91.1

M. Diagnosis

a. Complicated diverticulitis

N. Critical actions

a. Urine pregnancy test
b. IV fluid boluses
c. Antibiotics
d. Pain management
e. CT abdomen/pelvis with IV contrast
f. Admission

O. Examiner instructions

a. This is a case of complicated diverticulitis, an infection in the large intestine that typically needs admission with IV antibiotics. Complications include perforation of bowel and abscess formation. The patient's symptoms of abdominal pain that is constant and localizing to the left lower quadrant are consistent with diverticulitis. Important early actions include administering IV fluids, evaluating for gynecologic diagnoses with a urine pregnancy test and pelvic examination (since this patient is in the reproductive age). If fluids are not administered, the patient will become more tachycardic and eventually hypotensive. Her pain will continue to increase until an opioid medication (such as morphine) is administered. A CT abdomen/pelvis (preferably with IV contrast) is the diagnostic procedure of choice. Once the CT result is available, the patient should be started on IV antibiotics. In this case, admission is warranted given her inability to tolerate PO medications and persistent pain and tenderness despite treatment. In that setting, she should be made NPO and admitted to the hospital on either a medical or surgical service. Without these actions, the patient will decompensate with sepsis due to a perforated intraabdominal abscess. In cases where perforation is suspected, surgical evaluation is critical. If no operative intervention is anticipated, medical evaluation and antibiotics are generally sufficient.

P. Pearls
a. The most common symptom of diverticulitis is pain.
b. One-third of Americans have diverticulosis by age 60 and two-thirds by age 85.
c. Uncomplicated diverticulitis can potentially be treated as an outpatient. Complicated diverticulitis requires more aggressive treatment and hospitalization.
d. When younger patients develop diverticulitis, it tends to be more severe and require earlier surgical intervention.
e. Abdominal CT can show inflammation of pericolic fat, diverticuli, thickening of the bowel wall, or peridiverticular abscess.

Q. Figure legends
a. Figure 91.1 CT abdomen/pelvis without contrast: diverticulitis, with significant mesenteric stranding but without abscess.

R. References
a. *Tintinalli's Emergency Medicine: A Comprehensive Study Guide* (9th ed.): Chapter 71A, Acute Abdominal Pain. Chapter 82, Diverticulitis.
b. *Rosen's Emergency Medicine: Concepts and Clinical Practice* (10th ed.): Chapter 81, Large Intestine.

Seizure

Daniel Eraso, MD

A. Chief complaint
a. 37-year-old female brought in by EMS for seizure-like activity

B. Vital signs
a. BP: 190/100, HR: 100, RR: 16, T: 36°C, Sat: 98% on RA

C. What does the patient look like?
a. Patient appears stated age, resting on stretcher in no acute distress, appears confused

D. Primary survey
a. Airway: maintaining patent airway
b. Breathing: no apparent respiratory distress, breathing comfortably, no cyanosis
c. Circulation: warm, well perfused extremities; normal capillary refill

E. Action
a. Oxygen via NC or nonrebreather mask as needed to maintain O_2 saturation above 95%
b. Two large bore peripheral IV lines
c. Monitor: BP: 188/96, HR: 96, RR: 18, Sat: 100% on O_2
d. POCT glucose 110 mg/dL (must ask)
e. Labs
    i. CBC, BMP, LFT, type and cross, PT/PTT
    ii. Urinalysis, urine pregnancy
    iii. Lactic acid, uric acid, LDH, magnesium level

F. History
a. HPI: A 37-year-old G1P0 female brought in by EMS for seizure-like activity, accompanied by her husband. Husband states she is 28 weeks pregnant. Over the last 2 weeks she has been reporting generalized headaches and blurry vision, both of which have worsened over the last 2 days. While at home she became acutely confused and then started "convulsing" in all extremities; the episode lasted approximately 60 seconds, and she has remained confused since. He does not report recent fevers, infectious symptoms, or trauma.
b. PMHx: HTN, obesity
c. PSHx: none
d. Allergies: none

    e. Meds: amlodipine

    f. Social: lives with husband, no alcohol or drug use

    g. FHx: maternal history of lupus, no family history of seizure disorder

    h. PMD: Dr. Mauriceau

G. Nurse

    a. BP: 190/94, HR: 90, RR: 20, Sat: 98% on O_2

    b. If no magnesium immediately given: patient has another generalized tonic-clonic seizure lasting 2 minutes

H. Action

    a. Meds

        i. Magnesium sulfate IV 4–6 g over 15–20 minutes, followed by continuous infusion of 2 g/hr (reduce loading and infusion dose for renal insufficiency)

        ii. Lorazepam for refractory seizures or magnesium contraindication (decision made in conjunction with obstetrics team)

    b. Emergent obstetrics consultation call – OB will return call in "a few minutes"

I. Secondary survey

    a. General: appears confused, not following commands, repetitive questioning

    b. Head: normocephalic, atraumatic

    c. Eyes: extraocular movement intact, pupils 5 mm equal, reactive to light

    d. Ears: normal tympanic membranes, no hemotympanum

    e. Nose: no discharge

    f. Neck: full range of motion, no jugular vein distension, no stridor

    g. Pharynx: normal dentition, no lesions, no swelling

    h. Chest: nontender

    i. Lungs: clear bilaterally, no wheezing or rales

    j. Heart: regular rate and rhythm, no murmurs, rubs, or gallops, normal capillary refill

    k. Abdomen: obese, soft, mild tenderness in RUQ, no rebound or guarding, gravid abdomen with fundal height 4 cm above umbilicus

    l. Rectal: deferred

    m. Urogenital: normal external genitalia, no vaginal bleeding, no discharge, cervix closed

    n. Extremities: full range of motion, no deformity, normal pulses, 2+ bilateral pedal edema

    o. Back: nontender

    p. Neuro: grossly moving all four extremities, patellar tendon reflexes 4+, appears postictal, not fully cooperating with exam

    q. Skin: warm and dry

    r. Lymph: no lymphadenopathy

J. Nurse

    a. BP: 150/86, HR: 90, RR: 16, Sat; 98% on O_2

    b. Patient: resting comfortably, no additional seizures (if magnesium given), more alert, answering questions appropriately, no obvious focal neurologic deficit, no reported trauma

Case 92: Seizure

K. Results

Table 92.1 Results table

Test	Result	Test	Result
Complete blood count:		**Liver function panel:**	
WBC	$17.1 \times 10^3/\mu L$	AST	95 U/L
Hct	22.9%	ALT	64 U/L
Plt	$95 \times 10^3/\mu L$	Alk phos	165 U/L
		T bili	1.4 mg/dL
		D bili	0.4 mg/dL
Basic metabolic panel:		Albumin	4.1 g/dL
Na	139 mEq/L		
K	4.1 mEq/L		
Cl	101 mEq/L	**Urinalysis:**	
CO_2	20 mEq/L	SG	1.020
BUN	30 mEq/dL	pH	6
Cr	1.4 mg/dL	Prot	++
Gluc	110 mg/dL	Gluc	Neg
		Ketones	+
		Bili	Neg
Coagulation panel:		Blood	Neg
PT	13.1 sec	LE	Neg
PTT	26 sec	Nitrite	Neg
INR	1.0		

a. Lactic acid: 5.6 mmol/L
b. Uric acid: pending
c. LDH: 654 U/L

L. Action
a. Monitor for magnesium toxicity with serial exams
   i. Loss of deep tendon reflexes
   ii. Hypotension
   iii. Respiratory depression
   iv. Calcium gluconate IV 1 g can be administered for magnesium toxicity
b. Blood pressure control as needed
   i. Diastolic BP goal <105
   ii. Hydralazine IV, labetalol IV, with repeat doses as needed
c. CT head to exclude other causes of seizure, as needed if diagnosis is not certain
d. Reassess
   i. Patient's mental status continues to improve and blood pressure is adequately controlled after magnesium administration
e. Admission to the obstetrics service for monitoring

M. Diagnosis

a. Eclampsia

N. Critical actions

a. Large-bore IV access
b. POCT glucose
c. Pregnancy test
d. Magnesium administration
e. Blood pressure control
f. Emergent obstetric consultation

O. Examiner instructions

a. This is a case of third-trimester eclampsia. The pathophysiology is likely vasospastic, causing multiorgan dysfunction. There are multiple risk factors, including age (young and old), nulliparity, primigravida, obesity, chronic hypertension, and thrombotic conditions, among others. The vast majority of eclampsia cases occur in the third trimester and within 1 week postpartum, but they can occur later than 1 week. The crux of the diagnosis revolves around obtaining information relating to current pregnancy or recent delivery. Symptoms of preeclampsia with severe features include headaches, visual changes, abdominal pain, edema, and mental status changes. Important early actions including obtaining intravenous access, obtaining a fingerstick glucose, the administration of magnesium, and obstetrics consultation. If benzodiazepines are given instead of magnesium, the seizures will eventually cease; however, the blood pressure will remain elevated until antihypertensive medications are given.

P. Pearls

a. Eclampsia is the presence of seizure activity during pregnancy with signs or symptoms of preeclampsia.
b. Magnesium sulfate is usually sufficient for both seizure and blood pressure control; however, antihypertensives (such as IV labetalol, hydralazine, or oral nifedipine) may be required for persistently elevated blood pressures. Precipitous drops in blood pressure should be avoided in order to minimize risk of uteroplacental insufficiency.
c. The loading dose of magnesium sulfate IV is 4–6 g over 20 minutes, followed by an infusion of 2 g per hour.
d. If IV access is unavailable, an alternative route is magnesium sulfate 5 mg IM into each buttock, for a total of 10 mg.
e. Emergent obstetrics consultation is required for delivery management as well as fetal monitoring.
f. Delivery is the only definitive treatment.

Q. References

a. *Tintinalli's Emergency Medicine: A Comprehensive Study Guide* (9th ed.): Chapter 100, Maternal Emergencies after 20 Weeks of Pregnancy and in the Postpartum Period.
b. *Rosen's Emergency Medicine: Concepts and Clinical Practice* (10th ed.): Chapter 173, Complications of Pregnancy. Chapter 174, Medical Emergencies during Pregnancy.

Palpitations

Edward R. Melnick, MD, MHS and Jay Khadpe, MD

A. Chief complaint
a. 59-year-old male brought in by EMS with the complaint of palpitations

B. Vital signs
a. BP: 101/73, HR: 162, RR: 22, T: 36.0°C, Sat: 98% on RA, Wt (est.): 80 kg

C. What does the patient look like?
a. Patient appears older than stated age, pale, diaphoretic, and anxious.

D. Primary survey
a. Airway: speaking in full sentences
b. Breathing: tachypneic without apparent respiratory distress, no cyanosis
c. Circulation: pale and warm skin, normal capillary refill

E. Action
a. Oxygen via NC or nonrebreather mask as needed to maintain saturation >95%
b. Two large-bore peripheral IV lines
c. Point-of-care glucose: 167 mg/dL
d. 1 L NS bolus
e. Labs
   i. CBC, BMP, TSH, LFT, coagulation studies, blood type and crossmatch
   ii. Troponin
f. Monitor: BP: 110/78, HR: 164, RR: 18, Sat: 100% on O_2, rhythm strip (Figure 93.1)
g. Place defibrillator/cardioverter pads on patient with defibrillator/cardioverter in case of deterioration
h. EKG

F. History
a. HPI: A 59-year-old male with a history of coronary artery disease status post-myocardial infarction 2 years ago and hypertension, brought in by EMS with palpitations. He awoke from sleep 30 minutes earlier at 5 a.m. with palpitations, nausea, shortness of breath, and dizziness. EMS noted tachycardia on their monitor and gave a bolus of amiodarone 150 mg. The patient's symptoms and rhythm strip failed to respond to this treatment. Patient denies chest pain, fever, cough, and syncope.
b. PMHx: coronary artery disease status post-myocardial infarction 2 years ago, hypertension, hypercholesterolemia
c. PSHx: coronary artery bypass graft 2 years ago

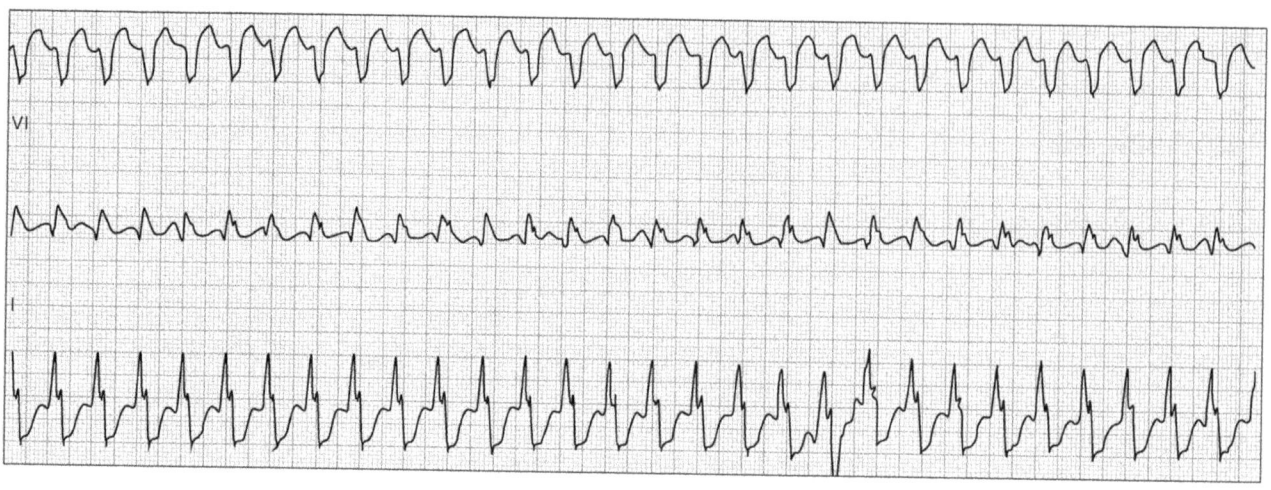

Figure 93.1

d. Allergies: none
e. Meds: hydrochlorothiazide, aspirin, losartan, atorvastatin
f. Social: lives with wife at home, quit smoking 20 years ago, denies alcohol or illicit drug use
g. FHx: father died of heart attack at age 53
h. PMD: Dr. Bern

G. Nurse
a. EKG (Figure 93.2)

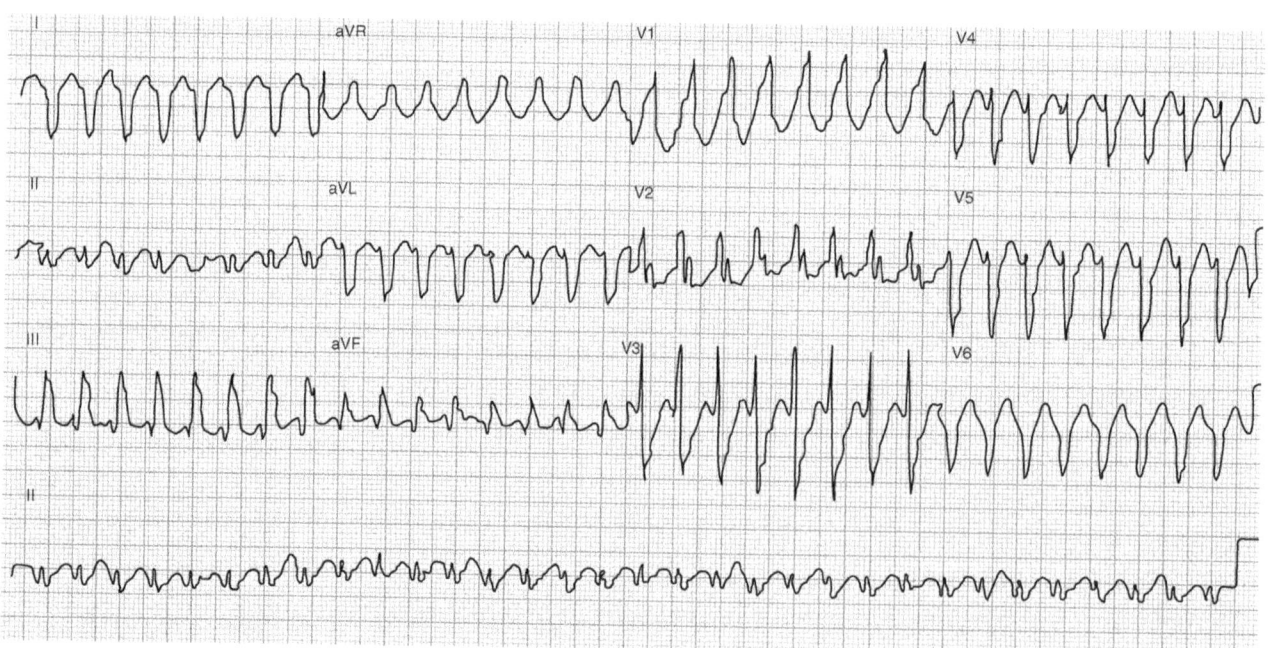

Figure 93.2

H. Action
a. Meds
   i.   Procainamide, 50 mg/min IV, up to 17 mg/kg (1360 mg) in normal patients
   ii. Alternative: amiodarone 150 mg IV bolus over 10 minutes

b. Reassess
   i. Rhythm strip unchanged from prior, with or without antiarrhythmic
   ii. BP: 106/71, HR: 162, RR: 20, Sat: 99% on O_2

I. Secondary survey

a. General: alert, oriented × 3, pale, anxious
b. HEENT: normal
c. Neck: normal
d. Chest: tachypneic, otherwise clear bilaterally and nontender, well-healed sternotomy scar
e. Heart: tachycardic rate, rhythm regular, no murmurs, rubs, or gallops
f. Abdomen: normal
g. Rectal: deferred
h. Urogenital: normal
i. Extremities: normal
j. Back: normal
k. Neuro: normal
l. Skin: normal
m. Lymph: normal

J. Action

a. Meds
   i. Amiodarone 150 mg IV bolus over 10 minutes (may repeat if given already)
   ii. Alternative: lidocaine 1.0–1.5 mg/kg (80–120 mg) IV push
b. Reassess
   i. Rhythm strip unchanged from prior, with or without antiarrhythmic
   ii. BP: 96/66, HR: 161, RR: 20, Sat: 99% on O_2
c. Consult
   i. Cardiology

K. Nurse

a. Patient: complaining of chest pain

L. Action

a. Reassess
   i. Rhythm strip unchanged from prior, with or without antiarrhythmic
   ii. BP: 90/52, HR: 166, RR: 24, Sat: 99% on O_2
   iii. Patient noted to be drowsy, cool, and diaphoretic
b. Synchronized cardioversion
   i. Midazolam (0.01–0.03 mg/kg; 1–2 mg) or equivalent for sedation. Use lower than usual procedural sedation dose due to low BP
   ii. 100 J biphasic
   ii. Rhythm strip converts to normal sinus rhythm after cardioversion
   iii. Order 12-lead EKG

M. Nurse

a. Patient
   i. If patient not cardioverted, patient noted to be pulseless and begin ACLS adult cardiac arrest algorithm. Any cardioversion from this point should be unsynchronized.

    ii. If patient is cardioverted, chest pain improves, no longer feeling palpitations, nausea, or dizziness.

b. EKG (Figure 93.3 if cardioverted; Figure 93.2 if not cardioverted and in ACLS)

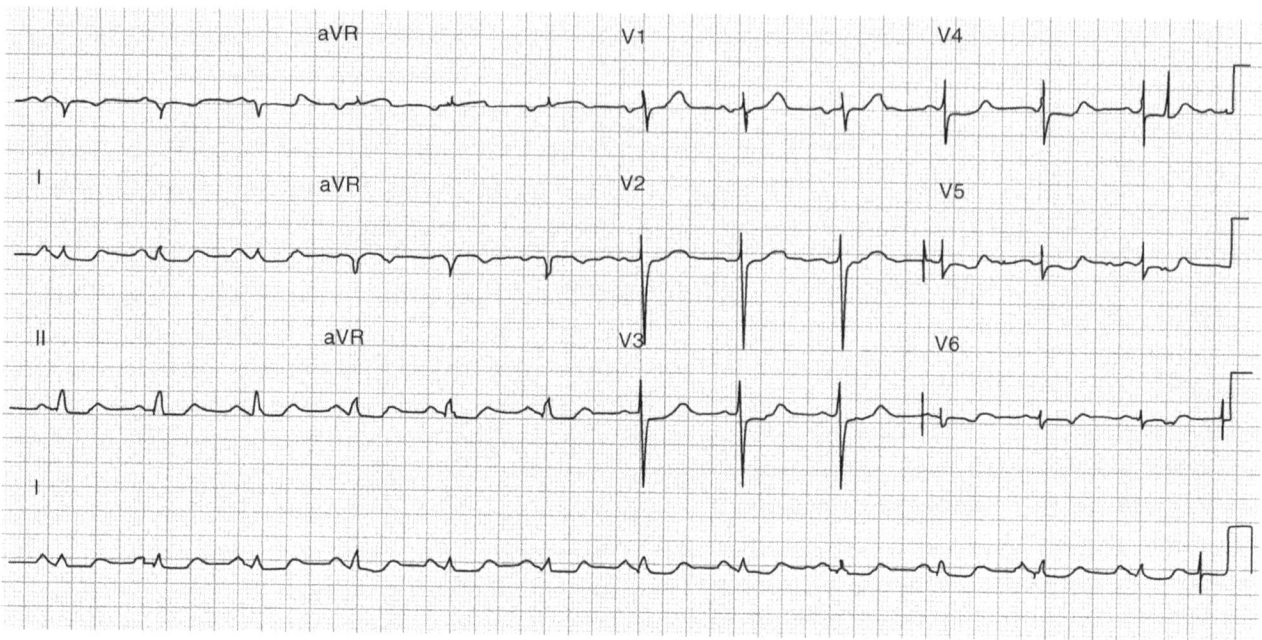

Figure 93.3

N. Results

Table 93.1 Results table

Test	Result	Test	Result
Complete blood count:		T bili	1.0 mg/dL
WBC	$6.4 \times 10^3/\mu L$	D bili	0.3 mg/dL
Hct	30.5%	Amylase	50 U/L
Plt	$250 \times 10^3/\mu L$	Lipase	25 U/L
		Albumin	4.7 g/dL
Basic metabolic panel:			
Na	138 mEq/L	**Urinalysis:**	
K	4.3 mEq/L	SG	1.020
Cl	105 mEq/L	pH	7
CO_2	30 mEq/L	Prot	Neg
BUN	12 mEq/dL	Gluc	Neg
Cr	1.1 mg/dL	Ketones	Neg
Gluc	100 mg/dL	Bili	Neg
		Blood	Neg
Coagulation panel:		LE	Neg
PT	12.6 sec	Nitrite	Neg

Table 93.1 (cont.)

Test	Result	Test	Result
PTT	26.0 sec	Color	Yellow
INR	1.0		
		Arterial blood gas:	
Liver function panel:		pH	7.4
AST	23 U/L	pO_2	95 mmHg
ALT	26 U/L	pCO_2	41 mmHg
Alk phos	42 U/L	HCO_3	24 mmol/L

a. Calcium 10.1 mg/dL
b. Magnesium 2.2 mg/dL
c. Phosphorous 3.8 mg/dL
d. Troponin I: 0.6 ng/mL

O. Action
a. Cardiology consult
   i. CCU admission
b. Discussion with patient ± family regarding patient status and need for CCU admission
c. Med
   i. Maintenance infusion of antiarrhythmic:
      1. Amiodarone (1 mg/min × 6 hours) or
      2. Lidocaine (1–4 mg/min)

P. Diagnosis
a. Ventricular tachycardia

Q. Critical actions
a. Rhythm strip/12-lead EKG
b. Confirm IV access
c. Amiodarone, procainamide, or lidocaine while stable
d. Synchronized cardioversion for instability
e. Cardiology consult

R. Examiner instructions
a. This is a case of a ventricular tachycardia, likely from myocardial ischemia or infarction. Ventricular tachycardia is a life-threatening irregularity of the heart's conduction system, which is often caused by reduced blood flow to the heart. The patient's symptoms of palpitations, nausea, and dizziness occurred spontaneously, awaking him from sleep. Important early actions include obtaining a 12-lead EKG and administering an antiarrhythmic medication. This patient's ventricular tachycardia is refractory to drug therapy and will persist regardless of treatment. Eventually, the patient becomes unstable, with chest pain, altered mental status, and hypotension. Without synchronized cardioversion at this point, the patient will become pulseless. After cardioversion, the patient will convert into normal sinus rhythm with a 12-lead EKG concerning for myocardial ischemia.

S. Pearls

a. Ventricular tachycardia is rare in patients without underlying heart disease. Patients with chronic ischemic heart disease and acute myocardial infarction are the most common.

b. It can be challenging to differentiate ventricular tachycardia from supraventricular tachycardia with aberrant conduction based on clinical symptoms, vital signs, and even using the 12-lead EKG. When in doubt, assume a ventricular origin.

c. Defibrillation and cardioversion simultaneously depolarize all cardiac tissue and terminate any sites of reentry, causing all cardiac cells to be in the same depolarized state. This allows a dominant pacemaker – usually the sinus node – to pace the heart.

d. Wolff–Parkinson–White syndrome, Brugada syndrome, and prolonged QT syndrome can also all cause fatal tachydysrhythmias.

T. Figure legends

a. Figure 93.1 (Rhythm strip) Monomorphic ventricular tachycardia.

b. Figure 93.2 (EKG) Monomorphic ventricular tachycardia.

c. Figure 93.3 (EKG) Normal sinus rhythm; lateral T wave changes.

U. References

a. *Tintinalli's Emergency Medicine: A Comprehensive Study Guide* (9th ed.): Chapter 18, Cardiac Rhythm Disturbances.

b. *Rosen's Emergency Medicine: Concepts and Clinical Practice* (10th ed.): Chapter 65, Dysrhythmias.

Seizure

Alexandra Mannix, MD

A. Chief complaint
a. 28-year-old female brought in by her boyfriend who states the patient "had a seizure"

B. Vital signs
a. BP: 92/68, HR: 125, RR: 25, T: 36.2°C, Sat: 98% on RA

C. What does the patient look like?
a. Patient appears stated age, drowsy but arousable to painful stimuli, supine on stretcher, vomitus noted on clothes. Male visitor in the room (boyfriend).

D. Primary survey
a. Airway: patent.
b. Breathing: tachypneic but no apparent respiratory distress
c. Circulation: dry and cool skin, normal capillary refill

E. Action
a. Monitor: BP: 85/63, HR: 130, RR: 28, Sat: 100% on O_2
b. Rectal temperature: 38.1°C
c. Oxygen via NRB mask (anticipate intubation)
d. Two large-bore peripheral IV lines
e. Finger stick blood glucose: 110 mg/dL (must ask)
f. Labs
   i. CBC, BMP, LFT, coagulation studies, blood type and crossmatch
   ii. Urinalysis, urine pregnancy test
   iii. Lactate, alcohol level, acetaminophen level, salicylate level, urine/serum toxicology screen, ABG
   iv. Blood cultures
g. 1 L NS bolus
h. EKG

F. History
a. HPI: A 28-year-old female with a history of depression.
   i. Patient unable to provide any history.
   ii. History obtained from boyfriend.
      1. Patient has been taking amitriptyline for the past 6 months, and today admitted to taking "a lot" of pills after a fight they had ~2 hours ago. Patient initially was nauseated, then vomited twice and then become "sleepy." Boyfriend states they got into an argument and he left the patient alone in the bedroom. He became concerned when she

did not come out after some time. He reports the patient was found lying in bed upon reentering the bedroom, was able to rouse her briefly, followed shortly by generalized shaking that lasted less than 1 minute. No prior suicide attempts as per boyfriend. No known fevers, chills, headaches, rashes, abdominal pain, diarrhea, dysuria. Currently menstruating. In usual state of health before argument.

   b. PMHx: depression

   c. PSHx: none

   d. Allergies: none

   e. Meds: amitriptyline

   f. Social: denies alcohol use, smoking, or illicit drug use; lives with boyfriend in apartment

   g. FHx: no relevant history

   h. PMD: Dr. Jung (psychiatrist)

G. Nurse

   a. EKG (Figure 94.1)

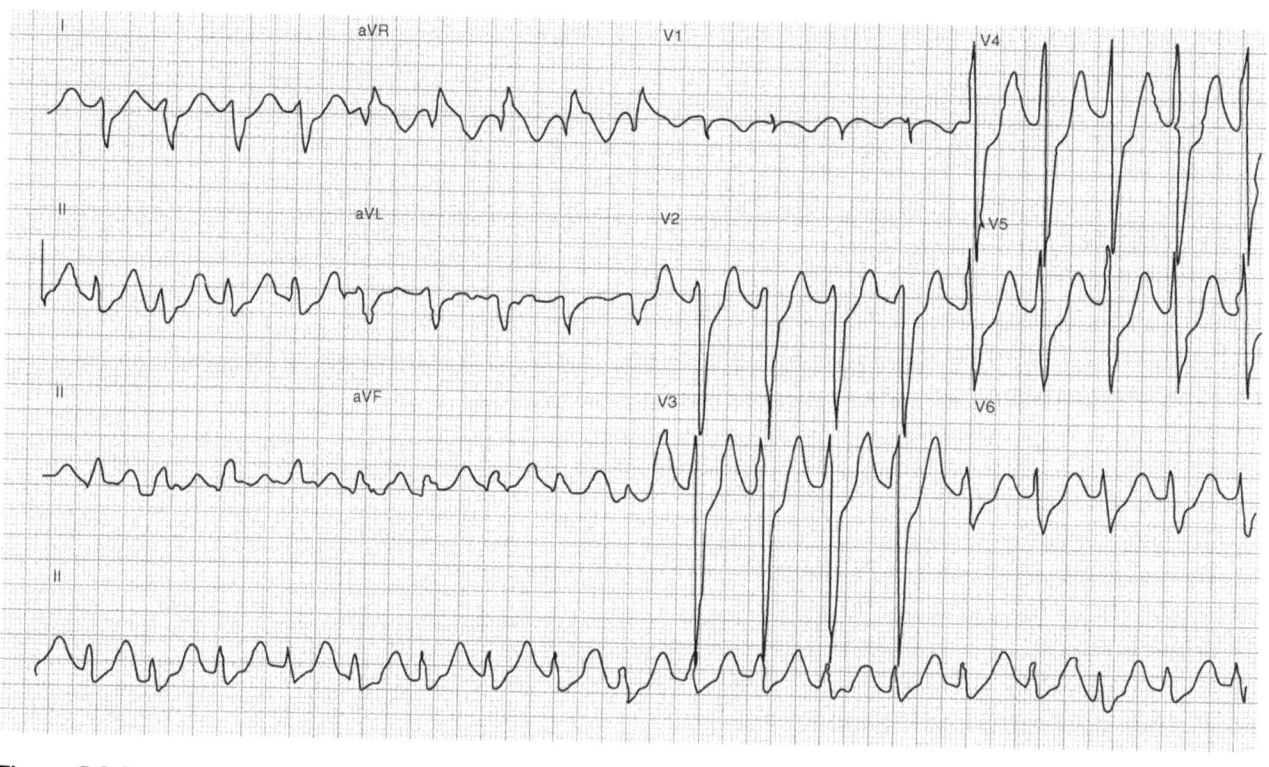

Figure 94.1

H. Secondary survey

   a. General: drowsy but arousable, oriented to person; unable to provide any additional history

   b. Head: normocephalic, atraumatic

   c. Eyes: opens eyes to name, 6 mm pupils, equal, sluggish to light

   d. Ears: normal tympanic membranes

   e. Nose: no discharge

   f. Neck: full range of motion, no jugular vein distension, no stridor

   g. Pharynx: normal dentition, no lesions, no swelling

   h. Chest: normal

   i. Lungs: normal

   j. Heart: tachycardic rate; rhythm regular; 2+ pulses in all extremities

k. Abdomen: mildly tender in epigastrium, decreased bowel sounds, no masses, no hernias, no rebound, no guarding, no rigidity
l. Rectal: normal tone, brown stool
m. Extremities: full passive range of motion, no deformity, 2+ pulses
n. Back: nontender
o. Neuro: eyes: opens eyes to voice; confused response; localizes pain – will not follow commands (GCS: 12)
p. Skin: warm and dry; no rashes
q. Lymph: no lymphadenopathy

I. Action

a. Meds
   i. Sodium bicarbonate:
      1. push 3 amps (150 mEq) immediately
      2. create a drip – 3 amps (150 mEq) in 1 L D5 W, run at 1 L/hr until patient consistently stabilized
      3. target: serum pH of 7.45–7.55
   ii. Consider vasopressor (e.g., norepinephrine 8–12 mcg/min) after bicarbonate bolus and infusion started
   iii. Isotonic IV fluids
   iv. Consider activated charcoal in consultation with Poison Center; intubate if used
b. Consult
   i. Poison Control Center
   ii. Medical ICU
c. Repeat EKG
   i. If bicarbonate given: Figure 94.2
   ii. If no bicarbonate given: Figure 94.1

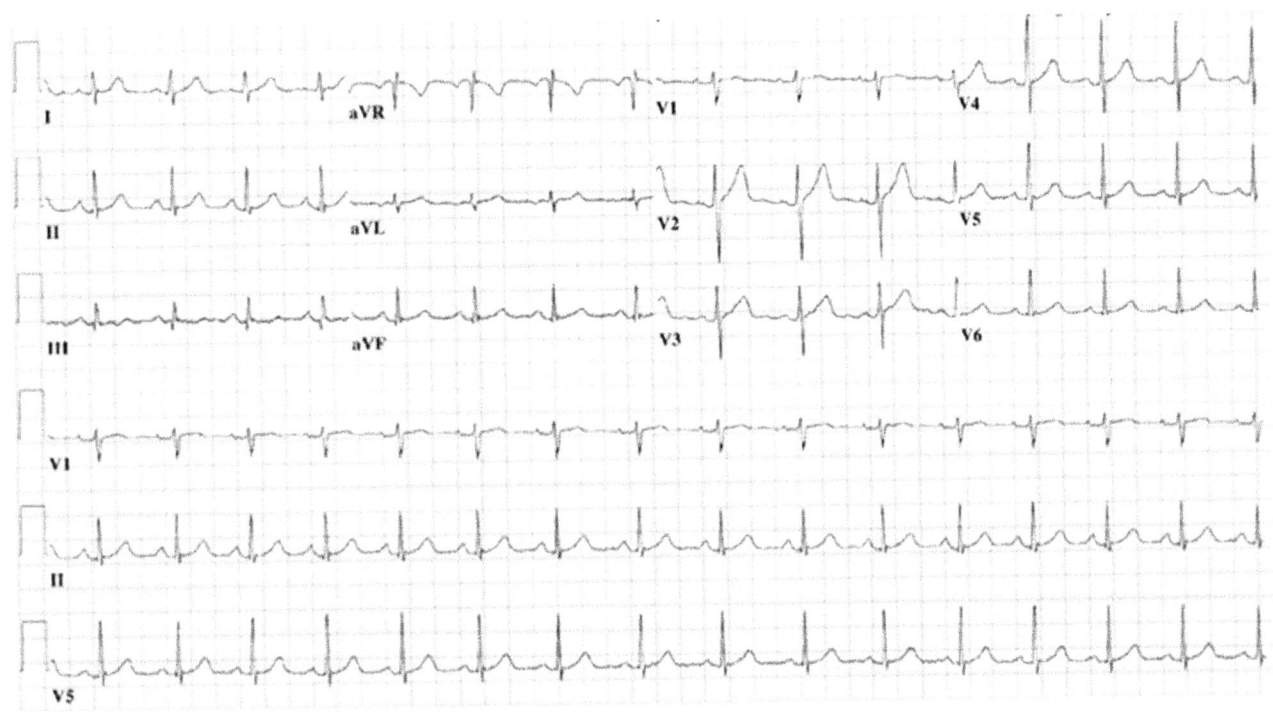

Figure 94.2

J. Nurse

a. Vitals

   i. With fluids and bicarbonate: BP: 100/75, HR: 105, RR: 22, Sat: 100% on O_2

   ii. With fluids without bicarbonate: BP: 85/62, HR: 135, RR: 25, Sat: 100% on O_2

   iii. Without fluids: BP 70/50, HR 145, RR 30, Sat 95% on 100% O_2

b. With or without acetaminophen/ibuprofen: core temperature 38.1°C

c. Patient: unresponsive, has repeat generalized tonic-clonic seizure lasting 30 seconds

K. Actions

a. Meds

   i. Sodium bicarbonate: repeat boluses in addition to drip

   ii. Lorazepam IV

b. Intubation/mechanical ventilation

L. Results

Table 94.1 Results table

Test	Result	Test	Result
Complete blood count:		Alk phos	42 U/L
WBC	$5.3 \times 10^3/\mu L$	T bili	1.0 mg/dL
Hct	41.5%	D bili	0.3 mg/dL
Plt	$350 \times 10^3/\mu L$	Amylase	50 U/L
		Lipase	25 U/L
Basic metabolic panel:		Albumin	4.7 g/dL
Na	138 mEq/L		
K	4.3 mEq/L	**Urinalysis:**	
Cl	10 mEq/L	SG	1.015
CO_2	18.9 mEq/L	pH	6
BUN	22 mEq/dL	Prot	Neg
Cr	1.1 mg/dL	Gluc	Neg
Gluc	100 mg/dL	Ketones	Neg
		Bili	Neg
Coagulation panel:		Blood	Neg
PT	12.6 sec	LE	Neg
PTT	26.0 sec	Nitrite	Neg
INR	1.0	Color	Yellow
Liver function panel:		**Arterial blood gas:**	
AST	23 U/L	pH	7.30
ALT	26 U/L	pCO_2	48
		pO_2	400

a. Lactate: 4.0 mmol/L
b. Urine pregnancy test: negative
c. Urine/serum tox screen: pending
d. EtOH: 6 mg/dL
e. Acetaminophen: <5 mcg/mL
f. Salicylate: <5 mg/dL

M. Action
a. Admit to medical ICU
b. Consider toxicology consultation

N. Diagnosis
a. Tricyclic antidepressant toxicity

O. Critical actions
a. Large-bore peripheral IV access
b. Fluid bolus
c. EKG
d. Sodium bicarbonate – bolus *and* drip
e. Repeat EKG after treatment
f. Intubation
g. Medical ICU consultation

P. Examiner instructions
a. This is a case of intentional tricyclic antidepressant (TCA) in a suicide attempt. Taking large doses of TCA is a medical emergency that can lead to life-threatening abnormalities in heart rhythm, seizures, and death if untreated. In this patient, the symptoms of nausea, vomiting, mental status changes, and seizures began within 2 hours of amitriptyline ingestion, signifying a large dose or co-ingestion of another drug. Important early actions include administering IV fluids, preferably crystalloid for hypotension, obtaining an EKG, alkalizing the serum for increased excretion and sodium loading to reduce risk of cardiac dysrhythmias, and management of TCA-induced seizures. If an EKG is not obtained early in the course of management, the patient should seize and decompensate.

Q. Pearls
a. Most Poison Control directors in the United States use a QRS of 100 ms or greater as the cutoff for IV sodium bicarbonate administration.
b. The greatest risk of seizures and arrhythmias occurs within the first 6–8 hours of TCA ingestion.
c. Crystalloid fluids such as normal saline are indicated for TCA-induced hypotension. For hypotension refractory to IV saline, vasopressors such as phenylephrine or norepinephrine, with α-agonist effect, may be used.
d. Once the patient is stabilized, activated charcoal can be considered for gastrointestinal decontamination.
e. The treatment of choice for prolonged or recurrent seizures in TCA toxicity is a benzodiazepine, though most are self-limited.

R. Figure legends

a. Figure 94.1 (EKG) Intraventricular conduction delay with QRS >100 ms and terminal R wave >3 mm in aVR.

b. Figure 94.2 (EKG) Normal sinus rhythm.

S. References

a. *Tintinalli's Emergency Medicine: A Comprehensive Study Guide* (9th ed.): Chapter 168, Altered Mental Status and Coma. Chapter 177, Cyclic Antidepressants.

b. *Rosen's Emergency Medicine: Concepts and Clinical Practice* (10th ed.): Chapter 141, Antidepressants.

Fever

Ryan McKenna, DO and Ram Parekh, MD

A. Chief complaint
a. 27-year-old female who presents with fever, foot and ankle pain and swelling

B. Vital signs
a. BP: 110/63, HR: 114, RR: 22, T: 38.9°C, Sat: 98% on RA, FS: 120 mg/dL (must ask)

C. What does the patient look like?
a. Patient appears stated age and in no acute distress.

D. Primary survey
a. Airway: speaking in full sentences
b. Breathing: tachypneic but in no apparent respiratory distress, no cyanosis
c. Circulation: warm to touch, well perfused

E. Action
a. Peripheral IV access
b. 1 L NS or LR bolus
c. Monitor: BP: 118/69, HR: 108, RR: 22, Sat: 98% on RA

F. History
a. HPI: A 27-year-old female with a history of adult polycystic kidney disease status post kidney transplantation 3 weeks ago, presents to the ED with fever to 38.9°C. Patient states that she has noticed over the last 2 days progressively worsening redness, swelling, warmth, and pain in her right foot and ankle. She states that she developed a fever and came to the ED for evaluation. Other than mild generalized malaise, she denies any other symptoms such as nausea, vomiting, diarrhea, dysuria, urinary frequency, headaches, cough, rhinorrhea, vision complaints, or neurological symptoms.
b. PMHx: adult polycystic kidney disease
c. PSHx: living donor kidney transplant 3 weeks ago
d. Allergies: none
e. Meds: cyclosporine, tacrolimus, prednisone
f. Social: married with two children, denies alcohol, smoking, or recreational drugs
g. FHx: not relevant

G. Nurse
a. Acetaminophen 1 g PO
   i. BP: 115/75, HR: 102, RR: 20, T: 37.6°C, Sat: 100% on O_2

H. Secondary survey

a. General: alert, oriented × 3, comfortable
b. Head: normocephalic, atraumatic
c. Eyes: extraocular movement intact, pupils equal, reactive to light, non-icteric sclera
d. Ears: normal tympanic membranes
e. Nose: no discharge
f. Neck: full range of motion, no jugular vein distension, no stridor
g. Pharynx: normal dentition, no lesions, no swelling
h. Chest: nontender
i. Lungs: clear bilaterally
j. Heart: tachycardic rate, rhythm regular, no murmurs, rubs, or gallops
k. Abdomen: surgical incision well-healed, mild incisional tenderness; no guarding, rebound, tenderness, or distension
l. Rectal: deferred due to concern for neutropenia
m. Urogenital: deferred
n. Extremities: full range of motion, no deformity, normal pulses
o. Back: nontender
p. Neuro: cranial nerves II to XII intact; normal sensation, strength; normal reflexes and gait
q. Skin: hot to touch diffusely; circumferential erythema and induration of all of right foot and ankle; warm, tender to touch; no abscess or fluctuance, no crepitus
r. Lymph: no lymphadenopathy

I. Action

a. X-rays:
    i. Foot
    ii. Chest
b. Labs
    i. CBC, BMP, LFT, coagulation studies, lactic acid, blood type and crossmatch
    ii. Blood cultures, urinalysis, urine HCG, urine culture
c. EKG (Figure 95.1)
d. 1 L bolus of lactated Ringer's or normal saline (attempting to reach 20–30 cc/kg)
e. Meds
    i. Piperacillin and tazobactam
    ii. Vancomycin
    iii. Fluconazole
f. Reassess
g. Consult
    i. Transplant nephrology

J. Nurse

a. BP: 85/59, HR: 128, RR: 22, Sat: 98% on O_2 (after 2 L bolus)
b. Patient: still complaining of foot pain

K. Actions

a. Obtain central access using aseptic technique
b. Repeat fluid bolus
c. Start norepinephrine (start 10 mcg/min; titrate to MAP >60 mmHg)

Case 95: Fever

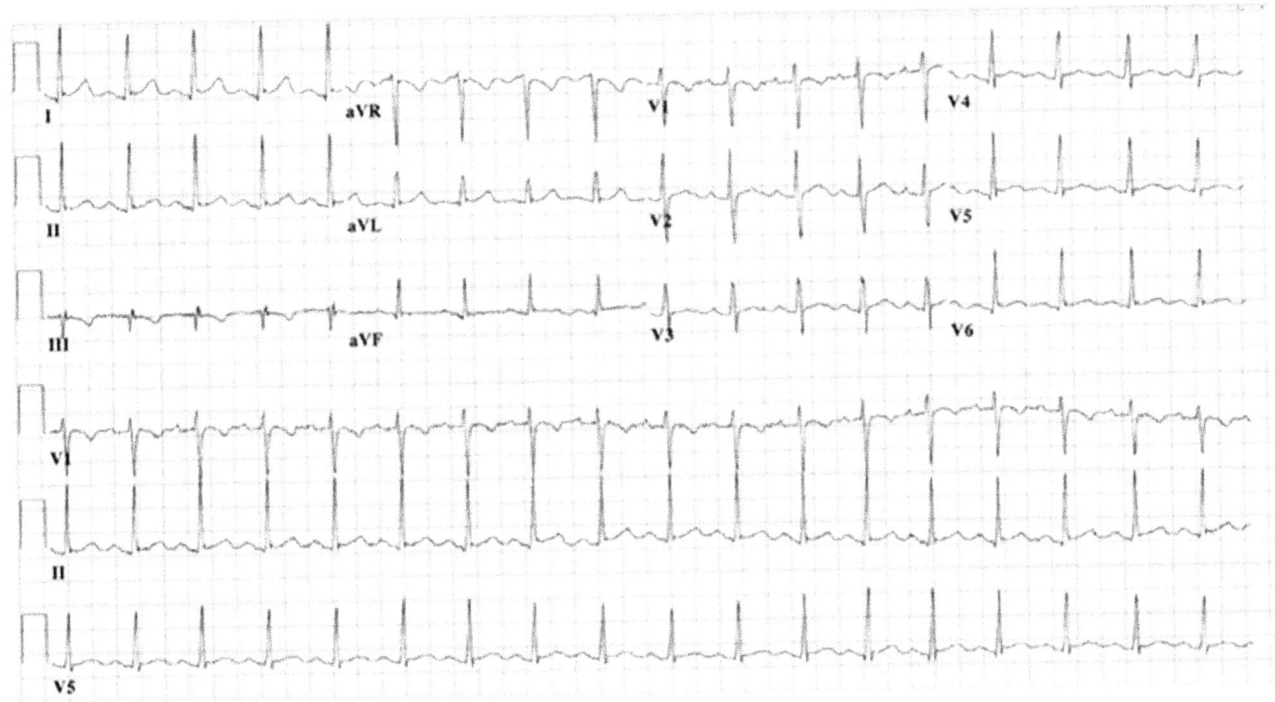

Figure 95.1

d. Reassess
e. Morphine IV

L. Nurse

a. BP: 119/70, HR: 98, RR: 22, Sat: 98% on O_2 (after 2 L bolus and norepinephrine)

M. Results

Table 95.1 Results table

Test	Result	Test	Result
Complete blood count:		**Liver function panel:**	
WBC	$1.1 \times 10^3/\mu L$	AST	23 U/L
Diff	45/9.4/1.2	ALT	26 U/L
Hct	41.5	Alk phos	42 U/L
Plt	$350 \times 10^3/\mu L$	T bili	1.4 mg/dL
		D bili	0.8 mg/dL
Basic metabolic panel:		Amylase	50 U/L
Na	138 mEq/L	Lipase	25 U/L
K	4.3 mEq/L	Albumin	3.9 g/dL
Cl	105 mEq/L		
CO_2	30 mEq/L	**Urinalysis:**	
BUN	12 mEq/dL	SG	1.020
Cr	1.1 mg/dL	pH	6

Table 95.1 (cont.)

Test	Result		Test	Result
Gluc	100 mg/dL		Prot	Neg
			Gluc	Neg
Coagulation panel:			Ketones	Neg
PT	14.0 sec		Bili	Neg
PTT	26.0 sec		Blood	Neg
INT	1.1		LE	Neg
			Nitrite	Neg
			Color	Yellow

a. Lactate: 4.2 mmol/L
b. Patient: return from radiology
c. BP: 103/54, HR: 112, RR: 22, Sat: 98% on O_2
d. X-rays (Figures 95.2 and 95.3).

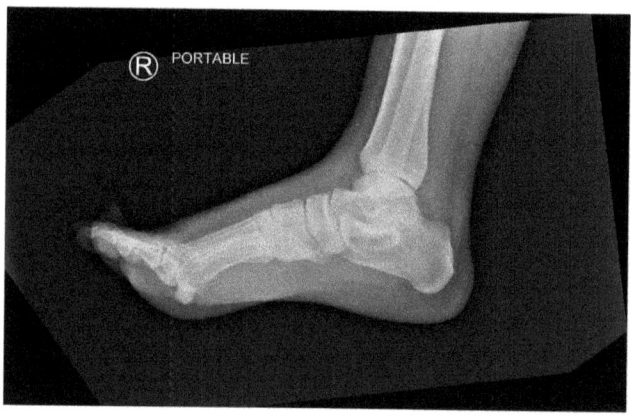

Figure 95.2

N. Action

a. Initiate sepsis bundle
   i. Give 30 mL/kg fluid bolus of normal saline or lactated Ringer's if not already given
   ii. Intravenous antibiotics
   iii. Trend lactate
b. Discussion with renal transplant team
   i. Admission, reverse isolation hospital bed/ICU

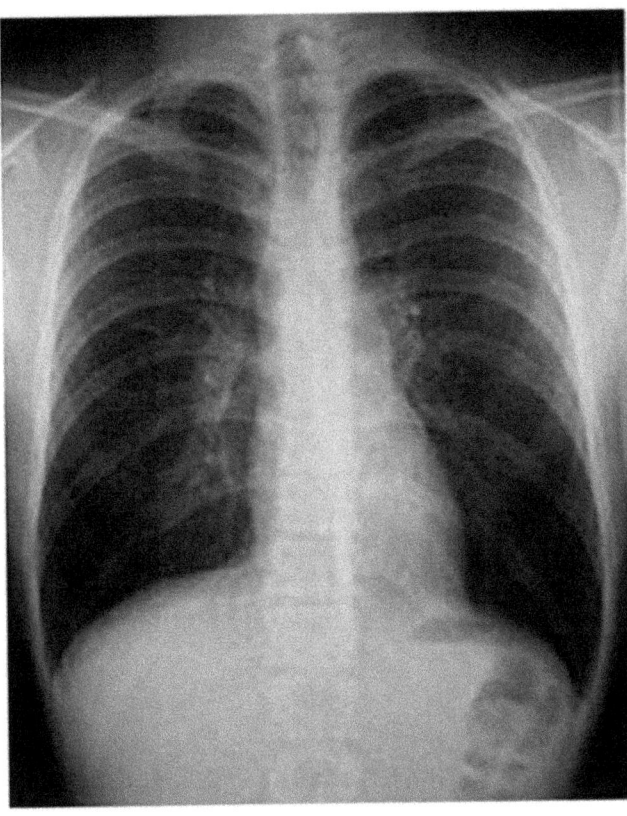

Figure 95.3

c. Discussion with family and PMD regarding need for hospitalization for IV antibiotics and to rule out rejection

O. Diagnosis
a. Post kidney transplant fever

P. Critical actions
a. IV access and fluid bolus
b. Cultures before antibiotics
c. Broad-spectrum antibiotics
d. Pain medication
e. Contacting appropriate consultant

Q. Examiner instructions
a. This is a case of a fever in a post-transplant patient, which is a serious concern because these patients are on multiple medications to suppress their immunity and are at high risk for serious infections. The patient's presenting signs and symptoms are consistent with right lower extremity cellulitis in the setting of immunosuppression. Important early actions include administering IV fluids for hypotension, obtaining cultures of blood and urine, early antibiotics, contacting the appropriate consultant (in this case the renal transplant team), and appropriate disposition to the ICU given elevated lactic acid and hypotension concerning for sepsis.

R. Pearls
a. Fever in transplant recipients should be considered an emergency.

b. Bacterial infection is most common in the first month post-transplant. Although Gram-negative organisms predominate (especially *Pseudomonas aeruginosa*), Gram-positive and anaerobic organisms are not uncommon.

c. Fungi are also common within the first month post-transplantation.

d. Although there is large regional variability, the incidence of tuberculosis in solid organ transplant recipients is 20–74 times the general population, with a mortality rate approaching 30%.

S. Figure legends

a. Figure 95.1 (EKG) Sinus tachycardia; minimal voltage criteria for LVH.

b. Figure 95.2 (X-ray) Normal right foot x-ray, no subcutaneous gas.

c. Figure 95.3 (CXR) Hyperinflation, otherwise normal chest x-ray.

T. References

a. *Tintinalli's Emergency Medicine: A Comprehensive Study Guide* (9th ed.): Chapter 297, The Transplant Patient.

b. *Rosen's Emergency Medicine: Concepts and Clinical Practice* (10th ed.): Chapter 183, The Solid Organ Transplant Patient.

Abdominal Trauma

Ram Parekh, MD and Carolina Pereira, MD

A. Chief complaint
a. 46-year-old male brought in by EMS on backboard and cervical collar with spinal immobilization after being involved in a high-speed motor vehicle collision

B. Vital signs
a. BP: 95/63, HR: 120, RR: 20, T: 36.2°C, Sat: 98% on RA

C. What does the patient look like?
a. Patient appears stated age, immobilized on backboard, moaning and complaining of abdominal pain.

D. Primary survey
a. Airway: speaking clearly in full sentences
b. Breathing: no apparent respiratory distress, unlabored breathing, no cyanosis
c. Circulation: diaphoretic and cool skin, normal capillary refill

E. Action
a. Two large-bore peripheral IV lines
b. Labs
    i. CBC, BMP, LFT, coagulation studies, and blood type
c. Crossmatch 2 units and/or call for uncrossed blood/massive transfusion
d. 1 L NS bolus
e. Monitor: BP: 98/69, HR: 112, RR: 22, Sat: 98%
f. Expose the patient to identify injuries

F. History
a. HPI: A 46-year-old male was the unrestrained driver in a motor vehicle collision, car versus tree, with significant front car damage including intrusion and steering wheel deformity. Airbags deployed. The patient required extrication by EMS and was not ambulatory on scene. EMS reports that patient was GCS of 15 throughout. The patient complains mainly of significant abdominal pain. Patient denies loss of consciousness, alcohol ingestion, head injury, headache, nausea, vomiting, neck pain, numbness, tingling, shortness of breath, dizziness, or chest pain.
b. PMHx: HTN
c. PSHx: none
d. Allergies: none
e. Social: married with two children, social EtOH, denies smoking and recreational drug use
f. FHx: no relevant history

G. Nurse
a. 1 L isotonic solution or empiric blood administration
   i. BP: 105/75, HR: 102, RR: 18, Sat: 100%
b. No fluid
   i. BP: 80/45, HR: 120, RR: 24, Sat: 98%

H. Secondary survey (must include use of logroll technique with spinal immobilization)
a. General: alert, oriented × 3, spinal immobilization, complaining of abdominal pain
b. Head: normocephalic, atraumatic
c. Eyes: extraocular movement intact, pupils equal, reactive to light, no raccoon eyes
d. Ears: normal tympanic membranes, no hemotympanum, no Battle's sign
e. Nose: no discharge, no deformity
f. Neck: cervical collar, no gross deformity or abrasion, nontender
g. Oropharynx: normal dentition, no lesions, no swelling
h. Chest: nontender, no seatbelt sign
i. Lungs: clear bilaterally
j. Heart: rate and rhythm regular, no murmurs, rubs, or gallops
k. Abdomen: horizontal abrasion to epigastrium, diffuse tenderness, moderately distended, left flank ecchymosis, bowel sounds mildly decreased, no masses, no hernias, no rebound, no rigidity
l. Pelvis: stable
m. Rectal: normal tone, brown stool, occult blood negative, normal prostate
n. Urogenital: normal male external genitalia
o. Extremities: full range of motion, no deformity, normal pulses
p. Back: nontender
q. Neuro: GCS 15, cranial nerves II to XII intact; normal sensation, strength; normal reflexes and gait
r. Skin: warm and dry, horizontal abrasion to epigastrium
s. Lymph: no lymphadenopathy

I. Action
a. Medication for pain (fentanyl, hydromorphone, morphine, etc.)
   i. Reassessment: patient still with significant pain
b. Consult: trauma or general surgery
c. Imaging
   i. CXR
   ii. Pelvic x-ray
d. FAST examination (Figure 96.1)
e. EKG

J. Nurse
a. CXR (Figure 96.2)
b. Pelvic x-ray (Figure 96.3)
c. EKG (Figure 96.4)
d. Vitals: BP: 89/59, HR: 128, RR: 22, Sat: 98% (after 1 L)
e. Patient: still complaining of abdominal pain, abdominal distension worsening

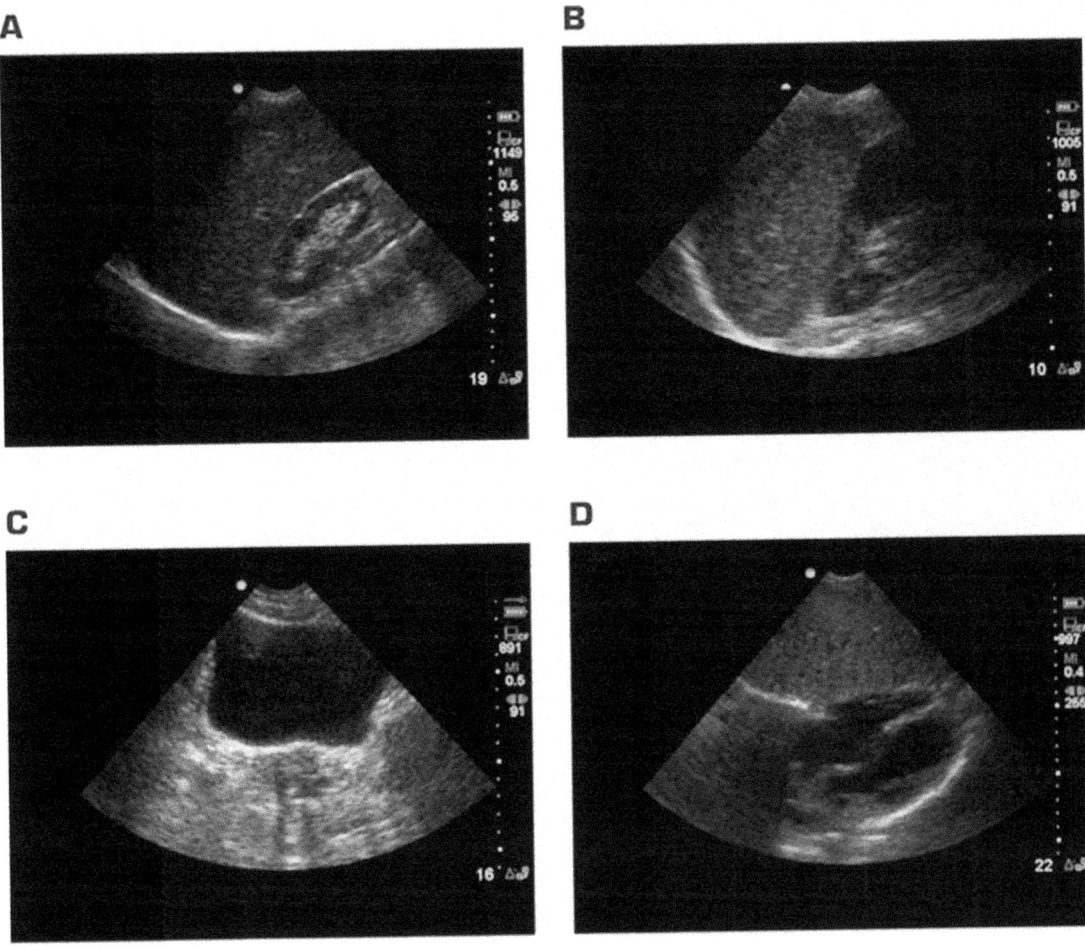

Figure 96.1

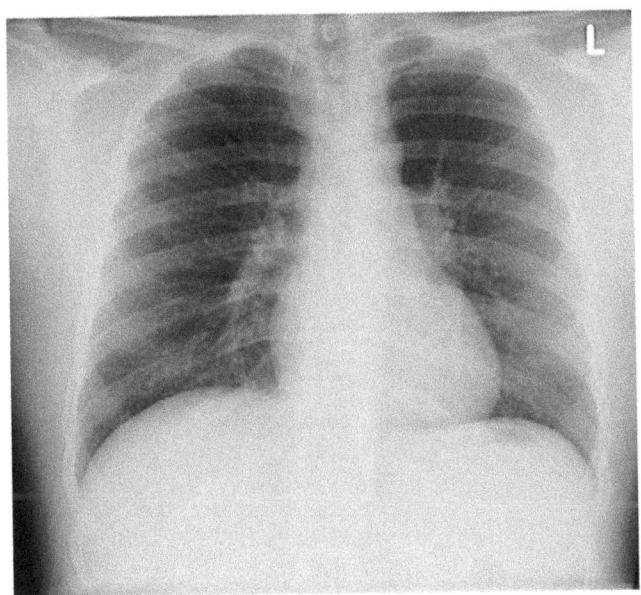

Figure 96.2

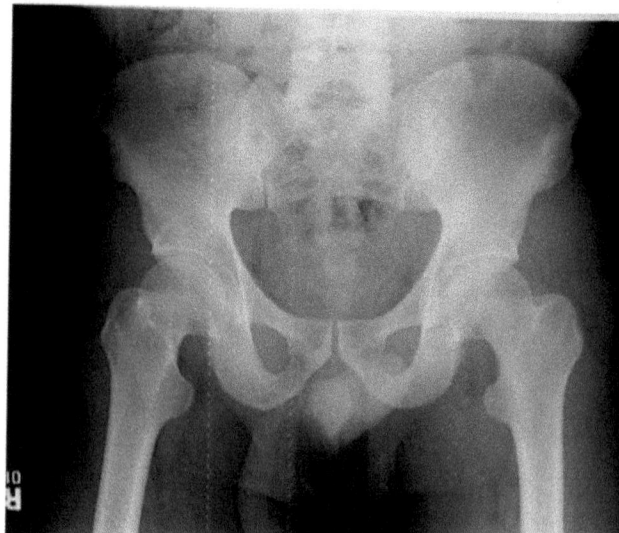

Figure 96.3

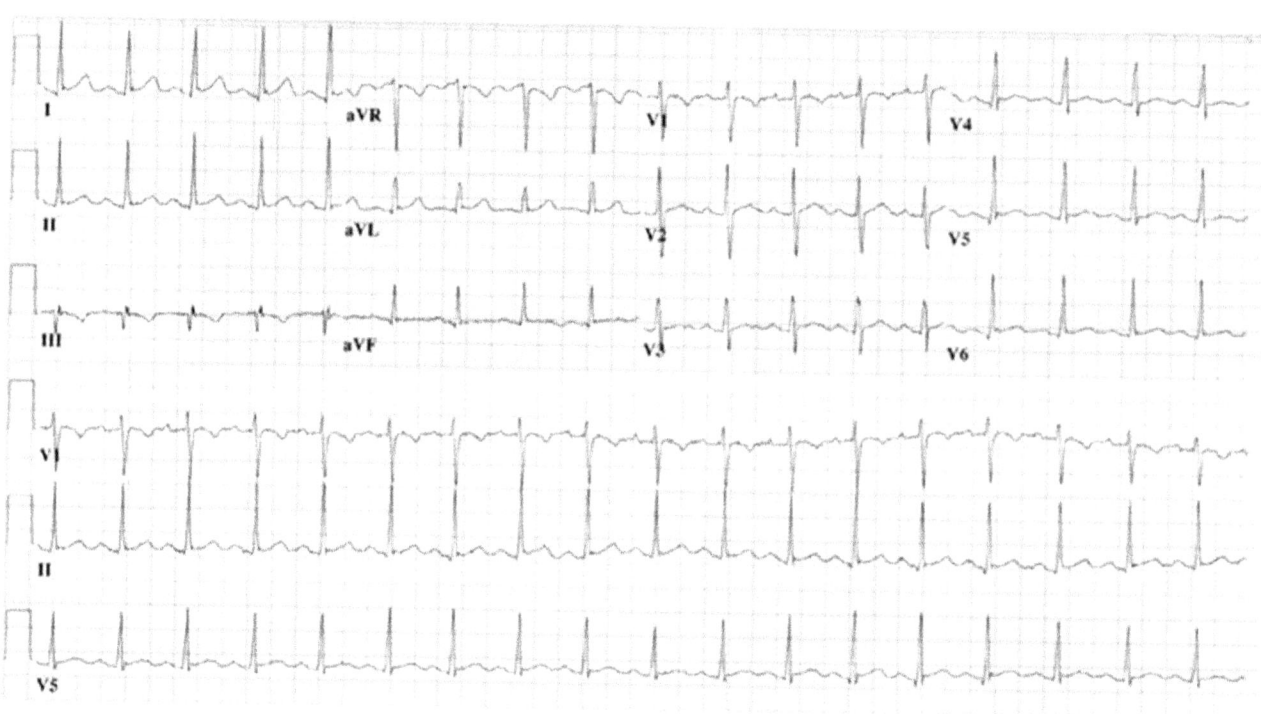

Figure 96.4

K. Action

a. Infuse O packed red blood cells 1 unit; awaiting 2 units crossmatched

   b. Imaging

i. Repeat FAST (Figure 96.1)

L. Nurse

a. Blood products given

   i. BP: 119/70, HR: 98, RR: 22, Sat: 98% (after 1 L isotonic solution or 1 unit pRBCs)

b. No blood or isotonic solution

   i. BP: 70/30, HR: 130, RR: 28, Sat: 96% on O_2

M. Action

a. Imaging
   i. CT head
   ii. CT cervical spine
   iii. CT chest/thoracic spine
   iv. CT abdomen/pelvis/lumbar spine

N. Results

Table 96.1 Results table

Test	Result	Test	Result
Complete blood count:		**Coagulation panel:**	
WBC	$5.3 \times 10^3/\mu L$	PT	12.6 sec
Hct	37.5%	PTT	26.0 sec
Plt	$350 \times 10^3/\mu L$	INR	1.0
Basic metabolic panel:		**Liver function panel:**	
Na	138 mEq/L	AST	23 U/L
K	4.3 mEq/L	ALT	26 U/L
Cl	105 mEq/L	Alk phos	42 U/L
CO_2	30 mEq/L	T bili	1.0 mg/dL
BUN	12 mEq/dL	D bili	0.3 mg/dL
Cr	1.1 mg/dL	Amylase	50 U/L
Gluc	100 mg/dL	Lipase	25 U/L

a. Lactate: 4.2 mmol/L
b. CT head (Figure 96.5): negative
c. CT cervical spine (Figure 96.6): negative
d. CT chest/thoracic spine (Figure 96.7): negative
e. CT abdomen/pelvis/lumbar spine (Figure 96.8): grade IV splenic laceration with rupture and retroperitoneal hemorrhage

Figure 96.5

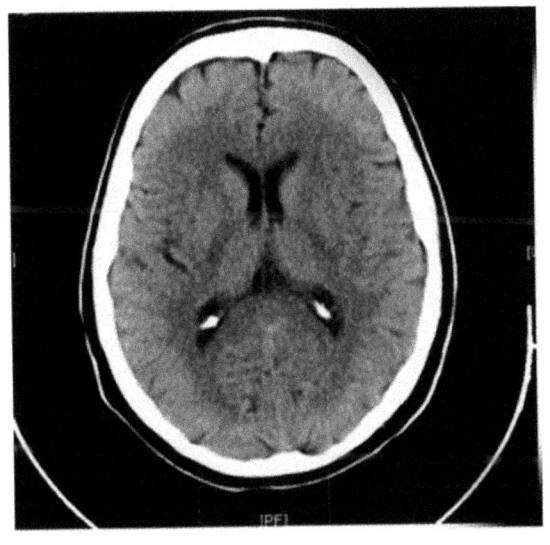

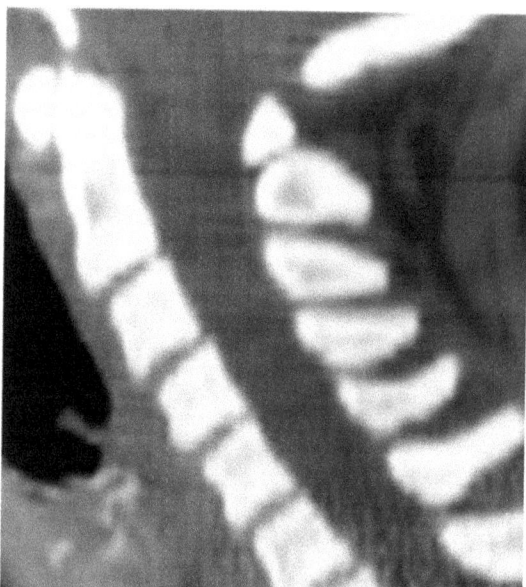

Figure 96.6

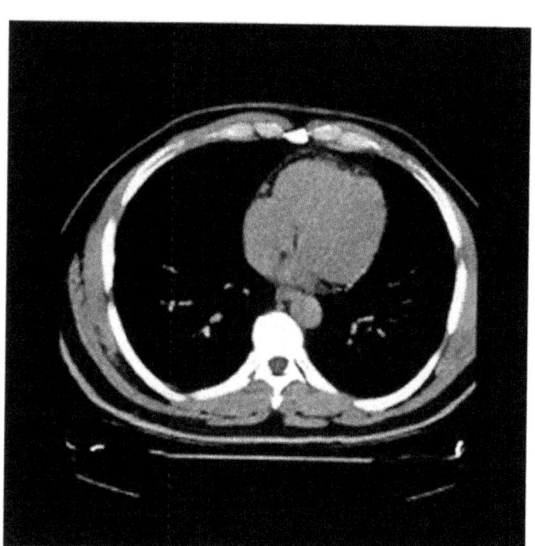

Figure 96.7

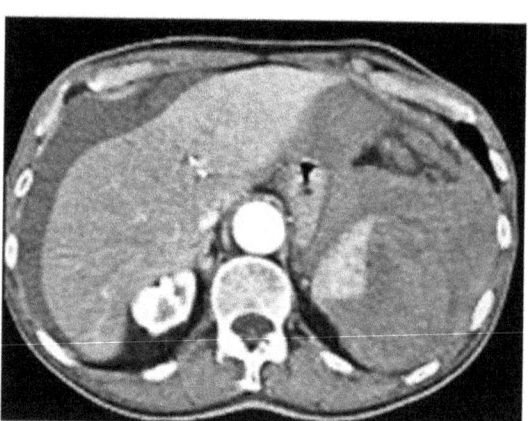

Figure 96.8

O. Nurse

a. Patient:
   i. Returns from radiology
   ii. BP: 83/54, HR: 132, RR: 22, Sat: 98%

P. Action

a. Discussion with trauma surgeon
   i. To operating room for laparotomy
b. Discussion with patient and family regarding need for emergent OR for hemostasis and splenectomy

Q. Diagnosis

a. Splenic rupture secondary to blunt abdominal trauma

R. Critical actions

a. Large-bore IV access
b. Blood type and crossmatch
c. Pain control
d. Trauma surgery or general surgery
e. FAST examination
f. Early pRBC transfusion or massive transfusion protocol in response to destabilization of vital signs
g. Advocate for laparotomy once the patient decompensates and diagnosis of splenic rupture is made

S. Examiner instructions

a. This is a case of splenic rupture from blunt abdominal trauma, an injury which can lead to significant bleeding when severe.
b. The patient's symptoms of abdominal pain, distention, hypotension, and tachycardia in the setting of a high-speed motor vehicle collision point to intra-abdominal injury with hemorrhage when other sources of bleeding (brain, chest, extremity) have been ruled out.
c. Important early actions include obtaining large-bore IV line access, administering initial IV fluid challenge, performing a FAST examination including thoracic views, early PRBC infusion once hemorrhage recognized, early trauma surgery involvement, pain control, and advocating for laparotomy given the patient decompensated twice with CT findings of splenic rupture.
d. If IV access is not obtained in a timely fashion, resuscitation will be slowed. If pain is not controlled, full evaluation of the patient's injuries will be difficult.

T. Pearls

a. Although protected under the bony ribcage, the spleen remains the most commonly affected organ in blunt injury to the abdomen in all age groups.
b. The spleen is a highly vascular organ that filters an estimated 10–15% of total blood volume every minute.
c. CT scanning has made conservative management more practical and safer for victims of splenic injury; however, unstable patients with presumed intraabdominal injury and clinical signs of hemorrhagic shock, including abdominal distension, peritoneal signs, and hypotension, require emergent operative intervention for hemostasis, especially high-risk patients such as those on anticoagulation.

d. The lethal triad of hypothermia, coagulopathy, and acidosis must be avoided with proper resuscitation to offer the patient the best chance of survival and minimal morbidity.

U. Figure legends

a. Figure 96.1 (a) (US) No free fluid in Morisson's pouch. (b) (US) No free fluid in splenorenal recess. (c) (US) No free fluid in pelvis. (d) (US) No pericardial effusion.
b. Figure 96.2 (CXR) Normal chest x-ray.
c. Figure 96.3 (X-ray) Normal pelvis x-ray.
d. Figure 96.4 (EKG) Sinus tachycardia; minimal voltage criteria for LVH.
e. Figure 96.5 (CT) Normal CT head.
f. Figure 96.6 (CT) Normal CT cervical spine.
g. Figure 96.7 (CT) Normal CT chest.
h. Figure 96.8 (CT) Splenic laceration with acute hemorrhage; perihepatic fluid suspicious for blood.

V. References

a. *Tintinalli's Emergency Medicine: A Comprehensive Study Guide* (9th ed.): Chapter 254, Trauma in Adults. Chapter 263, Abdominal Trauma.
b. *Rosen's Emergency Medicine: Concepts and Clinical Practice* (10th ed.): Chapter 32, Multiple Trauma. Chapter 38, Abdominal Trauma.

Hematochezia

Mariam Said, MD and Ram Parekh, MD

A. Chief complaint
a. 2-month-old male preterm infant brought in by parents for emesis and blood in diaper

B. Vital signs
a. BP: 50/27 (MAP 35), HR: 190, RR: 50, T: 36.0°C, Sat: 98% on RA, FS: 110 mg/dL, Wt: 3.5 kg

C. What does the patient look like?
a. Patient is a listless-appearing neonate with sunken eyes, intermittently crying without tear formation.

D. Primary survey
a. Airway: weak cry
b. Breathing: beginning to show signs of labored breathing and periodic apnea
c. Circulation: mucous membranes dry, no tears, thready brachial and femoral pulses, mottled skin, tachycardic

E. Action
a. Peripheral IV access, largest caliber possible
b. Labs
   i. CBC, BMP, LFT, coagulation studies, blood type and crossmatch
   ii. Lactate, blood cultures
   iii. Urine culture, CSF studies (baby is still less that 44 weeks corrected age, and full septic work-up would be indicated in this presentation)
c. 20 cc/kg NS bolus
d. Radiology
   Two-view abdominal x-ray (KUB and cross-table lateral or lateral decubitus)
e. Monitor: BP: 52/27 (MAP 35), HR: 192, RR: 44, T: 36.0°C, Sat: 99% on RA

F. History
a. HPI: A 2-month-old male neonate status post normal spontaneous vaginal delivery at 29 weeks' gestational age, with birth weight 975 g. He was recently discharged from the NICU, and presents with poor feeding and frequent emesis over the past 2 days. His NICU course was relatively unremarkable, and he was discharged home at 37 weeks corrected age in room air and taking full PO feeds with preterm infant formula. Mother reports the baby has had frequent small-volume emesis after feeds over the last 2 days, and has been more sleepy

than usual, not waking for feeds. This morning, she noticed bright red blood in the diaper, prompting her to bring him to the ED.

b. PMHx: 29-week preterm infant
c. PSHx: none
d. Allergies: none
e. Social: lives at home with mom and dad; no tobacco exposure
f. FHx: unremarkable

F. Nurse

a. 20 cc/kg NS bolus
   i. BP: 62/35 (MAP 44), HR: 170, RR: 45, Sat: 98%
b. No IV fluids
   i. BP: 50/30 (MAP 36), HR: 190, RR: 75, Sat: 98%

G. Secondary survey

a. General: awake, crying but lethargic, current weight 2175 g
b. HEENT: dry oral mucosa, sunken anterior fontanelle, sunken eyes
c. Neck: normal
d. Chest: shallow breathing, periodic apneas with associated bradycardia and desaturation
e. Heart: tachycardic, no murmurs
f. Abdomen: marked distension, diffusely tender, bowel sounds decreased, no masses, no hernias
g. Rectal: no anal fissures appreciated, stool positive for gross blood, yellow stool, hemoccult positive
h. Urogenital: normal, descended testes
i. Extremities: radial pulse rapid and weak, capillary refill 2 seconds
j. Back: normal
k. Neuro: lethargic, decreased responsiveness to examination
l. Skin: mottled, pale, delayed retraction on pinch

I. Action

a. Spinal tap, urine catheterization for culture, urinalysis
b. Meds
   i. Broad-spectrum antibiotics (Gram-negative, Gram-positive, and anaerobic coverage)
      1. Ampicillin, vancomycin
      2. Gentamicin, cefotaxime
      3. Piperacillin/Tazobactam
c. Reassess
   i. Neonate lethargic, less responsive
d. Consult
   i. Pediatric surgery
e. Imaging
   i. AP and cross-table lateral or left lateral decubitus x-ray

J. Nurse

a. BP: 62/35 (MAP 44), HR: 170, RR: 45, Sat: 98% (after 20 cc/kg bolus)
b. Patient: had brief period of bradycardia to 40 beats/minute

K. Results

Table 97.1 Results table

Test	Result	Test	Result
Complete blood count:		T bili	1.0 mg/dL
WBC	$12.1 \times 10^3/\mu L$	D bili	0.3 mg/dL
Diff	88.6/8.4/1.8	Amylase	50 U/L
Hct	31%	Lipase	25 U/L
Plt	$97 \times 10^3/\mu L$	Albumin	4.7 g/dL
Basic metabolic panel:		**Urinalysis:**	
Na	128 mEq/L	SG	1.020
K	4.3 mEq/L	pH	7
Cl	105 mEq/L	Prot	Neg
CO_2	15 mEq/dL	Gluc	Neg
BUN	22 mEq/dL	Ketones	+
Cr	0.8 mg/dL	Bili	Neg
Gluc	33 mg/dL	Blood	Neg
		LE	Neg
Coagulation panel:		Nitrite	Neg
PT	12.6 sec	Color	Yellow
PTT	66.0 sec		
INR	2.0	**Blood gas:**	
		pH	7.15
		pCO_2	66 mmHg
Liver function panel:		pO_2	88 mmHg
AST	23 U/L	HCO_3	16 mmol/L
ALT	26 U/L	BD	−10
Alk phos	42 U/L		

a. Lactate: 5 mmol/L
b. Abdominal x-ray (Figure 97.1)

L. Action
a. Pediatric surgery consult
   i. To admit for IV antibiotics and possible exploratory laparotomy OR
b. Discussion with family and PMD regarding need for admission for IV antibiotics, bowel rest with parenteral nutrition, and possible need for operative intervention

M. Diagnosis
a. Necrotizing enterocolitis

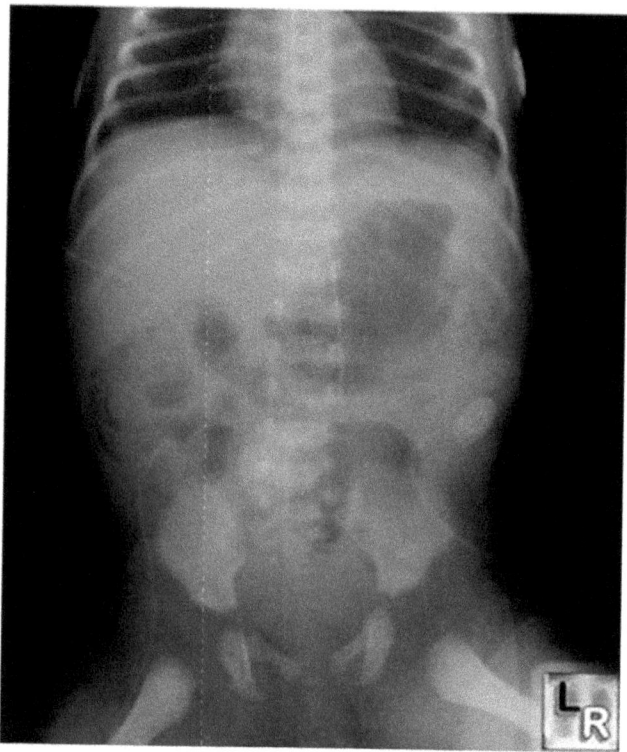

Figure 97.1

N. Critical actions

a. IV access and fluid bolus
b. Abdominal x-ray
c. Cultures/antibiotics for presumed sepsis
d. NPO and IV fluids
e. Place sump to low intermittent suction to decompress bowel
f. Pediatric surgery consult

O. Examiner instructions

a. This is a case of necrotizing enterocolitis (NEC), a serious condition characterized by intestinal inflammation, that in the most severe cases may lead to intestinal perforation, bowel necrosis, and/or death. This patient's presenting symptoms of poor feeding, emesis, lethargy, and bloody stools are concerning for sepsis. His physical exam findings of abdominal distension and tenderness accompanied by bloody stools point to an abdominal focus. Physical exam findings of weak pulses, shallow breathing, and delayed capillary refill are consistent with systemic illness. Vitals are notable for tachycardia, tachypnea, and hypotension, with apnea and bradycardia events. Laboratory findings are notable for leukopenia and thrombocytopenia, and prolonged coagulation studies are worrisome for sepsis with possible disseminated intravascular coagulation (DIC). Though the patient's symptoms appear indolent and mild initially, it is not uncommon for the condition to deteriorate rapidly, and progress to respiratory failure and shock. Care must be taken to initiate antibiotics and supportive care immediately, including respiratory support and volume resuscitation. Mainstays of therapy also include bowel rest, bowel decompression, and broad-spectrum antibiotics. The initial work up should include sepsis evaluation with blood, urine, and CSF cultures, as well as CBC, electrolytes, and blood gas. X-ray findings in this case include diffuse pneumatosis intestinalis and portal venous air. Pneumatosis intestinalis is pathognomonic for NEC. Pediatric surgery should be immediately consulted, with serial exams and x-rays to monitor for pneumoperitoneum.

P. Pearls
a. Blood in the diaper or stool can be a difficult complaint to evaluate in the ED. After the first few days of life, coagulopathies, NEC, anal fissures, allergic or infectious colitis, and congenital defects should be considered.
b. The pathogenesis of NEC remains incompletely understood, but is thought to be multifactorial in nature. It is characterized by inflammation of the intestine, and in severe cases may progress to a coagulation necrosis. There are many associations with NEC, including prematurity, intrauterine growth restriction, small for gestational age, infection, and hypoxic-ischemic insults. While NEC is a condition primarily afflicting preterm infants, up to 10% of cases may occur in term infants.
c. AP abdominal and cross-table lateral or left lateral decubitus x-ray are the mainstay of diagnostic imaging for pediatric abdominal complaints. Pneumatosis intestinalis is pathognomonic for NEC. Other findings may include bowel dilation, thickened bowel wall, ileus, portal venous air, and pneumoperitoneum.
d. Free air may be seen and is a surgical emergency. Initiate prompt antibiotics and fluids, along with other supportive care measures, and obtain surgical consultation.

Q. Figure legends
a. Figure 97.1 (X-ray) Dilated small bowel loops with pneumatosis

R. References
a. *Tintinalli's Emergency Medicine: A Comprehensive Study Guide* (9th ed.): Chapter 133, Acute Abdominal Pain in Infants and Children.
b. *Rosen's Emergency Medicine: Concepts and Clinical Practice* (10th ed.): Chapter 166, Pediatric Gastrointestinal Disorders.

Abdominal Pain

John Kiel, DO, MPH and Anita Vashi, MD

A. Chief complaint
a. 68-year-old male brought in by son with the complaint of worsening abdominal pain for the past 2 days

B. Vital signs
a. BP: 90/68, HR: 98, RR: 18, T: 39.2°C, Sat: 98% on RA, FS: 80 mg/dL

C. What does the patient look like?
a. Patient appearing uncomfortable secondary to pain in mild distress, lying still supine on stretcher.

D. Primary survey
a. Airway: speaking in full sentences
b. Breathing: no apparent respiratory distress, no cyanosis
c. Circulation: pale and cool skin, normal capillary refill

E. Action
a. Oxygen via NC or nonrebreather mask as needed to maintain saturation >95%
b. Two large-bore peripheral IV lines
c. 1 L NS bolus
d. Monitor: BP: 91/68, HR: 99, RR: 18, Sat: 100% on O_2
e. EKG or rhythm strip (Figure 98.1)

F. History
a. HPI: A 68-year-old male with a history of cirrhosis secondary to hepatitis C, esophageal varices, hypertension, and chronic renal insufficiency with the complaint of worsening abdominal pain over the past 2 days. Pain is constant, diffuse, and worse with movement. Symptoms are associated with fever and chills; denies nausea, vomiting, diarrhea, chest pain, or shortness of breath. Son notes patient seems more tired and slow to answer today compared to baseline.
b. PMHx: cirrhosis, hepatitis C, esophageal varices, hypertension, chronic renal insufficiency; denies any history of spontaneous bacterial peritonitis; has had paracentesis in past, last several months ago
c. PSHx: esophageal banding following an episode of upper gastrointestinal bleed several years ago
d. Allergies: none
e. Meds: noncompliant
f. Social: lives at home alone, alcohol use in the past (quit 10 years ago), ex-smoker (quit 5 years ago), remote history of IV drug use (1 year ago), not sexually active
g. FHx: no relevant history
h. PMD: Dr. Manoogian

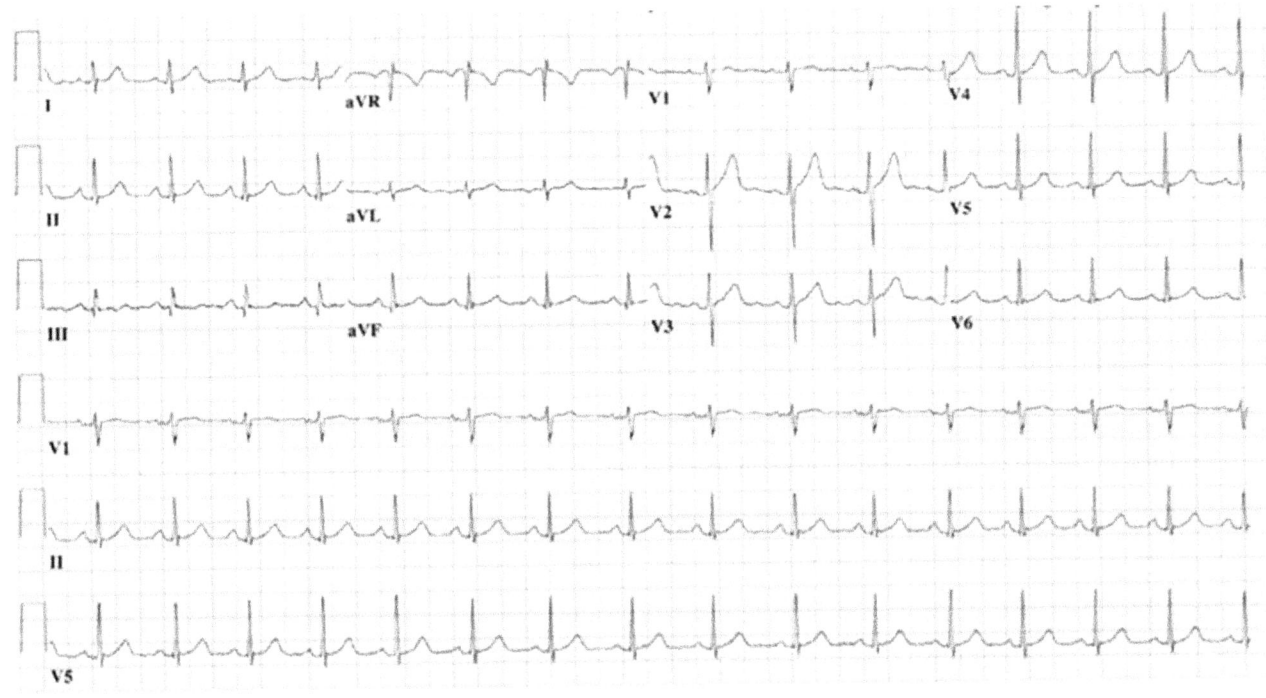

Figure 98.1

G. Nurse
a. EKG (Figure 98.1)
b. 1 L NS
   i. BP: 98/59, HR: 90, RR: 18, Sat: 98% on O_2
c. No fluids
   i. BP: 90/57, HR: 101, RR: 20, Sat: 98% on O_2

H. Secondary survey
a. General: alert, oriented × 3, comfortable
b. Head: mildly icteric conjunctivae, normocephalic, atraumatic
c. Eyes: extraocular movement intact, pupils equal, reactive to light
d. Ears: normal tympanic membranes
e. Nose: no discharge
f. Neck: full range of motion, no jugular vein distension, no stridor
g. Pharynx: normal dentition, no lesions, no swelling
h. Chest: nontender
i. Lungs: clear bilaterally
j. Heart: tachycardic rate, rhythm regular, no murmurs, rubs, or gallops
k. Abdomen: soft, distended, diffusely tender, with definite fluid wave and hepatosplenomegaly; no rebound, no guarding, no pulsatile masses, no hernias, bowel sounds normal
l. Rectal: normal tone, brown stool, occult blood negative
m. Urogenital: normal external genitalia
   i. Male: no discharge, normal testicular examination
n. Extremities: full range of motion, no deformity, normal pulses, 2+ pitting edema to knees
o. Back: nontender
p. Neuro: cranial nerves II to XII intact; normal sensation, strength; normal reflexes and gait, mild asterixis

   q. Skin: warm and dry, slightly jaundiced
   r. Lymph: no lymphadenopathy

I. Action

a. Procedures
   i. Bedside abdominal US (Figure 98.2)
   ii. Paracentesis
      1. Must send fluid for cell count, Gram stain, culture.
      2. Also helpful to check fluid protein, glucose, and LDH levels.
b. Blood cultures
c. Meds
   i. Cefotaxime or ceftriaxone
   ii. Morphine, fentanyl, or hydromorphone
d. Reassess
   i. Patient still with moderate discomfort

J. Nurse

a. BP: 98/59, HR: 90, RR: 18, Sat: 98% on O_2 (after 1 L fluids)
b. Patient: still with significant pain

A

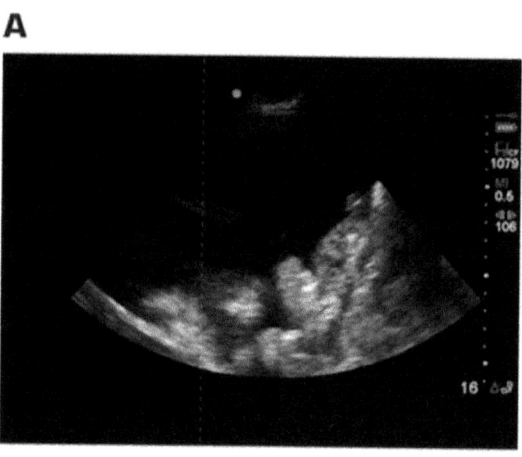

B

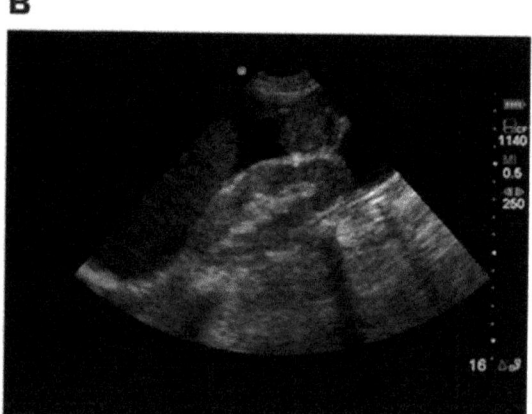

Figure 98.2

K. Results

Table 98.1 Results table

Test	Result	Test	Result
Complete blood count:		**Liver function panel:**	
WBC	$16.1 \times 10^3/\mu L$	AST	93 U/L
Diff	89.2/7.4/1.9	ALT	150 U/L
Hct	41.5%	Alk phos	153 U/L
Plt	$350 \times 10^3/\mu L$	T bili	4.3 mg/dL
		D bili	3.1 mg/dL
Basic metabolic panel:		Amylase	50 U/L
Na	138 mEq/L	Lipase	25 U/L

Table 98.1 (cont.)

Test	Result	Test	Result
K	4.3 mEq/L	Albumin	2.2 g/dL
Cl	105 mEq/L		
CO_2	30 mEq/L	**Urinalysis:**	
BUN	47 mEq/dL	SG	1.020
Cr	2.6 mg/dL	pH	7
Gluc	100 mg/dL	Prot	Neg
		Gluc	Neg
		Ketones	Neg
Coagulation panel:		Bili	+
PT	16.6 sec	Blood	Neg
PTT	26.0 sec	LE	Neg
INR	1.7	Nitrite	Neg
		Color	Yellow

a. Lactate: 2.2 mmol/L
b. Urine culture: in progress
c. Ascitic fluid: cloudy
   i. Cell count: 425 WBC, 90% PMNs
   ii. Albumin 0.5
   iii. Total protein 0.7
   iv. Gram stain/culture: pending
   v. Glucose: <50 mg/dL
   vi. LDH: elevated
d. Blood culture in progress
e. CXR (Figure 98.3)
f. Ammonia (if requested): 83

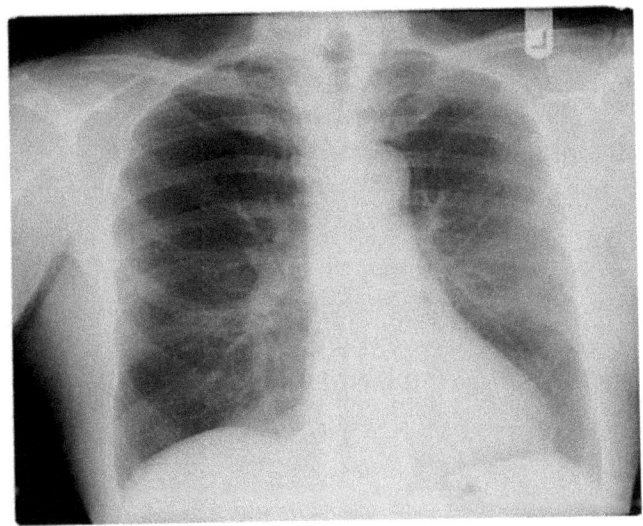

Figure 98.3

L. Action

a. IV fluid bolus – should receive total 20–30 cc/kg IV

b. Admit

c. Meds

    i. Morphine

    ii. Lactulose (optional)

M. Diagnosis

a. Spontaneous bacterial peritonitis

N. Critical actions

a. IV access and fluid bolus

b. Early paracentesis

c. Early antibiotics

d. Pain management

e. Admission to medical service

O. Examiner instructions

a. This is a case of spontaneous bacterial peritonitis (SBP) in a patient with cirrhosis. SBP is an isolated spontaneous infection of the abdominal fluid collection that often occurs in patients with end-stage liver disease. Critical early actions include initial resuscitation with IV fluids, pan-culturing, and most important, early antibiotics. If fluids and antibiotics are not given early, the patient's clinical course will deteriorate with a drop in blood pressure.

P. Pearls

a. Diagnosis of SBP requires paracentesis with a fluid polymorphonucleocyte count of greater than 250 cells/mm^3. Elevated protein, decreased glucose, and elevated LDH also support the diagnosis. However, when suspicion is high (unexplained fever, abdominal pain, or change in mental status) antibiotics should be started immediately after paracentesis, without waiting for results.

b. Fever is the most common presentation.

c. Findings of shock before antibiotic administration is an ominous sign.

d. The most frequent organism isolated in SBP is *Escherichia coli*, followed by streptococcal species.

e. Spontaneous peritonitis should be distinguished from secondary peritonitis.

Q. Figure legends

a. Figure 98.1 (EKG) Normal sinus rhythm.

b. Figure 98.2 (POCUS) Large hypoechoic fluid collection on abdominal ultrasound.

c. Figure 98.3 (CXR) No acute cardiopulmonary disease, no free air.

R. References

a. *Tintinalli's Emergency Medicine: A Comprehensive Study Guide* (9th ed.): Chapter 80, Hepatic Disorders, 3.

b. *Rosen's Emergency Medicine: Concepts and Clinical Practice* (10th ed.): Chapter 76, Liver and Biliary Tract Disorders.

Cough

Xiao Han, MD and Anita Vashi, MD

A. Chief complaint
a. 42-year-old male brought in by EMS with rapidly worsening cough and shortness of breath for the past 8 hours preceded by flu-like symptoms of fevers, cough, myalgia, and malaise over the past few days

B. Vital signs
a. BP: 90/50, HR: 107, RR: 34, T: 37.2°C, Sat: 85% on RA, FS: 90 mg/dL

C. What does the patient look like?
a. Patient appears stated age, diaphoretic, uncomfortable-appearing secondary to moderate respiratory distress.

D. Primary survey
a. Airway: speaking in full sentences
b. Breathing: tachypneic, mildly cyanotic
c. Circulation: pale, cool, diaphoretic skin, normal capillary refill

E. Action
a. Oxygen via NC or nonrebreather mask
b. Two large-bore peripheral IV lines
c. Labs
    i. CBC, BMP, LFT, BNP, troponin, VBG, lactate, coagulation studies, dimer, blood type and crossmatch
    ii. Blood cultures
d. 1 L NS bolus
e. Monitor: BP: 105/70, HR: 96, RR: 30, Sat: 90% on NRB
f. EKG
g. CXR

F. History
a. HPI: A 42-year-old male with no past medical history presents with 2 days of subjective fever and nonproductive cough, malaise, and myalgia. Today, the patient's symptoms worsened with additional shortness of breath. Patient denies chest pain, sore throat, abdominal pain, nausea, vomiting, diarrhea, urinary symptoms, or leg swelling. No sick contacts, no recent travel.
b. PMHx: none
c. PSHx: none

d. Allergies: none
e. Social: lives with wife at home. Works on a ranch taking care of cows (must inquire about nature of occupation), denies EtOH, smoking, drugs
f. FHx: no relevant history
g. PMD: Dr. Nicklaus

G. Nurse

a. EKG (Figure 99.1)

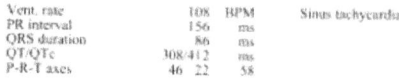

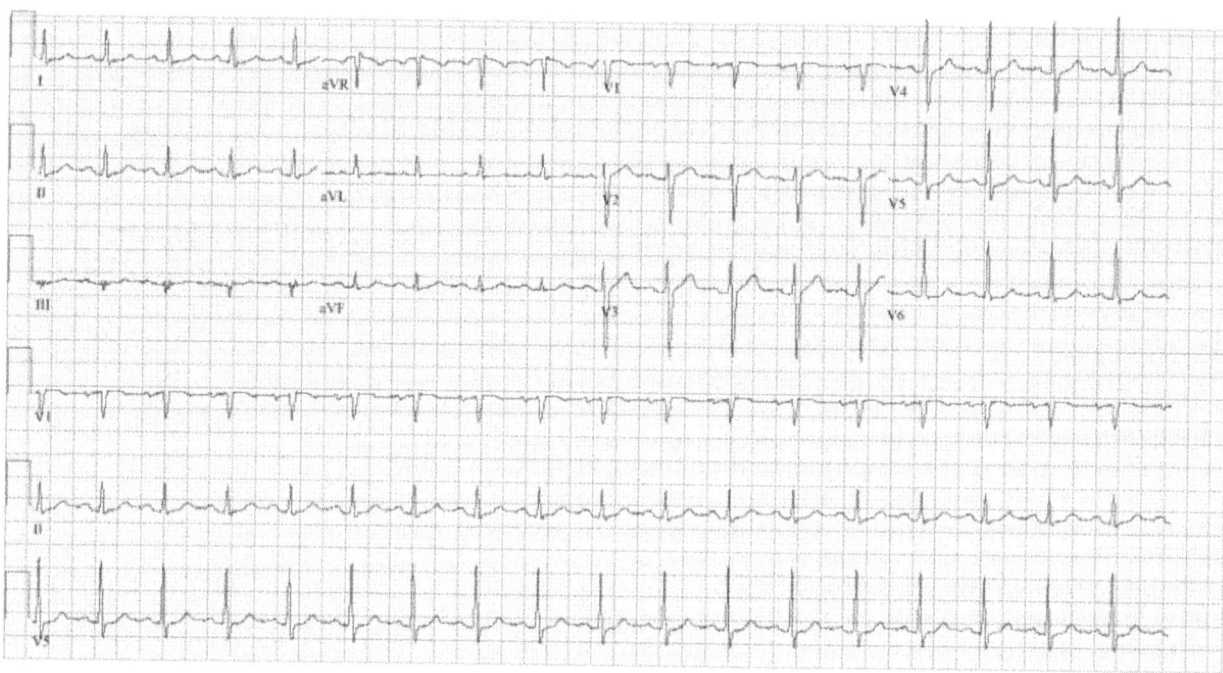

Figure 99.1

H. Secondary survey

a. General: alert, oriented × 3, moderate distress secondary to tachypnea
b. Head: normocephalic, atraumatic
c. Eyes: extraocular movement intact, pupils equal, reactive to light, conjunctiva – pink, sclera – anicteric (if asked)
d. Ears: normal tympanic membranes
e. Nose: no discharge
f. Neck: full range of motion, no jugular vein distension, no stridor
g. Pharynx: normal dentition, no lesions, no swelling
h. Chest: nontender
i. Lungs: scattered crackles at bilateral bases
j. Heart: tachycardia, regular rhythm, no murmurs, rubs, or gallops
k. Abdomen: normal bowel sounds, soft, nontender or distended
l. Extremities: full range of motion, no deformity, normal pulses, no leg swelling

m. Back: nontender
n. Neuro: cranial nerves II to XII intact; normal sensation, strength; normal reflexes and gait
o. Skin: pale, diaphoretic, no rashes, no open wound
p. Lymph: no lymphadenopathy

I. Action

a. Reassess
  i. Patient still looks uncomfortable and has difficulty breathing.

J. Nurse

a. BP: 110/79, HR: 120, RR: 38, Sat: 92% on O_2 (after 1 L)
b. Patient: notable increasing moderate to severe respiratory distress, no wheezing; patient appears to be tiring

K. Results

Table 99.1 Results table

Test	Result	Test	Result
Complete blood count:		T bili	1.0 mg/dL
WBC	13.0×10^3 /µL	D bili	0.3 mg/dL
Hct	41.5%	Amylase	50 U/L
Plt	350×10^3 /µL	Lipase	25 U/L
		Albumin	4.7 g/dL
Basic metabolic panel:			
Na	138 mEq/L	**Urinalysis:**	
K	4.3 mEq/L	SG	1.020
Cl	105 mEq/L	pH	7
CO_2	30 mEq/L	Prot	Neg
BUN	12 mEq/dL	Gluc	Neg
Cr	1.1 mg/dL	Ketones	Neg
Gluc	100 mg/dL	Bili	Neg
		Blood	Neg
Coagulation panel:		LE	Neg
PT	12.6 sec	Nitrite	Neg
PTT	26.0 sec	Color	Yellow
INR	1.0		
		Arterial blood gas:	
Liver function panel:		pH	7.50
AST	23 U/L	pO_2	66 mmHg
ALT	26 U/L	pCO_2	25 mmHg
Alk phos	42 U/L	HCO_3	22 mmol/L

a. Lactate: 4.5 mmol/L
b. Troponin: 0.02 ng/mL
c. BNP: 20 pg/mL
d. Dimer: 80 ng/mL
e. Portable CXR (Figure 99.2)

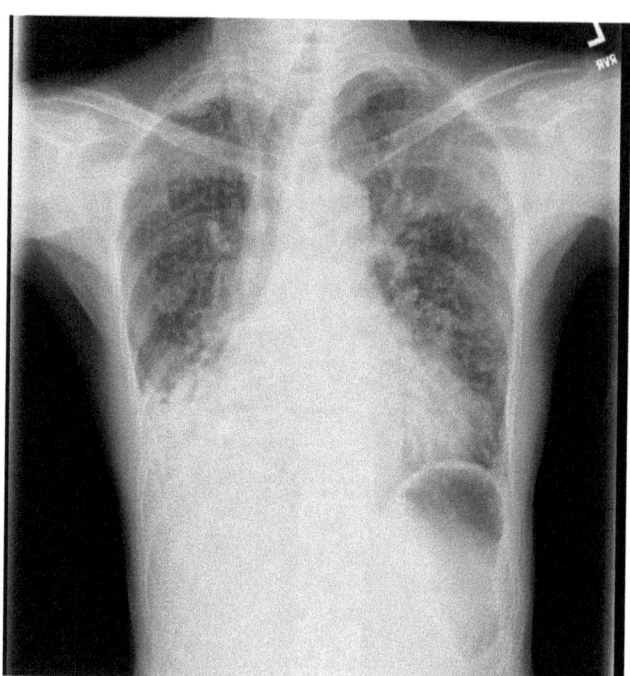

Figure 99.2

L. Action

a. Isolation
    i. Contact Centers for Disease Control
b. Intubation with rapid sequence intubation techniques
c. Admit to MICU for medical management
d. Meds
    i. Ciprofloxacin + clindamycin IV
    ii. Antitoxins (raxibacumab or obiltoxaximab)
e. Provision of ciprofloxacin to exposed health care providers and family members

M. Diagnosis

a. Pulmonary inhalation anthrax

N. Critical actions

a. Intubation
b. CXR
c. Early antibiotics
d. MICU admission
e. Isolation
f. Contact Centers for Disease Control
g. Prophylaxis for health care workers and family

O. Examiner instructions

a. This is a case of pulmonary anthrax from exposure to infected animal spores. Pulmonary anthrax is a fatal condition resulting in a severe hemorrhagic pneumonia. Important early actions include careful history, securing a definitive airway (especially when clinical picture worsens on NRB), obtaining blood cultures, recognizing pathognomonic CXR findings, administering high-dose penicillin, and medical ICU consult. If fluids are not administered, the patient's blood pressure will begin to drop. If airway is not secured, respiratory distress will worsen. A CXR can be readily obtained; if a CT scan is ordered, note that the scanner is busy, and it will "be a while" before the test can be performed. Once the diagnosis is realized by the candidate, they should isolate the patient with airborne precautions, give prophylaxis to health care workers and family, and contact the CDC.

P. Pearls

a. Manifestations of anthrax vary across cutaneous disease, pulmonary disease, and GI disease.
b. Transmission: exposure to spores from infected domestic and wild animals such as cattle, sheep, goats, or deer.
c. The course of inhalational anthrax can progress from initial nonspecific influenza-like symptoms to severe respiratory distress, hypotension, hypoxia, tachypnea, cyanosis, and hemorrhage within days.
d. Also check for signs of meningitis caused by anthrax, because the choice of antibiotics will change.
e. Pathognomonic CXR findings include mediastinal widening due to hemorrhagic mediastinitis, pleural effusion, and mediastinal lymphadenopathy. When diagnosis is suspected, CT of the chest is the test of choice.
f. Anthrax is highly susceptible to penicillin, amoxicillin, chloramphenicol, tetracycline, erythromycin, streptomycin, and ciprofloxacin. Anthrax is resistant to cephalosporins or trimethoprim–sulfamethoxazole.
g. ICU monitoring and care is necessary as inhalation anthrax progresses to septic and/or hemorrhagic shock.

Q. Figure legends

a. Figure 99.1 (EKG) Sinus tachycardia (copyright holder: Jacqueline Nemer).
b. Figure 99.2 (CXR) Mediastinal widening and pleural effusions (copyright holder: Jacqueline Nemer).

R. References

a. *Tintinalli's Emergency Medicine: A Comprehensive Study Guide* (9th ed.): Chapter 161, Zoonotic Infections.
b. *Rosen's Emergency Medicine: Concepts and Clinical Practice* (10th ed.): Chapter 15, Weapons of Mass Destruction.

Altered Mental Status

Nicole Munz, DO and Anita Vashi, MD

A. Chief complaint

a. 71-year-old male brought in by ambulance with wife for altered mental status and escalating headache for 7 hours

B. Vital signs

a. BP: 229/133, HR: 94, RR: 18, T: 36.9°C, Sat: 97% on RA, FS: 92 mg/dL

C. What does the patient look like?

a. Patient appears stated age, appears uncomfortable due to pain, lying supine on stretcher.

D. Primary survey

a. Airway: patent, speaking in full sentences
b. Breathing: unlabored, no apparent respiratory distress
c. Circulation: skin warm and dry, normal capillary refill

E. Action

a. Oxygen via NC or nonrebreather mask as needed to maintain saturation >95%
b. Two large-bore IV lines
c. Labs
   i. CBC, BMP, LFT, coagulation studies, blood type and hold, lactate, troponin, urinalysis
d. Monitor: BP: 232/128, HR: 92, RR: 18, T: 36.9°C, Sat: 99%
e. EKG

F. History

a. HPI: A 71-year-old male with a history of hypertension, coronary artery disease, and hypercholesterolemia who is complaining of a severe generalized headache that is associated with nausea, drowsiness, and difficulty concentrating for the past 7 hours. He describes a headache that was sudden in onset and increasing in intensity over the past few hours. Headache started at rest. He denies similar headaches in the past. He denies neck pain, fever, chills, sweats, photophobia, changes in vision or speech, or numbness of his face or extremities. He denies associated chest pain, shortness of breath, abdominal pain, vomiting, or diarrhea. Denies recent illness, travel, or trauma. Wife is at bedside and reports the patient has been confused since onset of headache.
b. PMHx: hypertension, hypercholesterolemia, coronary artery disease
c. PSHx: none
d. Allergies: none

e. Meds: patient cannot remember his meds, but wife provides a list – metoprolol, amlodipine, clonidine, hydrochlorothiazide, and simvastatin. Wife states they are visiting from out of town and patient has not taken his medications in 8 days because he forgot them at home (must ask about compliance).

f. Social: lives with wife at home, smokes one pack per day for 50 years, social drinker, denies drug use, sexually active only with wife

g. FHx: not relevant

h. PMD: Dr. Ray (who he sees annually)

G. Nurse

a. EKG (Figure 100.1)

b. Patient complaining of worsening headache and nausea. Wife concerned that patient is becoming more confused.

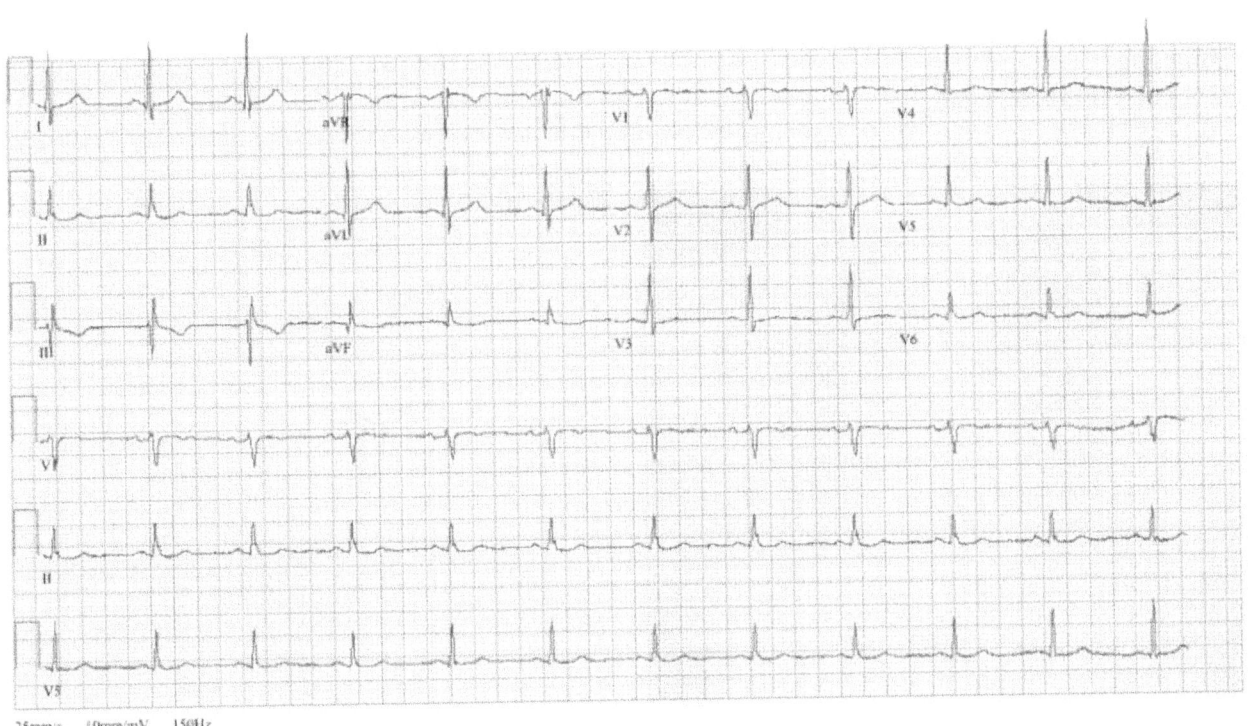

Figure 100.1

H. Secondary survey

a. General: alert and oriented × 1 (self), moderate distress due to pain

b. Head: normocephalic, atraumatic

c. Eyes: extraocular movements intact, pupils equal and reactive to light, unable to visualize fundus

d. Ears: normal tympanic membranes

e. Nose: normal

f. Pharynx: normal dentition, no lesions, no swelling
g. Neck: full range of motion, no tenderness, supple, no jugular venous distension
h. Lungs: clear bilaterally
i. Heart: regular rate and rhythm, no murmurs, rubs, or gallops
j. Abdomen: nontender, normal bowel sounds, no masses, no hernias, no rebound, no guarding
k. Rectal: hemoccult negative brown stool, normal rectal tone
l. Urogenital: normal
m. Extremities: full range of motion, no deformity, no edema, normal pulses
n. Back: normal
o. Neuro: cranial nerves II–XII intact, normal sensation and strength, normal reflexes and gait
p. Skin: warm and dry
q. Lymph: no lymphadenopathy

I. Action

a. Frequent BP checks and neurologic exam
b. Meds
    i. Antihypertensive: goal is for slow titratable medication to decrease blood pressure (i.e., labetalol IV). Nurse asks "What is the BP goal?" Should be 25% reduction of MAP.
    ii. Pain control
    iii. Antiemetic
c. Imaging
    i. CXR (Figure 100.2)
    ii. CT brain, noncontrast (Figure 100.3)

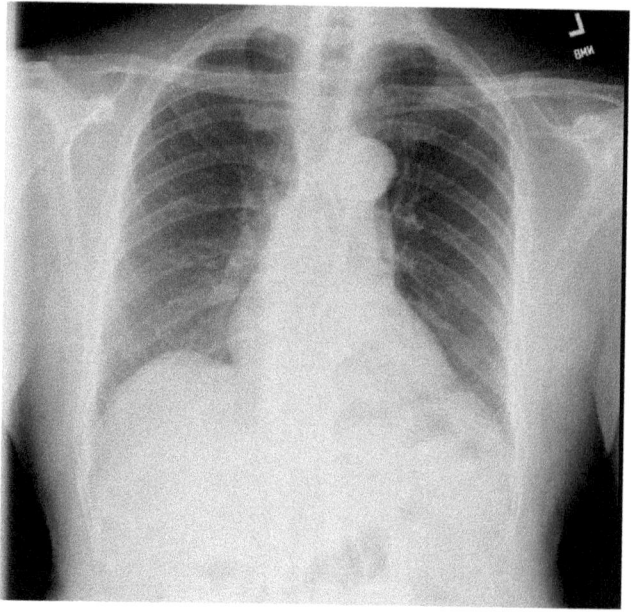

Figure 100.2

J. Nurse

a. If IV antihypertensives given
    i. BP: 185/92, HR: 70, RR: 18, Sat: 99% on RA
    ii. Patient has moderate improvement in symptoms
b. If IV antihypertensives not given
    i. BP: 245/122, HR: 90, RR: 18, Sat: 94% on RA
    ii. Patient has sudden decline in mental status, mumbling incoherently, and is responsive only to painful stimuli

Figure 100.3

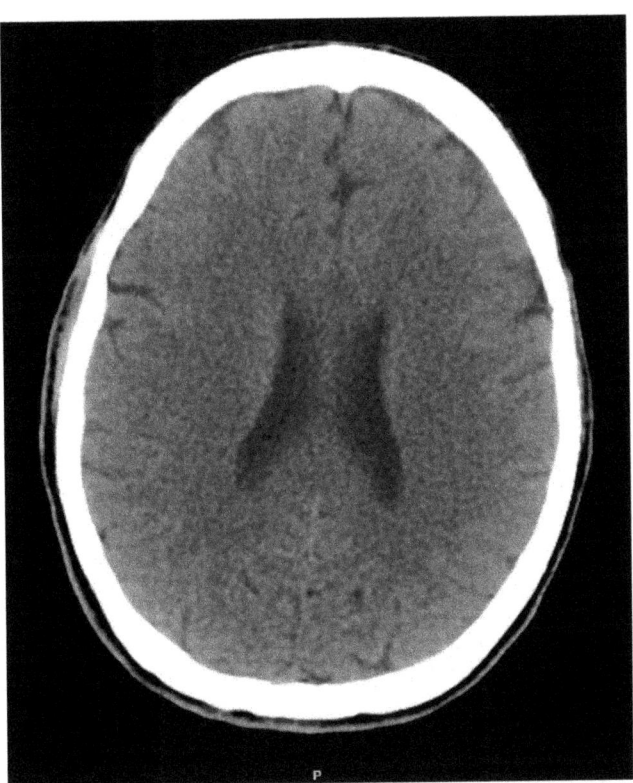

K. Results

Table **100.1** Results table

Test	Result	Test	Result
Complete blood count:		**Liver function panel:**	
WBC	$9.1 \times 10^3/\mu L$	AST	23 U/L
Hct	39.9%	ALT	19 U/L
Plt	$313 \times 10^3/\mu L$	Alk phos	47 U/L
		T bili	0.7 mg/dL
		D bili	0.1 mg/dL
Basic metabolic panel:		Amylase	40 U/L
Na	135 mEq/L	Lipase	22 U/L
K	4.4 mEq/L	Albumin	4.1 g/dL
Cl	108 mEq/L		
CO_2	30 mEq/L	**Urinalysis:**	
BUN	40 mEq/dL		
Cr	2.9 mg/dL	SG	1.020
Gluc	102 mg/dL	pH	7
		Prot	Neg
		Gluc	Neg
Coagulation panel:		Ketones	Neg
PT	13.1 sec	Bili	Neg
PTT	26 sec		

Table 100.1 (cont.)

Test	Result		Test	Result
INR	1.0		Blood	Neg
			LE	Neg
			Nitrite	Neg
			Color	Yellow

a. Lactate: 2.9 mmol/L
b. CXR (Figure 100.2)
c. CT brain (Figure 100.3)

L. Action

a. Lumbar puncture
    i. Results: RBC 0, WBC 0, glucose 45, protein 30, negative xanthochromia
b. Admit to monitored bed
c. Discussion with patient and wife regarding diagnosis and treatment plan

M. Diagnosis

a. Hypertensive emergency with hypertensive encephalopathy and acute kidney injury

N. Critical actions

a. IV antihypertensive medications (such as labetalol [20 mg IV q 10 minutes], nicardipine [5 to 15 mg/hr IV], or clevidipine [1 to 6 mg/hr IV])
b. Pain control
c. CT brain
d. Lumbar puncture after negative CT
e. Admission with telemetry

O. Examiner instructions

a. This is a case of hypertensive emergency with hypertensive encephalopathy and acute kidney injury in the setting of abrupt cessation of antihypertensive medications. Hypertensive emergency is an acute elevation of blood pressure (usually >180/110 mmHg) associated with end-organ injury (brain and kidney in this case). Hypertensive emergency can be present at lower blood pressures with hypertension-associated signs and symptoms. Critical early actions for this patient include frequent blood pressure monitoring and neurologic checks, administering IV antihypertensive medications, and evaluating for evidence of end-organ damage (EKG, CXR, labs, UA, and brain CT [given altered mental status]). If IV antihypertensive medications are not given early, the blood pressure will continue to increase and patient will have an acute deterioration in mental status.
The patient should have a lumbar puncture after the negative CT as subarachnoid and intracerebral hemorrhage are still within the differential. CT alone has adequate test characteristics to exclude subarachnoid hemorrhage within the first six hours of symptom onset, but sensitivity decreases after that and LP should be considered to effectively rule out the diagnosis.

P. Pearls

a. Treatment goal is to reduce mean arterial pressure (MAP) by a maximum of 20–25% in the first 1–2 hours and then, if clinically stable, reduce BP to 160/100 mmHg over the next 6–12 hours. (Notable exceptions: aortic dissection SBP goal 100–120 mmHg; neurocritical care patients may need higher MAP or SBP to maintain cerebral perfusion).

b. Aggressive reduction in blood pressure can lead to coronary, cerebral, or renal hypoperfusion.

c. Pharmacologic therapy should be used to provide a predictable, titratable, and transient effect on blood pressure. Commonly used medications include IV labetalol, esmolol, nicardipine, clevidipine, and nitroglycerin (for ACS and pulmonary edema).

d. If a patient presents with symptoms consistent with ischemic stroke, it is recommended to only treat BP if it exceeds 220/120 mmHg. In a patient *not* undergoing reperfusion therapy, treat with a goal to reduce BP by 10–15%. If patient is a candidate for reperfusion therapy, the BP should be lowered if it is above 185/110 mmHg.

e. SBP goal for subarachnoid hemorrhage is 140–160 mmHg and SBP goal for intracerebral hemorrhage is 140–180 mmHg based on patient's baseline BP and if there is evidence of increased ICP.

f. Headache alone is not evidence of end-organ damage or hypertensive emergency. However, headache is often present with hypertensive encephalopathy, subarachnoid hemorrhage, intracerebral hemorrhage, and posterior reversible encephalopathy syndrome (PRES).

g. Hypertensive emergency warrants medical admission with telemetry or ICU.

h. Management of "hypertensive urgency" differs from that of hypertensive emergency. Patients with elevated blood pressures but no symptoms and a normal physical examination may not require any specific work-up or treatment in the emergency department. Although there is increasing evidence that it is safe to discharge patients with asymptomatic hypertension, at the time of this writing the major EM texts still recommend EKG and laboratory evaluation but no mandate to rapidly lower the blood pressure. Patients with reliable follow-up can often be discharged home without any pharmacological intervention. If medication is used, oral antihypertensive medications are often sufficient.

Q. Figure legends

a. Figure 100.1 (EKG) Normal sinus rhythm; nonspecific lateral and inferior T wave changes.

b. Figure 100.2 (CXR) Normal chest x-ray.

c. Figure 100.3 (CT) Normal head CT.

R. References

a. *Tintinalli's Emergency Medicine: A Comprehensive Study Guide* (9th ed.): Chapter 57, Systemic Hypertension.

b. *Rosen's Emergency Medicine: Concepts and Clinical Practice* (10th ed.): Chapter 70, Hypertension.

Drowning

Anita Vashi, MD and Ariella Nadler MD

A. Chief complaint
a. 14-year-old girl brought in by EMS after falling into a partially frozen lake; required CPR on scene with return of spontaneous circulation; patient on backboard with C collar

B. Vital signs
a. BP: 72/43, HR: 42, RR: 10, T: 30.5°C, Sat: 97% on nonrebreather mask

C. What does the patient look like?
a. Patient appears wet, cold; not shivering; minimally responsive to sternal rub.

D. Primary survey
a. Airway: occasional groaning
b. Breathing: bradypneic, no cyanosis
c. Circulation: pale and cold skin
d. Disability: pupils 6 mm bilaterally and sluggish, no spontaneous movement
e. Exposure: removal of all clothes, no obvious injuries, deformities, bleeding, or bruising

E. Action
a. Intubation for airway protection using RSI and inline immobilization, warm humidified oxygen
b. Two large-bore peripheral IV lines
c. Warm blankets, external warmer
d. Labs
    i. Point of care glucose, VBG with lactate
    ii. CBC, BMP, LFT, coagulation studies, CK, blood type and crossmatch, alcohol level, acetaminophen level, salicylate level, urine toxicology screen, pregnancy test
e. 2 L warm (38–42°C) NS bolus
f. Monitor
g. Rectal temperature: 30°C
h. Temperature sensing Foley catheter (or temperature-sensing esophageal probe or rectal probe that reads temperatures <30°C, inserted to 15 cm)
i. EKG
j. POCUS eFAST: no free fluid identified in Morison's pouch, in the pelvis, in the perisplenic space, or in the pericardial sac. Cardiac motion identified. No pneumothorax identified.
k. Initial imaging

l. CXR

m. Cautious handling of patient to minimize movement

F. History

a. HPI: A 14-year-old girl with no past medical history was ice skating on a frozen pond when she suddenly fell through the ice and into the water. She remained submerged for ~8 minutes while a friend called EMS. On arrival to the scene, the patient had no detectable pulses. Compressions were started, pulse was quickly regained, and the patient was brought to the ED with a 5-minute transport time. The patient grimacing but not speaking or spontaneously moving extremities.

b. PMHx: none

c. PSHx: none

d. Allergies: none

e. Meds: none

f. Social: according to her friend, she lives with family at home, denies EtOH, smoking, or drug use, not sexually active

g. FHx: not relevant

h. PMD: Dr. Silverstein

G. Nurse

a. EKG (Figure 101.1)

b. After intubation:
    i. BP: 98/59, HR: 45, RR: 18, Sat: 98% on mechanical ventilation

c. If not intubated
    i. BP: 90/55, HR: 38, RR: 10, Sat: 85% on nonrebreather O_2
    ii. Will need intubation

d. CXR (Figure 101.2)

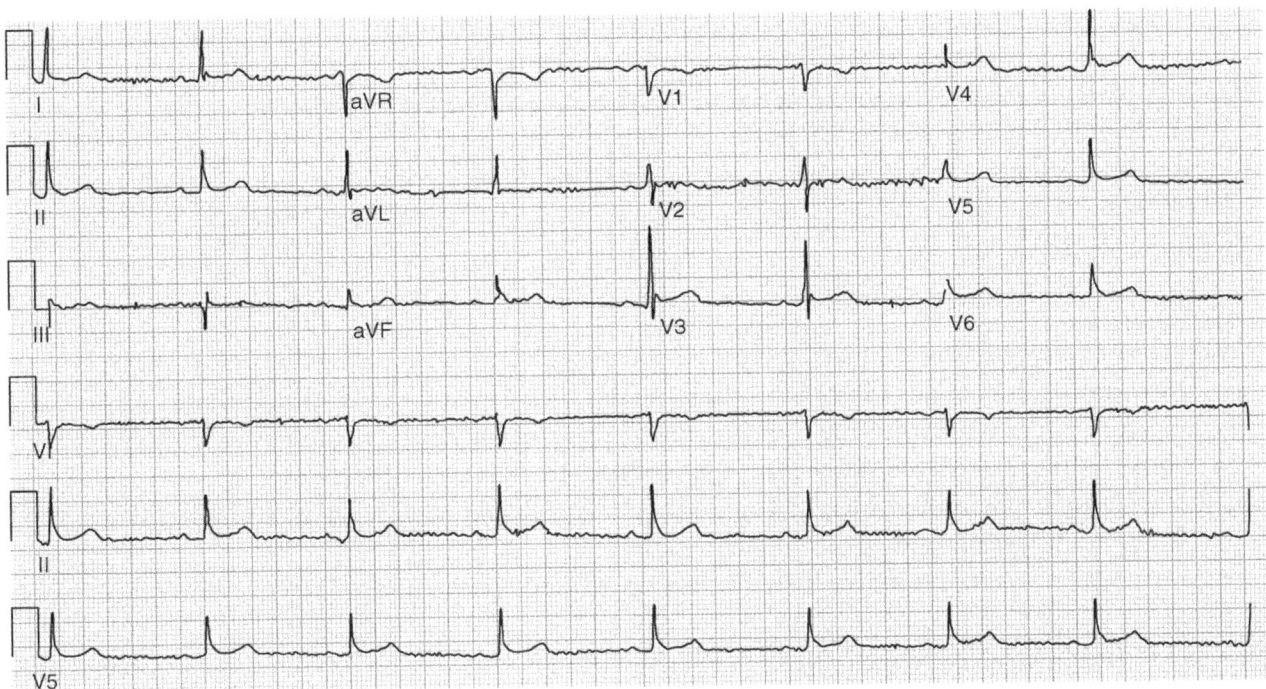

Figure 101.1

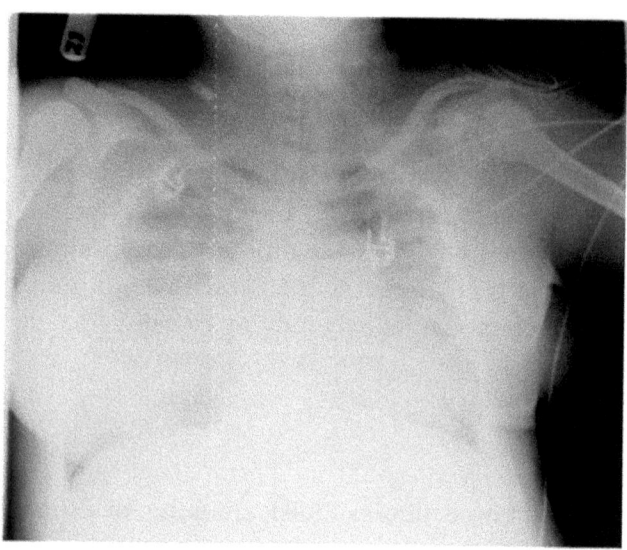

Figure 101.2

H. Secondary survey
a. General: alert and oriented × 0, intubated, no spontaneous movement
b. Head: normocephalic, atraumatic
c. Eyes: pupils 6 mm bilaterally and sluggish
d. Ears: normal tympanic membranes, no hemotympanum
e. Nose: no discharge
f. Neck: C collar in place, no obvious signs of trauma
g. Pharynx: normal dentition, no lesions, no swelling
h. Chest: nontender
i. Lungs: bilateral coarse breath sounds
j. Heart: bradycardic rate, rhythm regular, no murmurs, rubs, or gallops
k. Abdomen: decreased bowel sounds, soft, nontender, nondistended
l. Rectal: diminished tone, brown stool, occult blood negative
m. Extremities: full range of passive motion, no deformity, peripheral cyanosis
n. Back: no spinal tenderness, no stepoffs
o. Neuro: no spontaneous movements, hypoactive reflexes
p. Skin: pale, cool
q. Lymph: no lymphadenopathy

I. Action
a. Rewarming intervention
    i. Rewarming device (i.e., forced air warming device), warm IV fluids, warm humidified oxygen. Focus on rewarming the core, avoid rewarming the extremities while leaving the trunk exposed and cold when doing procedures or exam.
    ii. Nasogastric tube and urinary catheter placement. Consider infusion of warmed saline.
    iii. Consider warm pleural or peritoneal lavage.
    iv. If dialysis or cardiopulmonary bypass requested, unavailable at this time.
b. Reassess
    i. If warming intervention taken, temperature improves to 33°C (by internal sensing device).
    ii. If no warming intervention taken, patient's cardiac rhythm changes to ventricular fibrillation that does not respond to medications and/or defibrillation.
c. Pediatric ICU admission

d. Imaging
    i. C-spine x-ray or CT c-spine (Figure 101.3)
    ii. Head CT (Figure 101.4)

J. Nurse
a. BP: 98/59, HR: 65, RR: 18, Sat: 98% on mechanical ventilation
b. Patient: intubated, no spontaneous movement

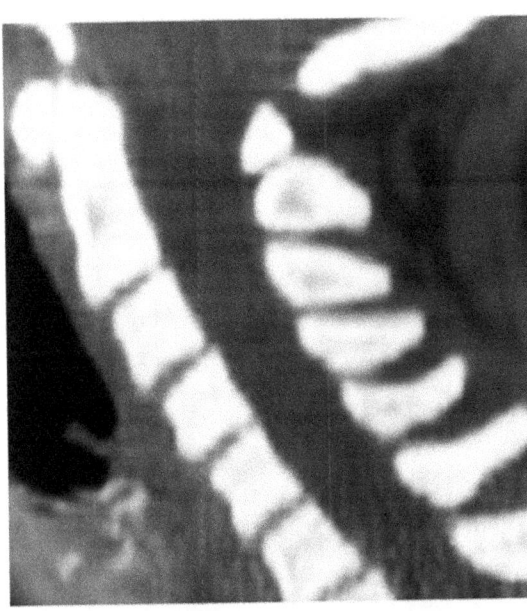

Figure 101.3

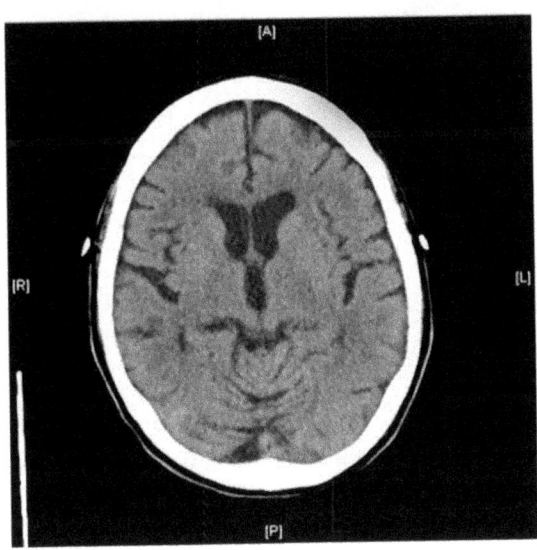

Figure 101.4

K Results

Table 101.1 Results table

Test	Result	Test	Result
Complete blood count:		D bili	0.3 mg/dL
WBC	$5.3 \times 10^3/\mu L$	Amylase	50 U/L
Hct	46.5%	Lipase	25 U/L
Plt	$350 \times 10^3/\mu L$	Albumin	4.7 g/dL
		CK	200 U/L
Basic metabolic panel:			
Na	138 mEq/L	**Urinalysis:**	
K	4.3 mEq/L	SG	1.005
Cl	105 mEq/L	pH	7
CO_2	20 mEq/L	Prot	Neg
BUN	12 mEq/dL	Gluc	Neg
Cr	0.6 mg/dL	Ketones	Neg
Gluc	120 mg/dL	Bili	Neg
		Blood	Neg
Coagulation panel:		LE	Neg
PT	12.6 sec	Nitrite	Neg
PTT	26.0 sec	Color	Clear
INR	1.0		
		Arterial blood gas (pre-intubation):	
Liver function panel:		pH	7.24
AST	23 U/L	pO_2	62
ALT	26 U/L	pCO_2	48
Alk phos	42 U/L	HCO_3	22
T bili	1.0 mg/dL		

a. FS: 125 mg/dL
b. Lactate: 5.2 mmol/L
c. CT head (Figure 101.4)
d. CT c-spine (Figure 101.3)
e. EtOH, aspirin, and acetaminophen levels, urine toxicology, urine pregnancy negative

L. Action

a. Continue rewarming

M. Diagnosis

a. Hypothermia secondary to cold-water immersion

N. Critical actions

a. Airway management
b. Undressing patient and assessing for any signs of trauma
c. Temperature monitoring via internal probe (esophageal, Foley, or rectal)
d. Point of care glucose
e. Aggressive rewarming
f. PICU admission

O. Examiner instructions

a. This is a case of hypothermia secondary to cold-water immersion. The patient was initially found in cardiac arrest due to hypothermia from extremely cold water or secondary to lack of oxygen supply to the brain, but was revived with CPR. It is critical to recognize the potential for hypothermia in cold-water immersion cases. Aggressive rewarming is vital. It is also important to intubate early for airway protection. Critical early actions include airway management, complete undressing of the patient, evaluating the patient for any associated trauma, placement of internal temperature-sensing device for constant temperature monitoring, and aggressive rewarming techniques, with a focus on rewarming the core. Because the circumstances are unclear, the candidate should consider potential head and neck injury.

P. Pearls

a. All near-drowning victims should be assessed for associated trauma.
b. In hypothermic patients, internal temperature-sensing devices such as rectal, esophageal, or bladder probes should be used for constant and accurate temperature monitoring.
c. Moderate hypothermia (between 28°C and 32°C) can present with loss of the shivering reflex, mild alteration in consciousness, bradycardia, and atrial fibrillation.
d. Patients with severe hypothermia (temperature below 28°C) can present with fixed, dilated pupils, diminished reflexes, coma, ventricular fibrillation, and/or asystole. The patient should be carefully handled to minimize movements that may lead to lethal arrhythmias.
e. Remember, no one is dead until they are "warm and dead."
f. An Osborne wave, or up-slurring of the QRS–ST junction, is the classic EKG finding for hypothermia (usually at temperatures <32°C).
g. Attempts at defibrillation are usually unsuccessful at temperatures below 28°C.
h. Vasopressors are usually not indicated in early resuscitation as hypothermia provides maximal vasoconstriction and vasopressors may increase the risk of arrhythmia.
i. Rewarming extremities prior to rewarming the core can lead to afterdrop, a decrease in core temperature after removal from the cold.
j. Rapid rewarming can cause lethal arrhythmias in hypothermic patients. Core rewarming (dialysis, cardiopulmonary bypass, thoracic and peritoneal cavity lavage) should be reserved for patients with severe cardiovascular instability (cardiac arrest, ventricular fibrillation). In milder cases of hypothermia, warm blankets, forced air blankets (such as a forced air warming device), warm humidified oxygen, and warm fluids are usually sufficient to safely rewarm the patient.
k. Initial CXR may grossly underestimate extent of pulmonary damage in near-drowning cases.
l. Antibiotics can be given on a case-by-case basis. Consider coverage if submersion occurs in grossly contaminated water or if aspiration is a concern.

Q. Figure legends

a. Figure 101.1 EKG with sinus bradycardia.
b. Figure 101.2 Chest x-ray with diffuse pulmonary edema.
c. Figure 101.3 Normal C-spine x-ray.
d. Figure 101.4 Normal CT head.

R. References

a. *Tintinalli's Emergency Medicine: A Comprehensive Study Guide* (9th ed.): Chapter 209, Hypothermia. Chapter 215, Drowning.
b. *Rosen's Emergency Medicine: Concepts and Clinical Practice* (10th ed.): Chapter 128, Hypothermia, Frostbite, and Nonfreezing Cold Injuries. Chapter 133, Drowning.

Pallor

Evelyn Chow, MD, Carrie Ng, MD, and Keegan Tupchong, MD

A. Chief complaint
a. 17-day-old male brought in by his mother for poor feeding and looking pale

B. Vital signs
a. BP: 100/80, HR 175, RR: 65, T: 37.1°C, Sat: 100% on RA (BP and pulse oximetry from right arm – only disclose this information if asked for)

C. What does the patient look like?
a. Tachypneic, pale, and lethargic infant being held by mother.

D. Primary survey
a. Airway: patent
b. Breathing: tachypneic, mild subcostal retractions, with crackles bilaterally, no cyanosis
c. Circulation: cool upper extremities and lower extremities with delayed capillary refill and thready pulses throughout

E. Action
a. Oxygen supplementation (nonrebreather)
b. Peripheral IV line placement
c. Labs: CBC, CMP, VBG, PT/PTT, type and screen, urinalysis
d. Check BP and pulse oximetry in all four extremities (lower extremities: BP 72/50, Sat 93%)
e. Cardiac monitor and EKG

F. History
a. HPI: A 14-day-old male, full term, normal spontaneous vaginal delivery without complications, presents with lethargy. Mother states that he has had poor feeding and becomes sweaty and starts to breath fast when he feeds. Otherwise, no fever, cough, or other URI symptoms; no vomiting or diarrhea; no change in the number of wet diapers.
b. PMHx: normal spontaneous vaginal delivery at 39 weeks, no complications
c. PSHx: none
d. Allergies: none
e. Meds: none
f. Social: lives at home with family
g. FHx: noncontributory
h. PMD: Dr. Han

G. Nurse

a. Repeat vital signs (unless prostaglandin E1 infusion is initiated)
   i. BP: 92/60 (upper extremities), BP 66/44 (lower extremities – do not give this unless specifically asked for), HR: 195, RR: 83, Sat: 100% (upper extremities), 93% (lower extremities)

b. EKG (Figure 102.1)

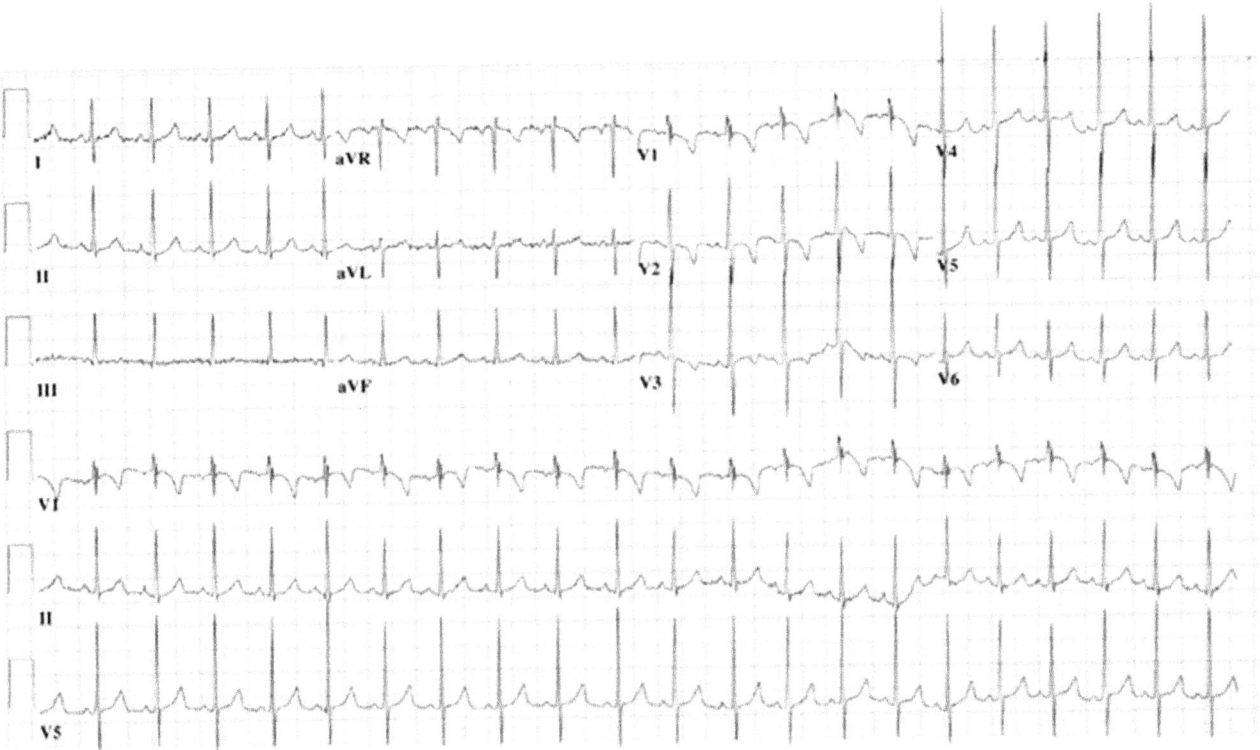

Figure 102.1

H. Secondary survey

a. General: lethargic but arousable, tachypneic
b. Head: anterior fontanelle flat, atraumatic
c. Eyes: pupils equal, reactive to light
d. Ears: normal tympanic membranes
e. Nose: no discharge
f. Neck: full range of motion, no stridor
g. Pharynx: no lesions, no swelling
h. Chest: nontender
i. Lungs: tachypneic, crackles bilaterally
j. Heart: tachycardic, rhythm regular, no murmur
k. Abdomen: normal bowel sounds, soft, nontender, nondistended
l. Rectal: brown stool, occult blood negative
m. Urogenital: normal external genitalia, no discharge, normal testicular examination
n. Extremities: cold, delayed capillary refill
o. Back: nontender

p. Neuro: minimally responsive
q. Skin: cold extremities, no rashes
r. Lymph: no lymphadenopathy

I. Action

a. Meds
   i. Prostaglandin E1 (alprostadil) IV infusion
   ii. Can start inotropic support (e.g., dobutamine) to improve contractility in patients with heart failure
b. Reassess
   i. Patient starts to improve a few minutes after starting prostaglandin E1
c. Consult
   i. Pediatric cardiology
d. Imaging
   i. CXR

J. Nurse

a. Prostaglandin E1 started
   i. HR: 141, RR: 48, Sat: 100% (all extremities regardless of oxygen supplementation)
b. No prostaglandin E1 started
   i. HR: 210, RR: 90, Sat: 100% (upper extremities), 93% (lower extremities) regardless of oxygen. Patient then develops pulseless electrical activity

K. Results

Table 102.1 Results table

Test	Result	Test	Result
Complete blood count:		T bili	1.0 mg/dL
WBC	$10.2 \times 10^3/\mu L$	D bili	0.3 mg/dL
Hct	51%	Amylase	50 U/L
Plt	$133 \times 10^3/\mu L$	Lipase	25/U/L
		Albumin	4.7 g/dL
Basic metabolic panel:			
Na	138 mEq/L	**Urinalysis:**	
K	4.3 mEq/L	SG	1.0.20
Cl	100 mEq/L	pH	7
CO_2	14 mEq/L	Prot	Neg
BUN	9 mEq/dL	Gluc	Neg
Cr	0.6 mg/dL	Ketones	Neg
Gluc	70 mg/dL	Bili	Neg
Lactate	4.5 mg/dL	Blood	Neg
		LE	Neg

Table 102.1 (cont.)

Test	Result	Test	Result
Coagulation panel:		Nitrite	Neg
PT	12 sec	Color	Yellow
PTT	26 sec		
INR	1.0	**Arterial blood gas:**	
		pH	7.30
Liver function panel:		pO_2	146
AST	23 U/L	pCO_2	30
ALT	26 U/L	HCO_3	35
Alk phos	42 U/L		

a. CXR (Figure 102.2)

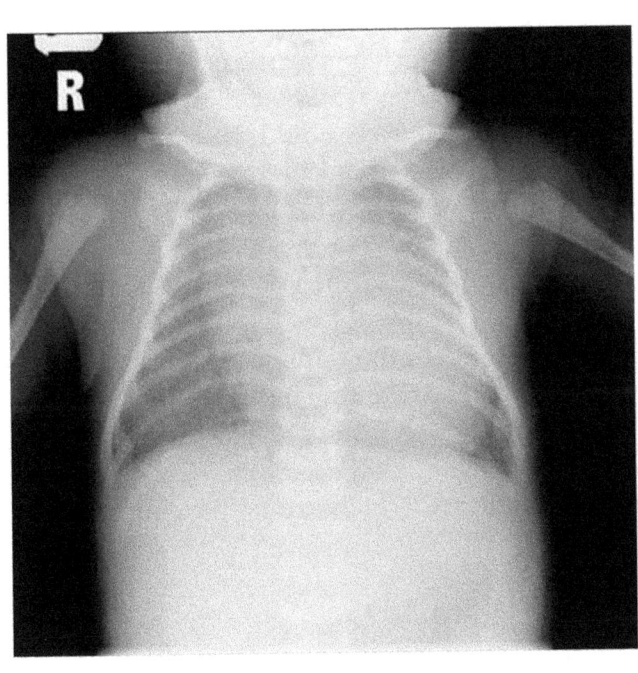

Figure 102.2

L. Action
a. Pediatric cardiology performs bedside echocardiogram, which confirms coarctation of the aorta.
b. Consult cardiothoracic surgery.
c. Discussion with parents regarding need for admission and surgical correction of the coarctation.

M. Diagnosis
a. Aortic coarctation

N. Critical actions
a. Check blood pressure and pulse oximetry in all extremities

b. Prostaglandin E1

c. Cardiology consult for emergent echocardiogram

O. Examiner instructions

a. This is a case of congenital critical coarctation of the aorta. This is a condition where there is discrete narrowing of the thoracic aorta usually distal to the left subclavian artery, near the insertion of the ductus arteriosus. This results in decreased blood flow to the lower body. Neonates try to increase systolic blood pressure proximal to the aorta to overcome the increased afterload from the outflow tract obstruction, leading to symptoms of heart failure. In this patient, the symptoms become more prominent in the second week of life as the ductus arteriosus closes. Stress, such as feeding, exacerbates the symptoms. Important early actions include checking the blood pressure in all extremities, recognizing shock, obtaining a chest x-ray, cardiology consultation, and prostaglandin E1 initiation. The chest x-ray will likely show cardiomegaly, hinting at congenital heart disease. Prostaglandin E1 is given to maintain patency of the ductus arteriosus. If prostaglandin E1 is not given, the patient will deteriorate. Labs generally are not helpful in the diagnosis of aortic coarctation. They may show a primary metabolic acidosis from shock. An echocardiogram should be obtained to definitively diagnose the coarctation. Importantly, this presentation may appear similar to a case of sepsis and the candidate should not be penalized for obtaining blood cultures or starting antibiotics. However, it is critical to check blood pressures and pulse oximetry readings in all extremities, note the upper and lower differential, and initiate prostaglandin E1. Should the candidate repeatedly fluid resuscitate this patient, then respiratory failure will occur.

P. Pearls

a. Dyspnea or diaphoresis during feeding can be a sign of heart failure due to a congenital heart defect.

b. Classic clinical findings in aortic coarctation are hypertension in the upper extremities (normally the blood pressure is 10 mmHg higher in the upper extremities) and diminished pulses in the lower extremities. They typically present with heart failure and shock (not cyanosis) when the PDA closes.

c. Prostaglandin E1 prevents closure of a patent ductus arteriosus, which can help stabilize the patient until definitive surgical repair can be performed.

Q. Figure legends

a. Figure 102.1 (EKG) Normal sinus rhythm; right ventricular hypertrophy.

b. Figure 102.2 (CXR) Cardiomegaly with pulmonary edema.

R. References

a. *Tintinalli's Emergency Medicine: A Comprehensive Study Guide* (9th ed.): Chapter 129, Congenital and Acquired Pediatric Heart Disease.

b. *Rosen's Emergency Medicine: Concepts and Clinical Practice* (10th ed.): Chapter 165, Pediatric Cardiac Disorders.

Diarrhea

Rijo Maracheril, MD

A. Chief complaint

a. 45 year-old male with bloody diarrhea

B. Vital signs

a. BP: 102/72, HR: 96, RR: 12, T: 37.5°C, Sat: 100% on RA

C. What does the patient look like?

a. Patient appears comfortable, lying supine on stretcher.

D. Primary survey

a. Airway: speaking in full sentences
b. Breathing: no respiratory distress, no cyanosis
c. Circulation: warm skin, normal capillary refill

E. Action

a. Peripheral IV access
b. Labs
  i. VBG with lactate, CBC, BMP, PT/PTT/INR, urinalysis
c. Monitor: BP: 102/68, HR: 106, RR: 14, T: 37.5°C, Sat: 100% on RA

F. History

a. HPI: A 45-year-old male with a history of hypertension complaining of diarrhea for the past 5 days. He notes 8–10 episodes per day, first watery, now bloody for the past day, and associated with mild lower abdominal pain and cramping, fever, chills, and malaise. Patient denies nausea, vomiting, hematuria; denies recent travel or antibiotic use. Patient lives alone, no known sick contacts.
b. PMHx: hypertension
c. PSHx: appendectomy
d. Allergies: none
e. Meds: amlodipine 5 mg daily
f. Social: lives alone, denies alcohol, smoking, or drug use, not sexually active for 5 years
g. FHx: not relevant
h. PMD: none

G. Nurse

a. If no fluids given
  i. BP: 100/68, HR: 111, RR: 14: Sat: 100%

b. If 1 L NS
   i. BP: 112/62, HR: 88, RR: 12, Sat: 100%

H. Secondary survey
a. General: alert, oriented × 3, comfortable
b. Head: normocephalic, atraumatic
c. Eyes: extraocular movement intact, pupils equal, reactive to light
d. Ears: normal tympanic membranes
e. Nose: no discharge
f. Neck: full range of motion, no jugular vein distension, no stridor
g. Pharynx: normal dentition, no lesions, no swelling, dry lips and mucosa (must ask)
h. Chest: nontender
i. Lungs: clear bilaterally
j. Heart: rate and rhythm regular, no murmurs, rubs, or gallops
k. Abdomen: hyperactive bowel sounds, mild diffuse tenderness, nondistended, no masses or organomegaly, no rebound or guarding (negative Murphy's sign, negative psoas sign, negative obturator sign, negative Rovsing sign – if asked)
l. Rectal: tenderness, grossly bloody stool in rectum
m. Urogenital: normal external genitalia
   i. Male: no discharge, normal testicular examination
n. Extremities: full range of motion, no deformity, normal pulses
o. Back: nontender
p. Neuro: cranial nerves II to XII intact; normal sensation, strength; normal reflexes and gait
q. Skin: decreased skin turgor (prior to IV fluids)
r. Lymph: no lymphadenopathy

I. Action
a. Meds
   i. Repeat 1 L NS IV bolus
   ii. BP: 112/76, HR: 85, RR 12, Sat 100%
b. Reassess
   i. Patient has one episode of bloody diarrhea in ED
c. Labs
   i. Stool culture/GI PCR

J. Nurse
a. Repeat vitals after second bolus
   i. BP: 126/72, HR: 72, RR: 12, Sat: 100%
b. Patient is stable and comfortable

Case 103: Diarrhea

K. Results

Table 103.1 Results table

Test	Result	Test	Result
Complete blood count:		T bili	1.0 mg/dL
WBC	$10.8 \times 10^3/\mu L$	D bili	0.3 mg/dL
Hct	41.8%	Amylase	50 U/L
Plt	$280 \times 10^3/\mu L$	Lipase	25 U/L
		Albumin	4.7 g/dL
Basic metabolic panel:			
Na	138 mEq/L	**Urinalysis:**	
K	3.3 mEq/L	SG	1.020
Cl	105 mEq/L	pH	7
CO_2	22 mEq/L	Prot	Neg
BUN	12 mEq/dL	Gluc	Neg
Cr	1.1 mg/dL	Ketones	Neg
Gluc	10 mg/dL	Bili	Neg
		Blood	Neg
		LE	Neg
Coagulation panel:		Nitrite	Neg
PT	12.6 sec	Color	Yellow
PTT	26.0 sec		
INR	1.0	**Venous blood gas:**	
		pH	7.38
Liver function panel:		pCO_2	45 mmHg
AST	23 U/L	pO_2	42 mmHg
ALT	26 U/L		
Alk phos	42 U/L		

a. Lactate: 2.3 mmol/L
b. Stool culture: pending

L. Action
a. Meds
    i. Ciprofloxacin
b. Add on lab study of magnesium level (if not ordered previously)
    i. 2.0 mEq/L
c. Replete K
    i. Potassium chloride

M. Nurse

a. Patient feeling significantly better

N. Action

a. Disposition
    i.   After rehydration with IV fluids, discharge from ED with prescription for ciprofloxacin and outpatient follow-up with PMD
b. Patient education regarding infectious diarrhea and prevention of spread/fecal oral contamination and importance of handwashing
c. Discussion about bland diet and the need for ongoing oral fluid repletion
d. Discussion about occupation/return to work

O. Diagnosis

a. Enteroinvasive diarrhea

P. Critical actions

a. Rehydration
b. Repletion of electrolytes
c. Antibiotics

Q. Examiner instructions

a. This is a case of enteroinvasive diarrhea from a bacterial infection. Viruses (especially norovirus) most commonly cause gastroenteritis leading to diarrhea. However, the bloody diarrhea in this case is suggestive of an invasive bacterial etiology. History of travel, antibiotic use, known sick contacts, or ingestion of contaminated food or water during an outbreak are also suggestive of bacterial infection. Key actions in this case are rehydration and repletion of electrolytes. With diarrhea, there is an expected loss of electrolytes, particularly potassium. However, the magnesium level must be assessed and corrected for since this will prevent absorption of potassium. Intravenous magnesium is preferred in this situation for repletion, as oral magnesium is known to worsen diarrhea.

R. Pearls

a. Infectious diarrhea is responsible for 85% of diarrhea.
b. Acute, infectious diarrhea is generally secondary to bacterial or viral causes, whereas enteroinvasive diarrhea is caused by invasive bacteria and parasites. These pathogens will often cause damage in the intestinal mucosa, causing water, electrolytes, blood, mucus, and plasma proteins to be secreted.
c. Most cases of infectious diarrhea are usually self-limited and require only supportive therapy. In the ED, mildly dehydrated patients will benefit from oral rehydration. Any patient with signs and symptoms of moderate to severe dehydration, such as dry mucous membranes, low blood pressure, or tachycardia, will benefit from IV rehydration with isotonic fluids. Urinary specific gravity can be followed during IV fluids treatment, with normal or dilute urine as the endpoint.
    i.   Oral rehydration should be taken by patients in small, frequent volumes and should include solutions with sodium, potassium, and glucose.
d. Patients may require antimicrobial therapy in severe cases, including fevers or bloody diarrhea.
    i.   Antibiotic therapy should be considered in travelers' diarrhea if patient is toxic, has fevers, or bloody diarrhea. Per the CDC, antibiotic choice is dependent on location of travel.

Fluoroquinolones are useful except when suspicious of *Campylobacter*, and should be considered particularly when traveling in South and Southeast Asia. Azithromycin is a good alternative, as well as rifaximin, particularly in cases of noninvasive *E. coli*.

e. Antidiarrheal agents are effective in symptom treatment; however, they should be avoided in patients with either bloody diarrhea or diarrhea and fever.

f. Culture should be sent in children, toxic patients, immunocompromised patients, or patients with history of travel. Culture for ova and parasites should be sent for high-risk patients.

   i. The CDC recommends stool cultures in the immunocompromised, febrile, bloody diarrhea, severe abdominal pain, and if the presentation of illness is considered by the practitioner to be severe/persistent or if the stool shows many leukocytes.

   ii. The CDC recommends stool should be investigated for parasites when patients have travel histories to endemic areas, are immunocompromised, have chronic diarrhea, or when the diarrhea does not resolve after antimicrobial therapy.

g. Typical viruses causing diarrhea are rotavirus, adenovirus, calicivirus, astrovirus, and Norwalk virus. Viruses typically affect the small intestine and do not present with bloody diarrhea.

h. Bloody diarrhea is suggestive of an invasive bacterial etiology. Bacteria causing bloody diarrhea include:

   i. Enterohemorrhagic *Escherichia coli* (*E. coli* 0157:H7)

   ii. Enteroinvasive *E. coli*

   iii. *Shigella* species

   iv. *Salmonella* species

   v. *Campylobacter* species

   vi. *Yersinia* species

   vii. *Aeromonas* species

   viii. *Plesiomonas* species

   ix. *Vibrio* species

i. Parasites causing bloody diarrhea include:

   i. *Giardia lambia*

   ii. *Cryptosporidium*

   iii. *Isopora* or *Cyclospora* spp.

   iv. *Entamoeba histolytica*

j. Thrombotic-thrombocytopenic purpura (TTP) and hemolytic-uremic syndrome (HUS) are complications of infectious diarrhea, usually caused by *E. coli* 0157:H7. These have been implicated especially when pediatric patients with severe gastroenteritis have been treated with antibiotics. HUS should be considered in children presenting with grossly bloody stool and oliguria or anuria, particularly when children with *E. coli* are treated with antibiotics. TTP/HUS have also been complications of patients infected with *Salmonella*, *Shigella*, and *Campylobacter*.

k. The CDC recommends all stool, even if not bloody, be tested for pathogens that are likely to cause TTP/HUS.

l. If TTP/HUS are suspected, CBC with blood smear, coagulation studies, BUN, Cr, and LDH are recommended for further risk stratification. HUS will have symptoms of fever, anemia, and thrombocytopenia. TTP can present with the pentad of anemia, thrombocytopenia, fever, renal dysfunction, and CNS dysfunction. Patients with HUS will often have worse renal dysfunction and little to no CNS dysfunction when compared to TTP.

m. First-line treatment for children with dehydration from diarrhea is oral rehydration therapy.

    n. Antibiotics should be considered in the pediatric patient if bloody diarrhea, severe watery diarrhea, or signs/symptoms of a systemic infection are present.
      i. Macrolides are the first-line treatment in the pediatric population
      ii. Rifaximin is approved in children greater than 11 years old
    o. In the setting of recent antibiotic use, stool specimen should be tested for the *Clostridium difficile* toxin. PO metronidazole is the treatment of choice if *C. diff* toxin is found on testing.
    p. In a patient presenting with bloody diarrhea, other conditions that should be considered include diverticulitis, mesenteric ischemia, gastrointestinal hemorrhage, and inflammatory bowel disease.
    q. Radiologic exams have low utility in these patients unless there is significant abdominal pain, signs of peritonitis on exam, or concern for abdominal perforation. In this situation, CT scan has the highest utility.

S. References

    a. *Tintinalli's Emergency Medicine: A Comprehensive Study Guide* (9th ed.): Chapter 73, Disorders Presenting Primarily with Diarrhea.
    b. *Rosen's Emergency Medicine: Concepts and Clinical Practice* (10th ed.): Chapter 27, Diarrhea.

T. Acknowledgements

    a. We would like to acknowledge Mieka Close for their contribution to this chapter in the previous edition of this book, which has been updated by Rijo Maracheril.

Cough

Jeanne Noble, MD

A. Chief complaint
a. 48-year-old male brought in by EMS from corrections facility with the complaint of cough, chest pain, and shortness of breath

B. Vital signs
a. BP: 106/62, HR: 125, RR: 26, T: 38.4°C, Sat: 87% on RA

C. What does the patient look like?
a. Patient is cachectic, appearing older than stated age, and in moderate respiratory distress, sitting forward on gurney.

D. Primary survey
a. Airway: normal phonation, speaking in four-word sentences
b. Breathing: tachypneic, symmetric chest rise, using accessory muscles
c. Circulation: warm skin, palpable distal pulses

E. Action
a. Airborne isolation
b. Place patient on monitor and oxygen supplementation via nonrebreather face mask (NRBFM)
c. Two large-bore peripheral IV lines
d. Labs
   i. CBC, BMP, LFT, LDH, coagulation studies, blood cultures
   ii. VBG or ABG with lactate
1 L NS bolus
e. Antipyretic (e.g., acetaminophen)

F. History
a. HPI: A 48-year-old male with a history of AIDS and nonadherence to antiretroviral therapy, complaining of 2–3 weeks of cough and now with worsening shortness of breath, chest pain, and subjective fevers. Patient denies headache, neck stiffness, abdominal pain, nausea, vomiting, diarrhea, or urinary symptoms. He has not been hospitalized in over one year.
b. PMHx: AIDS, last CD4 count 94, history of non-Hodgkin's lymphoma
c. PSHx: none
d. Allergies: none
e. Meds: unknown pills administered at corrections facility
f. Social: incarcerated × 1 month; active tobacco use with 40 pack per year history; denies alcohol or other drug use

g. FHx: no relevant history
h. PMD: corrections facility clinic

G. Nurse
a. EKG (Figure 104.1)
b. Fluids
   i. BP: 110/70, HR: 112, RR: 18, Sat: 93% on NRB
c. No fluids
   i. BP: 95/60, HR: 130, RR: 20, Sat: 93% on NRB

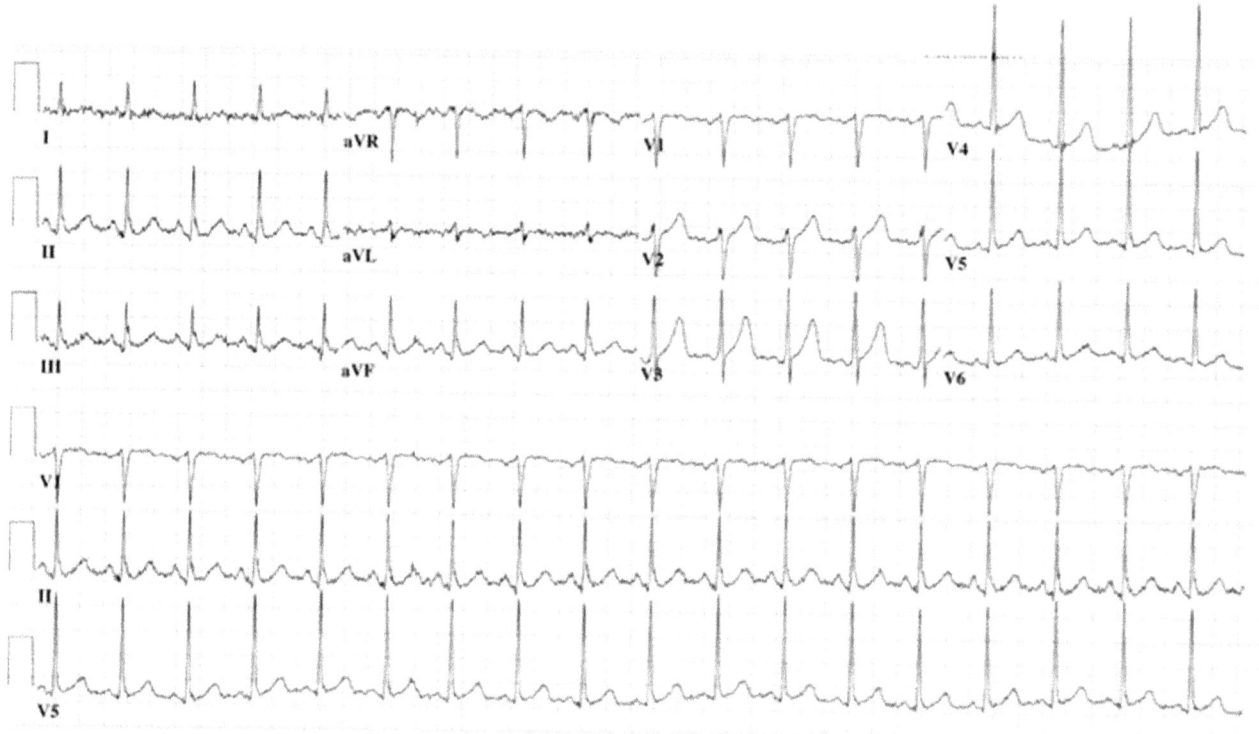

Figure 104.1

H. Secondary survey
a. General: alert, oriented × 3, cachectic, sitting upright on gurney with increased work of breathing
b. Head: normocephalic, atraumatic
c. Eyes: extraocular movement intact, pupils equal, reactive to light
d. Ears: normal tympanic membranes
e. Nose: no discharge
f. Neck: full range of motion, no jugular vein distension, no stridor
g. Pharynx: poor dentition, white plaques on posterior tongue and soft palate
h. Chest: nontender
i. Lungs: tachypneic, diffuse bilateral crackles, using accessory muscles
j. Heart: tachycardic, no murmurs, rubs, or gallops
k. Abdomen: soft, nontender, nondistended, normal bowel sounds
l. Rectal: normal tone, brown stool, occult blood negative
m. Urogenital: normal scrotum, no penile discharge

n. Extremities: no edema, full range of motion, normal pulses
o. Back: nontender
p. Neuro: cranial nerves II to XII intact; symmetric sensation, strength and coordination; normal reflexes and gait
q. Skin: warm, diaphoretic, no rash
r. Lymph: no lymphadenopathy

I. Action

a. Meds
   i. Antibiotics for bacterial pneumonia (e.g., ceftriaxone plus azithromycin or doxycycline)
   ii. Trimethoprim/sulfamethoxazole (Bactrim) for PCP coverage
   iii. Prednisone or IV methylprednisolone
b. Consider TB testing (e.g., Quantiferon-TB blood assay)
c. Reassess
   i. Patient still tachypneic but decreased work of breathing
      1. Consider high-flow nasal cannula or BiPAP
   ii. MICU
d. Imaging
   i. CXR

J. Nurse

a. BP: 118/76, HR: 106, RR: 18, Sat: 94% on NRB
b. Patient: mild respiratory distress, but improving

K. Results

Table **104.1** Results table

Test	Result	Test	Result
Complete blood count:		Alk phos	42 U/L
WBC	$3.1 \times 10^3/\mu L$	T bili	1.0 mg/dL
Hct	31%	Lipase	25 U/L
Hgb	10.3	Albumin	2.7 g/dL
Plt	$105 \times 10^3/\mu L$	LDH	490 U/L
Basic metabolic panel:		**Urinalysis:**	
Na	138 mEq/L	SG	1.030
K	4.3 mEq/L	pH	7
Cl	105 mEq/L	Prot	Neg
CO_2	18 mEq/L	Gluc	Neg
BUN	30 mEq/dL	Ketones	Neg
Cr	1.1 mg/dL	Bili	Neg
Gluc	100 mg/dL	Blood	Neg
		LE	Neg

Table 104.1 (cont.)

Test	Result	Test	Result
Coagulation panel:		Nitrite	Neg
PT	12.6 sec	Color	Yellow
PTT	26.0 sec		
INR	1.0	**Arterial blood gas:**	
		pH	7.34
Liver function panel:		pO_2	58 mmHg on RA
AST	35 U/L	pCO_2	30 mmHg
ALT	40 U/L	HCO_3	18 mmol/L

a. Lactate: 2.8 mmol/L
b. CXR (Figure 104.2)

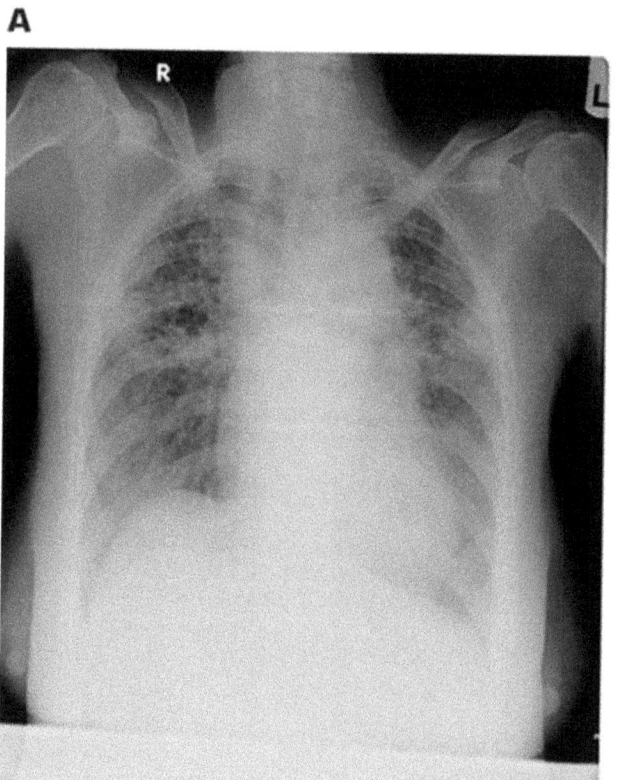
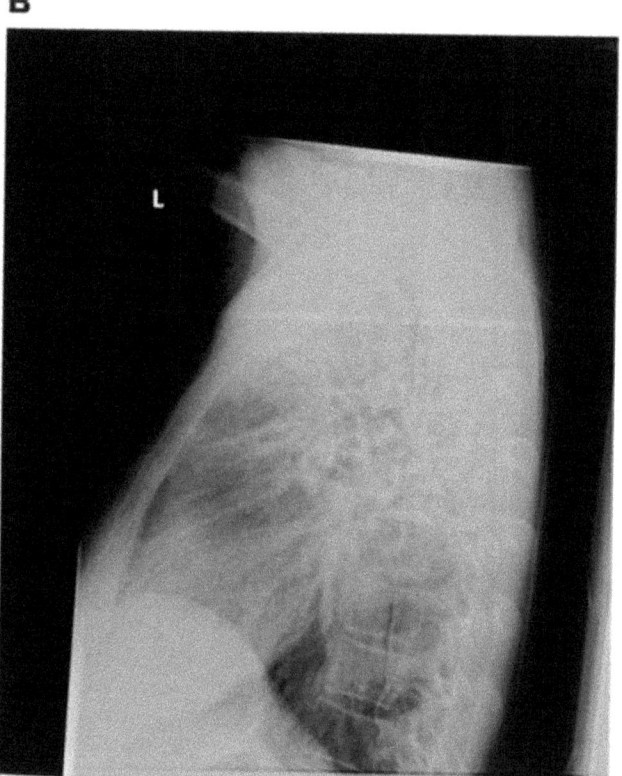

Figure 104.2

L. Action
a. Admit patient to MICU.
b. Discuss goals of care with patient and possible need for endotracheal intubation in case of worsening respiratory status.

M. Diagnosis
a. Pneumocystis pneumonia (PCP)

N. Critical actions

a. Airway management – supplemental oxygen via NRBFM, high-flow NC, or BiPAP
b. IV fluids
c. CXR
d. Antibiotics for both community-acquired pneumonia and PCP
e. Corticosteroids
f. Airborne isolation
g. MICU admission

O. Examiner instructions

a. This is a case of pneumonia in a patient with AIDS, likely due to *Pneumocystis jiroveci* (a ubiquitous fungus formerly identified as *Pneumocystis carinii*). Pneumocystis pneumonia (PCP) is seen in patients who are severely immunocompromised. Patients with AIDS have a CD4 cell count below 200, significantly increasing their risk for opportunistic infections such as PCP. In our patient, key actions are providing noninvasive airway support by NRB FM or BIPAP, obtaining a CXR, resuscitation with IV fluids, administering antibiotics for both community-acquired pneumonia (CAP) and PCP, and giving corticosteroids. The patient should also be placed in airborne isolation, given his risk factors for concurrent tuberculosis.

P. Pearls

a. The typical presentation of PCP is gradual onset of a nonproductive cough, followed by worsening shortness of breath, exertional hypoxia, chest discomfort, and fever.
b. Bacterial pneumonia remains the most common cause of respiratory failure in patients with HIV.
c. PCP is common in patients with CD4 counts <200.
d. Empiric PCP treatment is warranted in all patients with CD4 <200, hypoxemia, and interstitial infiltrates on CXR.
e. Co-infections are common: 15% of patients presenting with PCP also have acute bacterial pneumonia, TB, or Kaposi's sarcoma.
f. Up to 25% of patients with PCP have a normal CXR. High-resolution CT is highly sensitive for PCP and can be used to rule out the diagnosis.
g. Spontaneous pneumothorax in an HIV-infected patient should prompt consideration of PCP.
h. Corticosteroids are indicated in PCP for significant hypoxia, typically based on room air ABG results:
   i. PaO2 < 70 mmHg *or*
   ii. Alveolar-arterial gradient >35 mmHg
i. ICU admission should be considered for all PCP patients qualifying for steroids, as respiratory status may initially worsen with therapy.
j. Serum LDH has greater utility as a prognostic test rather than a diagnostic test (e.g., LDH levels may also be elevated in bacterial pneumonia). Persistently elevated LDH levels during PCP treatment are associated with higher mortality rates.

Q. Figure legends

a. Figure 104.1 (EKG) Sinus tachycardia
b. Figure 104.2 (CXR) Bilateral, patchy infiltrates. (b) Lateral also reveals patchy infiltrates.

R. References

a.   *Tintinalli's Emergency Medicine: A Comprehensive Study Guide* (9th ed.): Chapter 155, Human Immunodeficiency Virus Infection.

b.   *Rosen's Emergency Medicine: Concepts and Clinical Practice* (10th ed.): Chapter 62, Pneumonia. Chapter 121, HIV.

S. Acknowledgements

a.   We would like to acknowledge Mieka Close for their contribution to this chapter in the previous edition of this book, which has been updated by Jeanne Noble.

Vomiting and Altered Mental Status

Nicole Munz, DO

A. Chief complaint
a. 4-year-old male with vomiting and altered mental status

B. Vital signs
a. BP: 110/71, HR: 142, RR: 28, T: 37.1°C, Sat: 94% on RA, FS: 110 mg/dL (must ask)

C. What does the patient look like?
a. Patient appears stated age, no external evidence of trauma, no obvious evidence of congenital abnormality, weak cry, mumbling (according to mother who can usually understand him), vomitus around mouth.

D. Primary survey
a. Airway: crying and mumbling
b. Breathing: no apparent respiratory distress, no cyanosis
c. Circulation: warm skin, normal capillary refill

E. Action
a. Oxygen via NC or nonrebreather mask
b. Monitor: BP: 108/70, HR: 139, RR: 26, T: 37.1°C, Sat: 99% on 2 L
c. Two large-bore lines IV
d. Labs
    i. VBG or ABG with lactate, point of care glucose
    ii. CBC, BMP, LFT, coagulation studies, blood type and crossmatch, alcohol level, acetaminophen level, salicylate level, urine toxicology screen, urinalysis, blood cultures
e. IV bolus 20 mL/kg isotonic crystalloid
f. EKG

F. History
a. HPI: A 4-year-old male brought in by EMS with mother after collapsing at home. Per mother, the patient had been vomiting at home for the past hour, and was becoming progressively weaker and confused. Patient has no known medical problems and was asymptomatic when he woke up this morning. No recent trauma according to mother. Mother denies fever, rash, upper respiratory symptoms, diarrhea, or other infectious symptoms. No known sick contacts. Patient is up to date with his childhood immunizations (must ask). Mother doubts ingestion, but does state the patient was unsupervised for 10 minutes while she made lunch.
b. PMHx: none

    c. PSHx: none

    d. Allergies: none

    e. Meds: none; (must ask) meds in the home: father takes metoprolol and mother takes isoniazid for recent positive PPD (she works at a local prison).

    f. Social: lives with mother, father, and 8-year-old sister. Neither parent smokes or uses illicit drugs. Attends preschool.

    g. FHx: no relevant history

    h. PMD: Dr. Small (up to date with immunizations and well-child visits)

G. Nurse

    a. EKG : sinus tachycardia

    b. 20 mL/kg IV bolus given:

        i. BP: 106/68, HR: 135, RR: 26, Sat: 99% on O_2

    c. Patient is having a generalized tonic-clonic seizure

H. Action

    a. If lorazepam or other benzodiazepine given (no improvement in seizure)

        i. If one dose given

            1. Continued seizures

            2. BP: 99/61, HR: 123, RR: 20, Sat: 94% on O_2

        ii. If two or more doses given (or if additional, second-line medication given)

            1. Continued seizures

            2. BP: 88/55, HR: 109, RR: 10, Sat: 83% on O_2

            3. Patient loses airway protection reflexes, becomes bradypneic, and requires intubation for airway protection and hypoxia

    b. Seizures will continue until pyridoxine IV is given (70 mg/kg IV empirically)

I. Secondary survey (cannot be completed until pyridoxine is given)

    a. General: somnolent, no acute distress, confused (per mother), appears well nourished

    b. Head: normocephalic, atraumatic

    c. Eyes: extraocular movements intact, pupils 6 mm and reactive to light, normal conjunctiva

    d. Ears: normal tympanic membranes, no foreign bodies

    e. Nose: no discharge, no foreign bodies

    f. Neck: full range of motion, no tenderness, no lymphadenopathy, no stridor

    g. Throat: dentition appropriate for age, no trauma, no lesions, no swelling, no erythema of posterior pharynx or tonsillar enlargement

    h. Chest: nontender, no evidence of trauma

    i. Lungs: clear bilaterally

    j. Heart: tachycardic, no murmurs, rubs, or gallops

    k. Abdomen: normal bowel sounds, soft, nontender, no distention, rectal exam normal

    l. Urogenital: normal

    m. Extremities: full range of motion, no deformity, no tenderness, no edema, normal pulses

    n. Back: nontender

    o. Neuro: opens eyes spontaneously, moving all extremities spontaneously, withdraws from painful stimuli, mumbling (per mother), deep tendon reflex 2+ bilaterally, no clonus, negative Babinski sign

    p. Skin: no rash, warm, dry

    q. Lymph: no lymphadenopathy

J. Action

a. Meds
  i. Repeat 20 mL/kg IV bolus
b. Reassess
  i. No further seizure activity after pyridoxine, becoming more interactive with mother
c. Imaging
  i. CXR
  ii. Neuroimaging – CT or MRI

K. Nurse

a. BP: 94/68, HR: 112, RR: 22, Sat: 100% on O_2 NC

L. Results

Table 105.1 Results table

Test	Result	Test	Result
Complete blood count:		T bili	0.7 mg/dL
WBC	$18.3 \times 10^3/\mu L$	D bili	0.1 mg/dL
Hct	35.9%	Amylase	50 U/L
Plt	$350 \times 10^3/\mu L$	Lipase	20 U/L
		Albumin	4.7 g/dL
Basic metabolic panel:			
Na	139 mEq/L	**Urinalysis:**	
K	4.2 mEq/L	SG	1.020
Cl	101 mEq/L	pH	6
CO_2	14 mEq/L	Prot	Neg
BUN	13 mEq/dL	Gluc	Neg
Cr	0.5 mg/dL	Ketones	Neg
Gluc	95 mg/dL	Bili	Neg
		Blood	Neg
Coagulation panel:		LE	Neg
PT	12.6 sec	Nitrite	Neg
PTT	26 sec	Color	Yellow
INR	1.0		
		Arterial blood gas:	
Liver function panel:		pH	7.26
AST	23 U/L	pO_2	90 mmHg
ALT	19 U/L	pCO_2	28 mmHg
Alk phos	47 U/L	HCO_3	17 mmol/L

a. Lactate: 5.9 mmol/L
b. Aspirin level: negative
c. Acetaminophen level: negative
d. Alcohol level: negative
e. Urine toxicology screen: negative
f. CXR
    i. If intubated, portable CXR: endotracheal tube in place; no focal infiltrate
    ii. If not intubated, portable CXR (Figure 105.1)
g. Neuroimaging: CT/MRI
    i. If noncontrast brain CT head ordered (Figure 105.2)
    ii. If MRI brain ordered: normal

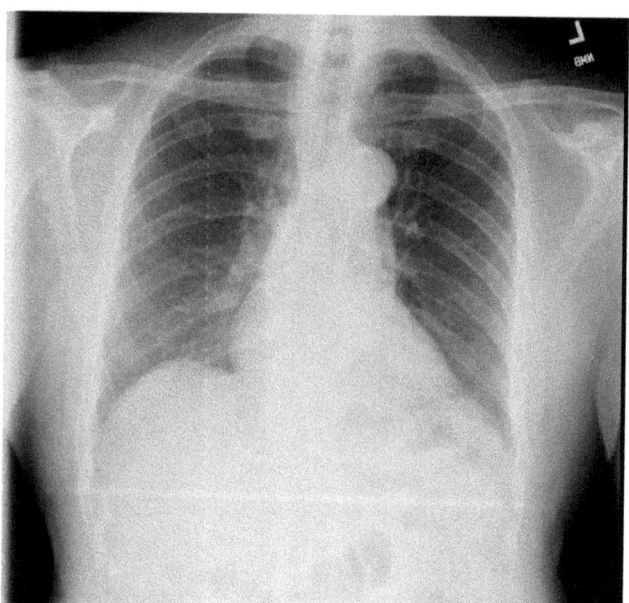

Figure 105.1

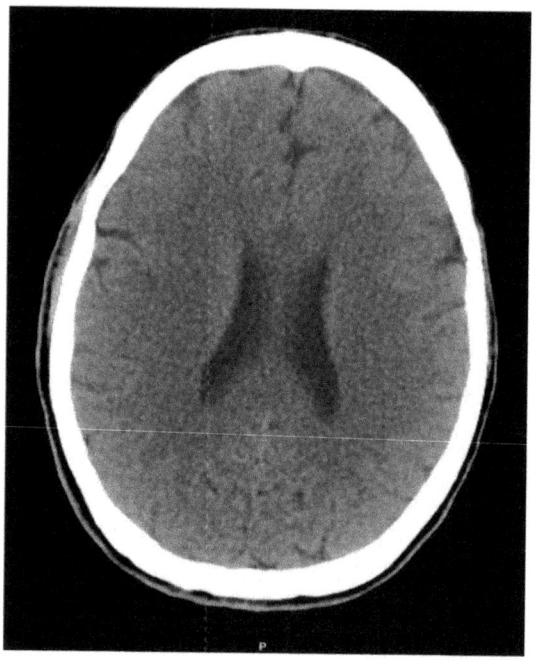

Figure 105.2

M. Action

a. Consults
   i. Toxicology
   ii. Neurology
   iii. Pediatric medical ICU
b. Discussion with family regarding diagnosis, treatment plan, and admission. Consider providing parental education on safe storage of medications and child-proofing cabinets.

N. Diagnosis

a. INH overdose

O. Critical actions

a. Airway management
b. Point of care blood glucose
c. Pyridoxine administration
d. Serum toxicology for aspirin, acetaminophen, and ethanol
e. Neuroimaging (evaluate for evidence of intercranial causes of vomiting and altered mental status: [nonaccidental] trauma, space-occupying lesion, congenital malformations, etc.)

P. Examiner instructions

a. This is a case on isoniazid (INH) toxicity due to accidental ingestion by a young child. This is not a febrile seizure as the child was not febrile, had no recent infectious symptoms, the seizure did not terminate spontaneously, and the seizure was refractory to anticonvulsants. In adults, INH toxicity can be due to INH overdose or noncompliance with the co-prescribed pyridoxine. INH is a first-line medication for prophylaxis and treatment of active tuberculosis. This presentation is a typical one, with nausea, vomiting, and mental status change. In the case of severe toxicity, patients will develop seizure, metabolic acidosis, coma, and even death. Seizures from INH toxicity are tonic-clonic in nature and refractory to standard seizure management. Key actions in this case are airway management and pyridoxine administration, as seizures caused by INH toxicity are likely refractory to standard anticonvulsants, including benzodiazepines, barbiturates, and phenytoin. The seizures in this patient will not stop until pyridoxine is given. If multiple doses of benzodiazepines are given, the patient will desaturate and require intubation.

Q. Pearls

a. Always consider and ask about ingestions in children presenting with altered mental status, seizure, vomiting, or any ill-appearing child without a clear etiology.
b. Consider INH toxicity as cause of seizures in cases of refractory seizures.
c. INH toxicity antidote is pyridoxine (vitamin B6). Treatment is 70 mg/kg IV empirically in children and adults. (Starting dose in adults is 5 g IV as this is based on a 70 kg adult.) If the amount of INH ingested is known, then the dose of pyridoxine is a gram-for-gram equivalent to the amount of INH ingested.
d. In acute overdose, typical presentation includes nausea, vomiting, mental status changes, and ataxia, which may progress to seizure, coma, and metabolic acidosis if more than 20–40 mg/kg is ingested.
e. INH toxicity occurs because INH inhibits the production of the inhibitory neurotransmitter GABA via vitamin B6 depletion.
f. Activated charcoal may be administered to decrease absorption of INH, if given within 1 hour of ingestion.

g. Metabolic acidosis may occur in severe overdose with seizure activity, due to production of lactic acid. Sodium bicarbonate is not recommended in treatment of acidosis. Hemodialysis may be required to correct acidemia and to remove INH from blood.

h. Most toxicity is manifested within 2 hours of ingestion. Patients who remain asymptomatic after 6 hours may be medically cleared for discharge from the ED.

R. Figure legends
a. Figure 105.1 (CXR) Normal chest x-ray.
b. Figure 105.2 (CT) Normal head CT.

S. References
a. *Tintinalli's Emergency Medicine: A Comprehensive Study Guide* (9th ed.): Chapter 206, Antimicrobials.
b. *Rosen's Emergency Medicine: Concepts and Clinical Practice* (10th ed.): Chapter 169, Pediatric Neurologic Disorders. Chapter 135, Care of the Poisoned Patient.

Weakness

Tomás Díaz, MD and Jacqueline Nemer, MD

A. Chief complaint
a. 94-year-old female brought in by EMS after found to be globally weak in bed by home health aide who last saw patient 1 week prior

B. Vital signs
a. BP: 104/61, HR: 120, RR: 20, T: 35.7°C, Sat: 93% on RA

C. What does the patient look like?
a. Patient appears cachectic, disheveled, clothing soiled with urine and dried feces.

D. Primary survey
a. Airway: alert and oriented × 3, speaking softly in full sentences
b. Breathing: no respiratory distress, although resting tachypnea, no cyanosis
c. Circulation: warm skin, normal capillary refill

E. Action
a. Oxygen via NC
b. Peripheral IV access
c. Labs
   i. Point of care glucose
   ii. VBG or ABG, CBC, BMP, LFT, coagulation studies, blood type and crossmatch, lactate, troponin, total CPK, urinalysis
d. Monitor: BP: 108/64, HR: 122, RR: 16, Sat: 96%, on 2 L NC, FS: 84 mg/dL
e. EKG

F. History
a. HPI: A 94-year-old female was brought in by EMS after being found by her home health aide. She was found in bed too weak to get up, and she was covered in urine and feces. The patient and aide both report that the patient lives alone in her apartment and her primary caretaker is her son, who is expected to visit her daily. The home health aide is her additional home support 1 day per week. Her son was unable to be reached by the patient's aide. The patient states that he has not stopped by the apartment in several days. As such, the patient has been unable to feed nor ambulate to the bathroom since her son's last visit. She ambulates with a walker at baseline, but has been too weak to get out of bed. She notes mild low back pain, decreased urination, and minimal stool output for the past few weeks. ROS otherwise negative.

b. PMHx: hypertension, osteopenia, mild cognitive impairment
c. PSHx: remote total abdominal hysterectomy
d. Allergies: none
e. Meds: losartan, calcium supplement
f. Social: lives alone in apartment, son is caretaker
g. FHx: not relevant
h. PMD: Dr. Nguyen

G. Nurse
a. EKG (Figure 106.1)
b. 1 L NS
   i. BP: 124/72, HR: 119, RR: 12, Sat: 96% on 2 L NC

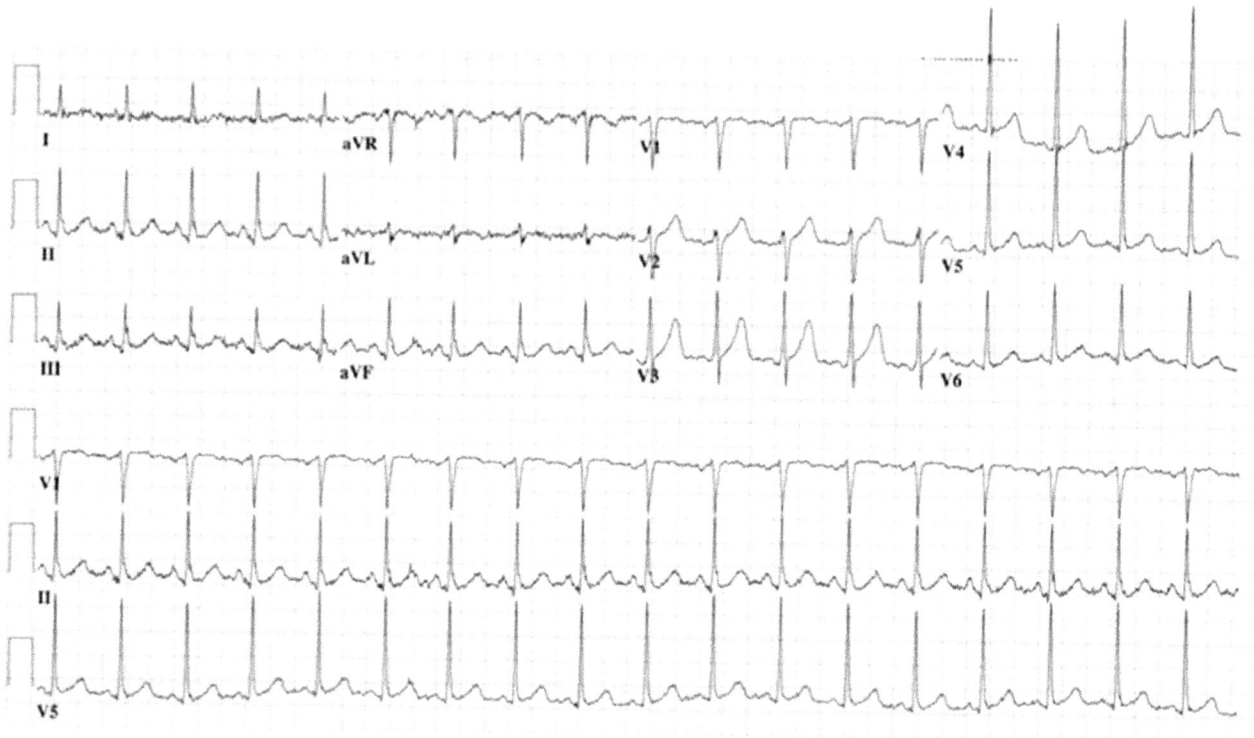

Figure 106.1

H. Secondary survey
a. General: alert, oriented to person and place, unsure of the day, cachectic, disheveled, covered in urine and dried feces
b. Head: normocephalic, atraumatic
c. Eyes: sunken eyes, extraocular movement intact, pupils equal, reactive to light, conjunctiva pale, sclera anicteric (if asked)
d. Ears: normal tympanic membranes
e. Nose: no discharge
f. Neck: full range of motion, no jugular vein distension, no stridor
g. Pharynx: dry mucous membranes, no lesions, no swelling
h. Chest: nontender

i. Lungs: diminished breath sounds, bibasilar crackles
j. Heart: tachycardic, no murmurs, rubs, or gallops
k. Abdomen: scaphoid, normal bowel sounds, soft, nontender or distended
l. Rectal: normal tone, brown stool, occult blood negative
m. Urogenital:
   i. Female: no discharge, normal external genitalia
n. Extremities: full range of motion, no deformity, normal pulses, circumferential ecchymosis around both upper arms
o. Back: nontender
p. Neuro: cranial nerves II to XII intact; clear speech, appropriate content, normal sensation; 4+/5 strength throughout, no focal motor deficits; normal reflexes, unable to ambulate secondary to global weakness
q. Skin: decreased skin turgor; two stage III pressure ulcers: sacrum and thoracic back
r. Lymph: no lymphadenopathy

I. Action
a. Point of care ultrasound: volume status, eFAST
b. Foley catheter placement
c. Skin and wound care – clean off skin for full exam, dressing applied to decubiti
d. Meds
   i. IV fluids: NS at 250 cc bolus, reassess and repeat 250 cc bolus
   ii. Oral hydration and easily digestible food for refeeding after starvation
e. Reassess
   i. Patient reports feeling better after IV fluids and PO nourishment
f. Consult: social work
g. Imaging
   i. CXR (Figure 106.2)

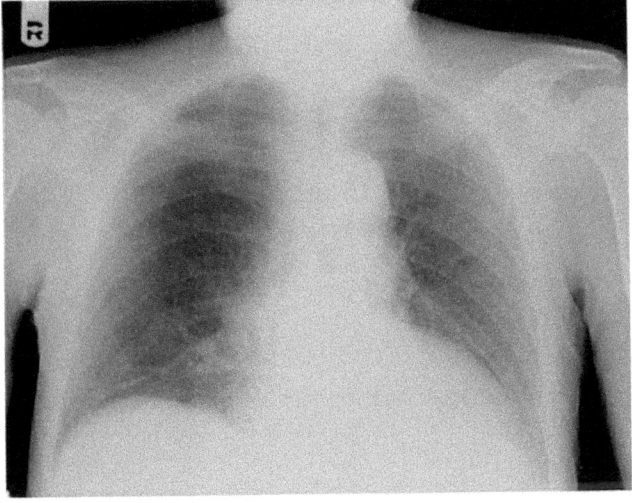

Figure 106.2

J. Nurse
a. BP: 126/68, HR: 97, RR: 14, Sat: 95% on 2 L NC
b. Patient: stable, no urine output

K. Results

Table 106.1 Results table

Test	Result	Test	Result
Complete blood count:		Alk phos	42 U/L
WBC	$5.3 \times 10/\mu L$	T bili	1.0 mg/dL
Hct	41.50%	D bili	0.3 mg/dL
Plt	$350 \times 10^3/\mu L$	Amylase	50 U/L
		Lipase	25 U/L
Basic metabolic panel:		Albumin	2.4 g/dL
Na	151 mEq/L		
K	5.3 mEq/L	**Urinalysis:**	
Cl	109 mEq/L	SG	>1.030
CO_2	15 mEq/L	pH	7.0
BUN	58 mEq/dL	Prot	+1 mg/dL
Cr	1.9 mg/dL	Gluc	Neg
Gluc	100 mg/dL	Ketones	+
		Bili	Neg
Coagulation panel:		Blood	Neg
PT	12.6 sec	LE	Neg
PTT	26.0 sec	Nitrite	Neg
INR	1.0	Color	Dark yellow
Liver function panel:		**Venous blood gas:**	
AST	23 U/L	pH	7.19
ALT	26 U/L	pCO_2	26
		pO_2	59

a. Lactate: 2.0 mmol/L
b. Portable CXR (Figure 106.2)
c. CPK: 60 U/L
d. Troponin: negative

L. Action
a. Admit patient to medicine
b. Report case of elder abuse to Adult Protective Services, or proper authorities as mandated by state

M. Diagnosis
a. Elder neglect
b. Dehydration with acute kidney injury

N. Critical actions
a. Reporting of case as mandated for elder abuse
b. Social work involvement
c. IV hydration

    d. Check CPK for rhabdomyolysis

    e. EKG

    f. Work-up for infection including urinalysis and CXR

O. Examiner instructions

a. This is a case of elder abuse in the form of neglect. The patient is in acute renal failure secondary to dehydration and has pressure ulcers from lying in bed unattended for several days. This patient cannot safely be discharged back to her home. She must be admitted for management of renal failure and social services assessment. Complete history, exposure, and thorough physical examination are the keys in exposing any signs of abuse or neglect. Circumferential bruising of the upper extremities is suggestive of the patient being grabbed or shaken; if this is found on the lower extremities, sexual abuse should be suspected. The clinician should look for signs of physical and sexual abuse, as well as neglect and abandonment.

P. Pearls

a. Elder abuse is defined as use of physical force that might result in bodily injury, physical pain, or impairment. Elder neglect is defined as failure of a caregiver to provide basic care to a patient and to provide goods and services necessary to prevent physical harm and emotional discomfort. Emotional or psychological abuse, financial or material exploitation, and abandonment are also forms of elder abuse/neglect.

b. The diagnosis of elder abuse is reliant on a clinician's assessment of the history, exam findings, recognition of risk factors, and any discovery of red flags that the patient has not been safely managed.

c. Elder abuse may present in the following forms (as defined by the National Center on Elder Abuse)

    i. Physical abuse

    ii. Sexual abuse

    iii. Emotional or psychological abuse

    iv. Financial or material exploitation

    v. Neglect

    vi. Abandonment

    vii. Self-neglect

d. Clinicians are required to report any suspicion of elder abuse to the appropriate hospital staff and to the proper authorities (e.g., Adult Protective Services) as mandated by the state.

Q. Figure legend

Figure 106.1 (EKG) Sinus tachycardia.

Figure 106.2 (CXR) Mild pulmonary vascular congestion, no focal infiltrate.

R. References

a. *Tintinalli's Emergency Medicine: A Comprehensive Study Guide* (9th ed.): Chapter 295, Abuse of the Elderly and Impaired.

b. *Rosen's Emergency Medicine: Concepts and Clinical Practice* (10th ed.): Chapter 181, Abuse and Neglect.

S. Acknowledgements

a. We would like to acknowledge Mieka Close for their contribution to this chapter in the previous edition of this book, which has been updated by Tomás Díaz and Jacqueline Nemer

Foot Pain

Marianne Juarez, MD

A. Chief complaint
a. 53-year-old male with left foot pain and swelling for the past 1 day

B. Vital signs
a. BP: 140/85, HR: 95, RR: 16, T: 36.5°C, Sat: 100% on RA

C. What does the patient look like?
a. Patient appears stated age, in moderate pain, sitting on the gurney.

D. Primary survey
a. Airway: speaking in full sentences
b. Breathing: no apparent respiratory distress, no cyanosis
c. Circulation: warm and dry skin, normal capillary refill

E. Action
a. One large-bore peripheral IV line
b. Labs
    i. CBC, BMP
    ii. Uric acid, ESR, CRP
c. Monitor: BP: 146/90, HR: 92, RR: 16, Sat: 100% on RA

F. History
a. HPI: A 53-year-old male with no significant history states he has had progressive left foot pain since waking yesterday morning. The pain is currently rated an 8/10, and is localized over the base of the great toe. It does not radiate and is worse with any movement or palpation. He is able to ambulate but with difficulty. The pain did not improve with a trial of acetaminophen. He denies any recent trauma or prior episodes. He denies fever or other systemic symptoms. He has no other complaints.
b. PMHx: none
c. PSHx: none
d. Allergies: none
e. Meds: none
f. Social: not sexually active; nonsmoker; drinks alcohol several times per week; denies illicit drug use; lives alone
g. FHx: diabetes, hypertension
h. PMD: none

G. Nurse

a. BP: 146/92, HR: 96, RR: 14, Sat: 98% on RA

b. Patient: reports 8/10 pain

H. Secondary survey

a. General: alert, oriented × 3, moderate pain

b. Head: normocephalic, atraumatic

c. Eyes: extraocular movement intact, pupils equal, reactive to light

d. Ears: normal tympanic membranes

e. Nose: no discharge

f. Neck: full range of motion, no jugular vein distension, no stridor

g. Pharynx: normal dentition, no lesions, no swelling

h. Chest: nontender

i. Lungs: clear bilaterally

j. Heart: rate and rhythm regular, no murmurs, rubs, or gallops

k. Abdomen: normal bowel sounds, soft, nontender, nondistended

l. Rectal: deferred

m. Urogenital: deferred

n. Extremities: left foot with warmth, erythema and swelling overlying the first metatarsal–phalangeal (MTP) joint; very tender to palpation with decreased ROM secondary to pain; able to bear weight; distal pulses normal, equal bilaterally; otherwise normal

o. Back: nontender

p. Neuro: cranial nerves II to XII intact; normal sensation, strength; normal reflexes and gait

q. Skin: warm and dry

r. Lymph: no lymphadenopathy

I. Action

a. Procedure

   i. Left foot arthrocentesis of first MTP joint

     1. Informed consent with explanation of risks, benefits, and alternatives

     2. Time out to identify site, done under aseptic conditions

     3. Clear fluid obtained – send for culture, cell count, Gram stain, crystals

b. Meds

   i. NSAIDs

   ii. ± Opioids

c. Reassess

   i. No pain meds: continues to have 8/10 pain

   ii. Pain meds given: pain is much improved but still present, now 4/10

d. Imaging

   i. X-ray left foot

J. Nurse

a. X-ray left foot (Figure 107.1)

b. BP: 130/75, HR: 88, RR: 12, Sat: 100% on RA

c. Patient: with mild pain

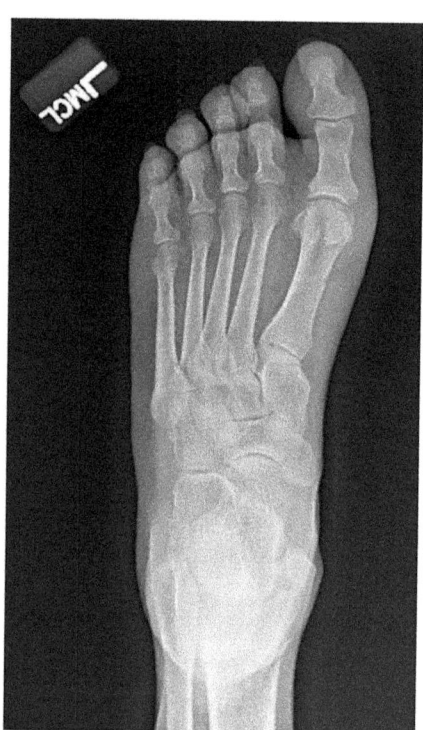

Figure 107.1

K. Results

Table 107.1 Results table

Test	Result	Test	Result
Complete blood count:		**Liver function panel:**	
WBC	$8.9 \times 10^3/\mu L$	AST	23 U/L
Hct	41.5%	ALT	26 U/L
Plt	$380 \times 10^3/\mu L$	Alk phos	42 U/L
		T bili	1.0 mg/dL
Basic metabolic panel:		D bili	0.3 mg/dL
Na	138 mEq/L	Amylase	50 U/L
K	4.3 mEq/L	Lipase	25 U/L
Cl	105 mEq/L	Albumin	4.7 g/dL
CO_2	24 mEq/L		
BUN	12 mEq/dL	**Urinalysis:**	
Cr	1.1 mg/dL	SG	1.020
Gluc	100 mg/dL	pH	7
		Prot	Neg
Coagulation panel:		Gluc	Neg
PT	12.6 sec	Ketones	Neg
PTT	26.0 sec	Bili	Neg

Table 107.1 (cont.)

Test	Result	Test	Result
INR	1.0	Blood	Neg
		LE	Neg
		Nitrite	Neg
		Color	Yellow

a. Serum uric acid: 9.0 mg/dL
b. ESR (if ordered): 4 mm/h
c. CRP (if ordered): 0.8 mg/L
d. Synovial fluid results
   i. Color: cloudy, WBC: 13,000/μL, PMN: 60%
   ii. Gram stain: no organisms seen
   iii. Crystals: negatively birefringent needle-shaped crystals present

L. Action

a. Meds
   i. NSAID and colchicine
b. Disposition
   i. Discharge home with instructions regarding gout

M. Diagnosis

a. Acute gout

N. Critical actions

a. Aspiration of joint to rule out septic arthritis
b. Pain management
c. Counseling on alcohol reduction

O. Examiner instructions

a. This is a case of acute gout of the first metatarsal–phalangeal joint of the left foot – an inflammatory reaction caused by the precipitation of uric acid crystals in the joint. This is a typical presentation of gout, with acute pain evolving over several hours, in a patient who is otherwise healthy and clinically appears well. In any patient presenting with pain and inflammation of a joint limiting ROM, it is imperative to rule out septic arthritis, which can lead to severe long-term joint damage if left untreated. This is accomplished by performing an arthrocentesis and confirming the presence of negatively birefringent crystals in the synovial fluid aspirate. Patients with crystal-induced arthropathy secondary to gout frequently have a normal serum uric acid level and may show a mild elevation of other serum inflammatory markers, including ESR and CRP. X-ray imaging will help to rule out other forms of arthritis, underlying trauma, or osteomyelitis. Patients may also present with low-grade fever and severely limited joint range of motion, further demonstrating the need for arthrocentesis to exclude septic joint and confirm the diagnosis.
b. Disposition is contingent on the exclusion of septic arthritis and adequate analgesia, with first-line medications including NSAIDs and colchicine in the acute setting.
c. Patient should be counseled on alcohol cessation as this is likely contributing to his gout.

P. Pearls

a. Gout occurs in middle-aged male patients much more frequently than in female patients. The majority of patients initially present with monoarticular disease, typically in the lower extremity. Polyarticular disease is more common in recurrences.

b. Acute attacks may be triggered by trauma, surgery, malnutrition, or overconsumption of meat, fish, and/or alcohol.

c. Microscopy of the joint aspirate is the key to diagnosis of gout or pseudogout. In both conditions, crystals are present. However, uric acid crystals in gout are needle-shaped and negatively birefringent, whereas the calcium pyrophosphate crystals of pseudogout are rhomboid-shaped and positively birefringent.

d. Serum uric acid levels are of low utility in the diagnosis of gout, as levels may be normal in many patients. Erythrocyte sedimentation rate is also low-yield in differentiating between crystal-induced arthropathy and septic arthritis, as levels may be elevated in both conditions.

e. NSAID treatment with indomethacin is first-line therapy for gout.

f. With pain refractory to NSAID therapy, colchicine may be administered. Higher doses of colchicine are associated with nausea, vomiting, and diarrhea. Dose reduction may be indicated in renal or hepatic impairment.

g. Prednisone is an option in patients with renal insufficiency where NSAIDs are contraindicated but should be avoided in patients with diabetes. Narcotics may be used as needed for additional pain control.

h. Patients who appear clinically toxic, in whom adequate analgesia is not achieved, or in whom a septic arthritis cannot be ruled out should be admitted for initiation of IV antibiotics until culture results become available.

i. If discharged from the ED, patient should have outpatient follow-up, as long-term therapy with allopurinol or probenecid may be necessary to prevent further attacks.

j. Patient should receive counseling regarding diet and lifestyle changes to reduce the chance of gout recurrence.

Q. Figure legends

a. Figure 107.1 (X-ray) Normal left foot x-ray.

R. References

a. *Tintinalli's Emergency Medicine: A Comprehensive Study Guide* (9th ed.): Chapter 284, Joints and Bursae.

b. *Rosen's Emergency Medicine: Concepts and Clinical Practice* (10th ed.): Chapter 102, Arthritis.

S. Acknowledgements

a. We would like to acknowledge Mieka Close for their contribution to this chapter in the previous edition of this book, which has been updated by Marianne Juarez

Neck Pain

Nicole Munz, DO and Evelyn Chow, MD

A. Chief complaint
a. 28-year-old female presents with headache, neck pain, and intermittent loss of vision in her right eye

B. Vital signs
a. BP: 124/73, HR: 86, R: 18, T: 36.9°C, Sat: 99% on RA

C. What does the patient look like?
a. Patient appears stated age, appears uncomfortable due to pain, in mild distress; lying supine on stretcher holding her head.

D. Primary survey
a. Airway: speaking in full sentences
b. Breathing: no apparent respiratory distress, no cyanosis
c. Circulation: dry and cool skin, normal capillary refill

E. Action
a. Oxygen via NC as needed to maintain saturation >95%
b. Peripheral IV access
c. Labs
    i. CBC, BMP, LFT, coagulation studies, blood type and crossmatch, lactate, urine hCG
d. Monitor: BP: 118/74, HR: 93, RR: 18, Sat: 100% on RA
e. EKG

F. History
a. HPI: A 28-year-old female who presents with 5 days of persistent right-sided neck pain and headache since participating in an advanced-level hot yoga class. Her class involved head stands and spine stretches with a partner. For the past two days, she has had intermittent painless darkening of the vision of her right eye lasting 10–30 minutes. She reports her vision is currently at baseline. She denies fever, photophobia, slurred speech, weakness, numbness, dizziness, nausea, vomiting, or bowel or bladder changes. She denies a history of migraines or similar headache in the past. Patient was seen at an outside hospital immediately after the yoga class for headache and had a normal head CT. She was discharged with concussion instructions.
b. PMHx: none
c. PSHx: appendectomy
d. Allergies: none

    e. Meds: none

    f. Social: social drinker, denies tobacco or drug use

    g. FHx: not relevant

    h. PMD: none

G. Nurse

    a. EKG (Figure 108.1)

    b. Urine pregnancy test negative

    c. Patient reporting worsening headache and another episode of darkening in her right eye with decreased vision

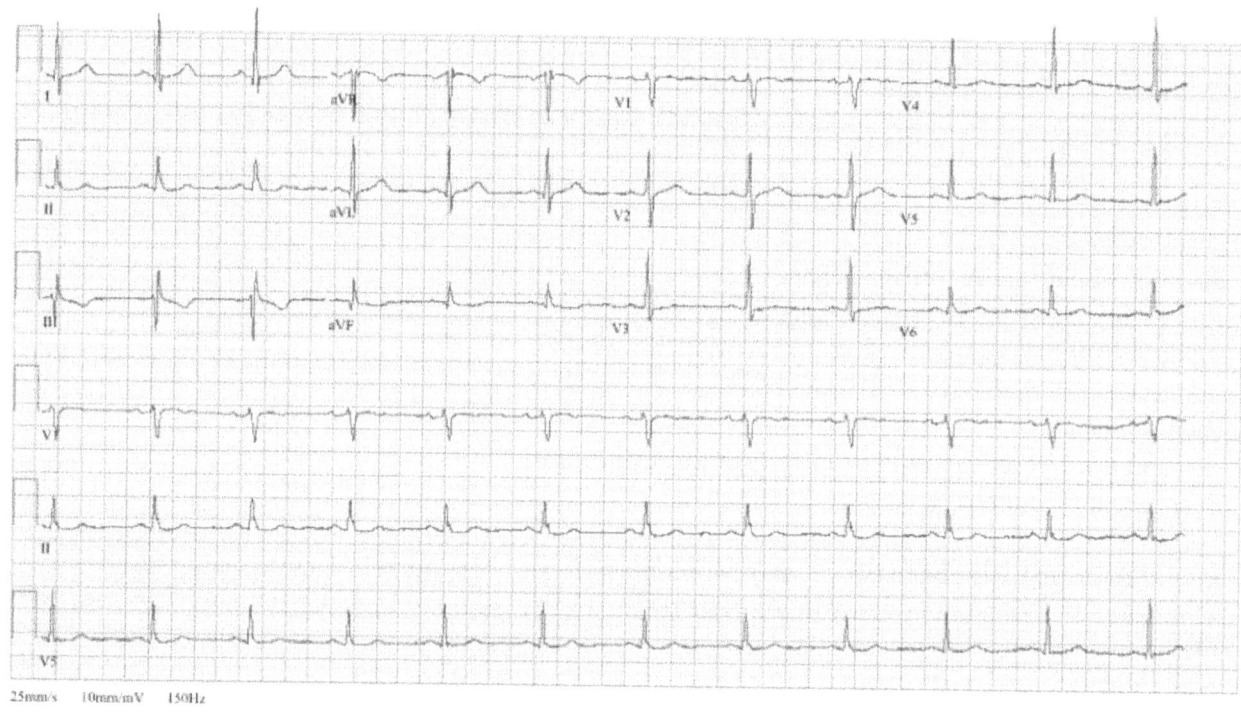

Figure 108.1

H. Secondary survey

    a. General: alert, oriented × 3, holding head and neck, in moderate distress due to pain

    b. Head: normocephalic, atraumatic

    c. Eyes: right ptosis, right pupil 2 mm, left pupils 4 mm, extraocular movements intact bilaterally, visually acuity 20/100 right eye and 20/20 left eye

    d. Ears: normal tympanic membranes

    e. Nose: normal

    f. Neck: right paraspinal neck tenderness, no midline tenderness, right carotid bruit (must ask)

    g. Pharynx: normal dentition, no lesions, no swelling

    h. Chest: nontender

i. Lungs: clear bilaterally
j. Heart: regular rate and rhythm, no murmurs, rubs, or gallops
k. Abdomen: soft, nontender, no rebound or guarding, no bruising, normal bowel sounds
l. Rectal: hemoccult negative brown stool, normal rectal tone
m. Urogenital: deferred
n. Extremities: full range of motion, no deformity, no edema, no tenderness, normal pulses
o. Back: nontender, no bruising
p. Neuro: alert, oriented × 3, right ptosis, right pupil 2 mm, left pupils 4 mm, extraocular movements intact bilaterally, no facial droop, sensation intact, 5/5 motor in all extremities, normal deep tendon reflexes, normal gait, no cerebellar findings
q. Skin: warm and dry
r. Lymph: no lymphadenopathy

I. Action
a. Meds
    i. Analgesia
b. Reassess
    i. Vision returning to baseline
c. Consult
    i. Neurology
d. Imaging
    i. CT brain noncontrast
    ii. CT cervical spine
    iii. CT neck with angiography or MRA neck

J. Nurse
a. Patient reports decreased pain after pain medication

K. Results

Table 108.1 Results table

Test	Result	Test	Result
Complete blood count:		**Liver function panel:**	
WBC	$9.1 \times 10^3/\mu L$	AST	23 U/L
Hct	42.9%	ALT	19 U/L
Plt	$345 \times 10^3/\mu L$	Alk phos	47 U/L
		T bili	0.7 mg/dL
		D bili	0.1 mg/dL
Basic metabolic panel:		Amylase	40 U/L
Na	139 mEq/L	Lipase	20 U/L
K	4.1 mEq/L	Albumin	4.1 g/dL
Cl	105 mEq/L		
CO_2	30 mEq/L		
BUN	13 mEq/dL	**Urinalysis:**	
Cr	1.1 mg/dL	SG	1.010

Table 108.1 (cont.)

Test	Result	Test	Result
Gluc	102 mg/dL	pH	7
		Prot	Neg
Coagulation panel:		Gluc	Neg
PT	13.1 sec	Ketones	Neg
PTT	26 sec	Bili	Neg
INR	1.0	Blood	Neg
		LE	Neg
		Nitrite	Neg
		Color	Yellow

a. Lactate: 1.5 mmol/L
b. CT brain (Figure 108.2)
c. CT cervical spine: normal
d. CTA neck or MRA neck: dissection of carotid artery on the right side

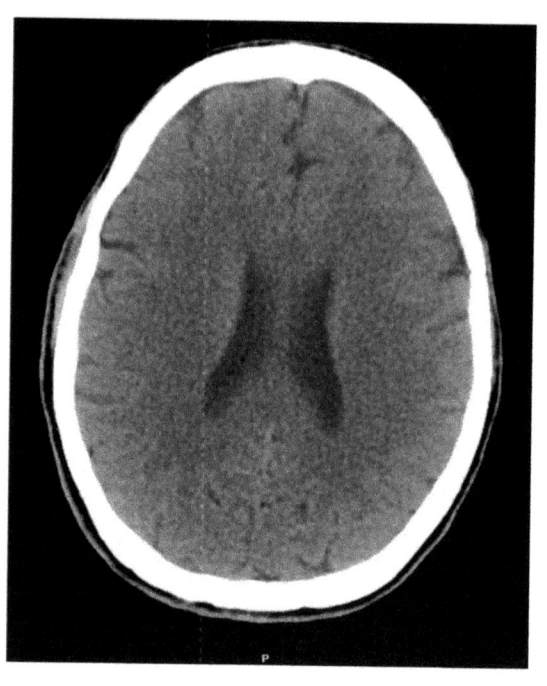

Figure 108.2

L. Action

a. Heparin
    i.   If patient is not started on anticoagulation, they will develop slurred speech and left-sided hemiparesis consistent with acute stroke in the right middle cerebral artery distribution.
    ii. If patient started on anticoagulation before obtaining CT brain, they will acutely deteriorate, becoming obtunded, nonverbal, and withdrawing only to painful stimuli, and the case diagnosis will be massive subarachnoid hemorrhage.
b. Admit patient to neurology or medicine service with frequent neurologic checks
c. Discussion with patient regarding diagnosis and treatment plan

M. Diagnosis

a. Carotid artery dissection

N. Critical actions

a. Pain control
b. CT head noncontrast
c. CT neck with angiography or MRA neck
d. Neurology consult
e. Heparin

O. Examiner instructions

a. This is a case of carotid artery dissection secondary to a neck injury from aggressive manipulation in stretching. The injury caused a tearing of the wall of the internal carotid artery that led to TIA/stroke symptoms with visual changes. Important actions in this case include imaging of the brain and cervical arteries (carotid and vertebral). If carotid artery dissection is not considered in the differential and the patient is not started on heparin, the patient will develop a right middle cerebral artery stroke with slurred speech and left-hemiparesis. If anticoagulation is started before obtaining a CT brain, patient will become obtunded.

P. Pearls

a. Cervical artery dissection (carotid artery and vertebral artery) is rare overall, but a common cause (10–25% of cases) of stroke in patients under 50 years old.
b. Dissection can occur spontaneously or secondary to neck trauma such as an auto collision, as well as minor trauma such as chiropractic manipulation of the neck.
c. Patients with internal carotid artery dissection often present with unilateral headache, face pain, or neck pain hours to days before developing neurologic deficits.
d. Neurologic signs and symptoms of carotid artery dissection can include transient monocular blindness, cranial nerve palsies, or partial Horner syndrome (ptosis and miosis without anhidrosis).
e. Vertebral artery dissection often presents with occipital headache and posterior neck pain preceding neurologic symptoms consistent with brainstem TIA or stroke.
f. Dissection can cause transient (TIA) or persistent (stroke) signs and symptoms.
g. If not treated, carotid artery dissection can progress to MCA territory stroke. Vertebral artery dissection can progress to a posterior circulation stroke.
h. If the dissection in extracranial, then treatment involves anticoagulation to prevent thrombotic events.
i. Do not start anticoagulation if the dissection is intracranial: this can lead to a subarachnoid hemorrhage. In that case, an antiplatelet agent should be started.
j. Subarachnoid hemorrhage must be ruled out prior to starting anticoagulation.

Q. Figure legends

a. Figure 108.1 (EKG) Normal sinus rhythm; nonspecific lateral and inferior T wave changes.
b. Figure 108.2 (CT) Normal head CT.

R. References

a. *Tintinalli's Emergency Medicine: A Comprehensive Study Guide* (9th ed.): Chapter 167, Stroke Syndromes.
b. *Rosen's Emergency Medicine: Concepts and Clinical Practice* (10th ed.): Chapter 87, Stroke.

Abdominal Pain

Jeanne Noble, MD and Evelyn Chow, MD

A. Chief complaint
a. 78-year-old male sent from nursing home for abdominal pain and constipation

B. Vital signs
a. BP: 137/78, HR: 98, RR: 22, T: 36.9°C, Sat: 96% on RA

C. What does the patient look like?
a. Patient is an elderly male, awake and alert, appearing uncomfortable.

D. Action
a. Large-bore peripheral IV access
b. Labs
  i. CBC, BMP, LFT, coagulation studies, blood type and crossmatch, urinalysis
  ii. Lactate – preferably as part of point of care blood gas for quick results.
c. Monitor: BP: 137/78, HR: 98, RR: 22, Sat: 96% on RA
d. EKG

E. Primary survey
a. Airway: speaking in full sentences
b. Breathing: no respiratory distress
c. Circulation: warm skin, normal capillary refill

F. History
a. HPI: A 78-year-old male with a history of Parkinson's and hypertension sent from nursing home for worsening abdominal pain and distension for 1 week. His pain is colicky and worsens with eating. Patient complains of nausea and has vomited once in the past 24 hours. Patient has a history of constipation and reports that his last bowel movement was at least 1 week ago. He denies fevers or chills or any urinary symptoms.
b. PMHx: Parkinson's disease, hypertension
c. PSHx: none
d. Allergies: none
e. Meds: carbidopa-levodopa, metoprolol, docusate, senna
f. Social: resides in nursing home
g. FHx: no relevant history
h. PMD: nursing home doctor

G. Nurse
a. EKG (Figure 109.1)

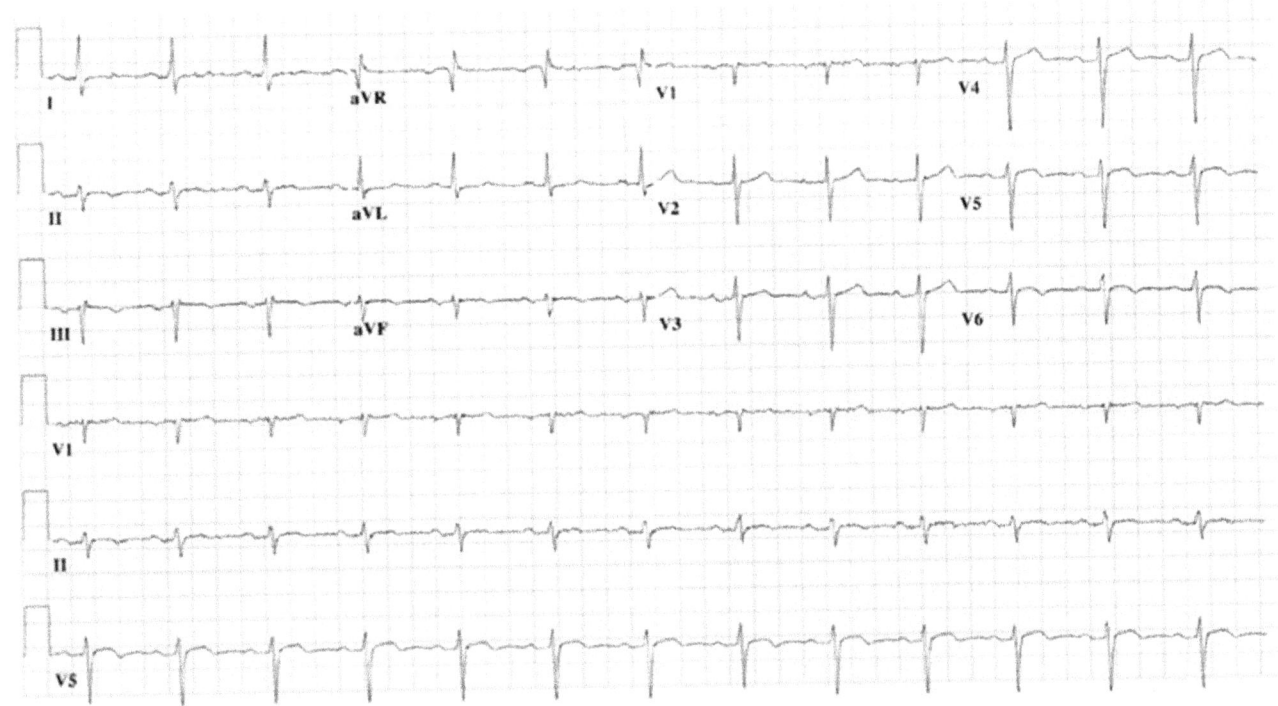

Figure 109.1

H. Physical examination
a. General: alert, oriented × 2 (baseline)
b. Head: normocephalic, atraumatic
c. Eyes: extraocular movement intact, pupils equal, reactive to light
d. Ears: normal tympanic membranes
e. Nose: no discharge
f. Neck: full range of motion, no jugular vein distension, no stridor
g. Pharynx: dry mucous membranes, normal dentition, no lesions or swelling
h. Chest: nontender
i. Lungs: clear bilaterally
j. Heart: mild tachycardia, regular rhythm, no murmurs, rubs, or gallops
k. Abdomen: soft but distended with tympanitic bowel sounds; diffuse tenderness to palpation without rebound or guarding
l. Rectal: normal tone, small amount of hard stool in rectal vault, occult blood negative
m. Urogenital: normal external genitalia
   i. Male: no discharge, normal testicular examination
n. Extremities: full range of motion, no deformity, normal pulses
o. Back: nontender
p. Neuro: cranial nerves II to XII intact; normal strength and sensation; bilateral resting tremor; normal reflexes
q. Skin: warm and dry
r. Lymph: no lymphadenopathy

I. Action
a. Meds
   i. Opioid analgesia (i.e., fentanyl for short-acting pain control during work-up)
b. Imaging: abdominal series (if CT abdomen/pelvis ordered, there is a delay in scanner)

J. Nurse

a. BP: 132/74, HR: 96, RR: 20, Sat: 96%

b. Abdominal series X-ray (Figure 109.2)

A

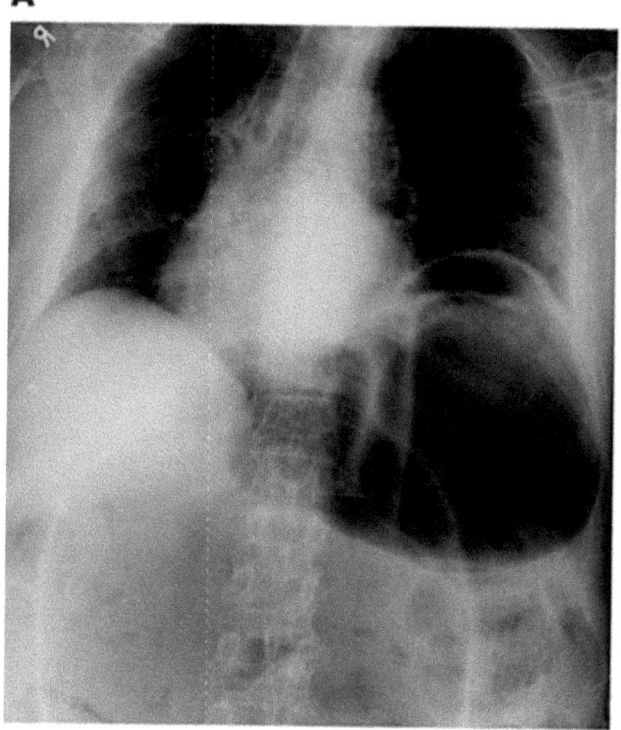

B

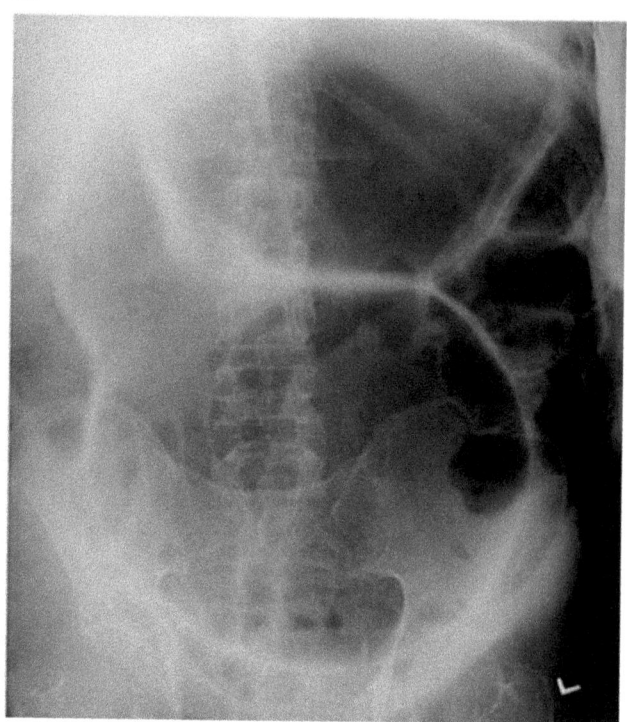

Figure 109.2

K. Action

a. Consult
  i. Gastroenterology
  ii. Surgery

b. Nasogastric tube

L. Results

Table 109.1 Results table

Test	Result	Test	Result
Complete blood count:		**Liver function panel:**	
WBC	$18 \times 10^3/\mu L$	AST	33 U/L
Hct	38%	ALT	42 U/L
Plt	$180 \times 10^3/\mu L$	Alk phos	42 U/L
		T bili	1.0 mg/dL
Basic metabolic panel:		D bili	0.3 mg/dL
Na	140 mEq/L	Amylase	50 U/L
K	4.3 mEq/L	Lipase	25 U/L
Cl	105 mEq/L	Albumin	4.7 g/dL

Table 109.1 (cont.)

Test	Result	Test	Result
CO_2	20 mEq/L	**Urinalysis:**	
BUN	29 mEq/dL	SG	1.030
Cr	1.2 mg/dL	pH	7
Gluc	75 mg/dL	Prot	Neg
		Gluc	Neg
Coagulation panel:		Ketones	Trace
PT	12.6 sec	Bili	Neg
PTT	26.0 sec	Blood	Neg
INR	1.0	LE	Neg
		Nitrite	Neg
		Color	Yellow

a. Lactate: 2.5 mmol/L

M. Action
a. Antibiotics (acceptable regimens include piperacillin/tazobactam or ciprofloxacin/metronidazole).
b. Gastroenterologist or surgeon performs decompressive sigmoidoscopy.
c. Patient is admitted for monitoring and bowel prep in anticipation of sigmoid resection by surgical service to prevent recurrence.

N. Diagnosis
a. Sigmoid volvulus

O. Critical actions
a. Pain control
b. IV line placement
c. Abdominal x-rays
d. Nasogastric tube
e. Consult gastroenterology and surgery

P. Examiner instructions
a. This is a case of sigmoid volvulus in a nursing home patient with chronic constipation. Volvulus is a twisting of the intestine, commonly occurring in the sigmoid colon, leading to severe pain and distension of the proximal bowel and ultimately to intestinal perforation if not treated. Important early actions include rapid imaging (abdominal plain films if CT is delayed), nasogastric tube placement, gastroenterology consult, and/or surgery consult for reduction by sigmoidoscopy or laparoscopy. If a CT scan is ordered, note that the scan will be delayed. If no alternative imaging is ordered, the patient will develop signs of perforation with worsening pain, guarding, and rebound on exam while awaiting CT. These peritoneal signs, suggestive of bowel necrosis, are a contraindication to sigmoidoscopy necessitating surgical intervention.

Q. Pearls

a. Sigmoid volvulus most commonly occurs in elderly, bedbound patients with psychiatric or neurologic disorders.

b. Chronic constipation and anticholinergic medications are risk factors for sigmoid volvulus.

c. Abdominal x-rays may demonstrate a distended U-shaped sigmoid colon extending from the pelvis to the upper quadrants, known as a "bent innertube" sign.

d. Given a high rate of recurrence (around 50%), most patients undergo definitive sigmoid resection even after successful endoscopic decompression.

e. Endoscopic decompression is contraindicated if signs of bowel necrosis are present (i.e., peritoneal signs, evidence of shock, WBC >20,000, elevated lactate); emergent operative resection is then indicated.

f. Mimics of sigmoid volvulus include colonic pseudo-obstruction (Ogilvie's syndrome), which typically lacks a transition point; toxic megacolon, usually accompanied by bloody diarrhea and a more toxic clinical picture; and small bowel obstruction, which is less well tolerated, having a more rapid time course and more prominent vomiting.

g. Small bowel obstruction is four times more common than large bowel obstruction.

R. Figure legends

a. Figure 109.1 (EKG) Normal sinus rhythm: nonspecific lateral and inferior T wave changes.

b. Figure 109.2 (a) (x-ray) Large bowel obstruction with massive dilation suggestive of volvulus. (b) Large bowel obstruction with massive dilation suggestive of volvulus

S. References

a. *Tintinalli's Emergency Medicine: A Comprehensive Study Guide* (9th ed.): Chapter 83, Bowel Obstruction.

b. *Rosen's Emergency Medicine: Concepts and Clinical Practice* (10th ed.): Chapter 81, Large Intestine.

Shortness of Breath

Jennifer Roh, MD

A. Chief complaint
a. 72-year-old man with shortness of breath

B. Vital signs
a. BP: 52/34 (MAP 40), HR: 110 (on the monitor), RR: 26, T: 36.6°C, Sat: 86% on room air

C. What does the patient look like?
a. The patient is a thin man, pale, diaphoretic, and sitting on a gurney. There is an alarm sound coming from a pack next to the patient (his left ventricular assist device [LVAD]).

D. Primary survey
a. Airway: speaking in full sentences
b. Breathing: tachypneic, in mild respiratory distress
c. Circulation: diaphoretic, cool, pale skin

E. Action
a. Oxygen via nonrebreather mask
b. Two large-bore peripheral IV lines
c. Manual MAP check using doppler/US
d. Labs
   i. CBC, BMP, LFT, coagulation studies, blood type and crossmatch
   ii. Troponin
   iii. BNP
e. Monitor: MAP: 40, HR: 110, RR: 26, T: 36.6°C
f. Order electrocardiogram
g. Order chest radiograph
h. Request bedside echocardiogram

F. History
a. HPI: A 72-year-old man presents with shortness of breath, lightheadedness, and generalized fatigue for the last 6 hours. He has associated diaphoresis. He denies nausea, vomiting, fevers, chills. He admits to a nonproductive cough for the same amount of time. He has noticed that his LVAD parameters have changed in the last 6 hours, with higher power readings and lower flow rates. He states he has been taking all his medications as prescribed.

    b. PMHx: congestive heart failure (if asked, the patient's wife will mention that she thinks that his last ejection fraction was 8%), coronary artery disease, hyperlipidemia

    c. PSHx: wife: "2 years ago he had a device placed in his chest to help his heart" (the candidate should ask specifically if it was a left ventricular assist device; if it is specifically asked, the proctor should answer yes, it was implanted 2 years ago). Two drug eluting stents were placed 3 years ago to the LAD and left circumflex arteries

    d. Allergies: none

    e. Meds: carvedilol, furosemide, enalapril, simvastatin, aspirin, warfarin

    f. Social: denies drug or alcohol use; quit tobacco 3 years ago

    g. FHx: father died of MI at age 60; mother died of MI at 55

    h. Cardiologist: Dr. Shah

G. Secondary survey

    a. General: alert, oriented × 3, diaphoretic, in mild respiratory distress

    b. Head: normocephalic, atraumatic

    c. Eyes: extraocular movement intact, pupils equal and reactive to light

    d. Ears: normal tympanic membranes

    e. Pharynx: no erythema or exudates

    f. Neck: soft, supple, moderate jugular venous distension to angle of the jaw

    g. Chest: nontender to palpation, well-healed sternotomy scar

    h. Lungs: crackles at bilateral bases to mid-lung fields

    i. Heart: mechanical whirring

    j. Abdomen: soft, nontender to palpation, LVAD catheter exiting at RUQ is clean, dry, and secure

    k. Extremities: full range of motion, no deformity, no palpable pulses, 2+ pitting edema to the thighs bilaterally

    l. Neuro: cranial nerves II–XII intact; normal sensation and strength, normal reflexes, gait not tested

    m. Skin: cool and diaphoretic, no rashes

    n. Lymph: no lymphadenopathy

    o. Rectal: brown stool, no gross blood, melena or hemorrhoids and fecal occult blood testing is negative

H. Action

    a. Electrocardiogram (Figure 110.1)

    b. Chest radiograph (Figure 110.2)

    c. Meds:

        i. Heparin drip

    d. Consult

        i. VAD coordinator

        ii. Cardiology or the heart failure service

        iii. Cardiothoracic surgery

Case 110: Shortness of Breath

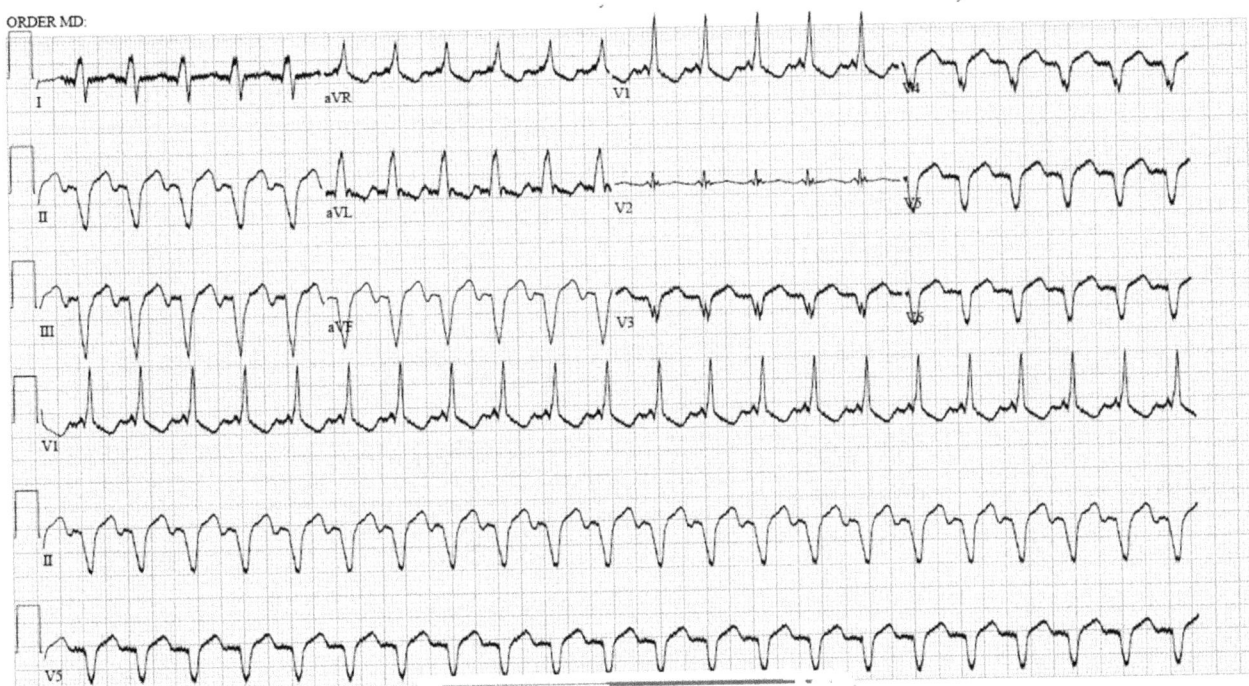

Figure 110.1

Figure 110.2

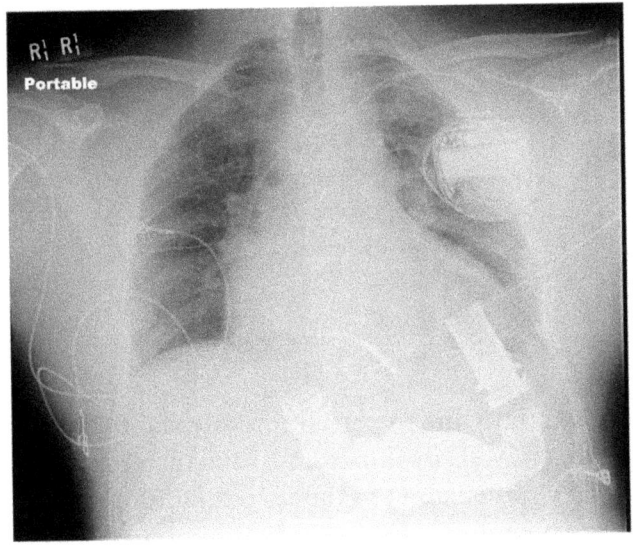

I. Results

Table 110.1 Results table

Test	Result	Test	Result
Complete blood count:		**Coagulation panel:**	
WBC	$11.1 \times 10^3/\mu L$	INR	1.7
Hgb	9.3		
Hct	28%	**Liver function panel:**	
Plt	$186 \times 10^3/\mu L$	LDH	3880 U/L

Table 110.1 (cont.)

Test	Result	Test	Result
		Albumin	3.8 g/dL
Basic metabolic panel:		D bili	0.5 mg/dL
Na	134 mEq/L	Indirect bili	2.5 mg/dL
K	3.5 mEq/L	AST	35 U/L
Cl	104 mEq/L	ALT	38 U/L
CO_2	24 mEq/L	Alk phos	106 U/L
BUN	20 mEq/dL		
Cr	1.7 mg/dL	**Urinalysis:**	
Glucose	96 mg/dL	Urobilinogen	+
		Color	Yellow

a. Troponin I: 0.143 ng/mL
b. BNP: 977 pg/mL
c. Portable echocardiogram demonstrates ejection fraction less than 15%, small pericardial effusion

J. Diagnosis
a. Cardiogenic shock due to partial pump thrombosis of the LVAD

K. Critical actions
a. Electrocardiogram
b. Bedside echocardiogram
c. Heparin drip
d. VAD coordinator or CT surgery consult or cardiology consult

L. Examiner instructions
a. This is a case of cardiogenic shock caused by LVAD failure due to partial thrombosis in the device pump. The candidate should recognize signs of LVAD dysfunction by the history and on the physical examination, and look for causes of hypotension as related to the LVAD. High power readings, low h/h and elevated LDH indicate hemolysis and possible thrombosis.
b. Absent peripheral pulses and mechanical whirring indicate that the LVAD is working enough to create flow, but not effectively enough to create a sufficient MAP. If a palpable pulse was present on exam this would indicate a much more significant thrombus was causing severe obstruction of the continuous flow of the LVAD, thus allowing the native heart conduction and contraction process to create a peripheral pulse.
c. A negative rectal and no history of melena should help rule out GI bleeding hypovolemic hypotension, which is a common LVAD complication.
d. The subtherapeutic INR puts the patients at risk for LVAD thrombosis and device failure. The candidate should also recognize laboratory findings consistent with hemolysis are a sign of pump thrombosis.
e. Once LVAD thrombosis or malfunction is recognized, the candidate should initiate anticoagulation with heparin and also alert the VAD coordinator (or alternatively contact the

heart failure or cardiology service). The candidate should also consult cardiothoracic surgery to request evaluation of lysing or extracting the pump thrombus.

M. Pearls

a. Patients with LVAD are at risk for thrombosis.
   i. Anticoagulated patients with therapeutic INR are still at risk for thrombosis.
   ii. Patients with VAD thrombosis will see an increase in device power readings but decreased flow readings on their device console.
   iii. Patients with pump failure will present with signs of heart failure.
   iv. Pump thrombosis may elicit elevated troponins and elevated BNP as well as laboratory findings consistent with hemolysis, including elevated LDH and indirect bilirubin.

N. Figure legends

a. Figure 110.1 (EKG) Right bundle branch block with left anterior hemiblock (courtesy of Atman P. Shah, MD).
b. Figure 110.2 (CXR) Cardiomegaly, VAD, implantable device with single RV lead, interstitial edema (courtesy of Atman P. Shah, MD).

O. References

a. *Tintinalli's Emergency Medicine: A Comprehensive Study Guide* (9th ed.): Chapter 297, The Transplant Patient.
b. *Rosen's Emergency Medicine: Concepts and Clinical Practice* (10th ed.): Chapter 66, Implantable Cardiac Devices.

P. Acknowledgements

a. We would like to acknowledge Tarlan Hedayati for their contribution to this chapter in the previous edition of this book, which has been updated by Jennifer Roh

Arm Pain

Kiyetta Alade, MD, MEd

A. Chief complaint
a. 3-year-old male with left arm pain

B. Vital signs
a. BP: 88/54, HR: 110, RR: 24, T: 37°C, Sat: 99% on RA, Wt: 15 kg

C. What does the patient look like?
a. Patient appears stated age, not using his left arm while exploring the exam room. No apparent distress.

D. Primary survey
a. Airway: speaking in full sentences
b. Breathing: no apparent respiratory distress, no cyanosis, clear lungs
c. Circulation: normal skin color, radial pulses 2+ bilaterally, normal capillary refill
d. Neuro: alert and oriented × 3, follows command

E. Action
a. Obtain history of events immediately preceding onset of pain.
b. Pain control with ibuprofen (10 mg/kg).
c. Radiography not necessary at this point.

F. History
a. HPI: A 3-year-old male with a history of reactive airway disease presents with parents to the ED, refusing to move his left arm and complaining of left wrist pain. Parents state they were at the park and when walking to the car the patient began to have a tantrum, trying to throw himself to the ground. Fortunately, dad was holding his left hand, so he did not hit the ground hard and there was no head injury. He immediately began to cry complaining of left wrist pain. No other trauma noted at the park.
b. PMHx: reactive airway disease, no previous history of broken bones or other similar events
c. PSHx: none
d. Allergies: none
e. Meds: albuterol as needed
f. Social: lives with both parents, no tobacco exposure in the home
g. FHx: no history of easily broken bones
h. PMD: local pediatrician that he sees annually
i. Immunizations: up to date

G. Nurse

a. No intervention

H. Secondary survey

a. General: awake, appropriate for age, cries only with exam of left arm
b. HEENT: oropharynx with 2+ tonsils but no exudate or erythema, otherwise normal
c. Neck: normal
d. Chest: normal
e. Heart: normal
f. Abdomen: normal
g. MSK: Left upper extremity adducted, slightly flexed at the elbow with forearm pronated. 2+ radial pulses. No visible swelling at elbow, wrist, or hand. Screams with attempts to examine left arm but no focal bony tenderness. Right arm and bilateral lower extremities, normal exam
h. Back: normal
i. Neuro: sensation normal for age; he refuses to participate in any movement of the left hand, wrist, elbow or shoulder
j. Skin: no rash or wounds noted
k. Lymph: normal
l. GU: deferred
m. Rectal: deferred

I. Action

a. Reduction maneuvers
   i. Ideally the candidate should be able to describe two reduction maneuvers (supination and flexion, as well as hyperpronation). The first attempt should fail, and the second attempt using a different approach should succeed (as long as it is described correctly).
   ii. If the second attempt is unsuccessful as well, the candidate may order imaging of left elbow and forearm (Figure 111.1).
   iii. The third attempted reduction (if imaging is ordered) is successful.
   iv. After successful reduction, re-evaluate function in 5–10 minutes (normal function now)
      1. Supination and flexion: Explain the procedure to the parent. The parent can gently restrain the patient in their lap. Grab the patient's affected hand as if going to shake it. Place your other hand on the patient's affected elbow with thumb over the radial head and annular ligament with the elbow slightly flexed. In a continuous motion, gently distract the elbow, supinate the hand, and flex the elbow until the hand is up to their shoulder. You should feel a "pop" during flexion, under your thumb that is over the radial head.
      2. Hyperpronation: Explain the procedure to the parent. The parent can gently restrain the patient in their lap. Grab the patient's affected hand as if going to shake it. Place your other hand on the patient's affected elbow with thumb over the radial head and annular ligament with the elbow slightly flexed. While applying pressure to the radial head, distract the elbow and hyperpronate by rotating the hand on the affected side medially. You should feel a "pop" under the finger that is over the radial head.

J. Diagnosis

a. Radial head subluxation (nursemaid's elbow)

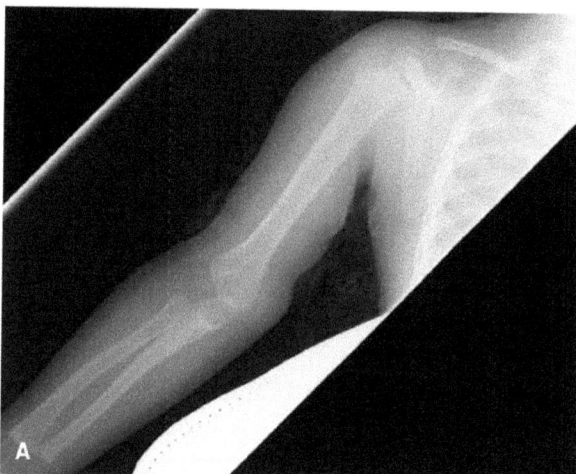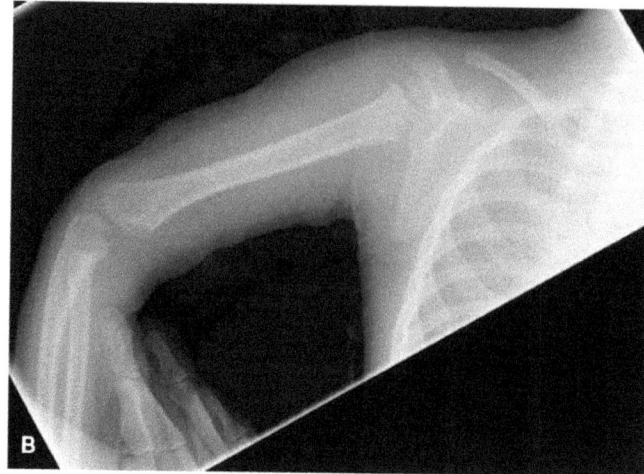

Figure 111.1

K. Critical actions

a. X-ray prior to attempted manual reduction is not necessary as long as the history and physical are consistent with radial head subluxation.
b. Attempt manual reduction.
c. Re-evaluate function 5–10 minutes after successful reduction.

L. Examiner instructions

a. This is a case of radial subluxation. This is one of the most common causes of traumatic injury to the upper extremity, occurring most often in children up to 5 years of age. It occurs by applying axial traction to the upper extremity and causes part of the annular ligament to slip over the radial head, where it gets trapped in the radiohumeral joint. This can occur by pulling, lifting, or swinging the patient by the hands. Radial head subluxation causes the child to refuse to move the affected extremity due to pain that they may localize anywhere between the elbow and the hand. The exterior exam of the affected extremity is normal. The child guards the affected extremity but is usually comfortable unless the affected arm is manipulated in any way. With a classic history like the one provided, there is no indication for labs or radiologic imaging prior to an attempt at manual reduction. There are two main maneuvers for attempted reduction that are described in detail above. If presenting within 4–6 hours of subluxation, function should return within 5–10 minutes after manual reduction. Recovery of function may be longer for those with greater than 4–6 hours of subluxation. If these methods of reduction fail, x-rays of the elbow and forearm may be obtained but will be normal in the setting of a nursemaid's elbow. Repeat attempts at manual reduction are appropriate after normal x-rays have ruled out a bony injury. When presented with a classic history for a radial head subluxation, failed manual reduction and normal x-rays, patients can be discharged home with a sling and follow-up as spontaneous reduction will likely occur. Recommend follow-up if patient refuses to use the arm the next day.

M. Pearls

a. Radial head subluxation (nursemaid's elbow) is a clinical diagnosis.
b. The classic presentation is a child refusing to move the arm, with the elbow pronated, slightly flexed, and held close to their side.

c. Radiologic imaging is not indicated when the history and clinical exam are classic, but imaging should be obtained if the history is unusual or proper attempts at manual reduction are unsuccessful.

d. The two most commonly used reduction techniques are supination and flexion or hyperpronation.

e. Hyperpronation has been found to be slightly less painful and more successful on the first attempt at reduction.

N. Figure legends

a. Figure 111.1 (X-ray) Right elbow x-ray.

O. References

a. *Tintinalli's Emergency Medicine: A Comprehensive Study Guide* (9th ed.): Chapter 143C, Pediatric Procedures: Nursemaid's Elbow Reduction.

b. *Rosen's Emergency Medicine: Concepts and Clinical Practice* (10th ed.): Chapter 44, Humerus and Elbow.

Altered Mental Status

Raashee Kedia, MD

A. Chief complaint

a. 88-year-old female with altered mental status

B. Vital signs

a. BP: 88/56, HR: 118, RR: 20, T: 38.6°C, Sat: 99% on RA

C. What does the patient look like?

a. Patient is a frail elderly female, eyes closed and not speaking

D. Primary survey

a. Airway: able to state her name and answer yes/no to questions
b. Breathing: no apparent respiratory distress, no cyanosis
c. Circulation: warm and diaphoretic skin, delayed capillary refill, equal peripheral pulses

E. History

a. HPI: An 88-year-old bed-bound female from a nursing home with decreased verbal responsiveness for 2 days. Decreased oral intake. Patient is usually talkative and able to feed herself.
b. PMHx: hypertension
c. PSHx: nonoperable left hip fracture 6 months earlier
d. Meds: lisinopril (held for last 2 days due to low blood pressure)
e. Allergies: none
f. Social: denies drug, alcohol, or tobacco use; good family support system
g. FHx: noncontributory
h. PMD: Dr. Marks

F. Secondary survey

a. General: lying with eyes closed, opens eyes to verbal stimulation, responds yes/no appropriately to questions
b. HEENT: atraumatic, no facial droop
c. Eyes: pupils equal, round, and reactive; sunken eyes; extraocular movements intact, fundi sharp, no papilledema
d. Ears: normal tympanic membranes
e. Nose: no discharge
f. Neck: full range of motion, supple, no jugular vein distension, no stridor
g. Pharynx: normal dentition, no lesions, no tonsillar swelling, dry mucosa
h. Chest: nontender, no crepitus
i. Lungs: clear bilaterally
j. Heart: tachycardic, regular rhythm, no murmurs, rubs, or gallops

k. Abdomen: normal bowel sounds, soft, nontender, nondistended
l. Rectal: normal tone, brown stool, occult blood negative
m. Back: stage 4 decubitus ulcer with purulent drainage and surrounding erythema
n. Extremities: left leg slightly shorter than right leg; full range of motion of upper and right lower extremities; equal strength in upper extremities; unable to move left hip but able to move left ankle and wiggle toes; mild tenderness over left hip, no overlying skin changes; pulses equal in all extremities
o. Neuro: cranial nerves II to XII intact; normal sensation
p. Skin: warm and diaphoretic
q. Lymph: no lymphadenopathy

G. Action
a. Two large-bore peripheral IV lines
b. Labs
   i. CBC, BMP, lactate, venous blood gas, PT/PTT/INR, blood culture, urinalysis, urine culture
   ii. Finger stick glucose: 125 mg/dL
c. Monitor: BP: 88/56, HR: 118, RR: 20
d. 2 L NS bolus
e. Imaging
   i. CXR (Figure 112.1)
   ii. X-ray left hip
   iii. CT head (patient too unstable to go to radiology)
f. Meds
   i. Vancomycin 1 g IV
   ii. Acetaminophen 650 mg PO

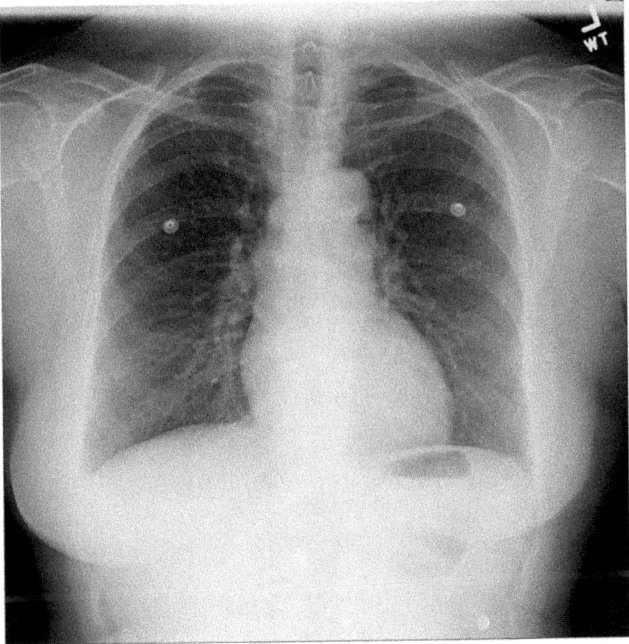

Figure 112.1

H. Nurse
a. EKG (Figure 112.2)
b. Foley catheter
c. Rectal temperature: 39.7°C

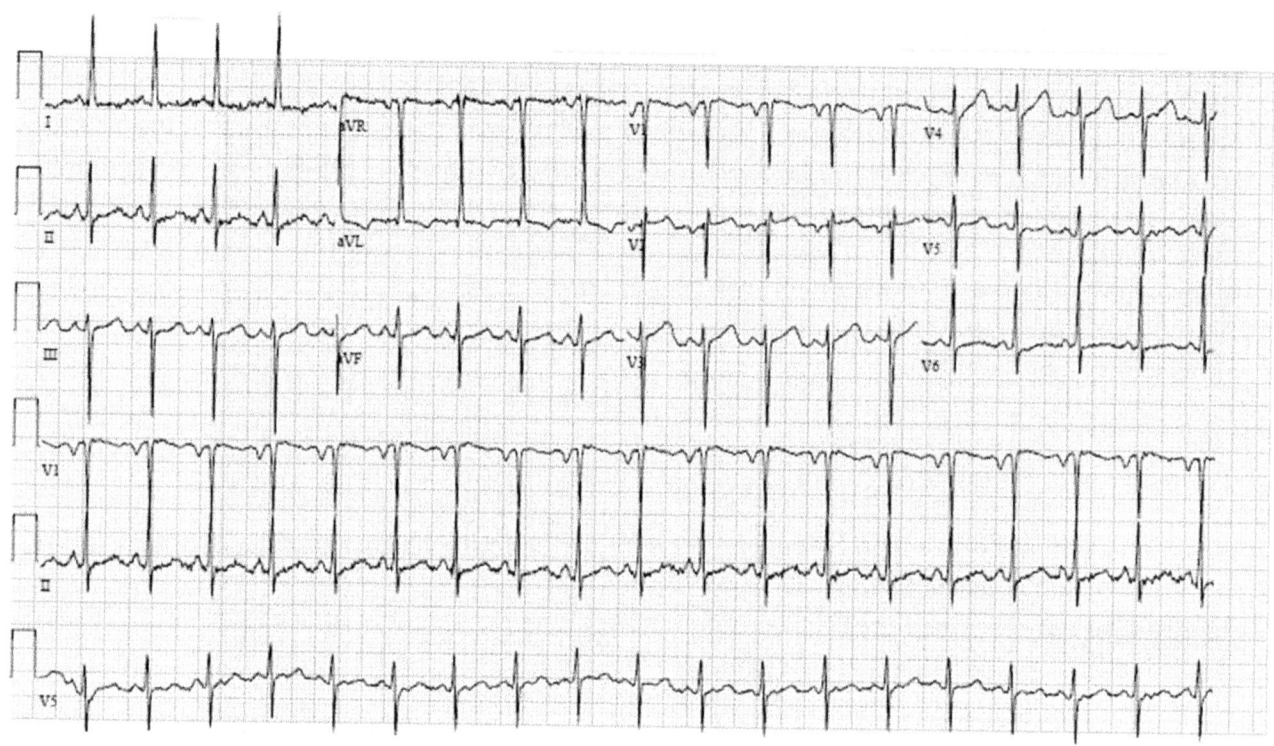

Figure 112.2

I. Results

Table 112.1 Results table

Test	Result	Test	Result
Complete blood count:		**Urinalysis:**	
WBC	$15.3 \times 10^3/\mu L$	SG	1.025
Hgb	8	pH	6
Hct	24.1%	Prot	Neg
Plt	$45 \times 10^3/\mu L$	Gluc	Neg
		Ketones	Neg
		Bili	Neg
Basic metabolic panel:		Blood	Moderate
Na	138 mEq/L	LE	Neg
K	3.8 mEq/L	Nitrite	Neg
Cl	100 mEq/L	Color	Yellow
CO_2	21 mEq/L		
BUN	38 mEq/dL		
Cr	2.0 mg/dL	**Blood gas:**	
Gluc	128 mg/dL	pH	7.30
		pCO_2	44 mmHg

Table 112.1 (cont.)

Test	Result	Test	Result
Coagulation panel:		pO_2	40 mmHg
PT	34 sec (10–12 sec)		
PTT	72 sec (30–45 sec)		
INR	1.3		

a. Hip X-ray: old left intertrochanteric fracture, no acute fracture

J. Action

a. Labs
   i. Recheck PT/PTT/INR, add fibrinogen, D-dimer
b. Reassess vitals
   i. If no IV fluids given: BP: 70/48, HR: 128, RR: 20
   ii. If 1 L IV fluids given: BP: 100/72, HR: 103, RR: 20
   iii. If 2 L IV fluids given: BP: 122/78, HR: 96, RR: 20
c. Recheck lactate
   i. If no IV fluids given: lactate = 6.5 mmol/L
   ii. If 1 L IV fluids given: lactate = 4.0 mmol/L
   iii. If 2 L IV fluids given: lactate = 2.5 mmol/L
d. Recheck mental status
   i. If no IV fluids given: patient more lethargic with decreased responsiveness
   ii. If IV fluids given: patient more alert and talkative

K. Results

Table 112.2 Coagulation panel results table

Test	Result
PT	34 sec (10–12 sec)
PTT	72 sec (30–45 sec)
INR	1.3
D-dimer:	>500 mmol/L
Fibrinogen:	<100 mmol/L

L. Action

a. Administer 1 unit platelets, 2 units FFP.
b. Administer vitamin K 10 mg subq and folate 1 mg IV.
c. Admit to ICU.

M. Diagnosis

a. Sepsis from decubitus ulcer causing disseminated intravascular coagulation (DIC)

N. Critical actions

a. Fluid resuscitation
b. Finding source of sepsis as decubitus ulcer
c. Antibiotic administration
d. Recheck lactate
e. Recognize DIC

O. Examiner instructions

a. This patient has an overwhelming systemic infection (sepsis) due to a skin infection on her back (decubitus ulcer). The ulcer developed from continued pressure on her skin from being immobile due to her hip fracture 6 months ago. This patient arrives already decompensated; she is tachycardic, febrile, hypotensive, and has altered mental status. She needs immediate care, including fluid and antibiotic administration.

P. Pearls

a. If there is no improvement in blood pressure after fluid administration (up to 3–5 L of crystalloid), dopamine should be titrated to appropriate blood pressure response.
b. In persistent hypotension despite fluid resuscitation, adrenal insufficiency should be suspected and glucocorticoid should be administered (hydrocortisone 100 mg IV).
c. When the source of sepsis is unknown, empiric antibiotic therapy against Gram-positive and Gram-negative organisms should be started.
d. Persistent severe acidosis can be treated with sodium bicarbonate 1 mEq/kg IV.
e. DIC is a possible complication of severe sepsis. DIC should be treated with fresh frozen plasma and platelets, keep PT 1.5–2 times normal and platelet counts to at least 50,000/µL.

Q. Figure legends

a. Figure 112.1 (CXR) Normal chest x-ray.
b. Figure 112.2 (EKG) Sinus tachycardia.

R. References

a. *Tintinalli's Emergency Medicine: A Comprehensive Study Guide* (9th ed.): Chapter 151, Sepsis. Chapter 233, Acquired Bleeding Disorders.
b. *Rosen's Emergency Medicine: Concepts and Clinical Practice* (10th ed.): Chapter 3, Shock.

Cardiac Arrest

Benjamin H. Slovis MD and Christopher McCoy, MD

A. Chief complaint
a. 56-year-old male is brought in by EMS after cardiac arrest

B. Vital signs
a. BP: 95/50, HR: 65 on monitor, RR: intubated, bagged at 8 breaths per minute, T: 36.7°C, Sat: 98% on 100% FiO_2

C. What does the patient look like?
a. Middle-aged male, intubated, pale, and unresponsive to painful stimuli.

D. Primary survey
a. Airway: endotracheal tube (ETT) in place, 23 cm at the teeth; otherwise patent
b. Breathing: no spontaneous breaths, respirations at 10 breaths per minute by EMS
c. Circulation: palpable radial and carotid pulses

E. Action
a. Confirm ETT placement (e.g., direct visualization, video laryngoscopy, $ETCO_2$, etc.)
b. Place patient on ventilator
c. Place patient on monitors (cardiac monitor and pulse oximetry)
   i. BP: 95/50, HR: 65, RR: 12 on vent, T: 36.7°C, Sat: 99% on 100% FiO_2
d. Finger stick blood glucose
e. Two large-bore IVs and/or IO access (if not already established by EMS)
f. ECG
g. Chest x-ray
h. Labs
   i. CBC, coagulation studies
   ii. CMP, magnesium, phosphorus, lactate
   iii. Troponin
   iv. Blood gas (venous or arterial acceptable), lactate
   v. Urinalysis, urine toxicology

F. History
a. HPI: The patient is a 56-year-old male presenting after cardiac arrest. According to EMS, the patient collapsed while eating dinner at a restaurant. No evidence of coughing or choking was witnessed prior to the event. The patient slumped over in his chair and bystanders promptly initiated CPR. Upon EMS arrival, the patient was found to be pulseless. The paramedics noted a wide complex tachycardic regular rhythm on their portable monitor and delivered a shock

(defibrillation) at 200 joules. After 2 minutes of CPR, the patient was found to be in the same dysrhythmia and subsequently shocked again. The patient was found to have a palpable pulse during the next pulse check, was given 1 mg epinephrine IV, intubated, and transported to the ED. The patient's wife is present to provide further past medical history if requested.

b. PMHx: hypertension, diabetes, coronary artery disease with stents 10 years ago
c. PSHx: cholecystectomy 15 years ago
d. Meds: clopidogrel, simvastatin, metformin
e. Allergies: ACE inhibitors
f. Social: smoker, 20 pack year history; social drinker; no illicit drug use
g. FHx: CAD and DM in both parents; father died of MI at 62

G. Paramedic

a. Rhythm strip (Figure 113.1)

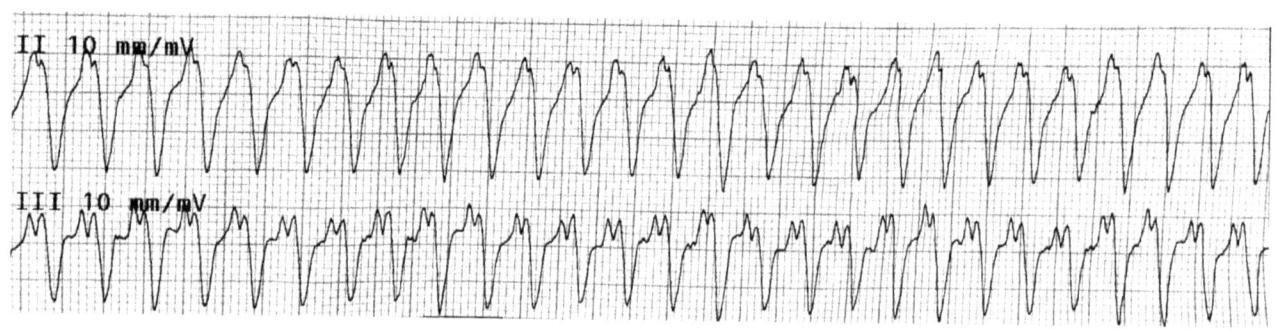

Figure 113.1

H. Secondary survey

a. General: intubated, unresponsive to painful stimuli
b. Head: normocephalic, atraumatic
c. Eyes: pupils equal, minimally reactive to light, no tracking noted, normal sclera
d. Ears: normal
e. Nose: normal
f. Oropharynx: intubated, no foreign bodies identified (if evaluated)
g. Neck: trachea midline, no bruit or jugular venous distension
h. Chest: bilateral chest rise on ventilator, no signs of trauma
i. Lungs: clear to auscultation bilaterally, no wheezes, rhonchi, or rales.
j. Heart: regular rate and rhythm, normal S1, S2, no murmurs, rubs, or gallops
k. Abdomen: normal bowel sounds, soft, nondistended
l. Rectal: normal tone, no gross blood
m. Urogenital: normal male external genitalia
n. Extremities: no obvious deformities, femoral pulses present
o. Back: no signs of trauma, no stepoffs
p. Neurologic: pupils minimally reactive, GCS: eyes: 1, motor: 1, verbal: T (patient is intubated), patient is unresponsive
q. Skin: cool and pale, no rashes noted
r. Lymphatic: no lymphadenopathy appreciated

I. Action

a. Airway
    i. End-tidal CO_2 monitoring

    ii. Ventilator set up
b. Begin antiarrhythmic (amiodarone or lidocaine) and/or synchronized cardioversion
c. ECG interpretation
d. Establish central venous access
e. Consider arterial line
f. Rectal temperature
g. Aspirin
h. Cardiology/ICU consult
i. Initiate targeted temperature management (TTM)
    i. Goal temperature of 32–36°C
    ii. Ice packs
    iii. 1–2 L 4°C chilled saline over 30 minutes
    iv. Cooling blankets
    v. Commercial cooling devices
    vi. Sedation and shivering inhibition
    vii. Esophageal or bladder temperature probe
j. Aspirin
k. Consider heparin (after confirming no hemorrhage exists and profound hypertension is absent)
l. Admit to appropriate service with ICU level of care

J. Nurse
a. If no sedation during TTM
    i. Patient is at 37°C and shivering
b. If patient is sedated with TTM
    i. Patient is at 36°C and comfortable

K. Results

Table 113.1 Results table

Test	Result	Test	Result
Complete blood count:		**Liver function panel:**	
WBC	$9.2 \times 10^3/\mu L$	AST	21 U/L
Hb / Hct	13.1/43.2%	ALT	45 U/L
Plt	$157 \times 10^3/\mu L$	Alk phos	104 U/L
		T bili	6.5 mg/dL
		D bili	0.1 mg/dL
Basic metabolic panel:		Amylase	56 U/L
Na	139 mEq/L	Lipase	100 U/L
K	4.9 mEq/L	Albumin	3.6 g/dL
Cl	91 mEq/L		
CO_2	21 mEq/L		
BUN	12 mEq/L	**Arterial blood gas:**	
Cr	1.1 mEq/dL	pH	7.12
Gluc	138 mEq/dL	pCO_2	52 mmHg

Table 113.1 (cont.)

Test	Result	Test	Result
Coagulation panel:		pO_2	96 mmHg
PT	15.0 sec (10–12 sec)	HCO3	21 mEq/L
PTT	29.8 sec (30–45 sec)		
INR	1.4		

a. ECG (Figure 113.2)
b. Lactate: 2.9 mmol/L
c. Troponin (hsTnI): 17 pg/mL

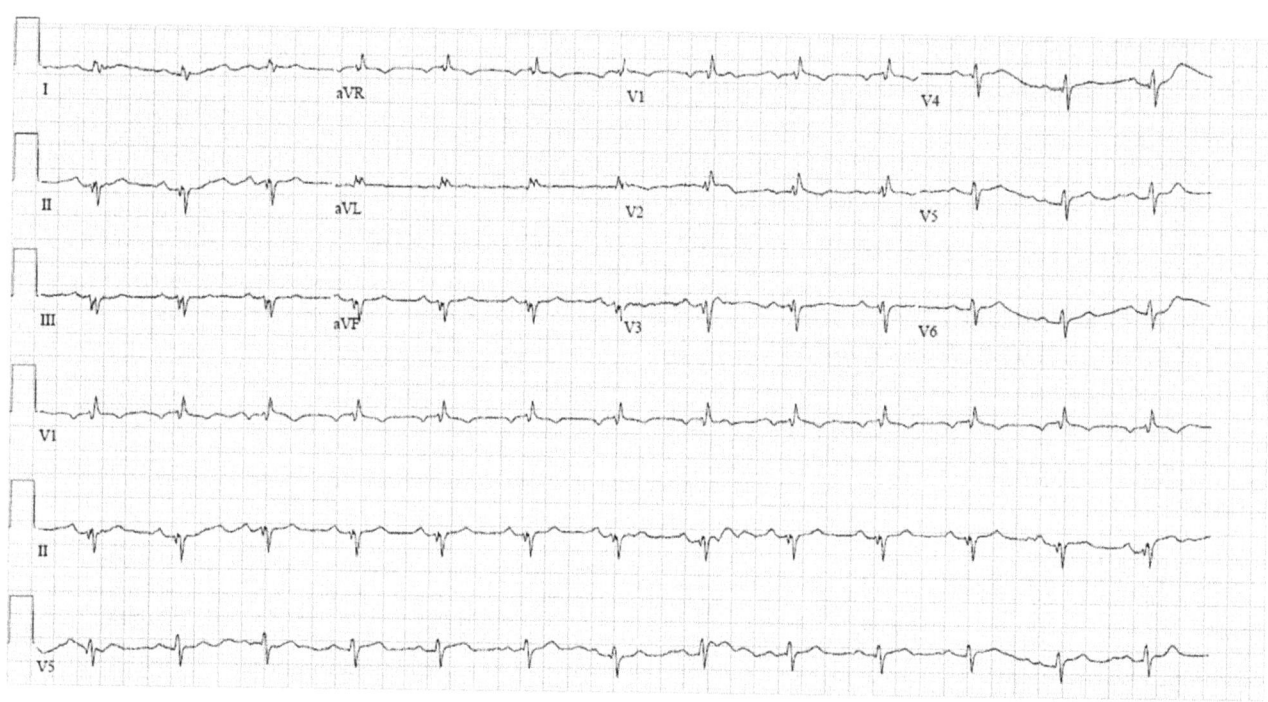

Figure 113.2

L. Action
a. Maintain hypothermia
b. Sign patient out to admitting service
c. Nursing phase of care
    i.   Eye lubrication
    ii. Glycemic control
    iii. NPO
    iv. Core temperature monitoring

M. Diagnosis
a. Pulseless ventricular tachycardia (pVT) – cardiac arrest

Case 113: Cardiac Arrest

N. Critical actions

a. Confirmation of airway
b. Establish two large-bore IVs
c. Place the patient on monitors (cardiac monitor and pulse oximetry)
d. Perform primary and secondary survey
e. Recognize pulseless VT arrest with return of spontaneous circulation (ROSC)
f. Begin antiarrhythmic (amiodarone or lidocaine)
g. Interpret ECG (with focus on presence or absence of STEMI)
h. Initiate targeted temperature management
i. Order sedation medications
j. Consult cardiology
k. Admit patient to appropriate service with ICU level of care

O. Examiner instructions

a. This is a case of pulseless ventricular tachycardia. In this scenario, the patient had a return of spontaneous circulation in the field after CPR and defibrillation. The patient was given 1 mg of epinephrine, intubated and transported to the ED. The participant is to recognize that the patient has a return of spontaneous circulation after cardiac arrest from pulseless ventricular tachycardia and begin appropriate management, including (but not limited to) confirmation of the endotracheal tube and assuring adequate ventilation and adequate circulation. After recognizing that the patient is unresponsive, targeted temperature management should be initiated. The participant should also begin an antiarrhythmic to prevent the patient from returning to a nonperfusing rhythm. If the participant does not start an antiarrhythmic (amiodarone or lidocaine), the patient will go into ventricular fibrillation and will need to be resuscitated. If defibrillated, the patient will convert to sinus tachycardia. If an antiarrhythmic is not given by this time, the patient will convert back to ventricular fibrillation and will expire regardless of therapies initiated. If managed appropriately, the cardiology service will take the patient on their service in the coronary care unit, with a plan for cardiac catheterization.

P. Pearls

a. Pulseless ventricular tachycardia (pVT) and ventricular fibrillation (VF) are nonperfusing rhythms for which early identification, high-quality CPR, and defibrillation are mainstays of treatment.
b. Decreased time to defibrillation improves the likelihood of successful conversion to a perfusing rhythm and patient survival.
c. ACLS guidelines recommend resumption of CPR immediately after defibrillation without checking for a pulse. The rhythm check should be done only after two minutes of CPR have been delivered, and not before the defibrillator is charged and ready for the next shock if indicated.
d. If VF or pVT persist after at least one attempt at defibrillation and two minutes of CPR, administration of epinephrine (1 mg IV or IO every 3–5 minutes) is advised while CPR is performed.
e. According to ACLS guidelines, amiodarone or lidocaine may be considered for VF/pVT that is unresponsive to defibrillation.
f. The recommended dose for amiodarone is an initial IV/IO dose of 300 mg with a second IV/IO dose of 150 mg if required.
g. The recommended dose for lidocaine is 1.0–1.5 mg/kg IV/IO for the first dose and 0.5–0.75 mg/kg IV/IO for a second dose if required.

h. An antiarrhythmic drug alone is unlikely to pharmacologically convert VF/pVT to an organized perfusing rhythm. Rather, the primary objective is to facilitate successful defibrillation and to reduce the risk of recurrent arrhythmias.

i. ROSC in VF/pVT hinges on early identification, high-quality CPR, and defibrillation (decreased mortality and improved neurologic outcomes have been reported in patients with out-of-hospital cardiac arrest who present with VF or pVT).

j. When combined with standard post–cardiac arrest care, lowering core body temperature to the range of 32–34°C during the first hours after cardiac arrest has been shown to improve neurologic outcome compared to not controlling body temperature.

k. A large randomized trial reports similar improvements in outcome whether temperature is maintained at 33°C or 36°C.

l. Hyperthermia must be avoided following cardiac arrest as it is associated with worse neurologic outcomes.

m. Overall, the data suggest that active control of the post–cardiac arrest patient's core temperature, with a target between 32°C and 36°C, followed by active avoidance of fever, is the optimal strategy to promote patient survival.

n. Regardless of the strategy selected, a cooling device with a feedback mechanism is necessary to actively control patient temperature.

o. Examples of cooling approaches/resources:
   i. Cold IV fluids (4°C)
   ii. Surface cooling (ice packs, cooling blankets, cooling vests, etc.)
   iii. Water baths ± fans

p. There is no evidence demonstrating the superiority of any cooling method and in clinical practice a combination of intravascular and surface cooling is commonly employed.

q. Sedation may need to be titrated to prevent shivering.

r. The core body temperature should be monitored continuously during targeted temperature management.
   i. Central venous temperature (gold standard, but several surrogates available)
   ii. Esophageal probe
   iii. Bladder probe
   iv. Rectal probe

s. Targeted temperature management should not delay other necessary interventions in the setting of cardiac arrest, such as emergent catheterization for ST-elevation myocardial infarction, but can be performed in conjunction with such procedures.

Q. Figure legends
a. Figure 113.1 EKG.
b. Figure 113.2 EKG.

R. References

a. *Tintinalli's Emergency Medicine: A Comprehensive Study Guide* (9th ed.): Chapter 18, Cardiac Rhythm Disturbances.
b. *Rosen's Emergency Medicine: Concepts and Clinical Practice* (10th ed.): Chapter 5, Adult Resuscitation. Chapter 65, Dysrhythmias.

Leg Pain

Mandy Pascual, MD and Jodi Jones, MD

A. Chief complaint
a. 45-year-old female with right leg pain

B. Vital signs
a. BP: 136/77, HR: 90, RR: 18, T: 37.3°C, Sat: 99% on RA, Wt: 80 kg

C. What does the patient look like?
a. Patient appears stated age, obviously uncomfortable; massaging right leg while on stretcher

D. Primary survey
a. Airway: speaking in full sentences
b. Breathing: no apparent respiratory distress, no cyanosis
c. Circulation: peripheral pulses equal

E. Action
a. Place on continuous telemetry monitor, including pulse oximetry
b. Establish IV access

F. History
a. HPI: A 45-year-old female presents with 1 day history of right lower extremity pain and swelling. Patient reports she began noticing pain shortly after awakening when she walked down her driveway this morning to check her mail. She reports subjective fever, but otherwise denies any headache, chest pain, shortness of breath, nausea, vomiting, or abdominal pain.
b. PMHx: type 2 diabetes mellitus, hypertension, and hypothyroidism
c. PSHx: perforated diverticulitis requiring bowel resection (3 weeks prior), cholecystectomy and hysterectomy (at age 40)
d. Meds: metformin, losartan, levothyroxine
e. Allergies: none
f. Social: married with two children; denies alcohol and drug use; smokes half-pack of cigarettes per day (25 pack per year history)
g. FHx: no pertinent history

G. Secondary survey
a. General: awake, alert, oriented
b. HEENT: pupils equal, round, reactive; oropharynx clear, mucous membranes moist
c. Neck: no appreciated lymphadenopathy or jugular vein distension
d. Heart: regular rate and rhythm, without murmurs, rubs, or gallops

e. Lungs: clear to auscultation, bilaterally
f. Abdomen: soft, nondistended, with normal bowel sounds; appropriately tender to palpation over well-healing surgical wound site without guarding or rebound tenderness
g. Extremities: right lower leg appears enlarged when compared to left; there is pain at rest that is augmented by palpation of extremity; dorsalis pedis and posterior tibial pulses are 2+ bilaterally
h. Neuro: no focal neurological findings
i. Skin: right lower extremity with mild diffuse erythema. No other abnormal skin findings

H. Action

a. Right lower extremity venous ultrasound
b. Provide analgesia
c. EKG
d. CXR
e. Labs
    i.   CBC with differential, BMP, PT/PTT/INR, D-dimer

I. Results

Table 114.1 Results table

Test	Result	Test	Result
Complete blood count:		CO_2	18 mEq/L
WBC	$12.3 \times 10^3/\mu L$	BUN	20 mEq/dL
Hgb	13.1 g/dL	Cr	0.8 mg/dL
Hct	39.3%	Gluc	129 mg/dL
Plt	$400 \times 10^9/L$		
		Coagulation panel:	
Basic metabolic panel:		PT	12.3 sec
Na	142 mEq/L	PTT	30 sec
K	4.1 mEq/L	INR	1.1
Cl	101 mEq/L		

a. D-dimer: 2250 ng/mL (normal <500 ng/mL)
b. Right lower extremity venous ultrasound. Figures 114.1 shows proximal common femoral vein before compression and Figure 114.2 shows the same with compression.

J. Action

a. Begin anticoagulation with oral anticoagulation such as rivaroxaban or apixaban.

K. Diagnosis

a. DVT after recent surgery and immobilization

L. Critical actions

a. Venous ultrasound of extremity

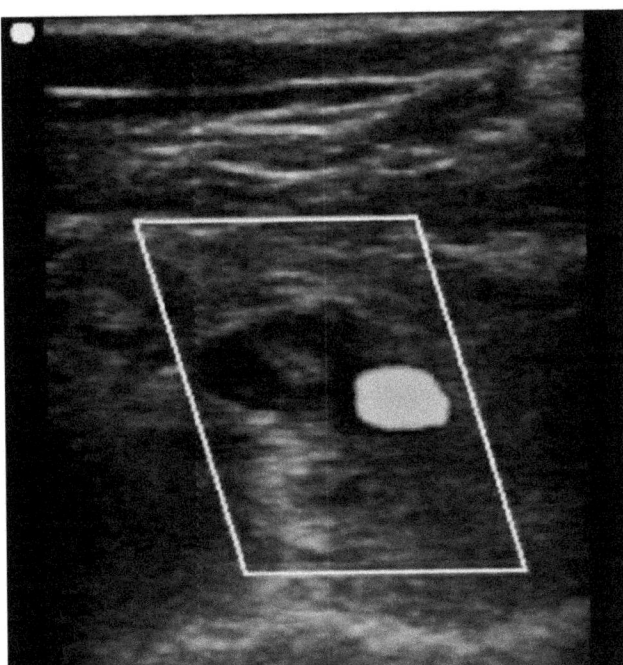

Figure 114.1

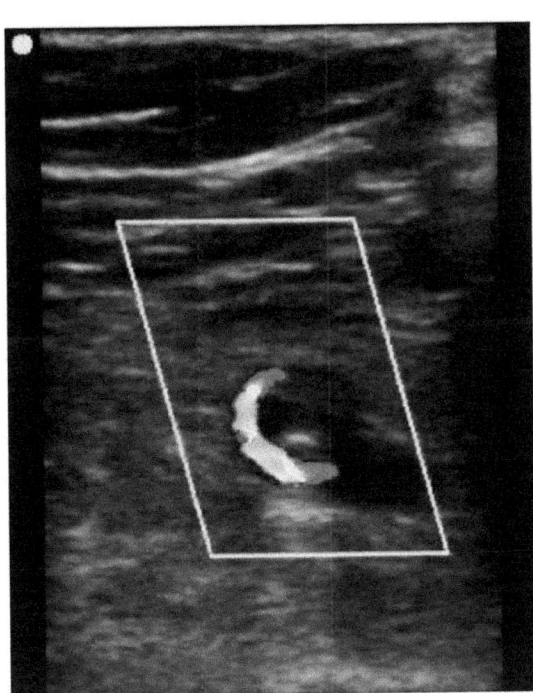

Figure 114.2

b. Anticoagulation
c. Pain management

M. Examiner instructions
a. This patient is suffering from a DVT after surgery, likely a combination of a pro-coagulable state post-surgery and prolonged immobilization. Common symptoms include pain and swelling of the affected extremity, which is most often a lower extremity. Compression ultrasonography is the key to diagnosis. The patient's recent history of surgery is a significant risk factor.

N. Pearls

a. Risk factors for DVTs include malignancy, recent surgery, history of DVT/PE, genetic predisposition to a hypercoagulable state, hospitalization, OCP/hormone replacement, pregnancy, and prolonged immobilization.

b. Symptoms include erythema, swelling, and pain of affected extremity with increased calf diameter in lower extremity DVTs increasing likelihood of its presence.

c. Differential diagnosis includes, but is not limited to, cellulitis, musculoskeletal injury, Baker's cyst, lymphangitis, chronic venous stasis without evidence of DVT.

d. D-dimer is useful to rule out DVT in those with low suspicion, but has limited utility if suspicion is moderate to high.

e. Compression ultrasonography is the most reliable diagnostic exam for DVT.

f. Outpatient treatment of DVT with oral anticoagulation such as rivaroxaban and apixaban is acceptable. Other options include LMWH, or LMWH bridge to warfarin.

g. Patients who present with signs/symptoms concerning for PE (chest pain, dyspnea, hypoxia, tachypnea, tachycardia) require further imaging such as CT scan or V/Q study.

O. Figure legends

a. Figure 114.1 (US) Common femoral vein before compression.

b. Figure 114.2 (US) Common femoral vein with compression, vein does not compress.

P. References

a. *Tintinalli's Emergency Medicine: A Comprehensive Study Guide* (9th ed.): Chapter 56, Venous Thromboembolism including Pulmonary Embolism.

b. *Rosen's Emergency Medicine: Concepts and Clinical Practice* (10th ed.): Chapter 74, Pulmonary Embolism and Deep Vein Thrombosis.

Q. Acknowledgments

a. We would like to acknowledge Sunil Aradhya for their contribution to this chapter in the previous edition of this book, which has been updated by Mandy Pascual and Jodi Jones.

Shortness of Breath and Swelling

Bashar A. Ismail, MD

A. Chief complaint
a. 60-year-old female complaining of shortness of breath with exertion and associated neck swelling for the last 3 weeks

B. Vital signs
a. BP: 100/90, HR 107, RR 22, T: 37.1°C, Sat: 94% on RA, Wt: 70 kg

C. What does the patient look like?
a. Patient appears stated age, uncomfortable, but not in distress; dyspneic with grossly obvious superficial vascular distention of neck veins.

D. Primary survey
a. Airway: patent airway, speaking in full sentences, no stridor
b. Breathing: no apparent respiratory distress, and no cyanosis
c. Circulation: warm, flushed skin, peripheral pulses equal

E. Action
a. Oxygen via nasal canula
b. Large-bore peripheral IV line (contralateral to swelling)
c. Monitor: BP: 100/90, HR 107, RR 22, T: 37.1°C, Sat: 93% on RA
d. Labs
   i. CBC, BMP, LFT, PT/PTT, TSH, blood type and crossmatch
e. EKG

F. History
a. HPI: A 60-year-old female with known history of small cell lung cancer, currently undergoing chemotherapy. She reports her last treatment was more than 8 weeks prior to her presentation, and presented to the ED complaining of dyspnea on exertion that started 3 weeks ago. The dyspnea is associated with facial and neck swelling which is more evident during early morning hours and seems to subside by mid-morning. She also reports decreased appetite and weight loss. No history of chest pain, no syncope, no fever or chills. Denies recent travel or sick contacts.
b. PMHx: small cell carcinoma of the lungs diagnosed 10 months ago
c. PSHx: none
d. Meds: none
e. Allergy: none

f. Social history: cigarette smoker since she was 16 years old, stopped last month; lives with her husband
g. FHx: none

G. Secondary survey

a. General: mildly obese, awake and alert, not in pain or distress
b. HEENT: pupils equal, round, reactive; facial and neck swelling are evident, no stridor or papilledema
c. Neck: swollen with obviously distended superficial veins
d. Chest: dilated superficial veins over upper chest; no rash or deformity
e. Lungs: clear to auscultation bilaterally, good air movement
f. Heart: tachycardic, no murmurs
g. Abdomen: no distension, no tenderness, no guarding or rebound tenderness; normal bowel sounds
h. Rectal: normal
i. Urogenital: normal
j. Extremities: normal
k. Back: normal, no CVA tenderness
l. Neuro: normal
m. Skin: distended superficial veins of the neck and upper chest; no ulcers
n. Lymph: normal

H. Action

a. Elevate the head of bed 45 degrees
b. Reassess oxygenation (100% on 2 L by NC)
c. Imaging
    i. CXR (Figure 115.1)
    ii. CT chest (unavailable due to scanner malfunction)

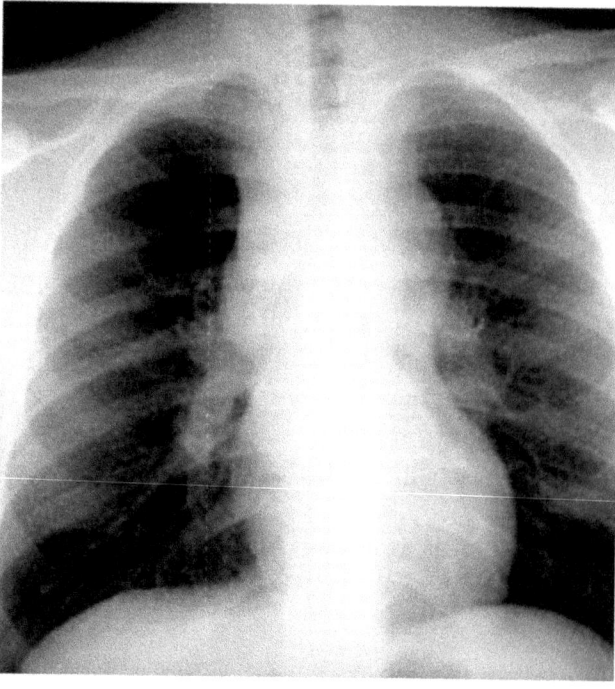

Figure 115.1

I. Nurse
a. Repeat vital signs: BP: 100/90, HR: 101, RR: 18, T: 37.1°C

J. Results

Table 115.1 Results table

Test	Result	Test	Result
Complete blood count:		**Coagulation panel:**	
WBC	9×10^9/L	PT	10–12 sec
Hb	15 g/dL	INR	1
Hct	40%	PTT	30–45 sec
Plt	350×10^9/L		
		Liver function panel:	
		AST	20 U/L
Basic metabolic panel:		ALT	15 U/L
Na	135 mEq/L	Alk phos	20 U/L
K	3.5 mEq/L	D bili	0.1 mg/dL
Cl	100 mEq/L	Albumin	3.9 g/dL
BUN	15 mEq/L		
Cr	1.0 mEq/L		
Mg	1.5 mEq/L	**Arterial blood gas:**	
Glucose	110 mg/dL	pH	7.45
		pCO_2	46 mmHg
		pO_2	95 mmHg

K. Action
a. Oncology consult: admission to ICU and arrange for tissue biopsy
b. Consult interventional radiologist for emergent percutaneous stent placement to SVC for symptomatic relief
c. Medications: Lasix

L. Diagnosis
a. Superior vena cava syndrome

M. Critical actions
a. Clinical identification of the diagnosis
b. Elevate the head and consider diuretics to avoid overhydration
c. Start supplemental oxygen and monitor closely
d. Consult oncology and interventional radiology

N. Examiner instructions
a. This patient is suffering from superior vena cava syndrome (SVCS), which can be an acute or subacute condition resulting from obstruction of the blood flow through the superior vena

cava (SVC). This can be a result of direct compression, infiltration, or thrombosis. Malignancy, specifically lung cancer, is the most common cause of SVCS. Early signs of SVCS can include periorbital edema and facial swelling, classically described as worse in the early morning hours with noted improvement throughout the day. Dyspnea and facial swelling are most commonly reported symptoms of SVCS. SVCS is not usually an immediately life-threatening oncological emergency, but careful and thorough work-up of potential etiology is warranted in all cases.

O. Pearls

a. Elevation of the head of the bed has been shown to be an effective and immediate therapeutic measure. Diuretics may also provide transient relief of symptoms, but should be used judiciously due to resulting hypovolemia. Steroids have shown limited effectiveness, but are occasionally used as part of standard therapy in patients presenting with respiratory compromise. More definitive management options include percutaneous transluminal stent placement or bypass surgery. The prognosis for treated patients varies by underlying tumor type, and overall survival is ~25% at 1 year.

b. Venography is relatively contraindicated due to associated bleeding complications, but other invasive procedures (bronchoscopy, mediastinoscopy, biopsy) are often required to establish diagnosis and underlying disease progression. Venous access is preferable on the contralateral side of the obstruction.

c. Emergency radiotherapy is recommended in patients with stridor due to central airway obstruction or severe laryngeal edema.

P. Figure legends

a. Figure 115.1 Chest x-ray.

Q. References

a. *Tintinalli's Emergency Medicine: A Comprehensive Study Guide* (9th ed.): Chapter 240, Emergency Complications of Malignancy.

b. *Rosen's Emergency Medicine: Concepts and Clinical Practice* (10th ed.): Chapter 112, Oncologic Emergencies.

Finger Pain

Alisa Wray, MD and Jeffrey R. Suchard, MD

A. Chief complaint
a. 35-year-old male with severe pain to right index finger for 4 hours

B. Vital signs
a. BP: 142/90, HR: 114, RR: 16, T: 37.1°C, Wt: 75 kg

C. What does the patient look like?
a. Patient appears in moderate distress secondary to right index finger pain, sitting up on the stretcher.

D. Primary survey
a. Airway: speaking in full sentences
b. Breathing: no apparent respiratory distress, no cyanosis
c. Circulation: peripheral pulses equal in bilateral upper and lower extremities

E. History
a. HPI: A 35-year-old male presents with complaints of right index finger pain. He reports that it started approximately 4 hours ago while he was at work and has progressively worsened. He describes the pain as throbbing and burning. He reports that he went home; however, the pain progressed to where he could not tolerate it any longer and he came to the ED. The patient doesn't recall any trauma to his finger.
    i. If asked, the patient should state that he works as a glass etcher.
    ii. If questioned about chemical exposures, the patient should state that he works with hydrofluoric acid, but wears gloves and eye protection. He is concerned that maybe there was a hole in his glove.
    iii. He denies pain elsewhere
b. PMHx: none
c. PSHx: appendectomy
d. Allergies: none
e. Social: lives with wife, drinks 1–2 beers per week, denies smoking or drug use
f. FHx: adopted, unknown family history

F. Action
a. Copious irrigation of the affected area
b. IV line placement
c. Labs: CBC, BMP, calcium, magnesium
d. EKG

G. Secondary survey

a. General: moderate distress, complaining of right index finger and hand pain
b. HEENT: normocephalic, atraumatic, pupils equal, reactive to light, normal tympanic membranes, no nasal discharge
c. Neck: full range of motion
d. Chest: heart tachycardic with regular rhythm, lungs clear bilaterally
e. Abdomen: soft, nontender, nondistended, normal bowel sounds
f. Extremities: right index finger with edematous, grayish, and blistered skin from the distal interphalangeal (DIP) joint to the tip of finger, including fingernail and cuticle. Pain out of proportion to examination. Full range of motion and normal strength to the affected digit. All other extremities within normal limits (Figure 116.1)
g. Back: nontender
h. Neuro: alert and oriented × 3, grossly normal sensation and strength, normal gait, cranial nerves II–XII intact
i. Skin: warm, well perfused, no other skin changes noted
j. Lymph: no lymphadenopathy

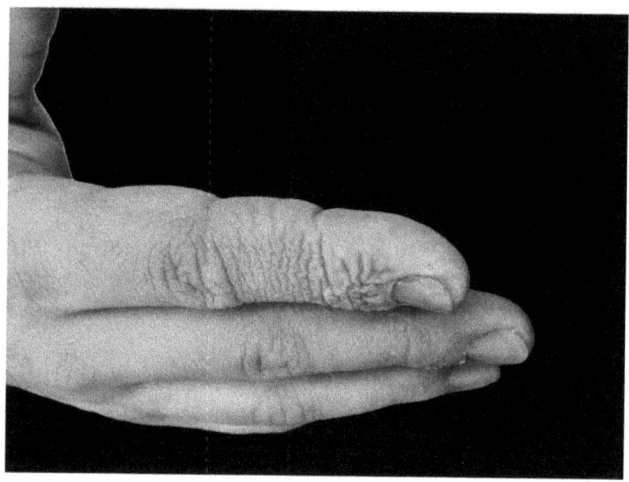

Figure 116.1

H. Meds

a. Calcium: application by any means: topical calcium gel application, 3.5 g of calcium gluconate powder in 150 mL of sterile water-soluble lubricant *or* 10% calcium gluconate in 75 mL of sterile water-soluble lubricant *or* intradermal injection of 5% calcium gluconate *or* IV calcium gluconate *or* intraarterial calcium gluconate
b. Pain control with IV or oral analgesics

I. Results

Table 116.1 Basic metabolic panel results table

Test	Result	Test	Result
Na	141 mEq/L	BUN	9 mEq/L
K	4.0 mEq/L	Cr	0.9 mg/dL
Cl	95 mEq/L	Ca	8.0 mg/dL
CO_2	22 mEq/L	Mg	1.9 mg/dL

a. iCa: 4.0 mg/dL
b. EKG: normal sinus rhythm
c. Patient reports no significant pain relief with topical, intradermal, or IV calcium therapy. Only intraarterial calcium therapy will reduce pain if initiated in the ED

J. Consult:
a. Burn specialist or toxicologist (or poison control center)

K. Diagnosis
a. Hydrofluoric acid exposure

L. Critical actions
a. Diagnose hydrofluoric burn.
b. Check labs, including calcium level, potassium level, magnesium level.
c. Check EKG for dysrhythmia.
d. Attempt calcium therapy (by any means possible).
e. Administer analgesics.
f. Consult a toxicologist or burn specialist.
g. Admit patient (when calcium therapy fails).

M. Examiner instructions
a. This patient is suffering from dermal exposure to hydrofluoric acid, a chemical commonly used in glass etching. It is important that the examinee makes the connection between glass etching and hydrofluoric exposure.

N. Pearls
a. Treatment of hydrofluoric acid burns depends on the exposure (ingestion, dermal, inhalation) and the strength of concentration of the acid (higher concentrations have worse outcomes). Hydrofluoric acid dissociates to H^+ and fluoride ions, which then bind Ca^{++} and Mg^{++}, leading to hypocalcemia, hypomagnesemia, and hyperkalemia (via efflux of intracellular K); this can cause cardiotoxicity manifesting with dysrhythmias, including VFib, VTach, or torsades de pointes (polymorphic VTach).
b. Dermal exposures: hydrofluoric acid concentrations of 50% and greater cause immediate pain and visible damage. Household products are typically 6–10% and cause delayed pain. Exposure to >2% of body surface area (BSA) with high concentration can cause life-threatening systemic toxicity. Treatment for dermal exposure is calcium gluconate gel or intradermal calcium gluconate injection. For serious exposures, intraarterial calcium gluconate is indicated.
c. Inhalation exposures: typically present with complaints of shortness of breath and throat burning. Treatment consists of nebulized calcium gluconate, typically 4 mL of 2.5–5% solution.
d. Gastrointestinal exposures: Ingestion of concentrated hydrofluoric acid causes significant gastritis, altered mental status, nausea, vomiting, airway compromise, severe hypocalcemia, and hyperkalemia. Management includes ABCs and resuscitation. NG tubes can be placed to drain the stomach (this should be done under great care) and oral or NG tube calcium or magnesium salts can be given. Ingestions of hydrofluoric acid can be fatal.
e. Ophthalmic exposures: These typically occur from splashes or exposure to hydrogen fluoride gas. This can cause corneal edema, conjunctival ischemia, sloughing, and chemosis. Treatment

includes irrigation with 1 L Ringer's lactate or normal saline and 1% calcium eye drops. Limited data suggest that prolonged irrigation can cause worse outcomes.

O. Figure legends
a.   Figure 116.1 (Photo) Hydrofluoric acid burn of a hand (courtesy of Dr. Watchorn).

P. References
a.   *Tintinalli's Emergency Medicine: A Comprehensive Study Guide* (9th ed.): Chapter 218, Chemical Burns.
b.   *Rosen's Emergency Medicine: Concepts and Clinical Practice* (10th ed.): Chapter 55, Chemical Injuries.

Dizziness

Robert Katzer, MD and Bharath Chakravarthy, MD, MPH

A. Chief complaint
a. 61-year-old male with dizziness since this morning

B. Vital signs
b. BP: 92/51, HR: 51, RR: 16, T: 37.4°C, Sat: 99% on RA, Wt: 85 kg

C. What does the patient look like?
a. Patient is lying on the bed quietly in no apparent distress, but appears fatigued.

D. Primary survey
a. Airway: speaking full sentences
b. Breathing: no apparent respiratory distress, no cyanosis
c. Circulation: peripheral pulses equal, warm extremities

E. History
a. HPI: A 61-year-old male presents with dizziness since this morning. He has had intermittent dizziness over the past week, but worse this morning. He describes his dizziness as "lightheadedness." He also endorses feeling "weak all over," but denies chest pain, shortness of breath, nausea, or vomiting. Denies headache.
b. PMHx: cannot recall his medical history
c. PSHx: denies
d. Meds: none since he lost his health insurance; cannot recall what his prior meds were
e. Allergies: penicillin – rash
f. Social: lives alone, no tobacco, alcohol, or drugs
g. FHx: father with myocardial infarction at age 55

F. Secondary survey
a. General: awake, alert, appropriate for age, appears fatigued
b. HEENT: pupils equal, round, reactive, no papilledema
c. Neck: no cervical adenopathy, no meningismus
d. Chest: clear to auscultation bilaterally, palpable implanted cardiac device to left chest (only given if a good skin exam is performed)
e. Heart: bradycardic, regular rate
f. Abdomen: soft, nontender, nondistended
g. Rectal: hemoccult negative
h. GU: no testicular masses or tenderness, no penile discharge
i. Extremities: normal

j.   Back: tenderness to L-spine and paralumbar regions bilaterally, no CVA tenderness
k.   Neuro: normal
l.   Skin: normal
m.   Lymph: normal

G. Action

a.   peripheral IV access
b.   Note implanted cardiac device to left chest wall
c.   Cardiac monitor: BP: 85/49, HR: 45, RR: 18, Sat: 98% on RA
d.   EKG: Sinus bradycardia, rate 33, no visualized pacer spikes
e.   Place magnet over site of pacemaker to attempt to set device in asynchronous, fixed rate pacing mode (does not work)
f.   Meds
     i.   Atropine 1 mg IV
     ii. 250 mL crystalloid bolus
g.   Apply transcutaneous pacing pads, pace, and ensure electrical and mechanical capture
h.   Imaging: CXR (evaluate type of implanted cardiac device and ensure the device leads are not fractured)
i.   Labs: CBC, BMP, troponin, BNP
j.   Consult
     i.   Cardiology
     ii. Pacemaker interrogation

H. Results

Table 117.1 Results table

Test	Result	Test	Result
Complete blood count:		**Coagulation panel:**	
WBC	$8.3 \times 10^3/\mu L$	PT	14 sec
Hct	36.1%	PTT	34 sec
Plt	$310 \times 10^3/\mu L$	INR	0.8
Basic metabolic panel:		**Liver function panel:**	
Na	139 mEq/L	AST	18 U/L
K	3.7 mEq/L	ALT	21 U/L
Cl	105 mEq/L	T bili	0.9 mg/dL
CO_2	27 mEq/L	D bili	0.2 mg/dL
BUN	19 mEq/dL	Albumin	3.9 g/dL
Cr	1.7 mg/dL		
Gluc	130 mg/dL		

a.   Troponin: <0.04 mg/mL
b.   BNP: 99 pg/mL

Case 117: Dizziness

I. Diagnosis
a. Malfunctioning pacemaker

J. Critical actions
a. Note pacemaker to left chest on physical exam
b. Obtain EKG
c. Atropine 1 mg IV
d. Apply transcutaneous pacemaker pads; ensure electrical and mechanical capture
e. Apply magnet over pacemaker
f. Consult cardiology and/or device manufacturer

K. Examiner instructions
a. This is a case of a malfunctioning pacemaker in which the set rate is too slow, resulting in decreased cerebral perfusion and dizziness. Specifically, the candidate should note on physical exam that the patient has had a cardiac device implanted (confirmed on CXR) and symptomatic bradycardia indicates it is a pacemaker and not just an automated implantable cardioverter defibrillator, even though the patient has neglected to volunteer this information in the past medical history. The candidate should address this issue in several ways: medically treat the bradycardia with atropine per ACLS, apply transcutaneous pacemaker pads and ensure mechanical capture, return the pacemaker to its default settings with a magnet. Lack of pacer spikes on the ECG indicate that the device has a fractured/displaced lead, dead battery, or is oversensing the native cardiac activity.

L. Pearls
a. Patients are often unaware of their own medical history, especially those who have been out of medical care.
b. Transcutaneous pacing can be initiated over an existing pacemaker.
c. Applying a magnet over a pacemaker will revert the pacemaker settings to an asynchronous, preset rate (the rate depends on the manufacturer). If this is unsuccessful, the pacemaker battery may be depleted or the device may be programmed to ignore the magnet. Alternative management, such as transcutaneous pacing, will then be required.

M. References
a. *Tintinalli's Emergency Medicine: A Comprehensive Study Guide* (9th ed.): Chapter 33, Cardiac Pacing and Implanted Defibrillation.
b. *Rosen's Emergency Medicine: Concepts and Clinical Practice* (10th ed.): Chapter 66, Implantable Cardiac Devices.

N. Acknowledgements
a. We would like to acknowledge Maxwell Jen for their contribution to this chapter in the previous edition of this book, which has been updated by Robert Katzer and Bharath Chakravarthy

Intoxication

Lars K. Beattie, MD and Henry Young, MD

A. Chief complaint
a. 47-year-old confused male found stumbling in a pile of beer cans by police, brought in by EMS

B. Vital signs
a. BP: 136/83, HR: 92, RR: 18, T: 37.1°C, Wt: 72 kg

C.What does the patient look like?
a. Patient appears older than stated age, disheveled

D. Primary survey
a. Airway: nonsensical speech, airway patent
b. Breathing: no apparent respiratory distress, no cyanosis
c. Circulation: pale, peripheral pulses equal

E. Action
a. Oxygen via NC or nonrebreather mask
b. Two large-bore peripheral IV lines
    i. CBC, BMP, LFT, coagulation studies, blood type and crossmatch
    ii. Alcohol level, acetaminophen level, salicylate level, urine toxicology screen, serum osmolality
c. Monitor: BP: 152/78, HR: 86, RR: 16, Sat: 100% on NC
d. Thiamine 100 mg IV
e. Dextrose 50% AMP (25 g) IV push
f. Naloxone 0.4 mg IV push

F. History
a. HPI: A 47-year-old male with a history of alcohol abuse known to EMS and triage nurse. The patient does not contribute to the history, and only stares at you upon questioning. The triage nurse states he is familiar with the patient and says "all he does is drink beer." EMS states they were called because of police concern about his mental status after they witnessed the patient shaking violently. There was no trauma, as the patient had already been placed in the police vehicle when the shaking started.
b. PMHx: alcoholism
c. Social: insecure housing
d. PSHx: Unknown
e. Meds: Unknown
f. Allergies: Unknown
g. FHx: Unknown

G. Secondary survey

a. General: lethargic, alert to self, urine-soaked pants
b. Head: normocephalic, atraumatic
c. Eyes: appear normal; pupils equal, normal conjunctiva, no nystagmus
d. Ears: normal
e. Mouth: tongue bite mark
f. Neck: supple, full ROM
g. Chest: no rashes
h. Lungs: normal air movement, clear breath sounds bilaterally
i. Heart: regular rate and rhythm, no murmurs
j. Abdomen: nontender, normal bowel sounds
k. Rectal: hemoccult negative
l. Urogenital: normal external genitalia
m. Extremities: full range of motion
n. Back: normal, no CVA tenderness
o. Neuro: alert to self, does not follow commands, no focal weakness, no tremors, no tongue fasciculations, no rigidity
p. Skin: ruddy, scattered abrasions
q. Lymph: no lymphadenopathy

H. Nurse

a. O_2, thiamine, naloxone, D50, IV push
   i. BP: 121/78, HR: 84, RR: 16, Sat: 100% on NC
   ii. No change in mental status
b. Labs drawn

I. Action

a. EKG, CXR
b. Noncontrast CT head

J. Results

Table 118.1 Results table

Test	Result	Test	Result
Complete blood count:		Alk phos	179 U/L
WBC	$5.9 \times 10^3/\mu L$	T bili	1.3 mg/dL
Hct	39.1%	D bili	0.2 mg/dL
Plt	$190 \times 10^3/\mu L$	Amylase	61 U/L
		Lipase	80 U/L
		Albumin	3.9 g/dL
Basic metabolic panel:			
Na	113 mEq/L		
K	2.9 mEq/L	Urinalysis:	
Cl	79 mEq/L	SG	1.003
CO_2	26 mEq/L	pH	5–8
BUN	15 mEq/dL	Prot	Neg

Table 118.1 (cont.)

Test	Result	Test	Result
Cr	0.9 mg/dL	Gluc	Neg
Gluc	71 mg/dL	Ketones	Neg
		Bili	Neg
Coagulation panel:		Blood	Neg
PT	13 sec	NH_4	30
PTT	25 sec	LE	Neg
INR	1.0	Nitrite	Neg
		Color	Yellow
Liver function panel:			
AST	80 U/L		
ALT	53 U/L		

a.   EtOH level: 122 mg/dL
b.   EKG (Figure 118.1)
d.   CXR (Figure 118.2)
d.   Noncontrast CT head (Figure 118.3)

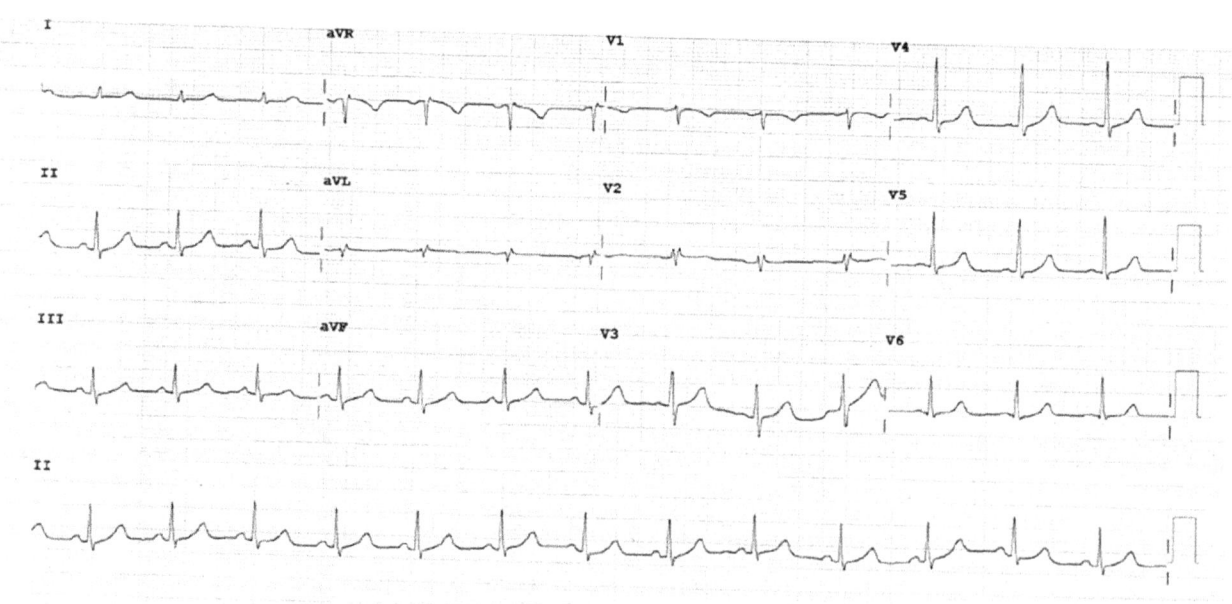

Figure 118.1

Figure 118.2

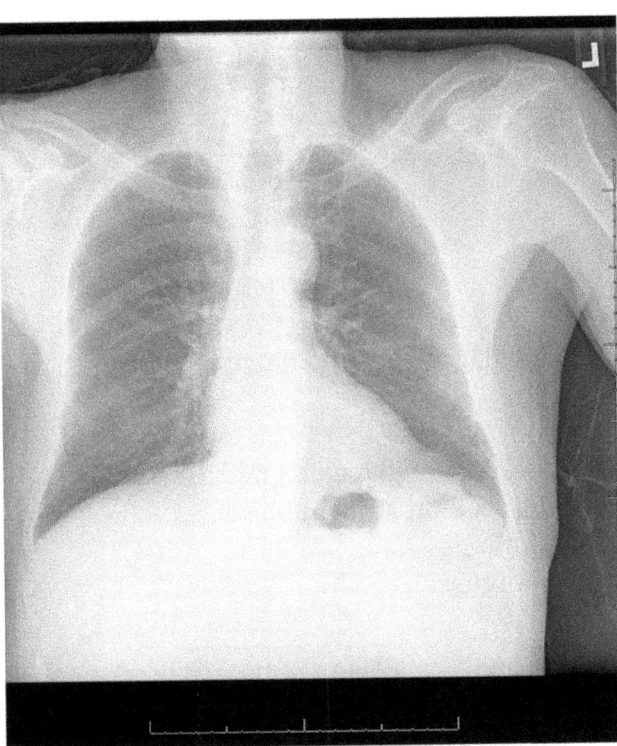

Figure 118.3

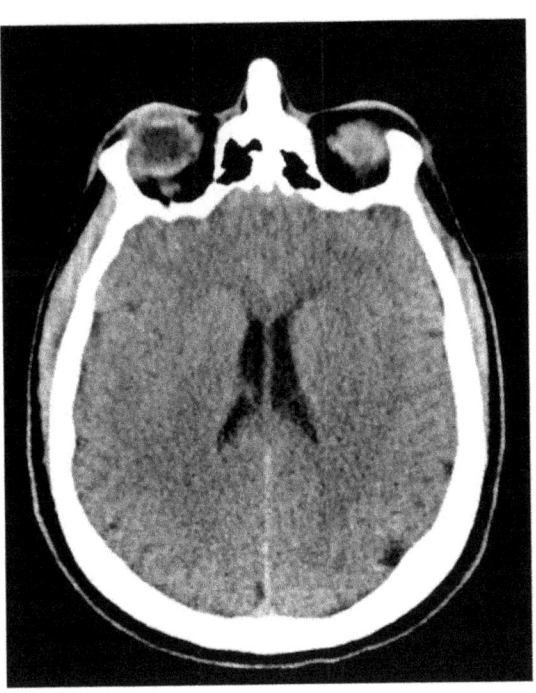

K. Action

a. 100 cc 3% hypertonic saline over 10 minutes
b. Serum osmolality
c. Urine osmolality
d. Nephrology consult

L. Nurse

a. Serum osmolality = 260 mOsm/kg
b. Urine osmolality = 59 mOsm/kg

M. Action

a. Serial BMP
b. Admission to ICU

N. Diagnosis

a. Hypo-osmolar hyponatremia with cerebral edema, secondary to beer potomania

O. Critical actions

a. Initial treatment of altered mental status (assess glucose, ABCs, give naloxone)
b. Recognition of altered mental status out of proportion to patient's alcohol level
c. Recognition of severe hyponatremia with neurologic findings
d. Up to 100 cc 3% hypertonic saline bolus over 10–15 minutes

P. Examiner instructions

a. This is a case of altered mental status and seizure secondary to hyponatremia. The patient has a hypo-osmolar hyponatremia with cerebral edema secondary to beer potomania. There are many potential causes for this patient's altered mental status and seizure. However, the constellation of normal vital signs, absent response to dextrose, oxygen, naloxone, and thiamine, absence of tremor/tongue fasciculations, and a low alcohol level should prompt the examinee to search for other causes. With the dangerously low serum sodium level on BMP, the etiology of the altered mental status and seizure should become clear. Failure to recognize and treat severe hyponatremia will result in a declining mental status and seizures, requiring intubation and treatment for status epilepticus. The goal of the case is to have the examinee work through an undifferentiated altered mental status case with seizure, then treat severe hyponatremia with cerebral edema.

Q. Pearls

a. Patients with sodium levels less than 120 mEq/L are more likely to exhibit symptoms of nausea, vomiting, anorexia, muscle cramps, confusion, and lethargy.
b. Altered mental status, seizures, and coma are serious sequelae of hyponatremia, caused by cerebral edema. Increasing the sodium level by 4–6 mEq/L will usually improve neurological sequalae from hyponatremia.
c. The rate of sodium repletion should be no greater than 0.5–1.0 mEq/L/hr in chronic severe hyponatremia, but may be increased to 1–2 mEq/L in the setting of acute severe hyponatremia. (No more than 10 mEq/L in 24 hours.)
d. In patients with severe neurologic symptoms (seizures, altered mental status), up to three boluses of 100 cc of 3% hypertonic saline bolus can be administered over 30–45 minutes (10–15 min/bolus), raising serum sodium to a level that improves neurologic symptoms or serum concentrations by 4–6 mEq/L.
e. Patients are at risk for central pontine myelinolysis, or osmotic demyelination syndrome, if serum sodium is too rapidly replaced (>12 mEq/L/24hr).
f. Hyponatremia due to "beer potomania" can occur in any patient with a very low intake of dietary solutes. Classically, this occurs in alcoholics whose sole nutrient is beer, hence the diagnostic label "beer potomania." Beer has low protein and salt content (1–2 mmol Na⁺

per liter). Reduced body solutes limit urinary water excretion and hyponatremia can ensue even after modest polydipsia.

R. Figure legends
a. Figure 118.1 (EKG) EKG showing normal sinus rhythm.
b. Figure 118.2 (CXR) Normal chest x-ray.
c. Figure 118.3 (Head CT) Normal computed tomography of head.

S. References
a. *Tintinalli's Emergency Medicine: A Comprehensive Study Guide* (9th ed.): Chapter 17, Fluids and Electrolytes.
b. *Rosen's Emergency Medicine: Concepts and Clinical Practice* (10th ed.): Chapter 114, Electrolyte Disorders.

T. Acknowledgements
a. We would like to acknowledge Desmond Fitzpatrick for their contribution to this chapter in the previous edition of this book, which has been updated by Lars K. Beattie and Henry Young

Altered Mental Status

Lars K. Beattie, MS, MD and Laura Scieszka, MD

A. Chief complaint

a. 64-year-old male with confusion

B. Vital signs

a. BP: 162/88, HR: 58, RR: 18, T: 37.0°C

C. What does the patient look like?

a. Patient is a thin man who is sleepy.

D. Primary survey

a. Airway: patient speaking in full sentences
b. Breathing: no apparent respiratory distress, no cyanosis
c. Circulation: warm and dry skin, normal capillary refill

E. Action

a. Oxygen via NC or nonrebreather mask as needed to maintain saturation >95%
b. Peripheral IV access
c. Labs
    i. CBC, BMP, LFT, coagulation studies, blood type and crossmatch
    ii. Finger stick glucose
d. Monitor: BP: 165/80, HR: 62, RR: 18, T: 37.0°C; Sat: 95%
e. CXR, EKG

F. History

a. HPI: A 64-year-old man who presents with confusion worsening over the last week. He has associated weakness. EMS states family lives in a cabin in "the sticks" (the deep woods). Per family, the patient has been having increasing weakness, itching, nausea, and abdominal cramps over the last week. He has also been exhibiting increasing confusion over the last 2 days. Today the patient was too weak to get out of bed and started speaking to "dead relatives." History is per EMS discussion with family.
b. PMHx: COPD
c. PSHx: none
d. Allergies: none
e. Meds: none
f. Social: 2.5 packs per day for 30 years, no drug or alcohol use
g. FHx: none
h. PMD: none

G. Nurse

a.   EKG (Figure 119.1)

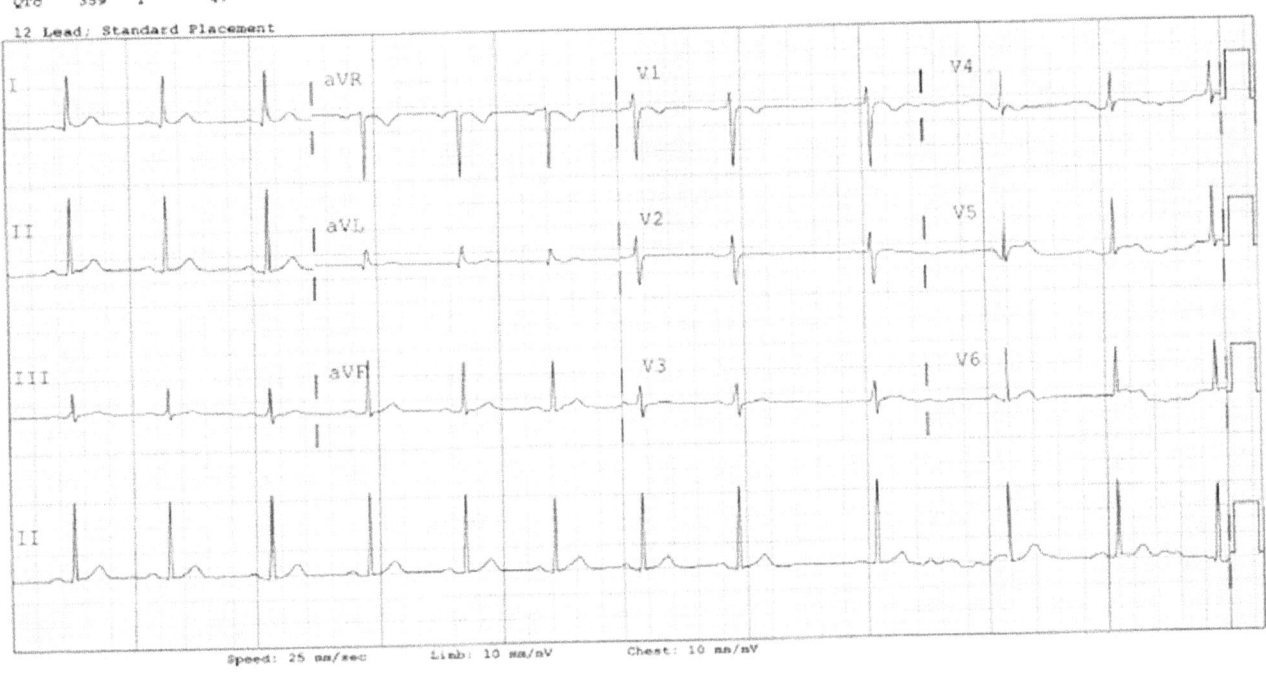

Figure 119.1

H. Secondary survey

a.   General: cachectic, disheveled man, oriented to self, sleepy but arousable
b.   Head: normocephalic, atraumatic
c.   Eyes: extraocular movement intact, pupils equal, reactive to light
d.   Ears: cerumen, normal tympanic membranes
e.   Nose: no discharge
f.   Neck: full range of motion, no jugular vein distension, no stridor
g.   Pharynx: edentulous, no lesions, no swelling
h.   Chest: cachectic chest, nontender
i.   Lungs: distant breath sounds, clear bilaterally
j.   Heart: rate and rhythm regular, no murmurs, rubs, or gallops
k.   Abdomen: normal bowel sounds, soft, (+) tender diffusely, no rebound
l.   Rectal: normal tone, brown stool, occult blood negative
m.   Extremities: full range of motion, no deformity, normal pulses
n.   Back: nontender
o.   Neuro: cranial nerves II–XII intact; normal sensation; 4/5 strength in all extremities; decreased reflexes; normal gait
p.   Skin: warm and dry
q.   Lymph: no lymphadenopathy

I. Nurse

a.   CXR (Figure 119.2)

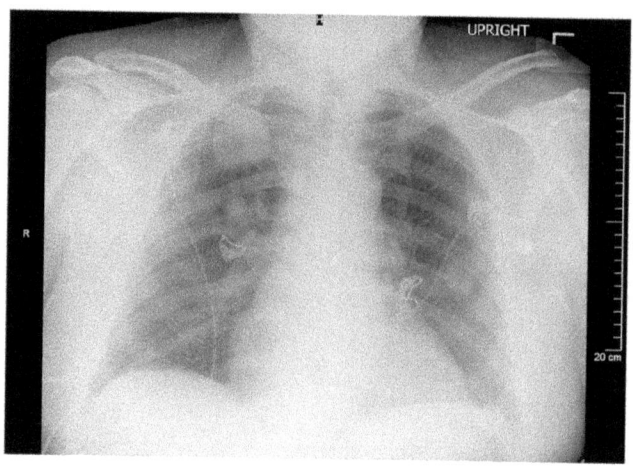

Figure 119.2

J. Action

a. Lipase
b. ABG
c. Ca, iCa, Mg

K. Results

Table 119.1 Results table

Test	Result	Test	Result
Complete blood count:		T bili	1.0 mg/dL
WBC	$7.3 \times 10^3/\mu L$	D bili	0.3 mg/dL
Hct	36.5%	Amylase	50 U/L
Plt	$330 \times 10^3/\mu L$	Lipase	25 U/L
		Albumin	3.2 g/dL
Basic metabolic panel:			
Na	141 mEq/L	**Urinalysis:**	
K	2.9 mEq/L	SG	1.010–1.030
Cl	105 mEq/L	pH	5–8
CO_2	24 mEq/L	Prot	Neg
BUN	29 mEq/dL	Gluc	Neg
Cr	2.2 mg/dL	Ketones	Neg
Gluc	89 mg/dL	Bili	Neg
		Blood	Neg
Coagulation panel:		LE	Neg
PT	12.6 sec	Nitrite	Neg
PTT	26 sec	Color	Yellow
INR	1.0		

Table 119.1 (cont.)

Test	Result	Test	Result
Liver function panel:		Arterial blood gas:	
AST	23 U/L	pH	7.38
ALT	26 U/L	pO_2	98 mmHg
Alk phos	42 U/L	pCO_2	36 mmHg
		HCO_3	23 mEq/L
		O_2 Sat	99%

a. Ca: 14.5 mg/dL
b. iCa: 3.9 mmol/L
c. Mg: 0.7 mg/dL

L. Action

a. 1–2 L NS bolus, then 200–300 cc/hr to urine output of 100–150 cc/hr
b. Bisphosphonate
   i. Zoledronic acid 4 mg IV over 15 minutes *or*
   ii. Pamidronate 90 mg IV over 2 hours
c. Calcitonin 4 IU/kg SC or IM
d. Potassium and magnesium replacement
e. Admission to ICU

M. Diagnosis

a. Hypercalcemia from squamous cell lung cancer

N. Critical actions

a. IV fluids
b. EKG: identification of short QTc
c. CXR: identification of pulmonary nodules
d. Identification of clinical hypercalcemia presentation
e. Ca, iCa levels
f. Bisphosphonate
g. ICU admission

O. Examiner instructions

a. This is a case of hypercalcemia secondary to squamous cell lung cancer. Cancer-induced hypercalcemia is a paraneoplastic syndrome caused by direct destruction of bone by tumor, and by tumor secretion of parathyroid hormone. The patient presents with moans (altered mental status and psychiatric complaints), groans (constipation and abdominal pain) in the setting of an EKG showing hypercalcemic changes (shortened QTc intervals), and a CXR showing multiple pulmonary nodules. If an abdominal CT is obtained during the case, an incidental nonobstructing kidney stone will be present in the renal calyx in an otherwise normal CT (Figure 119.3). Other findings consistent with hypercalcemia are hypertension, hypokalemia, hypomagnesemia, and renal insufficiency. Hypercalcemia is a common complication of many cancers, and is an oncologic emergency. The lung nodules seen on CXR should prompt the examinee to order calcium levels. If

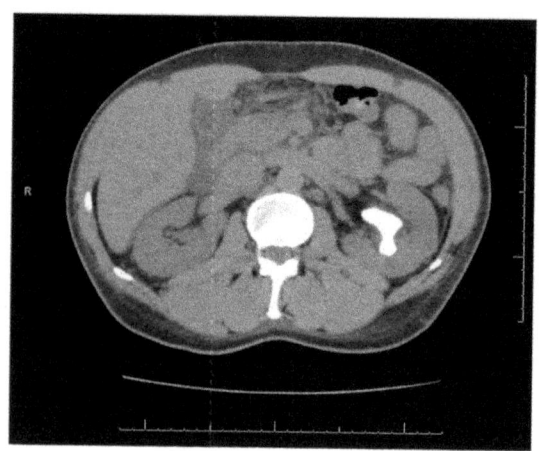

Figure 119.3

the examinee does not identify the clinical presentation of hypercalcemia, the patient will develop increasing lethargy that will progress to a comatose state, requiring intubation.

P. Pearls

a. Patients with hypercalcemia present with stones (renal calculi), bones (osteolysis), moans (altered mental status and psychiatric disorders), and groans (peptic ulcer disease, pancreatitis, or constipation).
b. From 20% to 40% of cancer patients develop hypercalcemia, and it is the most common life-threatening metabolic disorder in these patients.
c. The majority of patients presenting with hypercalcemia (90%) have associated malignancy or hyperparathyroidism.
d. EKG findings include short QTc intervals, short ST segments, depressed ST segments, and widened T waves. Bradyarrhythmia with bundle branch patterns can occur, and may progress to second-degree block, complete heart block, and even cardiac arrest.
e. Treatment consists primarily of fluid resuscitation followed by medically lowering calcium levels. Patients with severe symptomatic hypercalcemia should be admitted to the ICU until symptoms resolve and calcium levels return to normal.
f. Hypercalcemia may not always require treatment if the patient is asymptomatic and the serum calcium is less than 14 mg/dL (3.5 mmol/L).
g. Furosemide is not routinely recommended for hypercalcemia due to malignancy.
h. Clinical symptoms of hypercalcemia are correlated more with the rate of rise in calcium than the absolute number.

Q. Figure legends

a. Figure 119.1 (EKG) EKG showing short QTc.
b. Figure 119.2 (CXR) Chest x-ray showing pulmonary mass and nodules.
c. Figure 119.3 (CT) Noncontrast CT of abdomen showing left renal calculus.

R. References

a. *Tintinalli's Emergency Medicine: A Comprehensive Study Guide* (9th ed.): Chapter 240, Emergency Complications of Malignancy.
b. *Rosen's Emergency Medicine: Concepts and Clinical Practice* (10th ed.): Chapter 114, Electrolyte Disorders.

S. Acknowledgments

a. We would like to acknowledge Matthew Ryan for their contribution to this chapter in the previous edition of this book, which has been updated by Lars K. Beattie and Laura Scieszka.

Patient with Fatigue, Weight Gain, and Bruising

Victor Cisneros, MD, MPH, Mason Shieh, MD, MBA, and Thomas Nguyen, MD

A. Chief complaint
a. 38-year-old female with weight gain and fatigue over the last few months

B. Vital signs
a. HR: 88, BP: 136/90, RR: 18, T: 37°C, Sat: 99%, FS: 256 mg/dL, Wt: 10 kg

C. What does the patient look like?
a. Patient appears comfortable

D. Primary survey
a. Airway: speaking in full sentences
b. Breathing: spontaneous, nonlabored breathing
c. Circulation: peripheral pulses equal

E. History
a. HPI: A 38-year-old female presents with weight gain, amenorrhea, and generalized decrease in energy over the past 3 months. She also noticed easy bruising on her body. She denies any blood thinner use, increased sun exposure, new medications, recent illness, or recent trauma.
b. PMHx: none
c. PSHx: none
d. Meds: none
e. Allergies: no known drug allergies
f. Social: lives alone in apartment
g. FHx: family history of diabetes

F. Secondary survey
a. General: awake, alert, no distress
b. HEENT: pupils equal, round, reactive to light, slight puffiness around eyes, round cheeks
c. Neck: obese with moderate fat padding on posterior of neck
d. Chest: no rashes
e. Heart: regular rate and rhythm, no murmurs
f. Abdomen: obese, soft, no tenderness, no fluid wave, normal bowel sounds
g. Rectal: deferred
h. GU: normal
i. Extremities: no swelling
j. Back: no deformities, no CVA tenderness
k. Neuro: normal

l.   Skin: purple striae noted in abdomen, thighs, axillae, and buttocks; old bruises seen on the arm and leg

m.   Lymph: normal

G. Action

a.   IV

    i.   20-gauge peripheral IV

b.   Labs

    i.   CBC, BMP, PT/PTT, TSH, urine pregnancy

c.   Fluids

    i.   Not required, optional

d.   Monitor

    i.   Not required

e.   Consult

    i.   Endocrinology

f.   Medicines

    i.   None

g.   Additional labs

    i.   Random cortisol level.

    ii.   (If admitted) Order 24-hour cortisol urine, serum cortisol, serum ACTH, dexamethasone suppression test

h.   Imaging

    i.   CT abdomen/pelvis (can be ordered if there is a concern for primary adrenal tumor, based on exam and laboratory findings. This is more likely done as outpatient work-up or during hospital admission. If the examinee requests, radiologist asks, "What are you looking for?")

H. Results

Table 120.1 Results table

Test	Result	Test	Result
Complete blood count:		CO_2	25 mEq/L
WBC	$9.2 \times 10^3/\mu L$	BUN	16 mEq/dL
Hgb	14.3	Cr	0.81 mg/dL
Hct	42.7%	Glucose	270 mg/dL
Plt	$280 \times 10^3/\mu L$		
		Coagulation panel:	
Basic metabolic panel:		PT	12.3 sec
Na	138 mEq/L	PTT	31.2 sec
K	3.3 mEq/L	INR	0.9
Cl	102 mEq/L		

a.   Pregnancy test: negative

b.   Random serum cortisol: 54 mcg/dL (normal range 5–20 mcg/dL)

c.   If ordered, CT abdomen/pelvis: demonstrates adrenal tumor/hyperplasia

   d. If admitted, follow-up labs show 24-hour free urinary cortisol 318 mcg/24 h (normal range 10–150 mcg/24 h), serum ACTH < 4 pg/mL (normal range 10–60 pg/mL), dexamethasone suppression test – there is no drop in levels of blood cortisol following administration of dexamethasone.

I. Action

   a. Referral to endocrine and surgery for adrenal removal.

   b. Refer to primary care doctor for management of possible diabetes and hypertension.

J. Diagnosis

   a. Cushing syndrome from a cortisol-secreting adrenal mass

K. Critical actions

   a. Pregnancy test

   b. CBC to check platelets and coagulation profile

   c. Recognizes potential Cushing syndrome/endocrine etiology of the case presentation

   d. Endocrine consult or referral

   e. Orders random cortisol level

L. Examiner instructions

   a. The patient is suffering from Cushing syndrome, or hypercortisolism, due to excess secretion of cortisol (steroid hormone) from an adrenal gland tumor. She is presenting with very nonspecific complaints that could easily be missed in the ED setting. The key to the work-up is to ensure the examinee checks for non-immediate life-threatening etiologies, and ensures appropriate follow-up for work-up. Cushing syndrome can occur via any mechanism that increases cortisol levels in the body. This includes a cortisol-secreting adrenal tumor, an ACTH-secreting pituitary mass, an ectopic ACTH-secreting mass such as a lung cancer, or endogenous chronic steroid use such as prednisone for rheumatoid arthritis.

   b. Patients with suspected Cushing syndrome should get endocrine follow-up and/or consult. They may be discharged for outpatient work-up if stable.

M. Pearls

   a. The most specific lab test is the 24-hour free urinary cortisol, which should be elevated. Cortisol is released in spurts throughout the day, making random cortisol levels less reliable.

   b. Obesity, chronic illness, chronic alcoholism, and depression can cause false-positive results (pseudo-Cushing's syndrome) on the 1 mg dexamethasone suppression test and mildly elevated free cortisol values on the 24-hour urine collection.

   c. A midnight serum cortisol level of less than 7.5 mcg/dL is strongly suggestive of pseudo-Cushing's syndrome.

   d. Specific findings include easy bruising, purple striae, psychological changes, proximal myopathy, and fat deposition in the face and neck.

   e. Common nonspecific findings include central obesity, hypertension, osteoporosis, acne, hirsutism, amenorrhea, hyperlipidemia, and diabetes mellitus.

   f. Lung tumors account for over 50% of ectopic ACTH-secreting tumors, with small cell being the most common type.

   g. Dexamethasone suppression test and CRH stimulation test will help differentiate between pituitary ACTH-secreting adenoma, ectopic ACTH secretion, and cortisol-secreting adrenal tumors. Determining the type of tumor will dictate where to perform imaging studies as well as management.

h. Complications: If Cushing syndrome is left untreated, it can have high morbidity and even death. Patients may suffer complications from hypertension, diabetes mellitus, and osteoporosis.

i. Polycystic ovarian syndrome can mimic Cushing syndrome in females.

M. References

a. *Rosen's Emergency Medicine: Concepts and Clinical Practice* (10th ed.): Chapter 117, Thyroid and Adrenal Disorders.

b. *Tintinalli's Emergency Medicine: A Comprehensive Study Guide* (9th ed.): Section 17, Endocrine Disorders.

Toddler with Fever and Rash

Daniel Goldstein, MD and Michael Truax Jr., MD

A. Chief complaint
a. 3-year-old male with fever and rash

B. Vital signs
a. BP: 98/62, HR: 145, RR: 28, T: 39.1°C, Sat: 96%, Wt: 15 kg

C. What does the patient look like?
a. Patient is sitting in bed on mom's lap, crying, uncomfortable.

D. Primary survey
a. Airway: age-appropriate speech, answers questions when encouraged by mom
b. Breathing: no significant respiratory distress, no cyanosis, mildly tachypneic
c. Circulation: bounding peripheral pulses, equal bilaterally

E. History
a. HPI: A 3-year-old male with 3 days of tactile fever and nasal congestion, with patient developing rash to face earlier today. Mom was not concerned initially since fever was responding to acetaminophen, but concerned today given new rash. Per mom, no cough, vomiting, diarrhea, abdominal pain, urinary symptoms, headache, bone pain, neck stiffness, or recent travel. Patient attends daycare and has sick siblings at home.
b. PMHx: Sickle cell disease (type SC), baseline Hb 9; born full term, normal spontaneous vaginal delivery without complications; no hospitalizations within past 6 months
c. PSHx: circumcision
d. Meds: hydroxyurea, folate, penicillin
e. Social: lives at home with mom, grandparents, and two younger siblings; attends daycare
f. FHx: mom with sickle cell trait, father passed away in thirties from complications of sickle cell disease

F. Action
a. Oxygen via NC or nonrebreather mask as needed to maintain saturation at 95%
b. Peripheral IV access
c. Labs:
    i. CBC, blood cultures, BMP, LFT, reticulocyte count, group A Strep rapid and culture, type and cross, lactic acid
d. Monitor: BP: 92/60, HR: 138, RR: 30
e. IV fluids (amount and type of IV fluids may vary by institution/protocols)
f. CXR (Figure 121.1)

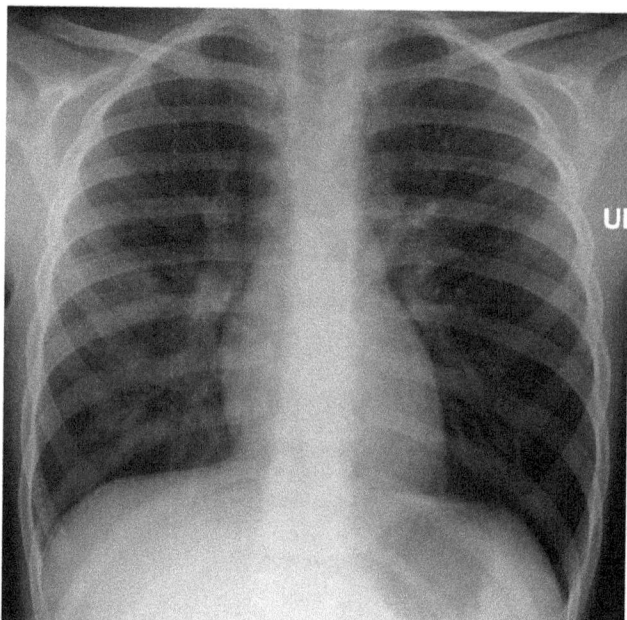

Figure 121.1

G. Secondary survey

a. General: awake, alert, answers questions appropriately, diaphoretic, uncomfortable
b. HEENT: normocephalic, atraumatic, jaundiced, conjunctival pallor, erythema of posterior oropharynx, no tonsillar exudate or petechiae, uvula midline, +rhinorrhea; tympanic membranes without erythema or bulging
c. Neck: bilateral, tender, anterior cervical lymphadenopathy, supple, nonmeningeal
d. Chest: nontender
e. Heart: tachycardic, no murmurs, rubs, or gallops
f. Lungs: clear, no crackles, no wheezing, no stridor, mildly tachypneic
g. Abdomen: normal bowel sounds, soft, nontender, no distention, no hepatosplenomegaly
h. Rectal: normal
i. GU: normal
j. Extremities: full passive and active range of motion of all extremities, no erythema or swelling, no focal bony tenderness
k. Back: nontender
l. Neuro: no focal cranial nerve or motor/sensory deficits; ambulates normally
m. Skin: maculopapular, fiery red rash along cheeks, no involvement of bridge of nose or forehead, no petechiae or purpura
n. Lymph: anterior cervical lymphadenopathy

H. Results

Table 121.1 Results table

Test	Result	Test	Result
Complete blood count:		**Liver function panel:**	
WBC	$5.2 \times 10^3/\mu L$	AST	42 U/L
Hgb	6.9 g/dL	ALT	36 U/L
Hct	17%	Alk phos	145 U/L
Plt	$150 \times 10^3/\mu L$	T bili	4.0 mg/dL
PMN	35%	D bili	0.3 mg/dL
Lymphs	60%	Amylase	76 U/L
Absolute neutro	$1.82 \times 10^3/\mu L$	Lipase	140 U/L
		Albumin	3.7 g/dL
Basic metabolic panel:		Lactic acid	1.5 mmol/L
K	138 mEq/L		
Cl	5.0 mEq/L	**Urinalysis:**	
Na	104 mEq/L	SG	1.010–1.030
CO_2	21 mEq/L	pH	5–8
BUN	19 mEq/dL	Prot	Neg
Cr	0.9 mg/dL	Gluc	Neg
Gluc	122 mg/dL	Ketones	Neg
		Bili	Trace
Coagulation panel:		Blood	Neg
PT	13 sec	LE	Neg
PTT	27 sec	Nitrite	Neg
INR	1.0	Color	Yellow
		Reticulocyte %:	2.5%
		Absolute retic. count	$1.0 \times 10^3/\mu L$

a. Rapid group A Strep: negative

I. Action
a. Meds
   i. Antipyretic
   ii. Ceftriaxone
b. Consultation
   i. Hematology
c. Transfuse 10 mL/kg pRBC and repeat CBC

J. Nurse

a. Transfusion of pRBC
   i. BP: 104/70, HR: 115, RR: 24
b. No transfusion of pRBC
   i. BP: 88/54, HR: 155, RR: 36
   ii. Nurse states patient now appears to have increased work of breathing

K. Action

a. Admission to monitored setting
b. Repeat CBC

L. Diagnosis

a. Aplastic crisis

M. Critical actions

a. CBC, reticulocyte count, blood cultures
b. Transfusion
c. CXR
d. Antibiotics
e. Admit

N. Examiner instructions

a. This is a case of a toddler with sickle cell disease, who presents with an aplastic crisis, when the bone marrow shuts down and does not produce red blood cells. In this case, the aplastic crisis is likely due to a viral infection caused by *Parvovirus* B19, which can present with fever, runny nose, headache, facial rash, and joint pain. Other causes of infection should be ruled out, and the patient started on broad-spectrum antibiotic coverage. The most important initial treatment is transfusion, antibiotics, and admission for hematology consultation and further monitoring of CBC.

O. Pearls

a. Aplastic crisis is when the bone marrow is unable to produce a sufficient number of new red blood cells as compared to aplastic anemia, which leads to pancytopenia.
b. In pregnant patients, *Parvovirus* B19 can cause hydrops of the fetus.
c. In most cases, *Parvovirus* B19 causes only a drop in the red cell line. This may go clinically unnoticed, as a short-lived aplastic episode may not cause a significant drop in red blood cells, which, on average, live for 120 days; however, in individuals with sickle cell disease, where a red blood cell only lives for 10–20 days on average, this can cause a profound drop in Hgb, leading to symptoms including pale skin or mucosa, fatigue, shortness of breath, fever, fast heart rate, weakness, headache, or agitation.
d. In the case of a patient with sickle cell disease, a transfusion can be lifesaving, as these individuals are unable to compensate for the temporary bone marrow suppression, which commonly lasts 5–10 days. The WBC and platelets are generally not affected.
e. Remember to calculate the reticulocyte index for all patients, as the reticulocyte count can be misleading in anemic patients. A value of 45% is used as the "normal hematocrit."
   i. retic index = retic count × (hematocrit/normal hematocrit)

    f. Reticulocyte index values with anemia
   i. Values <2 indicates loss of RBCs and a decreased production of new RBCs (an inadequate response to correct the anemia).
   ii. Values >3 indicate the appropriate response, with an increased compensatory production of RBCs to replace lost RBCs.

P. Figure legends
a. Figure 121.1 (CXR) Right middle lobe pneumonia in a child (https://commons.m.wikimedia .org/wiki/File:RtPneuKid.png; James Heilman, MD. CC BY-SA 4.0).

Q. References
a. *Tintinalli's Emergency Medicine: A Comprehensive Study Guide* (9th ed.): Chapter 142, Rashes in Infants and Children. Chapter 143, Sickle Cell Disease in Children.
b. *Rosen's Emergency Medicine: Concepts and Clinical Practice* (10th ed.): Chapter 109, Anemia and Polycythemia.

Arm Pain

Shahram Lotfipour, MD

A. Chief complaint
a. 28-year-old male who came to the ED with arm pain

B. Vital signs
a. BP: 90/65, HR: 125, RR: 16, T: 38.8°C, Sat: 98% on RA

C. What does the patient look like?
a. Patient is a muscular man, diaphoretic and anxious but in no apparent distress.

D. Primary survey
a. Airway: speaking in full sentences
b. Breathing: no apparent respiratory distress, no cyanosis
c. Circulation: warm, diaphoretic skin; diminished peripheral pulses with slightly delayed capillary refill (2–3 second)

E. Action
a. Peripheral IV access
b. Monitor: BP: 90/65, HR: 125, RR: 18, T: 38.8°C
c. Labs
    i. Urine analysis, CBC, BMP, LFT, CK, lactate
    ii. Optional: Troponin-I, CK-MB, coagulation studies
d. 1 L NS bolus
e. EKG

F. History
a. HPI: This is a 28-year-old man who presents with pain that started in his left arm 8 hours ago and has now spread to both arms as well as chest. The pain is currently starting in both of his legs. The pain is achy and he rates it as an 8 out of 10. The pain is worse with movement. He has had associated fever, nausea, and darker urine. He went to the gym yesterday and had a workout that lasted longer than usual. He went to work this morning as a demolition specialist in 95°F weather but left early because of the pain.
b. PMHx: occasional back pain from work
c. PSHx: none
d. Allergies: none
e. Meds: ibuprofen 800 mg PRN for back pain, he has been taking "a lot" recently (4–5 doses a day for last 3 days for back pain)

f. Social: uses cocaine "occasionally," last used yesterday, smokes tobacco – one pack per day for 10 years, no alcohol use; works as demolition specialist

g. FHx: father with MI at 50 years old; mother with a stroke at 72 years old

h. PMD: Dr. Steinberg

G. Secondary survey

a. General: alert, oriented × 3, uncomfortable, diaphoretic

b. Head: normocephalic, atraumatic

c. Eyes: extraocular movements intact, pupils equal and reactive to light

d. Ears: normal ear canals and tympanic membranes

e. Nose: no discharge

f. Neck: full range of motion, no jugular vein distension, no stridor

g. Pharynx: normal dentition, no lesions, no swelling, no erythema

h. Chest: nontender

i. Lungs: clear and equal bilaterally

j. Heart: tachycardic, rhythm regular, no murmurs, rubs, or gallops

k. Abdomen: normal bowel sounds, soft, nontender, nondistended

l. Rectal: normal tone, brown stool, occult blood negative

m. Extremities: mild tenderness on palpation of extremities but no joint findings, full range of motion, no deformity, diminished pulses

n. Back: nontender, no deformity

o. Neuro: cranial nerves II to XII intact; normal sensation, strength; normal reflexes, stable gait, negative cerebellar testing

p. Skin: warm and diaphoretic, no rashes or ecchymosis

q. Heme: no lymphadenopathy

H. Action

a. Second 1 L NS IV bolus

b. Meds:
    i. Morphine or hydromorphone (NSAIDs should be avoided due to renal damage from rhabdomyolysis and dehydration)

c. Cool patient with ice packs or cooling device

d. Bicarbonate therapy (not vital to patient's care)

e. Mannitol therapy (not vital to patient's care)

I. Nurse

a. EKG (Figure 122.1)

b. Fluid resuscitation
    i. 2 L IV fluids given
        1. BP: 110/80, HR: 95
    ii. Less than 2 L IV fluids given
        1. BP: 90/65, HR: 130

c. Analgesics
    i. Pain improves to 3/10 and patient appears more comfortable

d. Cooling with ice packs
    i. Temperature improves to 38.0°C

e. Bicarbonate and/or mannitol therapy
    i. No effect on patient

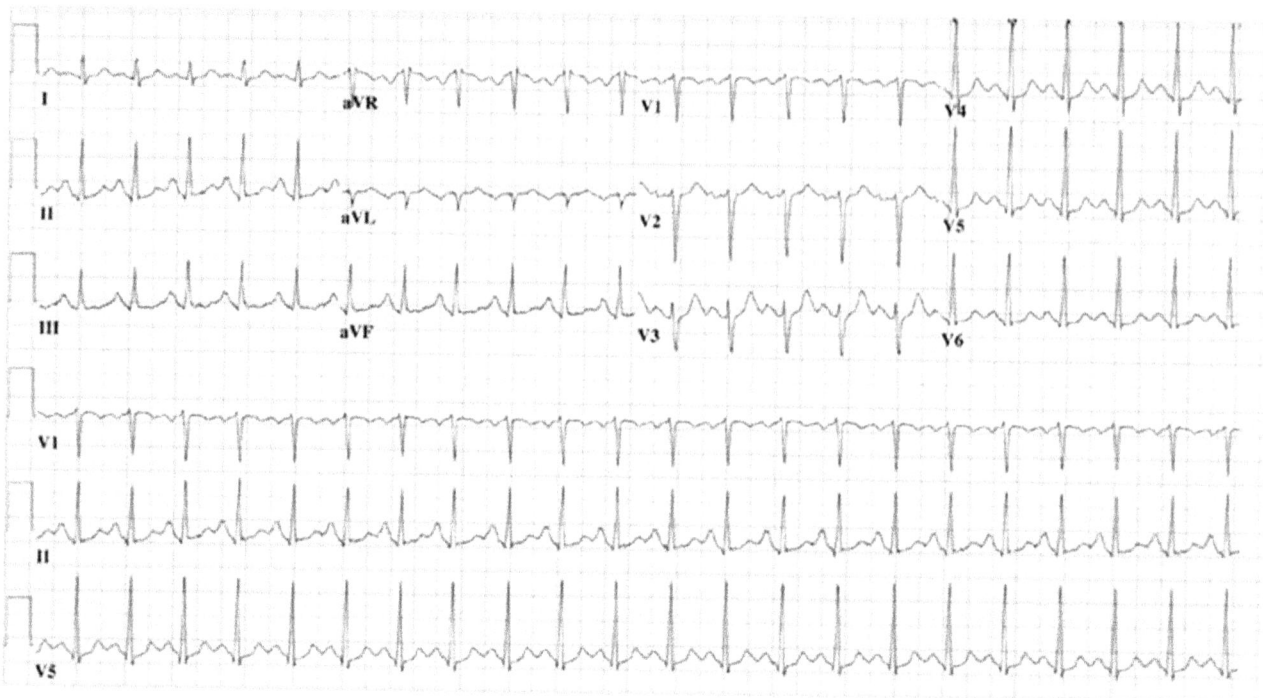

Figure 122.1

J. Results

Table 122.1 Results table

Test	Result	Test	Result
Complete blood count:		Creatinine kinase	12,000 U/L
WBC	$9 \times 10^3/\mu L$	Lactate	2.4 mmol/L
Hct	47%		
Plt	$150 \times 10^3/\mu L$	**Urinalysis:**	
		SG	1.015
Basic metabolic panel:		pH	6.2
Na	132 mEq/L	Prot	Trace
K	4.9 mEq/L	Gluc	Neg
Cl	99 mEq/L	Ketones	Present
CO_2	17 mEq/L	Bili	Neg
BUN	85 mEq/dL	Blood	+
Cr	4.8 mg/dL	LE	Neg
Glu	110 mg/dL	Nitrite	Neg
		Color	Tea-colored
Liver function panel:		RBCs	0
AST	32 U/L	WBCs	0
ALT	38 U/L	Casts	Pigmented, brown

Table 122.1 (cont.)

Test	Result	Test	Result
Alk phos	98 U/L	Blood gas:	
T bili	0.7 mg/dL	pH	7.32
D bili	0.1 mg/dL	pCO_2	35 mmHg
Albumin	5.5 g/dL	HCO_3	15 mEq/L
Total protein	7.4 g/dL		

K. Diagnosis
a. Primary: rhabdomyolysis
b. Secondary:
   i. Heat exhaustion
   ii. Acute kidney injury due to combination of:
      1. Dehydration/heat exhaustion
      2. Rhabdomyolysis (myoglobin effect on kidney)
      3. High-dose ibuprofen use (decreases GFR)

L. Critical actions
a. Cardiac monitoring
b. IV fluid administration
c. EKG within 10 minutes of arrival (due to chest pain and cocaine)
d. Pain control with opiates or other appropriate analgesic
e. Obtain cardiac history and/or ROS
f. Consult nephrology
g. Admit the patient to the hospital

M. Examiner instructions
a. This is a case of rhabdomyolysis, a breakdown of muscle tissue, which in this patient was caused by cocaine use and heavy workout. Rhabdomyolysis is defined as a CK level 5–10 times normal. The rhabdomyolysis, coupled with heat exhaustion, dehydration, and high-dose ibuprofen use, ultimately led to the patient's acute kidney damage, exacerbating the patient's condition.
b. The candidate should recognize the pathology that the patient has and aggressively hydrate him. Hyperthermia should also be treated. The candidate should obtain renal consultation for optimal renal resuscitation and possible dialysis. Intravenous bicarbonate therapy could be considered as it may provide benefit to decrease development of acute renal dysfunction in cases with a creatinine over 2 mg/dL and creatine kinase of greater than 10,000 IU/L. With bicarbonate, it is important to avoid hypokalemia and metabolic acidosis. A urinary catheter can be placed to monitor urine output. Cardiac monitoring might be needed due to metabolic and electrolyte complications. In patients with significant comorbid conditions, hemodynamic monitoring might be indicated to avoid fluid overload. Hyperkalemia after muscle injury, which can be most significant in the first 12–36 hours, can be difficult to treat and may require ion-exchange resin therapy. Severe hyperphosphatemia can be treated with oral phosphate binders.
c. Mannitol therapy has been suggested, but the data on its use in the treatment of rhabdomyolysis indicate it may be harmful as it may cause osmotic diuresis in hypovolemic patients.

N. Pearls

a. Dehydration causes a pre-renal/volume depleted state, creating clinically significant rhabdomyolysis with early renal dysfunction at lower CK levels.

b. Aggressive IV hydration improves the glomerular filtration rate (GFR), which reduces renal injury and improves outcomes in patients with rhabdomyolysis.

c. A significant complication of rhabdomyolysis is electrolyte abnormalities due to acute kidney injury, as well as skeletal muscle damage.

d. NSAIDs should be avoided because they can cause renal artery vasoconstriction (via prostaglandin inhibition), which reduces GFR, and makes patients more prone to renal injury from rhabdomyolysis.

O. Figure legends

a. Figure 122.1 (EKG) Sinus tachycardia.

P. References

a. *Tintinalli's Emergency Medicine: A Comprehensive Study Guide* (9th ed.): Chapter 89, Rhabdomyolysis.

b. *Rosen's Emergency Medicine: Concepts and Clinical Practice* (10th ed.): Chapter 116, Rhabdomyolysis.

Q. Acknowledgements

a. We would like to acknowledge Michael A.Cole for their contribution to this chapter in the previous edition of this book, which has been updated by Shahram Lotfipour.

Headache

Elisabeth Lessenich, MD, MPH

A. Chief complaint
a. 26-year-old female with headache, worsening since this afternoon

B. Vital signs
a. HR: 69, BP: 131/76, RR: 16, T: 36.0°C, Sat: 100% on RA

C. What does the patient look like?
a. Patient appears stated age, appears uncomfortable, resting her head on the stretcher with her eyes closed.

D. Primary survey
a. Airway: speaking quietly, but in full sentences
b. Breathing: no apparent respiratory distress, good air entry bilaterally
c. Circulation: intact peripheral pulses bilaterally, capillary refill normal

E. History
a. HPI: This is a 26-year-old female who presents with a throbbing headache, rated 8/10 and worse on the right side, which started this morning. She has associated nausea but has not vomited. She feels the pain is worsened by sunlight or room lights. She took acetaminophen and ibuprofen, which usually helps her by lunchtime, but the headache has progressed. She denies fevers, recent travel, fall or head trauma, neck or back pain, speech changes, visual changes, focal weakness, numbness, or trouble walking. She reports a history of 1–2 migraine episodes per month, which typically respond to over-the-counter medication and rest. Over the past 2 weeks she has had increased stress and workload at her job and has not been sleeping well.
b. PMHx: paroxysmal SVT, migraines
c. PSHx: status post SVT ablation 4 months prior
d. Medications: oral contraceptive pill daily; acetaminophen and ibuprofen prn
e. Allergies: none
f. Social: denies smoking or illicit drug use; 3–4 alcoholic drinks per week. She lives with roommates and works in the music industry doing concert promotion
g. FHx: mother has a history of migraines; brother also has a history of undifferentiated headaches

F. Action
a. Large peripheral IV
b. 1 L NS bolus intravenously
c. Urine pregnancy test
d. EKG (candidate may request given the history of SVT, although not required)

G. Secondary survey

a. General: obese, uncomfortable, resting with eyes closed, holding her head
b. Head: normocephalic, atraumatic
c. Eyes: extraocular movements intact without nystagmus, fundi unremarkable (must ask), pupils equal and reactive to light
d. Ears: normal ear canals and tympanic membranes
e. Nose: no discharge
f. Pharynx: clear without exudates or erythema
g. Neck: supple with full range of motion (must ask), no jugular vein distension
h. Cardiovascular: regular rate and rhythm, no murmurs or rubs
i. Lungs: clear to auscultation bilaterally, no wheezing or crackles
j. Abdomen: bowel sounds present, soft, nondistended, nontender
k. Back: nontender, normal range of motion
l. GU: deferred
m. Extremities: no edema, 2+ radial and DP pulses bilaterally
n. Neuro: alert and oriented × 3, intact concentration and short-term memory, cranial nerves II–XII intact, visual fields full, speech fluent, 5/5 strength in all extremities with normal tone and bulk, light touch sense intact bilaterally, no pronator drift, 2+ reflexes in upper and lower extremities, finger-to-nose and heel-to-shin intact without dysmetria, Romberg negative, normal gait
o. Skin: warm, dry, well perfused, without rashes
p. Lymph: no cervical or axillary lymphadenopathy

H. Results

a. Negative urine pregnancy test
b. EKG (Figure 123.1)

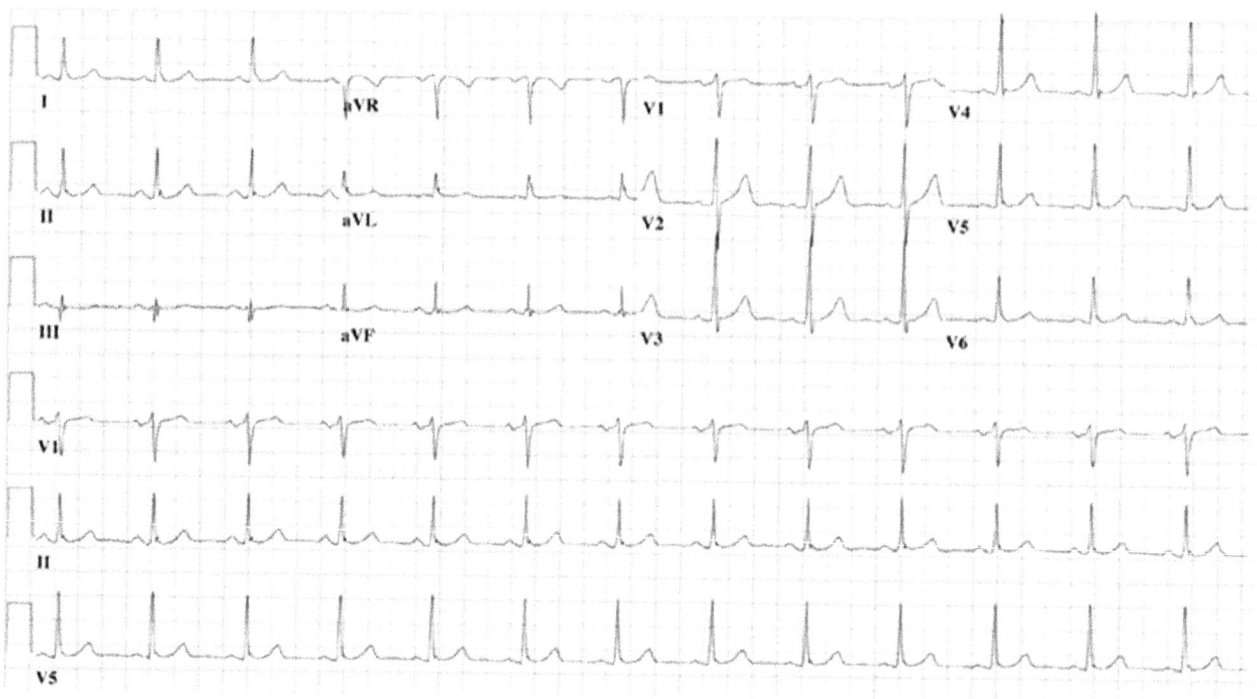

Figure 123.1

I. Action

a. Meds
   i. Prochlorperazine or metoclopramide 10 mg IV (or IM)
   ii. Benadryl 25 mg IV – may give with prochlorperazine
   iii. Sumatriptan 6 mg SC (or IM)

J. Nurse

a. Headache now minimal (should not improve sufficiently until sumatriptan given); patient feels improved and ready to go home

K. Action

a. Arrange neurology outpatient follow-up for patient to discuss possible prophylactic migraine therapy if episodes remain severe or become more frequent.

L. Diagnosis

a. Migraine without aura ("common migraine")

M. Critical actions

a. Full neurological exam
b. Fluids and medication administration for migraine management
c. Consideration of neuroimaging if the patient has abnormalities/deficits on neurologic examination, or if headaches were more sudden in onset

N. Examiner instructions

a. This is a case of a patient suffering from a migraine headache without aura, or common migraine, which accounts for about 80% of migraine cases. Migraine is a chronic neurovascular disorder that manifests with severe headache episodes and, in the case of "classic migraine," is also associated with auras of particular neurologic symptoms like visual scotomas, photopsias, or transient motor deficits. Migraines have been noted to be triggered or exacerbated by such elements as stress, disturbances of sleep pattern, menstrual cycles in women, and weather – some of which could be elicited in this patient's history.
b. Given that the patient has already tried over-the-counter medications unsuccessfully at home, she should be treated with IV medications. She should not improve sufficiently until the candidate administers, or at least considers a triptan medication such as sumatriptan or a dopamine agonist. The candidate should demonstrate consideration of other neurological entities by questions asked to obtain patient history.

O. Pearls

a. In the evaluation of patients with headache in the ED, the provider must first distinguish between primary headache entities (such as migraines, tension headaches, and cluster headaches) and secondary headaches (where the headache is a manifestation of another insult or underlying abnormality, such as hemorrhage, infection, or malignancy).
b. Migraine treatment involves acute or abortive therapies as well as preventive or prophylactic regimens.
c. Common analgesics such as acetaminophen and NSAIDs are considered first-line therapies for mild to moderate migrainous headache. Combinations of acetaminophen, aspirin, and caffeine have also been shown to be effective, and can be tried if the patient has not already used them prior to arrival.

d. For moderate to severe migraine pain, the triptan medications (which act specifically on the 5-HT1 serotonin receptors) are recommended as first-line treatment. Triptans may diminish migraine pain by constricting dilated cerebral vessels and can be given subcutaneously or intranasally (or orally, if the patient has no associated nausea or vomiting). They are contraindicated in patients with coronary artery disease, peripheral vascular disease, pregnancy, or recent use of ergotamine-type medications.

e. Other first-line treatment options include dopamine antagonist antiemetics, such as metoclopramide and prochlorperazine.

f. Second-line parenteral medications include dihydroergotamine and magnesium.

g. Opioids are preferably avoided in migraine headache cases, given the risk of abuse or addiction (if used frequently), higher frequency of adverse effects, and study results indicating that other medication types are more effective for symptom relief.

h. Regardless of therapy choice, positive response to medication administration should not be used as an indication of headache etiology (as secondary headaches may also be alleviated by standard analgesics).

i. Because frequent severe migraine attacks can have a negative effect on patients' quality of life and productivity, patients with multiple episodes that do not respond to their usual analgesic regimen, or that require ED treatment, should be referred to a neurologist for discussion of the risks and benefits of prophylactic medication for their migraines (such as β-blockers, TCAs, or antiepileptics).

P. Figure legends

a. Figure 123.1 (EKG) Normal sinus rhythm.

Q. References

a. *Rosen's Emergency Medicine: Concepts and Clinical Practice* (10th ed.): Chapter 16, Headache. Chapter 89, Headache Disorders.

b. *Tintinalli's Emergency Medicine: A Comprehensive Study Guide* (9th ed.): Chapter 164, Neurologic Examination. Chapter 165, Headache.

Dizziness

Anne Chipman, MD, MS

A. Chief complaint
a. 72-year-old female with dizziness

B. Vital signs
a. BP:180/105, HR: 62, RR: 16, T: 37.4°C, Sat: 98% on RA

C. What does the patient look like?
a. The patient appears her stated age, lying supine, in no acute distress.

D. Primary survey
a. Airway: speaking in full sentences
b. Breathing: breathing comfortably
c. Circulation: normal capillary refill

E. Action
a. Two large-bore peripheral IVs
b. Labs:
    i.   Bedside glucose 175 mg/dL (must ask)
    ii. CBC, BMP, LFT, coagulation studies, troponin
c. Monitor
d. EKG

F. History
a. The patient reports that she awoke from sleep this morning and felt dizzy, as though the room was swaying. She attempted to get out of bed but was unable to walk because of the dizziness. She describes the dizziness as constant since waking (approximately 6 hours ago) and not affected by change in position. She also notes some incoordination with her left arm. She reports a mild headache and nausea. She denies other symptoms of vision or hearing changes, fevers, chills, confusion, chest pain, or palpitations.
b. PMHx: type 2 DM, HTN
c. PSHx: none
d. Allergies: penicillin
e. Medications: metformin, hydrochlorothiazide, lisinopril
f. Social: lives alone; does not smoke, drink, or use drugs
g. FHx: mother with CVA at age 65, father with MI at 70

G. Nurse

a. EKG (Figure 124.1)

b. BP: 195/110, HR: 65, RR: 18, Sat: 98% on RA

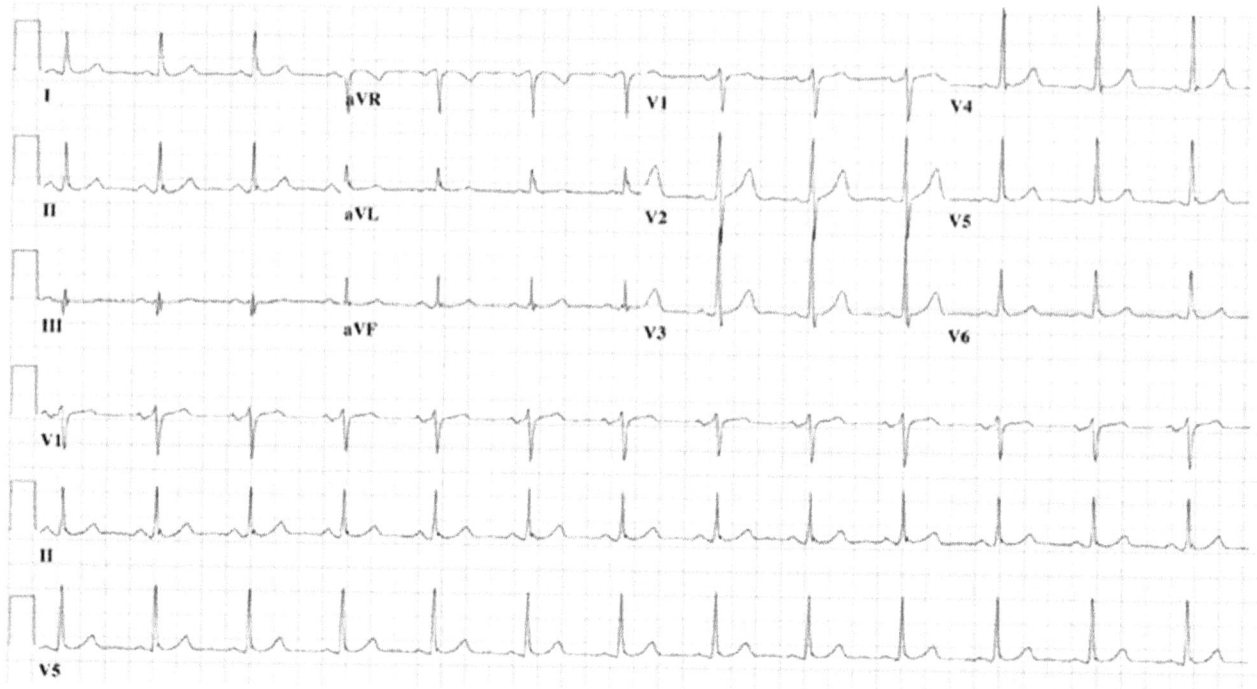

Figure 124.1

H. Secondary survey

a. General: NAD, lying in bed with eyes closed

b. Head: normocephalic, atraumatic

c. Eyes: pupils equal, round, and reactive to light; extraocular movements intact with bidirectional horizontal nystagmus; visual acuity normal

d. Ears: normal tympanic membranes

e. Nose: no nasal discharge

f. Neck: supple, with full range of motion; no carotid bruits

g. Pharynx: normal dentition, no lesions, no swelling

h. Lungs: clear bilaterally

i. Heart: rate and rhythm regular, no murmurs, rubs, or gallops

j. Abdomen: soft, nontender, nondistended, normal bowel sounds

k. Rectal: normal rectal tone

l. Extremities: no deformities, normal pulses

m. Back: nontender

n. Neuro: alert and oriented × 3; cranial nerves intact. Speech is clear. Left upper extremity with intention tremor, dysmetria and dysdiadochokinesia with testing. Strength difficult to assess in the left upper extremity due to intention tremor. Right upper extremity has normal motor and cerebellar findings. Significant truncal ataxia. Gait is wide-based and unsteady. She is unable to tandem walk. Sensation intact throughout the upper and lower extremities. Positive Romberg. See below for HINTS testing

o. Skin: warm and dry

I. Action

a. Imaging
   i. Head CT without contrast (negative)
   ii. Stroke protocol MRI/MRA of the brain or CT/CTA head and neck
b. Meds
   i. Aspirin should not be given until after negative CT
   ii. Antiemetic (patient will vomit if not given)
c. Additional testing
   i. HINTS testing (if requested, should be described): head impulse is with no corrective saccade; nystagmus horizontal and bidirectional, changes direction with gaze; positive for skew deviation.
   ii. Dix–Hallpike maneuver is not indicated. However, if done, should produce no change in nystagmus or experience of vertigo.

J. Nurse

a. BP: 232/130, HR: 80, RR: 17, Sat: 98% on RA
b. Patient continues to appear comfortable

K. Results

Table 124.1 Results table

Test	Result	Test	Result
Complete blood count:		T bili	1.0 mg/dL
WBC	$6.4 \times 10^3/\mu L$	D bili	0.3 mg/dL
Hct	40.5%	Amylase	40 U/L
Plt	$400 \times 10^3/\mu L$	Lipase	20 U/L
		Albumin	4.3 g/dL
Basic metabolic panel:			
Na	137 mEq/L	**Urinalysis:**	
K	4.5 mEq/L	SG	1.010–1.030
Cl	105 mEq/L	pH	5–8
CO_2	30 mEq/L	Prot	Neg
BUN	15 mEq/dL	Gluc	Neg
Cr	1.2 mg/dL	Ketones	Neg
Glucose	170 mg/dL	Bili	Neg
		Blood	Neg
Coagulation panel:		LE	Neg
PT	12.5 sec	Nitrate	Neg
PTT	26.0 sec	Color	Yellow
INR	1.0		

Table 124.1 (cont.)

Test	Result	Test	Result
Liver function panel:		Arterial blood gas:	
AST	24 U/L	pH	7.4
ALT	26 U/L	pO_2	95 mmHg
Alk phos	45 U/L	pCO_2	40 mmHg
		HCO_3	25 mmol/L

a. Troponin: <0.03 ng/mL
b. MRI/MRA brain (Figure 124.2): area of abnormal signal intensity in the left superior cerebellum. No hydrocephalus or brain herniation. Left vertebral artery occlusion.

A
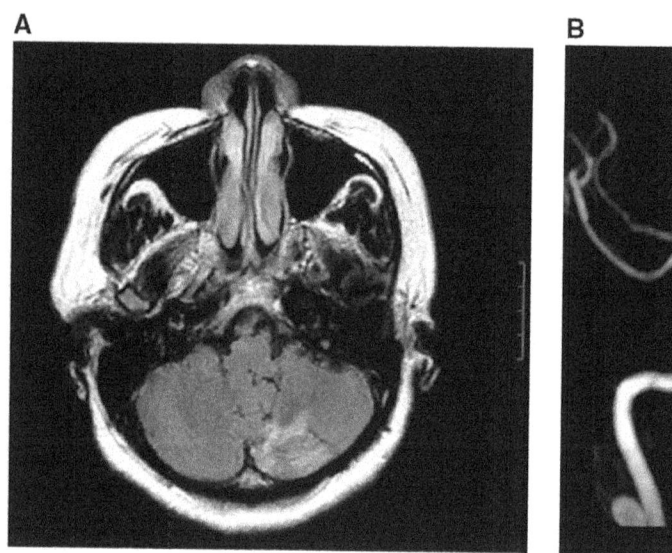

B
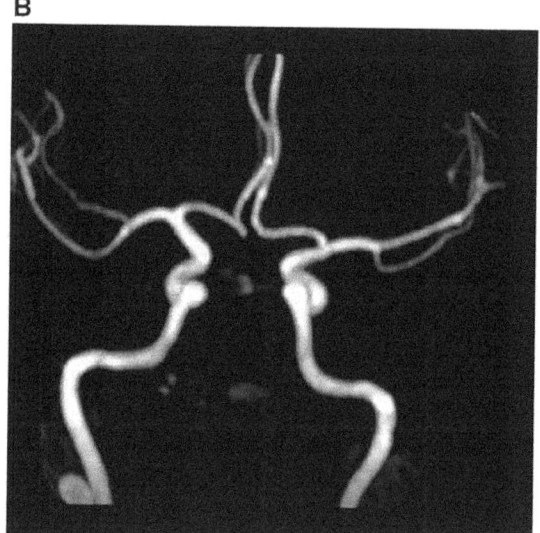

C
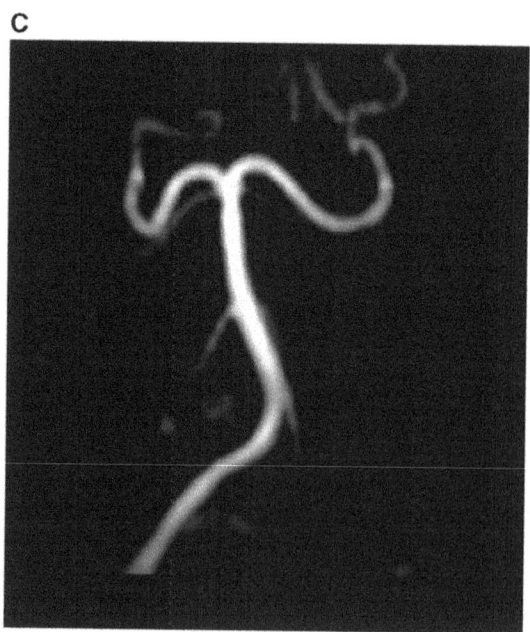

Figure 124.2

L. Actions

a. Consults:
   i. Neurology consult: admission
   ii. Neurosurgery consult: consultation for the possibility of progression of edema and herniation
b. Discussion with patient about findings
c. Meds
   i. Aspirin PO
   ii. Blood pressure control: indicated now given sBP > 220 and dBP >120. Preferred treatment is with easily titratable IV options (labetalol, esmolol, nitroprusside) to reduce the risk of hypotension and decreased cerebral perfusion pressure.

M. Diagnosis

a. Acute cerebellar stroke

N. Critical actions

a. Establishing time of onset of symptoms
b. Detailed neurological examination
c. MRI/MRA brain
d. Neurology and neurosurgery consultation
e. BP control with IV agents
f. Aspirin within 24 hours

O. Examiner instructions

a. This is a case of an acute cerebellar infarction. The clinical features can be subtle and may include vertigo, gait instability, limb ataxia, headache, nausea, vomiting, dysarthria, and cranial nerve abnormalities. Early critical actions in this case include assessing for central causes of vertigo with a thorough history and neurologic exam, establishing time of onset, obtaining IV access and hemodynamic monitoring, ordering a noncontrast head CT and MRI/MRA of the brain, and obtaining immediate neurology and neurosurgery consultations. Blood pressure management with the goal of permissive hypertension (<220/120) is important. Once an ischemic infarction has been diagnosed, antiplatelet therapy with aspirin should be initiated. Because of the unknown time of onset (certainly more than 4.5 hours) this patient is not a candidate for thrombolytic treatment.

P. Pearls

a. Cerebellar infarction tends to present with vague symptoms, including vertigo, ataxia, headache, nausea, and vomiting.
b. It is imperative to determine whether vertigo has features of a central etiology (disorders affecting the brainstem and cerebellum) or a peripheral etiology (disorders affecting the vestibular apparatus and eighth cranial nerve). Older adults and those with stroke risk factors are at increased risk for central causes of vertigo. Peripheral vertigo may be intermittent, provoked by position changes, reproducible, and fatigable. Central vertigo tends to be more constant, and relatively unaffected by positional changes. Headache or neck pain should raise concern for a central etiology. Hearing loss or tinnitus usually indicates a peripheral cause, though may also be seen with ischemia. Any abnormality on neurologic exam suggests a central cause of vertigo. HINTS testing (**H**ead–**I**mpulse–**N**ystagmus–**T**est of **S**kew) is a

three-step bedside oculomotor examination that is a useful screening tool in differentiating central and peripheral vertigo.

c. MRI/MRA is the best imaging to assess cerebellar and posterior circulation pathology. CT is useful in acute stroke for identifying hemorrhage; however, in posterior circulation stroke is often inadequate due to the artifact from posterior fossa bone.

d. Cerebellar infarction may result in cerebellar edema, followed by herniation and rapid clinical deterioration. Therefore, all patients with cerebellar infarction must have frequent neurologic exams and early neurosurgical consultation.

e. Current guidelines in the management of ischemic stroke call for permissive hypertension with blood pressure control only indicated if the systolic BP rises above 220 or the diastolic blood pressure above 120. Aspirin should be given to all ischemic stroke patients within 24–48 hours unless they have received thrombolytics, in which case aspirin administration should be delayed until more than 24 hours after initiation of thrombolytic therapy. This patient is not a candidate for thrombolytics, given the onset of symptoms over 4.5 hours from presentation. Endovascular thrombectomy is recommended in patients with large anterior circulation artery occlusions; however, the benefit in posterior circulation occlusion and appropriate timing is unclear.

Q. Figure legends

a. Figure 124.1 (EKG) Normal sinus rhythm.

b. Figure 124.2 (MRI/MRA) Brain area of abnormal signal intensity in the left superior cerebellum. No hydrocephalus or brain herniation. Left vertebral artery occlusion.

R. References

a. *Tintinalli's Emergency Medicine: A Comprehensive Study Guide* (9th ed.): Chapter 167, Stroke Syndromes. Chapter 170, Vertigo.

b. *Rosen's Emergency Medicine: Concepts and Clinical Practice* (10th ed.): Chapter 9, Weakness.

Weakness

Bonnie Lau, MD

A. Chief complaint
a. 29-year-old female with weakness

B. Vital signs
a. BP: 117/70, HR: 85, RR: 14, T: 37°C, Sat: 92% on RA

C. What does the patient look like?
a. Patient appears stated age, sitting up.

D. Primary survey
a. Airway: speaking in full sentences
b. Breathing: no apparent distress, no cyanosis
c. Circulation: dry and warm skin, normal capillary refill

E. Action
a. Oxygen via 2 L NC or nonrebreather mask
b. Two peripheral IV lines
c. Monitor: BP: 117/70, HR: 85, RR: 14, T: 37°C, Sat: 98% if placed on O_2 (if not placed on O_2, will remain 92% on RA)
d. EKG (Figure 125.1)

F. History
a. HPI: A 29-year-old female with 1 week of generalized weakness, worsened over the past day. She is having difficulty studying due to double vision and feeling like her eyelids droop, especially at night. Denies headache, fevers/chills, cough, chest pain, abdominal pain, nausea, vomiting, diarrhea, urinary symptoms, numbness. Reports occasional shortness of breath.
b. PMHx: denies
c. Allergies: none
d. Meds: none
e. Social: denies tobacco, illicit drug use; social EtOH; pharmacy student.
f. FHx: denies
g. PMD: Dr. Bond

G. Secondary survey
a. General: alert, oriented × 3, appears fatigued
b. Head: normocephalic, atraumatic

c. Eyes: pupils equal, reactive to light, bilateral ptosis, weak cranial nerves III, IV, VI, end-gaze nystagmus, diplopia
d. Ears: normal tympanic membranes
e. Nose: no discharge
f. Neck: full range of motion, no jugular vein distension, no stridor
g. Pharynx: normal dentition, no lesions, no swelling
h. Lungs: clear bilaterally
i. Heart: rate and rhythm regular, no murmurs, rubs, or gallops
j. Abdomen: normal bowel sounds, soft, nontender
k. Rectal: normal tone, brown stool, occult blood negative
l. Extremities: no deformity, normal pulses
m. Back: nontender
n. Neuro: bilateral ptosis, end-gaze nystagmus, diplopia, weak cranial nerves III, IV, VI; other cranial nerves intact, 4/5 proximal strength of bilateral upper extremities (UEs) and lower extremities (LEs), 5/5 distal strength UEs and LEs; normal sensation, reflexes, cerebellar testing
o. Skin: warm and dry
p. Lymph: no lymphadenopathy

H. Action
a. Labs
   i. CBC, BMP, LFT, coagulation studies, TSH
   ii. Urinalysis, urine hCG, urine toxicology screen
b. Imaging:
   i. CXR (Figure 125.2)
   ii. Noncontrast head CT (Figure 125.3)
c. Neurology consult

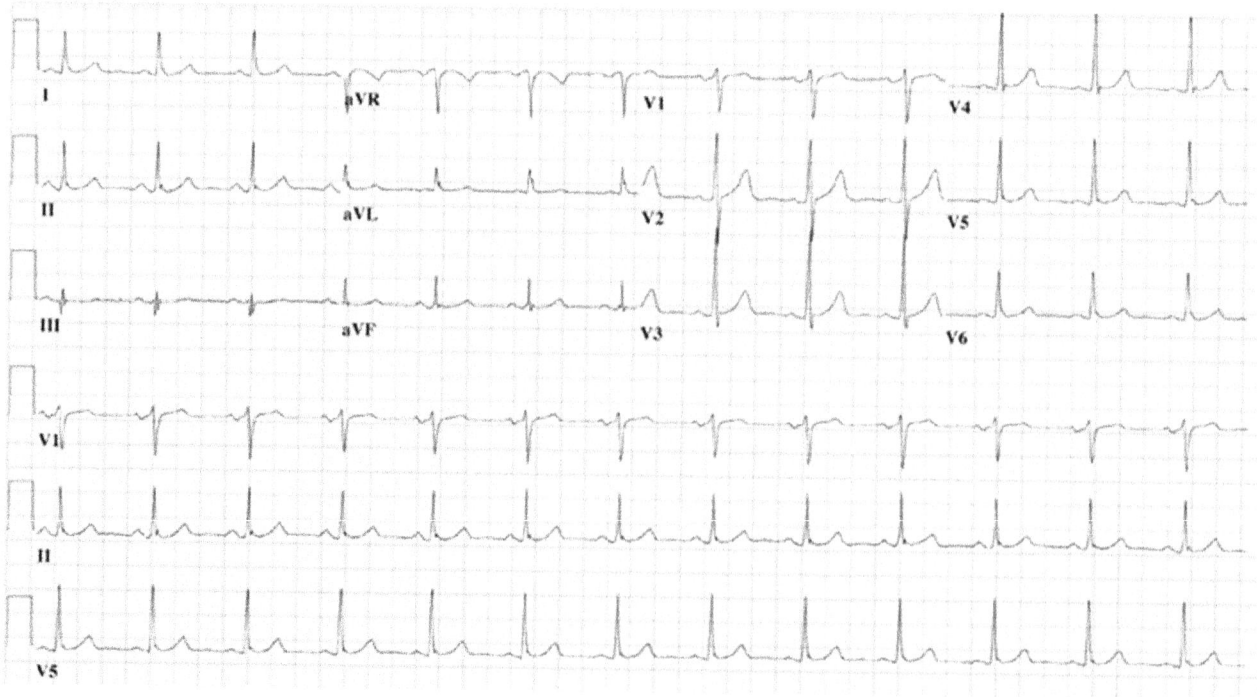

Figure 125.1

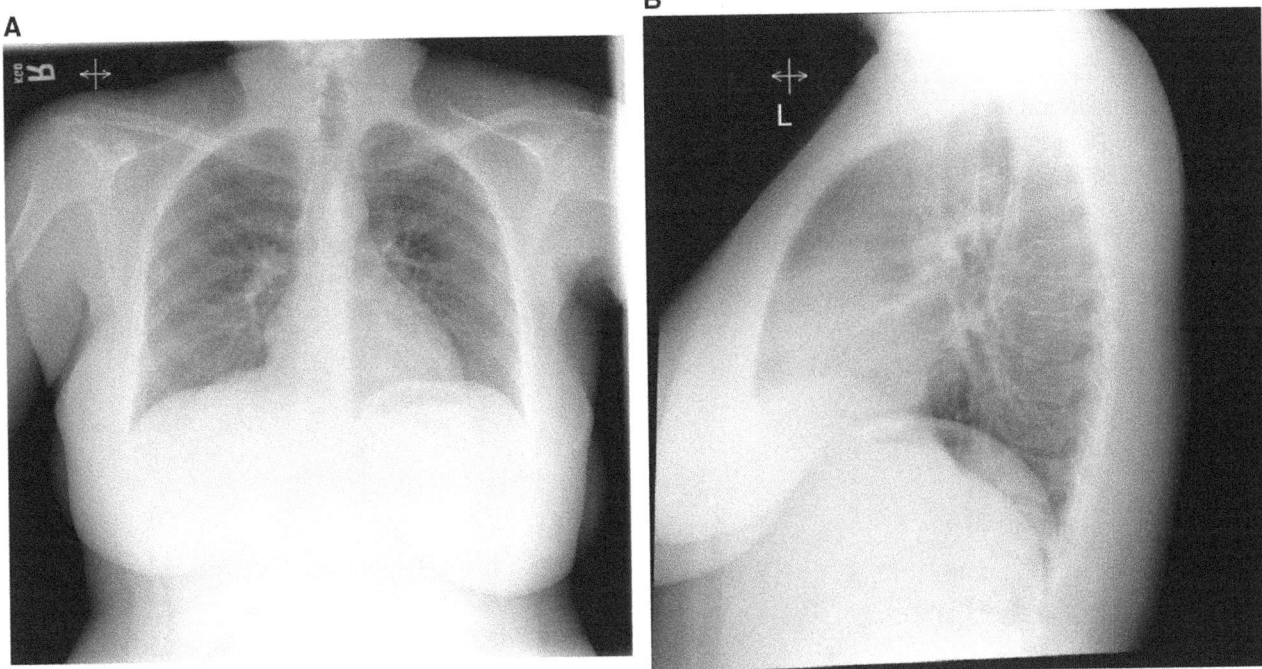

Figure 125.2

Figure 125.3

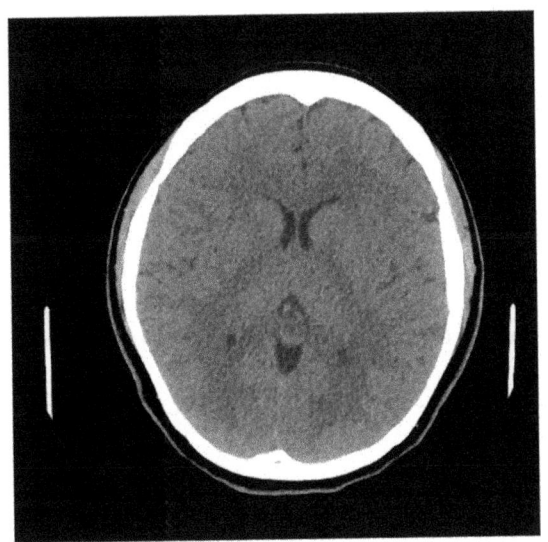

I. Results

Table 125.1 Results table

Test	Result	Test	Result
Complete blood count:		**Liver function panel:**	
WBC	$5.0 \times 10^3/\mu L$	AST	22 U/L
Hct	40.5%	ALT	27 U/L
Plt	$350 \times 10^3/\mu L$	Alk phos	88 U/L
		T bili	1.0 mg/dL

Table 125.1 (cont.)

Test	Result	Test	Result
Basic metabolic panel:		D bili	0.2 mg/dL
Na	137 mEq/L	Lipase	21 U/L
K	3.9 mEq/L	Albumin	4.9 g/dL
Cl	101 mEq/L		
CO_2	25 mEq/L	**Urinalysis:**	
BUN	15 mEq/dL	SG	1.020
Cr	0.9 mg/dL	pH	7
Glucose	129 mg/dL	Prot	Neg
		Gluc	Neg
Coagulation panel:		Ketones	Neg
PT	11.8 sec	Bili	Neg
PTT	29.0 sec	Blood	Neg
INR	1.1	LE	Neg
		Nitrite	Neg
		Color	Yellow

a. TSH: normal
b. Urine toxicology and urine pregnancy test: negative

J. Action

a. Ice-pack testing (examinee must describe test) confirms diagnosis of myasthenia gravis
b. Meds
    i.   Acetylcholinesterase inhibitor (pyridostigmine or neostigmine)
    ii. Consider corticosteroids, plasma exchange, or IVIG
c. Admission to ICU

K. Diagnosis

a. Myasthenia gravis

L. Critical actions

a. Obtain detailed history and examination
b. Consult neurology
c. Preparation for airway support during neurology testing
d. If paralytic is needed for RSI, nondepolarizing agent is preferred over a depolarizing agent at a significantly reduced dosage
e. Admit to ICU

M. Examiner instructions

a. This is a case of newly diagnosed myasthenia gravis (MG). MG is an autoimmune disease characterized by muscle weakness and fatigue, especially of proximal extremity, facial, and bulbar muscles. A detailed history and physical examination are key in making the clinical diagnosis. The diagnosis is confirmed with bedside testing (the ice bag test) and serologic testing . If paralytic is needed for RSI, a nondepolarizing agent is preferred over a depolarizing agent at a significantly reduced dosage. MG treatment involves administration of acetylcholinesterase inhibitors (pyridostigmine or neostigmine).

N. Pearls

a. In MG, there is a marked decrease in the number and function of muscle fiber acetylcholine receptors (AChRs) due to autoantibodies. Autoantibodies also compete with acetylcholine for binding at the remaining receptors. Decreased response to acetylcholine stimulation causes decreased muscle strength, including the diaphragm.

b. MG is called the "great imitator" since it may mimic the symptoms of many other chronic neurologic disorders. Ptosis and diplopia are the most common presenting symptoms. Other MG findings may include: limb weakness, oropharyngeal symptoms (such as dysphagia and dysarthria, dysphonia), cranial nerve III, IV, or VI weakness, gaze palsies, and dyspnea. There is usually no deficit in sensory, reflex, or cerebellar functioning.

c. Symptoms fluctuate throughout the day, usually worsening later in the day or with prolonged muscle group use (e.g., prolonged reading or prolonged chewing).

d. Myasthenic crisis may be seen prior to the diagnosis of MG, with infections, surgery, pregnancy, or as a result of inadequate drug therapy. It is characterized by respiratory failure due to extreme weakness in the muscles of respiration.

e. If ventilatory support is needed, noninvasive ventilation should be attempted first, as there are specific medication considerations for intubation.

f. Depolarizing or nondepolarizing paralytic agents should be avoided if possible in MG patients because the paralytic effects may persist two to three times longer than in normal patients. If paralytic agents are necessary, some support using half the dose, although no clinical studies support this practice, favoring nondepolarizing agents over depolarizing agents. Also consider using short-acting induction agents (such as etomidate or propofol) in smaller doses.

g. The diagnosis of MG requires strong clinical suspicion and confirmation through the administration of the ice bag test, electromyography, and serologic testing for acetylcholine receptor antibodies.

h. Treatment of MG involves administration of acetylcholinesterase inhibitors (pyridostigmine or neostigmine), chronic immune suppression with corticosteroids or azathioprine, and thymectomy. Severe symptoms may require high-dose corticosteroids, plasma exchange, or IV immunoglobulin.

O. Figure legends

a. Figure 125.1 (EKG) Normal sinus rhythm.
b. Figure 125.2 (CXR) Normal chest x-ray.
c. Figure 125.3 (Noncontrast head CT) Normal head CT.

P. References

a. *Tintinalli's Emergency Medicine: A Comprehensive Study Guide* (9th ed.): Chapter 173, Chronic Neurologic Disorders.
b. *Rosen's Emergency Medicine: Concepts and Clinical Practice* (10th ed.): Chapter 94, Neuromuscular Disorders.

Altered Mental Status

Michael Cassara, DO, MSEd

A. Chief complaint
a. 35-year-old man "found drunk" by police, demonstrating altered mental status and signs and symptoms of acute intoxication from an unknown substance

B. Vital signs
a. BP: 120/60, HR: 102, RR: 30, T: 36.5°C, Sat: 96%

C. What does the patient look like?
a. Thin, disheveled man with poor personal hygiene; demonstrates moaning and slurred speech with incomprehensible words in response to painful stimuli. He has abrasions to the face and head.

D. Primary survey
a. Airway: patent airway; gag reflex present; no pooling of secretions; no drooling; no stridor
b. Breathing: tachypnea and hyperpnea (e.g., "Kussmaul respirations") (represent to candidate as "breathing quickly and deeply")
c. Circulation: tachycardia
d. Disability: lethargy and obtundation; opens eyes only to painful stimuli; withdraws to painful stimuli; no posturing; no focal weakness; demonstrates moaning and slurred speech with incomprehensible words in response to painful stimuli
e. Exposure: no rashes, no lesions, no "track marks," abrasions to face and head but without other evidence of trauma

E. Action
a. Apply cervical collar (if candidate expresses concern over occult traumatic injury)
b. Administer supplemental oxygen (although the patient is not hypoxic, the candidate may elect to provide supplemental oxygen in preparation for an advanced airway maneuver)
c. Order placement of two large-bore peripheral venous catheters
   i. Administer isotonic crystalloid fluid bolus (0.9% sodium chloride or lactated Ringer's solution)
   ii. Order laboratory tests
      1. Point-of-care testing: ABG, serum glucose concentration
      2. CBC, CMP, hepatic function tests, PT/INR/PTT, urinalysis, serum toxicology panel (acetaminophen, salicylate, ethanol)
      3. Serum osmolarity
      4. At faculty discretion, allow ordering ethylene glycol and methanol

   d. Place on continuous cardiac monitoring and obtain 12-lead ECG
      i. BP: 120/60, HR: 102, RR: 30, T: 36.5°C
   e. Place on continuous pulse oximetry and end-tidal capnography/capnometry
      i. SaO_2: increases to 100% with supplemental oxygen; $ETCO_2$: 22 mmHg
   f. Consider administration of thiamine and naloxone

F. History

Item a is provided only if the candidate requests that EMS or police "stay" at the beginning of the case; items b-h should be provided by examiner only if candidate requests access to an old medical record and specifically asks for the item; otherwise, any attempts to obtain this information should be answered with "unknown" or "unable".

   a. HPI: A 35-year-old man presenting with altered mental status and clinical intoxication. He was "found drunk" by police on one of the benches in the village park in the center of town. He had been seen earlier in the evening at a local bar, where he was seen to drink an unknown amount of alcohol but was "thrown out following an argument with his significant other." He is known to the ED staff as a frequent ED utilizer. The patient is unable to provide any HPI or past medical/surgical history because of his altered mental status/level of intoxication.
   b. PMHx: chronic alcohol use disorder (medical records demonstrate over 15 ED visits for "intoxication"); depression (medical records demonstrate two admissions for "major depressive disorder" and "suicidal ideation")
   c. PSHx: appendicitis (22 years ago)
   d. Allergies: none
   e. Meds: none
   f. Social: excessive ethanol use; regular tobacco use (one pack per day for 20 years); occasional marijuana use
   g. FHx: mother deceased at age 54, metastatic breast cancer; father deceased at age 62, cirrhosis
   h. PMD: Dr. Brewer (noncompliant with visits to the local medical clinic)

G. Nurse

   a. Provide 12-lead ECG (Figure 126.1)
   b. Place patient on supplemental high-flow oxygen
   c. Perform peripheral venous catheter placement and phlebotomy; start IV fluids as ordered
      i. No change in patient's vital signs with these interventions
   d. Provide thiamine and naloxone if ordered
      i. No change in patient's mental status with these interventions

H. Secondary survey

   a. General: disheveled, thin 35-year-old man demonstrating somnolence, lethargy, and obtunded mental status; disoriented; demonstrates moaning and slurred speech with incomprehensible words (patient only responsive to painful stimuli)
   b. Head: normocephalic; abrasions to face and scalp
   c. Eyes: pupils symmetrically equal (4 mm), sluggishly reactive to light; extraocular muscles intact; horizontal nystagmus; normal optic disk margins
   d. Ears: normal
   e. Nose: normal
   f. Neck: full range of motion, no jugular vein distension; no stridor; midline trachea

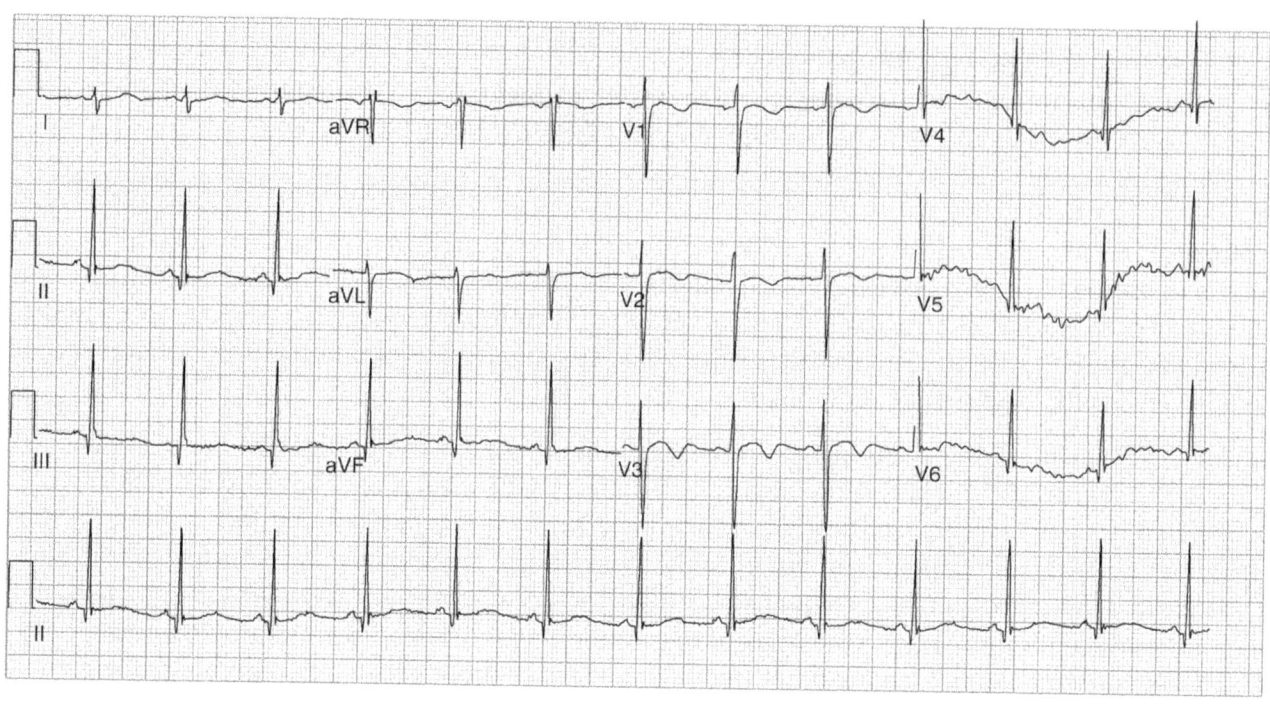

Figure 126.1

g. Pharynx: dry mucous membranes, lips, and tongue; no drooling; intact gag reflexes
h. Chest: nontender to palpation
i. Heart: rate and rhythm regular; no murmurs, rubs, or gallops
j. Lungs: tachypnea and hyperpnea (Kussmaul respirations); clear bilaterally; no wheezing
k. Abdomen: normal bowel sounds, soft, nontender, nondistended
l. Rectal: normal tone, brown stool, occult blood negative
m. Extremities: full range of motion, no deformities or evidence of trauma; normal pulses
n. Back: nontender to palpation
o. Neuro: cranial nerves II to XII intact; horizontal nystagmus; normal reflexes; unable to comply with most elements of the neurologic exam because of intoxication; cannot stand/walk (ataxia); disoriented; demonstrates moaning and slurred speech with incomprehensible words in response to painful stimuli
p. Skin: cool, dry skin; no rashes, lesions, petechiae, purpura, or "track marks"
q. Lymph: no lymphadenopathy

I. Action
a. Order CT head

J. Results

Table 126.1 Results table

Test	Result	Test	Result
Complete blood count:		D bili	0.3 mg/dL
WBC	$10.3 \times 10^3/\mu L$	Amylase	50 U/L
Hct	35.7%	Lipase	25 U/L
Plt	$150 \times 10^3/\mu L$	Albumin	4.7 mg/dL
Basic metabolic panel:		**Urinalysis:**	
Na	148 mEq/L	SG	1.010
K	4.9 mEq/L	pH	5
Cl	108 mEq/L	Protein	1+ (trace)
CO_2	5 mEq/L	Glucose	Neg
BUN	10 mEq/L	Ketones	1+ (trace)
Cr	1.1 mg/dL	Bili	Neg
Glucose	146 mg/dL	Blood	1+ (trace)
Ca	7 mEq/L	LE	Neg
		Nitrites	Neg
Coagulation panel:		Color	Yellow
PT	12.6 sec	Micro	Calcium oxalate crystals
PTT	26 sec		
INR	1.0	**Arterial blood gas:**	
		pH	6.95
Liver function panel:		FiO_2	1.0
AST	23 U/L	pCO_2	16 mmHg
ALT	26 U/L	pO_2	425 mmHg
Alk phos	42 U/L	HCO_3	5 mmol/L
T bili	1.0 mg/dL		

a. Lactate: 16 mmol/L (normal: <2 mmol/L)
b. Anion gap: 35 (normal: < 12)
c. Serum osmolarity (calculated): 311 mOsm/kgH$_2$O (normal: 285–295 mOsm/kgH$_2$O)
d. Serum osmolarity (measured): 350 mOsm/kgH$_2$O (normal: 285–295 mOsm/kgH$_2$O)
e. Osmolal gap: 39 mOsm/kgH$_2$O (normal: −14 to 10 mOsm/kgH$_2$O)
f. Acetaminophen: undetectable (normal: undetectable)
g. Salicylate: undetectable (normal: undetectable)
h. Ethanol: 14 mg/dL (normal: undetectable)
i. Methanol: 0 mg/dL (normal: undetectable)
j. Ethylene glycol: 170 mg/dL (normal: undetectable)
k. CT brain (Figure 126.2)

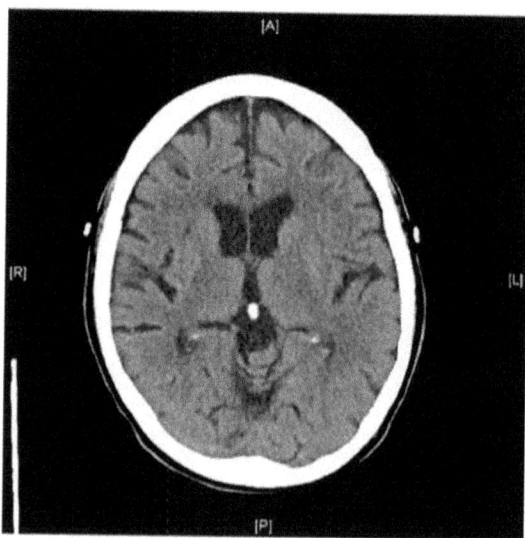

Figure 126.2

K. Action

a. Meds
   i.   Fomepizole or alternative antidote (e.g., ethanol)
   ii. Pyridoxine (vitamin B6)
   iii. Calcium chloride or calcium gluconate (to correct hypocalcemia)
b. Consult nephrology (for hemodialysis)
c. Admit to ICU

L. Diagnosis

a. Ethylene glycol poisoning
b. Hypocalcemia causing prolonged QT

M. Critical actions

a. Obtain EKG.
b. Order bedside serum glucose testing.
c. Administer sodium bicarbonate (bolus and/or continuous infusion).
d. Correct hypocalcemia.
e. Administer fomepizole or equivalent antidote (e.g. ethanol).
f. Arrange for hemodialysis.
g. Admit to the ICU.

N. Examiner instructions

a. This is a case of ethylene glycol toxicity. The patient intentionally ingested antifreeze after getting intoxicated at a local bar, arguing with his girlfriend (he got "dumped"), and getting "thrown out." The candidate should perform the primary survey and suspect an elevated anion gap metabolic acidosis is present by observing the signs (altered mental status, Kussmaul respirations) and interpreting the ABG results. The candidate should perform a diligent search for the causes ("MUDPILES") while attempting to stabilize the patient. Stabilization measures include reversal of acidosis, electrolyte correction, blockade of alcohol dehydrogenase (to decrease toxic metabolite production), and elimination of ethylene glycol (with hemodialysis).

O. Pearls

a. Toxic alcohol poisoning should be considered in any patient with altered mental status, evidence of acute intoxication, an elevated anion gap metabolic acidosis, and an elevated measured serum osmolarity with a significant osmolal gap. Toxic alcohol poisoning should be suspected when other causes for the findings above (e.g., diabetic ketoacidosis with hyperglycemia) are absent.

b. Fomepizole (4-methylpyrazole) and ethanol work by (competitively) inhibiting alcohol dehydrogenase and preventing the metabolism of ethylene glycol into multiple toxic metabolites (glycoaldehyde, glycolate, glyoxalate, and oxalate). These toxic metabolites cause direct tissue destruction, hypocalcemia, and elevated anion gap metabolic acidosis. If ethanol is used, the desired target serum ethanol concentration is 100–150 mg/dL.

c. Hemodialysis is the definitive management. There is no role for gastrointestinal decontamination in this patient.

d. Sodium bicarbonate, pyridoxine, thiamine, and calcium administration may be helpful. Sodium bicarbonate may enhance toxic metabolite excretion with acidosis correction, but may complicate hypocalcemia and cause other electrolyte abnormalities (e.g., hypokalemia). Pyridoxine may inhibit the metabolism of glycolate to oxalate. Thiamine may promote the conversion of glyoxylate to alpha-hydroxy-beta-ketoadipate. Calcium correction will correct ECG abnormalities related to hypocalcemia (prolonged QT interval), but may result in calcium oxalate crystal precipitation.

e. A dangerous commission during this case is to perform endotracheal intubation with sedation without recognizing and acknowledging the compensatory respiratory alkalosis (e.g., Kussmaul respirations) inherent in this situation. If the decision is made to intubate the patient, the candidate must order mechanical ventilation settings that maintain the patient's pre-intubation level of hyperventilation. The acidosis will rapidly worsen, and the patient will arrest if this is not done.

P. Figure legends

a. Figure 126.1 (EKG) Normal sinus rhythm.

b. Figure 126.2 (CT) Normal head CT.

Q. References

a. *Tintinalli's Emergency Medicine: A Comprehensive Study Guide* (9th ed.): Chapter 185, Alcohols.

b. *Rosen's Emergency Medicine: Concepts and Clinical Practice* (10th ed.): Chapter 136, Toxic Alcohols.

c. *Goldfrank's Toxicologic Emergencies* (10th ed.): Chapter 109, Toxic Alcohols.

Fever

Julie Tokarski, MD

A. Chief complaint
a. 13-month-old female brought in with fever and rash

B. Vital signs
a. BP: 90/54, HR: 152, RR: 28, T: 38.7°C, Sat: 99% on RA

C. What does the patient look like?
a. Patient appears well developed for age, fussy, consolable by mother, nontoxic.

D. Primary survey
a. Airway: patient crying, no stridor
b. Breathing: easy work of breathing
c. Circulation: brisk capillary refill, skin warm and dry

E. History
a. HPI: A 13-month-old female with no significant medical history is brought to the ED by her mother with chief complaint of fever and rash. She was well until 5 days ago, when she had a fever of 39.6°C, fussiness, and malaise. The following day she developed a cough, runny nose, and some eye redness. She was drinking well and breathing comfortably, so her mother assumed she "caught a cold on the airplane" while traveling home from Europe the week prior. The fever, cough, and congestion continued, and today the patient woke up with a rash on her face, which is what prompted their visit to the ED. The rash is not itchy or painful. Review of systems is also notable for fussiness and decreased appetite, but the child has been drinking well, has normal urinary output, and has had no difficulty breathing. No one else in the household has been sick with these symptoms.
b. PMHx: none; uncomplicated, full-term pregnancy
c. PSHx: none.
d. Allergies: none.
e. Meds: acetaminophen as needed
f. Social: lives at home with mother, father, and 4-year-old brother; family recently returned from a 6-week trip to Europe; no daycare
g. FHx: noncontributory
h. PMD: academic general pediatric clinic – individual physician varies with each visit; missed her 1-year well-child visit while traveling

F. Secondary survey
a. General: awake, appears tired, nontoxic. Fussy, cries throughout the physical examination. Consolable by mother
b. HEENT: clear rhinorrhea, mild conjunctival injection without discharge, moist mucous membranes, buccal mucosa with scattered 1–2 mm white lesions with erythematous base
c. Neck: supple
d. Chest: clear lungs, no retractions
e. Heart: tachycardic, regular, no murmurs, rubs, or gallops
f. Abdomen: soft, no tenderness, no hepatosplenomegaly
g. Urogenital: tanner 1 female, no lesions
h. Extremities: normal
i. Back: normal
j. Neuro: normal
k. Skin: maculopapular rash on face, neck, upper chest; no rash on palms or soles
l. Lymph: normal

G. Action
a. Isolation with airborne precautions
b. Meds
   i. antipyretic PO
c. Monitor
d. Labs:
   i. CBC, measles IgM, measles PCR nasopharyngeal swab
e. Consultation with local health department or pediatric infectious disease specialist

H. Nurse
a. BP: 92/57, HR: 126, RR: 25, T: 37.6°C, Sat: 99% on RA

I. Results

Table **127.1** Complete blood count results table

Test	Result
WBC	$4.3 \times 10^3/\mu L$
Hgb	12.5 g/dL
Plt	$376 \times 10^3/\mu L$

a. Measles IgM: pending
b. Measles PCR nasopharyngeal swab: sent out, pending

J. Action
a. Discharge home
   i. Home quarantine as per health department recommendations, typically 4 days after rash onset
b. Meds:
   i. Antipyretics as needed

   c. Return precautions:
      i. Monitoring for signs or symptoms of measles complications
      ii. Monitoring of hydration status, oral intake
   d. Post-exposure prophylaxis for close contacts as per local health department
      i. Healthy, immunocompetent contacts
         1. MMR vaccine within 72 hours of exposure, *or*
         2. Measles immune globulin 0.25 mL/kg within 6 days of exposure
      ii. Immunocompromised
         1. Measles immune globulin 0.5 mL/kg within 6 days of exposure

K. Diagnosis
a. Measles

L. Critical actions
a. Recognition of the classic presentation of measles.
b. Recognition of individuals at risk for measles infection.
c. Prompt airborne isolation.
d. Post-exposure prophylaxis for close contacts.

M. Examiner instructions
a. This is a case of measles, a highly contagious infection caused by a paramyxovirus. The patient in this case had a classic presentation of this illness and presented for care after the onset of the typical measles rash. The most important action in such scenarios is early recognition of potential measles cases with appropriate isolation of the patient until they can be further evaluated. In this case, the patient was at risk for measles as she was unvaccinated and had traveled to a high-risk area. The diagnosis of measles is a clinical one but can be confirmed or excluded with PCR or antibody testing. The next key step in patients like these is thorough history and physical exam to assess for common complications of measles, such as acute otitis media or pneumonia. Lastly, it is critical to consult with the local health department or pediatric infectious disease specialists to guide further testing, proper quarantine, and recommendations for close contacts of the patient.

N. Pearls
a. The measles virus is a highly contagious paramyxovirus that is spread by droplet transmission. Because of its long incubation period (average 10 days, range 7–21 days), infected individuals may have difficulty identifying the source of illness.
b. The classic presentation of measles is high fever (often greater than 40°C) and malaise, followed by cough, coryza, and nonpurulent conjunctivitis. Koplik spots, which are pathognomonic for measles but do not occur in all cases, are pinpoint white lesions with a red base ("grains of sand") that appear on the buccal mucosa within 2–3 days of symptom onset. The rash begins on the head on day 4–5 of the illness, spreads craniocaudally, then coalesces over the following 4–5 days. The rash spares the palms and soles.
c. Atypical presentation of measles is common in immunocompromised hosts or in patients who are previously vaccinated. Additionally, fever and a faint measles rash can occur 7–10 days after measles vaccination.
d. Measles is a clinical diagnosis, but can be confirmed by IgM antibody, which is detectable 2 weeks after onset of illness, or at onset of rash. PCR testing by nasopharyngeal swab can be

sent to the CDC for confirmation of acute illness. A CBC, if obtained, may show leukopenia and/or lymphopenia.

e. Complications of measles, which are more common in children <5 years of age, are rare but can be serious. These include viral pneumonia, acute encephalitis (1 in 1000 cases with mortality of 15%), or secondary bacterial infections (AOM, cervical adenitis, bacterial pneumonia). Subacute sclerosing panencephalitis is a rare but fatal complication that occurs remote from the acute infection (average 7 years).

f. Measles was one of the most common viral rashes before measles vaccination but was declared eliminated in the US by the CDC in 2000. Due to increased international travel and decreased vaccination rates, there has been increased incidence of measles in the United States. At the time of this publication, the incidence of measles infection in the United States is at its highest since 1992.

O. References

a. *Rosen's Emergency Medicine: Concepts and Clinical Practice* (10th ed.): Chapter 107, Dermatologic Presentations.

b. *Tintinalli's Emergency Medicine: A Comprehensive Study Guide* (9th ed.): Chapter 83, Rashes in Children.

LVAD Emergency

Giuliano De Portu, MD, FACEP and Michael Chami, MD

A. Chief complaint
a. 66-year-old male brought in by EMS obtunded

B. Vital signs
a. BP: "unable to detect," HR: 100, RR: 25, Sat: 98% on RA, FS: 100 mg/dL (must ask)

C. What does the patient look like?
a. Male, appears older than stated age, holding a bag with emesis. He has a harness over his lateral chest and EMS brings a backpack with them. There is an intermittent beeping sound coming from the harness. You see a small "computer-like device" connected to the patient.

D. Primary survey
a. Airway: speaking in full sentences
b. Breathing: slightly tachypneic but in no distress
c. Circulation: tachycardic and diaphoretic with increased capillary refill

E. History
a. HPI: A 66-year-old male with history of congestive heart failure who was doing well until earlier in the day, when he started to have numerous episodes of emesis and diarrhea. He states that he became progressively weaker and called EMS. He thinks that he ate a chicken sandwich that "had been in the fridge for too long." He denies any bloody emesis and reports no changes in stool color. He denies fevers, chills, shortness of breath, chest pain, or recent travel. He also reports no back pain and no weakness on the upper or lower extremities. He has had no loss of consciousness.
b. PMHx: congestive heart failure, hypertension
c. PSHx: left ventricular assisted device (LVAD) 1 year ago
d. Allergies: none
e. Meds: coumadin 5 mg once a day
f. Social: lives alone, denies tobacco, alcohol, recreational drugs, or alternative medicines; not sexually active
g. FHx: family history of HTN
h. PMD: none

F. Action
a. Oxygen via NC as needed to maintain saturation >95%
b. Two large-bore peripheral IV lines

c. Labs:
    i. CBC, BMP, LFT, coagulation studies, blood type and crossmatch, troponins, BNP
d. 1 L NS bolus
e. Cardiac monitor
    i. BP: "not obtainable," HR: 90, RR: 22, Sat 100% on O²
    ii. Attempt to obtain manual MAP with doppler/US
f. EKG
g. Call LVAD coordinator

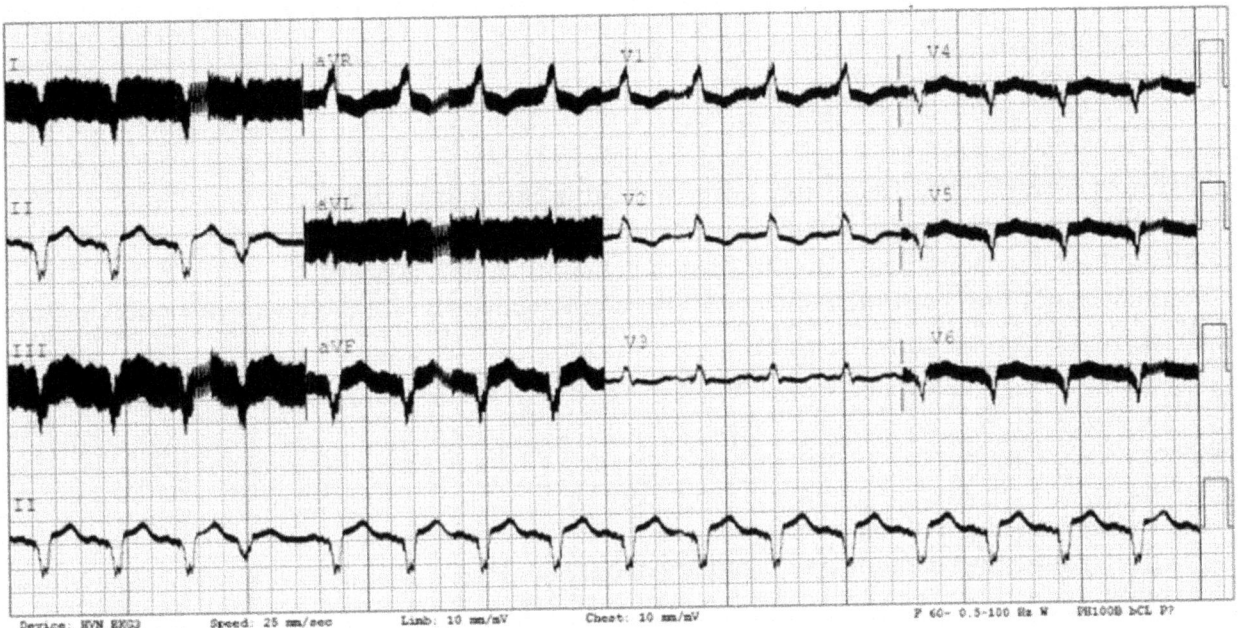

Figure 128.1

G. Nurse

a. EKG (Figure 128.1)
b. After 1 L of NS, BP still not obtainable

H. Secondary survey

a. General: appears weak, but alert, oriented × 3, slow to respond, vomited once since arrival but comfortable
b. Head: normocephalic, atraumatic
c. Eyes: extraocular movement intact, pupils equal, reactive to light
d. Ears: normal tympanic membranes
e. Nose: no discharge
f. Neck: full range of motion, no jugular vein distension, no stridor
g. Pharynx: normal dentition, no lesions, no swelling
h. Chest: nontender, midline sternotomy scar. There is a line coming out of the right abdomen, which connects to the LVAD controller. There is a Biopatch in place, no signs of erythema, area not warm to the touch (candidate needs to ask about erythema and warm area)
i. Lungs: clear bilaterally
j. Heart: you hear a continuous mechanical hum when you auscultate the chest

k. Abdomen: no distension, mild epigastric discomfort but tenderness, bowel sounds normal, no masses, no hernias, nontender at McBurney's point, negative Murphy's sign, no rebound, no guarding, no rigidity
l. Rectal: normal tone, very little stool, occult blood negative
m. Extremities: full range of motion, no deformity, normal pulses
n. Back: nontender
o. Neuro: cranial nerves II to XII intact; normal sensation, strength; normal reflexes and gait (unable to assess due to patient's condition); mental status: oriented to person, not place or time, appears confused, but responding
p. Skin: diaphoretic, capillary refill 3–5 seconds (must ask), cool (must ask), pallor over face and palms (must ask)
q. Lymph: no lymphadenopathy

I. Action

a. Second 1 L bolus of NS (will show improvement in the mental status)
b. Auscultation of LVAD with BP taken via Doppler device with "return to flow" technique: inflate the sphygmomanometer cuff, then deflate until sound is heard
c. Evaluation of LVAD controller: ensure all lines are connected on LVAD controller, note battery charge level and any ongoing alarms
d. Evaluation of LVAD bag to ensure additional controller and batteries are available

J. Nurse

a. Return to flow BP after second 1 L of NS = 70s (MAP)
b. Controller showing "low battery alarm"
c. Controller showing "suction event" but green light

K. Results

Table **128.1** Results table

Test	Result	Test	Result
Complete blood count:		Alk phos	42 U/L
RBC	$10.0 \times 10^3/\mu L$	T bili	2.0 mg/dL
WBC	$6.4 \times 10^3/\mu L$	D bili	0.2 mg/dL
Hct	40%	Amylase	280 U/L
Plt	$186 \times 10^3/\mu L$	Lipase	265 U/L
Basic metabolic panel:		**Urinalysis:**	
Na	142 mEq/L	Specific gravity	1.030
K	4.2 mEq/L	pH	7.3
CL	98 mEq/L	Protein	Neg
CO_2	30 mEq/L	Glucose	Neg
BUN	22 mEq/L	Ketones	Neg
Cr	1.0 mg/dL	Bilirubin	Neg
Glucose	mg/dL	Blood	Neg

Table 128.1 (cont.)

Test	Result	Test	Result
Coagulation panel:		LE	Neg
PT	12 sec	Nitrite	Neg
PTT	25 sec	Color	Yellow
INR	2.5		
		Arterial blood gas:	
Liver function panel:		pH	7.55
AST	20 U/L	pO_2	95mm/Hg
ALT	25 U/L	pCO_2	42mm/Hg
		HCO_3	30mm/L

a. Troponins: <0.04 ng/mL
b. BNP: 200 ng/mL

L. Action
a. Change battery on LVAD.
b. Continue with IV fluids NS.
c. Transfer to higher level of care with LVAD capabilities or consult cardiac surgery/cardiology if LVAD hospital for observation and monitoring and for LVAD device interrogation.
d. Consider head CT once stabilized, given altered mental status and potential for spontaneous intracranial hemorrhage.

M. Diagnosis
a. Acute emesis and diarrhea (most likely from food poisoning) with subsequent LVAD "suction event" due to dehydration and decreased mental status that led to inability to take care of device appropriately.

N. Critical actions
a. Large-bore IV access and fluid bolus
b. BP evaluation via "return to flow"
c. LVAD evaluation via auscultation
d. LVAD controller evaluation (make sure all of the lines are connected, green light, check RPM) and changing of battery

O. Examiner instructions
a. This is a case of an LVAD patient that has fallen ill due to a common issue of food poisoning, but the dehydration has been severe enough to lead to a problem with the mechanics of the LVAD. The patient had symptoms of emesis and diarrhea. This led to a "suction" event. These tend to occur when there is low volume state and the ventricular cannula moves onto the interventricular septum. These suction events are usually corrected when the patient receives adequate volume, or in the event of mild changes in volume (not this case) the controller will change the RPM on the device so the ventricular cannula goes back into place within the left ventricle and no occlusion occurs.

P. Pearls

a. The LVAD is a device that helps circulate blood from the failing left ventricle to the aorta. It bypasses the aortic valve (sometimes sutured to prevent backflow). Common uses for ventricular assisted devices are bridge to transplant, and destination therapies in patients who are not candidates for transplantation.

b. The LVAD pumps via a continuous flow mechanism powered by an external source of batteries and a controller that connects via a driveline to the patient. When auscultating a patient, you should hear the "hum" of the device. The absence of a "hum" is an indication that the LVAD has a major malfunction.

c. LVAD patients and their families have great insight into their disease process and are extremely compliant with their care and devices.

d. Usually, the LVAD is not the main culprit of a patient's complaint. Common issues with LVAD patients are

    i. Gastrointestinal hemorrhages occur due to anticoagulation (supratherapeutic) and due to an acquired von Willebrand's factor platelet dysfunction as the rotational forces of the LVAD will cleave vWF.

    ii. Infections of the drive line are also common, but patients usually are compliant with their care and are careful when changing their driveline area. In case of sepsis, treat with volume resuscitation and antibiotics, like any other infection.

e. EKGs of LVAD patients can demonstrate electromagnetic interference (like the one in this case). They can show ST-segment elevations and arrythmias (ventricular tachycardia, ventricular fibrillation, etc.) normally incompatible with adequate perfusion. In the case of LVAD patients, the device will generally preserve perfusion even in the presence of a malignant arrythmia.

f. Another cause of poor perfusion that should be considered is pump thrombosis of the inflow or outflow cannula; heparin should be considered in these patients. It is unlikely in this case since the patient was properly anticoagulated. Any treatment of LVAD patients should be done with consultation to the LVAD team or a cardiothoracic surgeon as you need to discuss risk benefits of therapy

h. Figure 128.2 shows a HeartMate II controller with the green circular arrows that indicate that the pump is operating with no intrinsic issues.

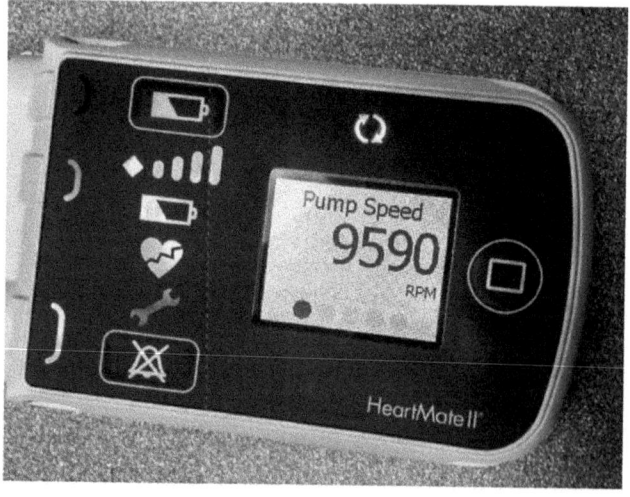

Figure 128.2

Q. Figure legends
a. Figure 128.1 (EKG) Normal EKG for LVAD patient showing interference.
b. Figure 128.2 (Photo) LVAD controller showing normal function (courtesy of Dr. Giuliano De Portu/University of Florida).

R. References
a. *Tintinalli's Emergency Medicine: A Comprehensive Study Guide* (9th ed.): Chapter 55, Cardiomyopathies and Pericardial Disease.
b. *Rosen's Emergency Medicine: Concepts and Clinical Practice* (10th ed.): Chapter 66, Implantable Cardiac Devices.
c. *Journal of the American College of Cardiology* 71(11) Supplement, March 2018.

The Chest Pain Patient: Five Life-Threatening Causes and Critical Actions

Elaine Rabin, MD and Luke Hermann, MD

THE APPROACH TO THE CHEST PAIN PATIENT

Place every patient on a cardiac monitor and establish IV access. Administer oxygen if the patient is in respiratory distress or has an oxygen saturation <94%.

Symptom descriptors and the differentials they suggest are as follows:

1. Abrupt onset:
   a. Severe intensity, ripping or tearing, radiation to back: aortic dissection or esophageal rupture
   b. Maximal at time of onset: aortic dissection
   c. Sharp pleuritic pain with dyspnea: pulmonary embolism or spontaneous pneumothorax
2. Gradual onset:
   a. Pressure-like, tight/squeezing, worse with exertion, radiation to arm or jaw: myocardial infarction
   b. Pleuritic, ± cough, fever: pneumonia, pleural effusion

Essential examination features and what they suggest are as follows:

1. Look:
   a. Significant tachypnea or respiratory distress: pulmonary embolism, significant myocardial infarction, or spontaneous pneumothorax
   b. Diaphoresis, clutching chest: myocardial infarction
2. Listen:
   a. Unilateral breath sounds: spontaneous pneumothorax
   b. Diastolic murmur: aortic dissection
   c. S3 gallop: myocardial infarction
3. Examine
   a. Subcutaneous emphysema: ruptured esophagus or large pneumothorax
   b. Pulse deficit, BP differential >20 mmHg, or neuro deficit: aortic dissection
   c. Unilateral leg swelling, warmth, redness, or palpable cord: pulmonary embolus

Essential EKG findings and what they suggest are as follows:

1. ST elevations: myocardial infarction or (rarely) aortic dissection
2. Right heart strain (prominent S wave in lead I) or sinus tachycardia: pulmonary embolus

Essential CXR findings and what they suggest are as follows:

1. Widened mediastinum: aortic dissection
2. Pleural edge: spontaneous pneumothorax

3. Pulmonary congestion: acute myocardial infarction
4. Small pleural effusion: pulmonary embolism

Myocardial Infarction (ST Segment Elevation)

- High-yield risk factors: diabetes, hypertension, smoking, family history
- High-yield history: substernal pain, gradual onset, pressure sensation

Essential Work-Up

- EKG: ideally obtain within 10 minutes of arrival. ST elevations in two or more contiguous leads ± reciprocal changes. If inferior leads involved, obtained right-sided EKG.
- CXR: typically nonspecific, obtain to evaluate for widened mediastinum. Pulmonary congestion may suggest heart failure secondary to MI.
- Troponin: send but may be negative within first few hours.

Treatment

1. Antiplatelet
   a. Aspirin 325 mg
   b. Clopidogrel if allergic to aspirin
2. Anti-ischemic
   a. β-blockers no longer recommended as part of initial management of STEMI
   b. Nitroglycerine (avoid if right ventricular infarct)
3. Anticoagulation
   a. Heparin or low molecular weight heparin
4. Reperfusion
   a. Cardiac catheterization if available, ideally in <90 minutes (<120 minutes if transfer to a capable center is required) (thrombolytics as alternative, within 30 minutes of arrival)

PULMONARY EMBOLISM

- High-yield risk factors: cancer, recent surgery, long trip, history of deep vein thrombus (DVT), oral contraceptives, or other exogenous hormone therapy
- High-yield history: dyspnea, cough, pleuritic pain, unilateral leg swelling
- High-yield examination: tachypnea, tachycardia, clear lungs, signs of DVT

Essential Work-Up

- EKG: typically nonspecific. Sinus tachycardia is the most common finding. Look for right axis deviation (prominent S in lead I).
- CXR: typically nonspecific, primary purpose is to evaluate for pneumothorax.
- Pulmonary embolism rule-out criteria (PERC): if negative in patients with low pretest probability, very low risk of PE.
- Well's score and revised Geneva score: use to risk-stratify.
- D-dimer: can use for rule out in stable, low-to-intermediate risk patients. Nonspecific.

- CT angiogram: preferred modality for definitive testing.
- VQ scan: alternative to CT when IV contrast contraindicated (allergy, renal insufficiency, etc.).

Treatment

1. Anticoagulation: low molecular weight heparin or unfractionated heparin

AORTIC DISSECTION

- High-yield risk factors: poorly controlled hypertension, known aortic aneurysm, Marfan syndrome or other connective tissue disease, family history of dissection, aortic instrumentation (i.e., cardiac catheterization or valve surgery)
- High-yield history: pain that is abrupt in onset, severe intensity, ripping or tearing, maximal at onset
- High-yield examination: pulse deficit, differential blood pressures, focal neurologic deficit, new diastolic murmur, ischemic limb

Essential Work-Up

EKG: typically nonspecific, look for concomitant STEMI or T-wave changes.
CXR: often nonspecific, look for widened mediastinum.
CT angiogram: most commonly used study.
Bedside transesophageal echocardiography: preferred if patient is unstable.

Treatment

1. Initiate rate control with β-blocker – titrate to pulse <60.
2. Initiate pain control with IV morphine.
3. If systolic BP still >120 mmHg, add nitroprusside.
4. Stat surgical evaluation for operative intervention.

SPONTANEOUS PNEUMOTHORAX

- High-yield risk factors: tall, thin, young patients, especially male, history of heavy smoking or COPD, history of Marfan syndrome
- High-yield history: sudden onset pleuritic pain with dyspnea
- High-yield examination: decreased or absent breath sounds on affected side (not always)

Essential Work-Up

CXR: if difficulty visualizing pleural edge, get end expiratory film.

Treatment

1. Stable patient with small pneumothorax (<3 cm between lung and chest wall):
   a. Supplemental O2 and repeat film in 6 hours
2. Stable patient with larger pneumothorax:
   a. Tube thoracostomy

3. Unstable patient:
    a. Immediate decompression with 14-gauge angiocatheter, second intercostal space, followed by tube thoracostomy

RUPTURED ESOPHAGUS

- High-yield risk factors: alcohol abuse, caustic ingestion
- High-yield history: retrosternal pain following vomiting or retching
- High-yield examination: typically not helpful, check for ill appearance, subcutaneous air in chest wall

Essential Work-Up

- CXR: screen for pneumomediastinum or pneumoperitoneum. Pleural effusion and pneumothorax may be seen.
- CT of chest or gastrografin swallow study: to confirm diagnosis. Use water-soluble contrast in case of extravasation into mediastinum.

Treatment

1. Broad-spectrum antibiotics
2. Surgical consult

The Confused Patient: Ten Most Common Causes and Critical Actions

Denise Nassisi, MD, FACEP

ALTERED MENTAL STATUS

- Common ED presentation with extensive possible underlying etiologies.
- Recognition:
  - May present as decreased responsiveness with obvious coma or more subtle lethargy or confusion.
  - Alternatively, may present hyperactively with agitation or combativeness.
  - Subtle presentations must not be missed as delirium is associated with high morbidity and mortality.
- Need for expedient targeted evaluation for serious and potentially life-threatening etiology.

IMMEDIATE ACTIONS AND STABILIZATION FOR ALTERED MENTAL STATUS

Must rapidly identify and intervene to reverse immediately life-threatening etiologies.

- Assess ABCs and initiate resuscitation with CPR and ACLS/ATLS as needed:
  - Airway: protect and secure airway.
  - Breathing: check oxygenation and adequacy of ventilation.
  - Circulation: check blood pressure and pulse, fluid and pressor support as needed.
- Check vital signs, place on cardiac and pulse oxygen monitors, evaluate pupillary response.
- Check finger stick glucose and administer glucose if low (add thiamine if malnourished or alcoholic).
- Administer naloxone if concern for opiate overdose.

KEY HISTORY FOR ALTERED MENTAL STATUS

Obtain a thorough history from all available sources to uncover the likely etiology.

- Recent symptoms and complaints
- Recent trauma
- Substance abuse and toxin exposures
- Medications
- Underlying medical conditions
- Baseline mental status
- Check for medic alert tag, EMS and bystander history, information from family or caregiver, medication list and contact information in wallet, check electronic medical record for medical history, medication list, and prior visits

KEY PHYSICAL ASSESSMENT AND TESTS FOR ALTERED MENTAL STATUS

Physical examination and targeted work-up should search for evidence of medical or surgical causes, including trauma, infection, or focal neurologic deficits.

- Vital signs including accurate temperature measurement
- Oxygen saturation
- Rapid glucose determination
- Physical examination with thorough neurologic examination
- Chemistry, including lactate, electrolytes, renal function, liver function panels
- Complete blood count
- Urinalysis
- Chest x-ray
- Electrocardiogram
- Target work-up dependent upon the clinical scenario; consider: head CT, lumbar puncture, blood cultures, toxicology screening, thyroid function
- Head CT: obtain when scenario suggests CNS etiology but also obtain if no other etiology for the altered mental status is uncovered

DIFFERENTIAL DIAGNOSIS OF ALTERED MENTAL STATUS

There are many possible etiologies for altered mental status and the differential diagnosis is extensive.

O_2/CO_2

Hypoxemia

- Pneumonia, pneumothorax, pulmonary embolism, asthma or COPD exacerbation, congestive heart failure
- Monitor with pulse O_2
- Provide supplemental O_2

Hypercarbia

- Acute rise may cause lethargy and coma.
- May occur in COPD patient placed on supplemental oxygen with loss of hypoxic drive.
- Hypoventilation from any cause.
- Measure with bedside capnography or blood gas analysis.
- Provide ventilatory support when needed.

Glucose

Hypoglycemia
- May present with confusion, agitation, or focal neurologic deficit; if untreated, severe coma or seizures may ensue.
- Immediate treatment with glucose bolus (add thiamine if malnourished or alcoholic).

Hyperglycemia

- Both diabetic ketoacidosis and hyperosmolar nonketotic state can present with altered mental status, lethargy, and coma.
- May or may not have prior diabetes history.
- Often with polyuria and polydipsia.
- Search for an underlying precipitant or stressor, especially infection.
- Treat with IV fluids and insulin.

Fluid/Electrolyte Disturbance

Hypoperfusion/Hypotension

- Volume loss, for example from severe gastroenteritis
- Acute hemorrhage
- Shock from any cause including sepsis
- Treat with fluids, transfusion, pressors as needed

Dehydration
- More likely etiology in elderly and debilitated patients

Hypernatremia

- Usually due to inadequate thirst mechanism or inability to respond to thirst.
- May also be due to diabetes insipidus (urine concentrating defect).
- Chronic hypernatremia, if corrected too rapidly, can lead to cerebral edema and brain damage.

Hyponatremia

- Degree of mental status change related to absolute degree and also the rate of reduction; sudden decrease is more likely to induce seizures.
- Syndrome of inappropriate antidiuretic hormone (SIADH): consider in patient with malignancy, more common with lung cancer and brain metastases.
- Hypertonic (3%) saline is administered in severe cases (obtundation, seizures); if corrected too rapidly, can lead to osmotic demyelination syndrome.

Hypercalcemia

- Malignancy
- Hyperparathyroidism
- Renal failure
- Associated symptoms include nausea, vomiting, abdominal pain, joint pain, polyuria, and constipation
- Treat initially with IV fluids, additional adjunct therapies may be necessary

Infection/Sepsis

- Pneumonia
- Urinary tract infection

- Meningitis
- Encephalitis
- Intraabdominal infection
- Skin/soft tissue infection
- Sepsis
- Common cause of mental status change, particularly in the elderly
- Check lactate
- Start empiric broad-spectrum antibiotic therapy as quickly as possible to cover likely pathogens
- Treat severe sepsis with crystalloid bolus, add vasopressors if needed

Drugs/Toxins

Alcohol and Drug Toxicity

- Acute intoxication with alcohol or drugs.
- Wernicke–Korsakoff syndrome: deficiency of thiamine (vitamin B_1), found in malnourished patients and chronic alcoholics; check for ataxia and ophthalmoplegia.
- Administer thiamine with glucose if at risk, to prevent precipitating Wernicke–Korsakoff syndrome.

Alcohol and Drug Withdrawal

- Alcohol and benzodiazepine withdrawal can cause delirium and may cause seizures.
- Delirium tremens from alcohol withdrawal – classical findings of tachycardia, elevated blood pressure, tremor and mydriasis.
- Must be treated with benzodiazepines.

Medication

- The elderly are particularly susceptible to polypharmacy and adverse drug effects.
- Medications with sedative and anticholinergic properties are common culprits.

Poisoning/Toxins

- Evaluate for potential toxidrome
- Consider accidental poisoning particularly in young children
- Opiate: pinpoint pupils and respiratory depression
- Anticholinergic: mydriasis, hyperthermia, anhidrosis, hyperemia
- Sympathomimetics and hallucinogens: increased heart rate and blood pressure; possible increased temperature, agitation, diaphoresis
- Carbon monoxide: flu-like symptoms, headache; if possible exposure check carboxy-hemoglobin (COHgB) level
- Pesticides
- Cyanide
- Methemoglobinemia
- Poisonous envenomation
- Occupational exposure

CNS Pathology

Head Trauma

- Altered mental status from diffuse axonal injury or intracranial bleed (subdural hematoma, epidural hematoma, traumatic subarachnoid hemorrhage)
- Elevated ICP, evaluate for Cushing's triad of bradycardia, HTN, irregular breathing
- Obtain stat head CT and neurosurgical consultation
- Protect airway and perform rapid sequence intubation (pretreat with fentanyl if hemodynamically stable)

Nontraumatic CNS Causes

- Cerebrovascular accident (CVA) – check for focal neurologic signs
- Subarachnoid hemorrhage (SAH) – headache, nuchal rigidity
- Lumbar puncture needed if CT negative
- Meningitis – lumbar puncture for diagnosis, early empiric antibiotics with steroids added for adults
- Encephalitis
    - Treat empirically with acyclovir for herpes simplex virus while awaiting confirmatory testing
    - High index of suspicion in HIV/immunocompromised host for uncommon infections (e.g., toxoplasmosis, cryptococcal meningitis)
- Brain tumor

Seizure or Postictal State

- History of seizures, witnessed seizure activity
- Postictal state following a generalized seizure should resolve in a few hours
- Absence seizures – brief altered mental status without motor activity, more common in children
- Nonconvulsive status epilepticus – may present with confusion, personality changes, hallucinations, delusions, nonfocal examination
- EEG is needed

Endocrinopathies

Thyroid

- Hypothyroid – gradual alteration in mental status, lethargy, bradycardia, hypotension. Severe = myxedema coma
- Hyperthyroid – agitated and tremulous, tachycardia, fever. Severe = thyroid storm
- Check serum TSH level, supportive care, β-blocker for thyroid storm

Adrenal

- Adrenal insufficiency
- Cushing syndrome – round full face, skin changes, hump on back of neck

Encephalopathies and Organ Failure/Damage

Hypertensive Encephalopathy

- Elevated blood pressure
- Check for evidence of end-organ damage (e.g., heart failure, kidney failure)

Liver Disease/Hepatic Encephalopathy

- History of liver disease, physical stigmata of chronic liver disease, and specifically history of prior hepatic encephalopathy
- Treat with lactulose
- Search for underlying precipitant, particularly spontaneous bacterial peritonitis (SBP) or GI bleeding

Renal Disease/Uremia
- Inquire about dialysis schedule and compliance

Cardiac Disease

- Arrhythmia
- Myocardial infarction
- Congestive heart failure, cardiogenic shock

Acute Abdomen

- Ischemic bowel
- GI obstruction, volvulus, incarceration, or perforation
- Infection (appendicitis, diverticulitis, cholecystitis)

Extremes of Temperature

Hyperthermia

- Temperature greater than 40°C
- Confusion, tachycardia, tachypnea
- Immediately initiate cooling interventions; evaporative cooling with water mist and fan is most effective

Hypothermia

- Temperature less than 35°C
- Apathy, slurred speech
- When severe loss of shivering ensues
- Immediately begin rewarming with blankets, warming blanket, warm IV fluids

Psychiatric

- Exacerbations of a psychiatric disorder or the first presentation of psychiatric illness may present with altered mental status.

- This should be a diagnosis of exclusion; psychiatric etiology is more likely in younger patients with prior psychiatric history.
- Exclude medical and reversible causes of altered mental status before transferring patient to a psychiatrist.

Dementia

- Do not assume that altered mental status in an elderly patient is just chronic dementia. Delirium must not be missed and should be ruled out.
- Search for a reversible medical etiology in all patients with abnormal mental status.
- Ascertain what the patient's usual baseline mental status is.

MNEMONIC FOR ALTERED MENTAL STATUS: AEIOU TIPS

A Alcohol
E Electrolytes, endocrine, encephalopathy
I Insulin (glucose)
O Oxygen, opiates, overdose
U Uremia
T Trauma, temperature, toxin
I Infection, intracranial process
P Pharmacology, poisoning, psychiatric
S Seizure, stroke, subdural, shock

SEDATION OF SEVERELY AGITATED AND UNCOOPERATIVE PATIENTS

Sedation may be necessary for agitated patients to proceed with necessary stabilization, evaluation, and treatment.

- Try to reassure and verbally deescalate whenever possible.
- Pharmacologic sedation is needed for agitated patients if there is a potential for the patient to harm himself or others or if agitation is impeding medical evaluation and treatment.
- Use an antipsychotic such as haloperidol or a benzodiazepine, such as lorazepam or midazolam.
  - With benzodiazepines, monitor for respiratory depression, particularly in elderly or debilitated patients.
  - With antipsychotics, beware of potential for QT prolongation (may rarely result in torsades de pointes), extrapyramidal side effects (e.g., dystonic reaction), potential lowering of seizure threshold.

The Poisoned Patient: Most Common Toxidromes and Treatments

Ruben Olmedo, MD

STABILIZATION

The clinical management of the overdosed or poisoned patient is underscored by the basic principle of treating the patient and not the poison. In following this clinical tenet, the critically ill poisoned patient is rapidly stabilized during the primary survey, emphasizing the ABCs to correct airway, breathing, and circulatory problems. Abnormalities in the patient's vital signs (heart rate, blood pressure, temperature, respiratory rate, pulse oximetry, and finger stick glucose) are also corrected at this time.

HISTORY

As with other patients, a key element in the approach to the poisoned patient is in obtaining a history of present illness. The presentation of the overdosed/poisoned patient will depend on both the patient and the toxin. Therefore, it is important to ask about the patient's general medical condition, medications, allergies, and the circumstances surrounding the overdose/poisoning. It is also important to inquire about what toxin(s) the patient may have access to, the dose, route, and time of overdose/poisoning. When inquiring about the circumstances surrounding the event, it is important to ask what signs and symptoms were experienced, their onset, and if anything has been done about them.

As there are many toxins, there are many toxidromes to be identified. This undertaking may seem daunting. However, it is simplified by classifying the toxidromes into categories that correspond to large pharmacological classes of agents (opioids, sympathomimetics, cholinergics, etc.). This is important as a specific agent may give you most, but not all, the signs and symptoms of that particular class of toxin. However, this information may be enough to suggest the correct implicated agent.

The physical examination is one of the most important tools that a physician has during the medical assessment; it provides supporting information in making the correct diagnosis. This is especially important in toxicology. The name given to the constellation of signs and symptoms that a patient may have after an exposure to a specific toxin (or class of toxin) is called the toxidrome. The finding of a specific toxidrome during a focused physical examination gives a clue to the type of toxin ingested.

It is important to note that many patients may ingest more than one toxin. As such, the physical examination will manifest mixed signs and symptoms of the agents involved. In a mixed overdose, therefore, the toxidromes may be obscured.

The toxicological physical examination begins with careful evaluation of the vital signs. These include pulse, blood pressure, respiratory rate, temperature, and pulse oximetry. Since normal vital signs are influenced by age and general state of health, attention should be paid to these parameters during the clinical assessment. Vital signs should be monitored for further clues to temporal changes of end-organ manifestations since this may be relevant to a specific toxin. Abnormalities in vital signs detected during a physical examination may also point to the involvement of specific toxins (Box C.1).

To quickly identify common toxidromes, the physical examination in toxicology is simplified. Conducting an assessment of the mental status first is important, especially for toxins that cause mental disturbances. For ease of determination, this assessment may be described as normal, depressed (lethargy or comatose), or agitated (hyperdynamic). In the following part of the physical assessment, the size and reactivity of the pupils should be noted. The abdominal examination should note the presence or absence of bowel sounds, including hyperactivity. The bladder should be percussed for urinary retention. The skin examination should similarly note whether it is dry, normal, or wet. Lastly, a neurological examination is performed to assess for any focal deficits.

Table C.1 describes the physical examination findings of some of the most common toxidromes encountered in an overdose. It is important to note that the sudden discontinuation of a medication/toxin may produce clinical manifestations that may be opposite to those manifested during an acute ingestion. In such a case, the constellation of signs and symptoms will be categorized as a withdrawal toxidrome (Table C.2). Tables C.3 and C.4 give examples of agents that cause common toxidromes.

Box C.1 Toxin-Associated Vital Sign Abnormalities

- Temperature: hypothermia
  - Ethanol
  - Sedative hypnotics
  - Barbiturates
  - Oral hypoglycemics
  - Opioids
  - General anesthetics
  - Carbon monoxide
  - BBs
  - α-blockers
- Temperature: hyperthermia
  - Cocaine
  - Amphetamines
  - Neuroleptics
  - Anticholinergics
  - Salicylates
  - PCP
- Respiratory rate: hyperventilation
  - Sympathomimetics
  - Anticholinergics
  - Caffeine
  - Seizuregenic agents (e.g., INH, *Gyromitra*)
  - Agents causing AG (i.e., salicylates, electron transport inhibitors [CO, cyanide], toxic alcohols)

- Cocaine
- Amphetamines
- Neuroleptics
- Anticholinergics
- Salicylates
- Dinitrophenol
- Respiratory rate: Hypoventilation
  - Barbiturates
  - Neuromuscular blockers (botulism, nicotine, organophosphates, elapid envenomation)
  - Opioids, clonidine
  - Tetrodotoxin
  - Poison hemlock
  - Strychnine
  - Colchicine
- Blood pressure: hypertension
  - Sympathomimetics
  - Cocaine
  - PCP
  - Lead
  - MAOI overdose
  - MAOI interaction
- Blood pressure: Hypotension
  - CCBs
  - BBs
  - Antihypertensives
  - TCAs
  - Barbiturates
- Pulse: tachycardia
  - Anticholinergics
  - Sympathomimetics
  - Cocaine
  - TCAs
  - Theophylline
  - Iron
  - Diuretics
- Pulse: bradycardia
  - CCBs
  - BBs
  - Digoxin
  - Clonidine
  - Opioids

AG, anion gap; BB, β-blocker; CCB, calcium channel blocker; CO, carbon monoxide; MAOI, monoamine oxidase inhibitor; PCP, pentachlorophenol; TCA, tricyclic antidepressant.

Table C.1 Common toxidromes

| Toxidromes | Vital signs | | | | Physical examination | | | |
	BP	HR	RR	T	MS	Pupils	Abdomen (BS)	Skin
Sympathomimetic	↑	↑	↑	↑	Agitated	Dilated	↑	Wet
Cholinergic (nicotinic)	↔	↑	↑	↔	Agitated	↔	↑	No change
Cholinergic (muscarinic)	↔	↔	No change	No change	Agitated	↔	↑	Wet
Anticholinergic	↔	↑	↔	↑	Agitated	Dilated	↓	Dry

BP, blood pressure; BS, bowel sounds; HR, heart rate; MS, mental status; RR, respiratory rate; T, temperature.

Table C.2 Common toxidromes and their respective withdrawal toxidromes

| Toxidromes | Vital signs | | | | Physical examination | | | |
	BP	HR	RR	T	MS	Pupils	Abdomen (BS)	Skin
Sedative hypnotic (SH)	↓	↓	↓	↓	Depressed	Dilated	No change	No change
SH withdrawal	↑	↑	↑	↑	Agitated	No change	No change	Wet
Opioid	↓	↓	↓	↓	Depressed	Pinpoint	↓	No change
Opioid withdrawal	↑	↑	No change	No change	Anxious	Dilated	↑	Wet

Abbreviations: BP, blood pressure; BS, bowel sounds; HR, heart rate; MS, mental status; RR, respiratory rate; T, temperature.

Table C.3 Examples of toxins that cause common toxidromes [1]

Sympathomimetics	Cholinergics (nicotinic)	Cholinergic (muscarinic)	Anticholinergic
Cocaine	Organophosphates	Organophosphates	Antihistamines
Amphetamines	Nicotine	Carbamates	Antipsychotics
Theophylline		Physostigmine	Selective serotonin
Epinephrine		Pyridostigmine	reuptake inhibitors
Norepinephrine		Neostigmine	(SSRIs)
Levothyroxine			Tricyclic antidepressants
Albuterol			(TCAs)
Ephedra			Atropine
Caffeine			Hyoscyamine
Guarana			Scopolamine
Yohimbine			Glycopyrrolate
Adderall (dextroamphetamine)			Benztropine
Atomoxetine			Glutethimide
Methylphenidate			
Phentermine			
Terbutaline			

Table C.4 Examples of toxins that cause common toxidromes (2)

Sedative hypnotics	Sedative hypnotic withdrawal	Opioid	Opioid withdrawal
Benzodiazepines	Benzodiazepine withdrawal	Heroin	In opioid-dependent person: opioid antagonists
Barbiturates	Barbiturate withdrawal	Codeine	
Ethanol	Ethanol withdrawal	Hydromorphone	
Alcohols	In sedative-hypnotic-dependent person: flumazenil	Oxycodone	
Carisoprodol		Methadone	
Flexeril		Fentanyl	
Chloral hydrate		Hydrocodone	
Buspirone		Propoxyphene	
Propofol		Clonidine	
Zolpidem			
Zaleplon			
Ethchlorvynol			
Meprobamate			
Glutethimide			
Bromides			
Kava kava			

The Trauma Patient: The Approach and Important Principles

David Cherkas, MD, FACEP

Questions to ask for **every** trauma victim:

- "When I walk into the room, what do I see?"
- "Is there any more information from EMS about the scene or mechanism?" If the answer seems long or they have lists of the patient's medications or past medical history, ask them to stay and get back to them later.
- ABCDE: "I would like to assess the patient's airway, breathing, and circulation; have the patient exposed and placed on a monitor, have two large-bore IVs placed, and see the patient's vital signs."

The initial assessment will drive the first big decisions:

Intubation: GCS <8, combative, airway protection, injury with likelihood of airway compromise later (burns, neck, or facial trauma). Use rapid sequence intubation (RSI) unless difficulty is predicted – then be prepared for surgical airway and consider awake or fiberoptic intubation. The simplest approach is to use etomidate as an induction agent and rocuronium as a paralytic for all traumatic RSI cases. Deviation from the standard may cause unnecessary extra questions. Don't forget to consider premedication with lidocaine and/or fentanyl for patients with head injury.

Tube thoracostomy: Decreased breath sounds on initial evaluation, asymmetrical chest movement (flail segment). Unless you are asked to describe the procedure, keep it simple.

Next, do an e-FAST exam and be ready to describe what it includes if asked. Take other obvious steps – staunch arterial bleeding, assess the abdomen and pelvis, and bind the pelvis if unstable.

For tachycardic or hypotensive patients you will want to start 1 L of crystalloid resuscitation at this point. It is reasonable but not critical to state that your goal is a hypotensive resuscitation where you maximize perfusion but minimize bleeding risk.

Order basic trauma labs and studies: CBC, chemistry, alcohol, coagulation studies, type and cross-match for two units, C spine (cross-table if high suspicion for injury, otherwise defer to CT scan), chest and pelvis x-ray.

While those are pending, verbalize your *complete* secondary survey, including potential repeat FAST examination and *complete* medical history, including *allergies*.

Now ask for the trauma team to be activated or the trauma surgeon to be notified and for the repeat vital signs after initial resuscitation.

Now you will come to the next big decisions:

Transfusion: You are expected to transfuse all patients that are hypotensive after appropriate initial resuscitation.

Central access: This is of less value than most people think in initial resuscitation in the real world and unlikely to win you any points – stick with multiple large-bore peripheral IVs or proximal IO access unless the patient has multiple limb injuries or if the examiner describes a problem in obtaining peripheral IV access.

Invasive monitoring: Unlike the place where you work, the monitoring devices at ABEM General "work flawlessly." Don't worry about invasive monitoring unless you are specifically told there is an issue with monitoring.

Next, fully define the patient's injuries and begin to order appropriate subspecialty consultations:

"Pan scan" may be common clinical practice for some emergency physicians, including those seeking greater security and less thought at the expense of greater radiation exposure. The oral boards are not the place to debate the relative merits of this approach. Simply order the tests that are appropriate for the patient's suspected injuries.

Disposition in the real world can be a difficult and cumbersome task. At ABEM General, the inpatient services are extremely compliant with whatever disposition you want for the patient. Put whatever institutional factors you may consider in your real job out of your mind and simply disposition the patient to the level of care that you think is most appropriate.

Completion: The case should end when you have completed the treatment and disposition expected by the examiner. Most of the critical steps will be resuscitation with blood products or crystalloid, procedures, or diagnostic testing, but don't forget to complete routine treatments such as giving antibiotics or updating tetanus.

PITFALLS

- Expecting someone to help you – that is, thinking the case will likely end when the surgeon, neurosurgeon, or other consultant shows up.
- Expecting anesthesia to assist with the intubation – again, at ABEM General you are expected to handle all the EM procedures yourself.
- Attempting to skip to sophisticated resuscitation before the appropriate initial evaluation steps have been taken. For example, attempting to push the patient to the operating room or admission before a reasonable primary and secondary survey has been completed or appropriate diagnostic tests and ED therapy have been initiated.

Addressing variations in the standard of care: There are areas of clinical controversy that remain. They will likely not be heavily weighted in your evaluation, but they can hinder your thought process and rhythm in the heat of a case. For example:

- Is it your responsibility to give phenytoin to every patient with a head injury?
- Should you administer high-dose steroids to patients with spinal cord injury?

One way around this is to ask/tell your consultant what your plan is and ask if they have any specific objections or suggestions. For example:

Jane Doe has a moderate right subdural hematoma with shift, her initial GCS was 7 and she was intubated on arrival for airway protection. Since arrival, her left pupil has become fixed and dilated. I was planning on initiating Dilantin and mannitol (or hypertonic saline). Do you have any objections or other suggestions? It is imperative that you evaluate the patient soon. Thank you.

Advanced Cardiac Life Support Review

Thomas Nguyen, MD and Avir Mitra, MD

CPR: EMPHASIS ON HIGH-QUALITY CPR

- Always find your landmarks (lower half of sternum).
- Push hard (adequately compress the chest **at least** 2.0 inches).
- Push fast (100–120 compressions per minute).
- Allow the chest to recoil after each compression.
- Compression to ventilation ratio is 30:2 (one cycle) for one and two rescuers for adult CPR.
- Ventilations should be given over about 1 second; sufficient just to cause the chest to rise.
- Continuous compressions: providers must minimize interruptions in chest compressions for rhythm check, shock delivery, advanced airway insertion, or vascular access.

Sequence for Bystander CPR

Call for help and defibrillator immediately
- **CAB is the New ABC.** The sequence of basic life support has changed: CAB, chest compressions, airway, breathing, has replaced ABC, airway, breathing, chest compressions.
- CPR (five cycles or 2 minutes) or until defibrillator or automatic external defibrillator (AED) arrives.
- For AED, turn power on first, and then attach pads.
- No CPR during the analyze mode of AED.
- Shock if indicated.
- Continue CPR (2 minutes) then do a pulse check.
- Repeat sequence as needed.
  - Consider naloxone 0.4–2.0 mg intranasal, SC, IM, IV in suspected opioid overdose

Sequence to Activate EMS for Out-of-Hospital Cardiac Arrest

- Call first: activate emergency response system for adult victims found unresponsive.
- If asphyxia arrest (drowning, choking) is likely, call after five cycles (or 2 minutes) of CPR.
- Call for an AED or defibrillator as soon as possible.
- If with another person, send that person for help and make sure they come back to assist.

Defibrillation Plus CPR

- Whenever defibrillator or AED is available, it should be used as soon as possible when indicated.
- For out-of-hospital *unwitnessed* arrests, providers/EMS should give five cycles of CPR in about 2 minutes before checking ECG and defibrillator (especially if wait time is greater than 4–5 minutes).

- Charge for all shockable pulseless VF/VT.
- One shock only.
- Energy level 360 J for monophasic and whatever is recommended by manufacturer with biphasic (200 J is default if unknown).
- The one shock is followed immediately with 2 minutes of CPR (five cycles) beginning with chest compressions; start thinking about pushing meds.
- If an organized rhythm is apparent during rhythm checks after 2 minutes (five cycles) of CPR, the provider checks a pulse; if still in VF/pulseless VT, shock again at 360 J or biphasic equivalent and continue with CPR sequence.

Airway and Ventilation

- Avoid prolonged interruptions of CPR when inserting an advanced airway device.
- Once airway device is in place, deliver 1 breath every 6 seconds (10 breaths per minute).
- The breaths are given asynchronously while the compressions are being done continuously at a rate of 100–120 per minute.
- Insertion of an advanced airway device should not take precedence over good-quality CPR.
- Use of endotracheal intubation or supraglottic device is limited to providers with adequate training and opportunities to practice or perform them.
- No cricoid pressure: not recommended as an aid to ventilation.

Post-Arrest Care

- Manage airway, consider early placement of ET.
- Manage respiratory parameters: start 10 breaths/min, SpO_2 92–98%, $PaCO_2$ 35–45 mmHg.
- Manage hemodynamic parameters: keep SBP > 90 mmHg, MAP > 65 mmHg.
- Consider targeted temperature management (32–36°C) in all comatose patients regardless of presenting rhythm or whether the arrest was out of hospital or in hospital.
- Obtain 12-lead EKG.
- Consider emergent cardiac intervention for STEMI, unstable cardiogenic shock: mechanical circulatory support.
- Consider CT brain and EEG monitoring.

Other Points to Remember

- Pacing: considered for symptomatic bradycardia with a pulse; *not* recommended for asystolic cardiac arrest.
- Vascular access: IV or IO (intraosseous) *preferred* to endotracheal. ETT dose is two times the IV/IO dose.
- There is an increased emphasis on physiologic monitoring to optimize CPR quality and detect ROSC (e.g., if $ETCO_2$ is decreasing or <10 mmHg, attempt to improve CPR quality).
- Drugs: timing of drug delivery is less important than the need to minimize interruptions in chest compressions. Give drug during CPR immediately following rhythm check; that is, have drugs prepared before rhythm check.
- Vasopressin is no longer recommended.
- For persistent VF/VT pulseless arrest, epinephrine 1 mg IV can be given as soon as possible after the rhythm check either during the CPR that precedes (until the defibrillator is charged) or after the shock.

Pulseless Arrest

Call for help, perform CPR until defibrillator/monitor arrives.

- Shockable rhythm (VF/pulseless VT):
  - Give one shock (360 J monophasic or 200 J biphasic or manufacturer's recommended dose).
  - Resume CPR (no pulse check) five cycles of CPR or 2 minutes.
  - Monitor check and pulse check.
  - Give another shock (if no pulse); if pulse is present begin post-resuscitation care.
- Give drugs:
  - Epinephrine 1 mg IV/IO (each round) every 3–5 minutes
  - Amiodarone 300 mg IV/IO once over 2 minutes then consider additional 150 mg IV/IO next round or consider
  - Lidocaine 1–1.5 mg/kg, IV/IO. May give second dose 0.5–0.75 mg/kg
- Repeat from the top, starting with CPR.
- Not shockable (asystole/PEA):
  - CPR for five cycles or 2 minutes
  - Epinephrine 1 mg IV/IO (may repeat each round)
  - Check for pulses/rhythm
  - Repeat cycle
  - Look for reversible causes
    - Hypovolemia
    - Hypoxia
    - Hydrogen ion (acidosis)
    - Hypo-/hyperkalemia
    - Hypothermia
    - Tension pneumothorax
    - Tamponade, cardiac
    - Toxins
    - Thrombosis – pulmonary and coronary

Bradycardia

- Maintain airway, give oxygen
- Monitor rhythm, blood pressure, oximetry
- Signs of adequate perfusion (good mentation, no chest pain, no hypotension, no signs of shock, no CHF)
  - Observe/monitor
- Signs of poor perfusion (altered mental status, chest pain, hypotension, no signs of shock, no CHF)
  - Prepare for transcutaneous pacing
  - Consider atropine 0.5 mg IV (may repeat to a total of 3 mg)
  - Consider epinephrine drip (2–10 mcg/min) or dopamine drip (2–20 mcg/kg/min)
  - Consider transvenous pacing

Tachycardia (with Pulse)

- Monitor, support ABCs, give oxygen
- Is patient stable or unstable?

- Unstable
  - Perform synchronized cardioversion
    - o Atrial fibrillation: 120–200 J biphasic or monophasic
    - o Atrial flutter/SVT: 50–100 J biphasic or monophasic
    - o Stable monomorphic VT: 100 J biphasic or monophasic
  - Consider sedation if patient is conscious
- Stable
  - Narrow QRS
    - a. Regular narrow (SVT, atrial flutter, junctional rhythm)
      Attempt vagal maneuvers
      Adenosine 6 mg IVP (may repeat 12 mg IVP × 2)
      Consider rate control with calcium channel blocker or β-blockers IV
    - b. Irregular narrow (rapid atrial fibrillation, multifocal atrial tachycardia)
      Rate control with calcium channel blocker or β-blockers IV
  - Wide QRS
    - a. Regular wide: VT, SVT with aberrancy
      VT: give amiodarone 150 mg IV over 10 minutes (repeat up to 2.2 g/24 hr) or procainamide 20–50 mg/min (max. 17 mg/kg) or sotalol 1.5 mg/kg IV over 5 minutes, or lidocaine 1–1.5 mg/kg IV (repeat 0.5–0.75 mg/kg IV every 5–10 minutes, max. total 3 mg/kg)
      SVT with aberrancy: give adenosine 6 mg IVP (may repeat 12 mg × 2). Consider β-blocker, diltiazem, amiodarone, digoxin
    - b. Irregular wide QRS: atrial fibrillation with aberrancy, WPW, polymorphic VT, torsades
      Atrial fibrillation with aberrancy: rate control with diltiazem or β-blocker. WPW – consider amiodarone 150 mg IV 10 minutes (avoid AV node blockers adenosine, diltiazem, digoxin)
      Polymorphic VT: seek expert consultation. Consider amiodarone 150 mg IV or magnesium 1–2 g IV
      Torsades de pointes: Shock immediately (see pulseless section above). Magnesium 1–2 g over 5–6 minutes, then infusion. Consider overdrive pacing

ACLS DRUG LIST: ANTIARRHYTHMICS

Adenosine

Action: Briefly suppresses AV and sinus node activity.

Use in ACLS

1. Drug of choice for stable, narrow-complex regular tachycardias (AV nodal or sinus nodal reentrant tachycardias) or wide-complex regular tachycardias confirmed as supraventricular.

Dose

- 6 mg IV push rapidly over 1–3 seconds, followed by a 20 mL saline flush. May give 12 mg if does not convert within 1–2 minutes. A second 12 mg bolus can be given if does not convert after the first 12 mg bolus.

Adverse effects: Transient flushing, dyspnea, chest pain; risk of acceleration of accessory conduction.

Amiodarone

Action: Class II antiarrhythmic; acts on blocking sodium, potassium, and calcium channels; also has α- and β-adrenergic blockade properties.

Use in ACLS

1. Narrow complex tachycardias originating from a reentry mechanism if uncontrolled by adenosine, vagal maneuvers, and AV nodal blockade in patients with preserved or impaired ventricular function.
2. In cardiac arrest with VT or VF after defibrillation and epinephrine.
3. Control of hemodynamically stable VT, polymorphic VT, and wide-complex tachycardia of uncertain origin.
4. Control of rapid ventricular rate due to accessory pathway conduction in pre-exited atrial arrhythmias.

Dose

- For pulseless VT or VF: can give 300 mg. Take two 10 mL syringes. Draw up 150 mg of amiodarone and 7 mL NS into each syringe for a total of 300 mg amiodarone. Give each over 1 minute if refractory or recurrent VT. Initial dose of 300 mg may be followed by one dose of 150 mg IV/IO.
- For VT with a pulse: can give 150 mg IV over 10 minutes which can be repeated if ineffective. Maintenance infusion: 1 mg/min infusion × 6 hours. Then 0.5 mg/min infusion × 18 hours.

Note that bolus doses can be given without using a glass bottle. A glass bottle and an in-line filter should be used for infusions. The amiodarone infusion is best given in a central line but a peripheral line can be used until a central line is available in an emergency.

Adverse effects: Hypotension and bradycardia.

Lidocaine

Action: Class Ib antiarrhythmic; sodium channel blocker.

Use in ACLS

May be considered, but not the treatment of choice, for:

1. stable monomorphic VT with preserved heart function
2. polymorphic VT with normal baseline QT interval
3. polymorphic VT with prolonged QT interval that suggests torsades
4. alternative treatment to amiodarone in VF/pulseless VT cardiac arrest

Dose

- 1–1.5 mg/kg IV push in VT/VF cardiac arrest; 1.5 mg/kg preferable in adults. Additional 0.5–0.75 mg/kg for refractory VT/VF at 5–10 minute intervals to a maximum dose of 3 mg/kg.
- *Reduce dose* or use amiodarone in low cardiac output states, such as in AMI with hypotension or shock, CHF, >70 years, or hepatic dysfunction.
  Adverse effects: Hypotension; CNS effects

Procainamide

Action: Class Ia antiarrhythmic; sodium channel blocker

Use in ACLS
1. One of several drugs for stable monomorphic VT with preserved heart function.
2. One of several drugs that may be used to restore sinus rhythm for atrial fibrillation or atrial flutter in patients with preserved ventricular function.
3. One of several drugs that can be used for acute control to restore normal sinus rhythm in atrial fibrillation or atrial flutter in patients with known WPW and preserved heart function.
4. One of several drugs that can be used for AV reentrant, narrow-complex tachycardias such as reentry SVT if rhythm is uncontrolled by adenosine and vagal maneuvers in patients with preserved heart function.

Dose
- 20 mg/min infusion until arrhythmia suppressed, hypotension, prolonged QRS by 50% from its original duration or total of 17 mg/kg; maintenance infusion is 1–4 mg/min.
- In refractory VF/VT or urgent situation, infusion rate can be increased up to 50 mg/min to a total of 17 mg/kg.

Adverse effect: Hypotension

Magnesium

Action: A vasodilator and a cofactor in the regulation of sodium, potassium, and calcium across membranes. It also corrects magnesium deficiency, which is associated with arrhythmias, cardiac insufficiency, and cardiac death.

Use in ACLS
1. Torsades de pointes
2. Magnesium deficiency

Dose
- Torsades with pulses: 1–2 g in 50–100 D_5 W over 5–60 minutes, followed by infusion of 0.5–1 g over 5–60 minutes.
- Torsades with VF/pulseless VT cardiac arrest: defibrillate, then give magnesium 1–2 g diluted in 10 mL D_5 W.

Adverse effects: If given too rapidly, hypotension or asystole.

Calcium Channel Blocker: Diltiazem or Verapamil

Action: Slows conduction and increases refractoriness in the AV node.

Use in ACLS
1. Stable, narrow-complex, reentry mechanism tachycardias (reentry SVT) if uncontrolled or unconverted by adenosine or vagal maneuvers.
2. Stable, narrow-complex, automaticity mechanism tachycardias (junctional, ectopic, multifocal) if rhythm not controlled or converted by adenosine or vagal maneuvers.

3. Control rate of ventricular response in patients with atrial fibrillation or atrial flutter; may be harmful in patients with WPW or similar syndrome.

Dose

- Diltiazem: 0.25 mg/kg followed by second dose of 0.35 mg/kg if no response in 10–15 minutes; maintenance of 5–15 mg/hr to control ventricular rate in atrial fibrillation or atrial flutter.
- Verapamil: 2.5–5 mg IV given over 2 minutes; can give repeated doses of 5–10 mg every 15–30 minutes to a total dose of 20 mg.

Adverse effects: May decrease myocardial contractility and exacerbate CHF in patients with severe LV dysfunction; hypotension, bradycardia.

β-Adrenergic Blockers

Use in ACLS

1. Narrow complex tachycardias from reentry mechanism, for example, reentry SVT or automatic focus (junctional, ectopic, or multifocal tachycardia) uncontrolled by vagal maneuvers and adenosine in the patient with preserved ventricular function.
2. Rate control in atrial fibrillation and atrial flutter in patients with preserved ventricular function.

Dose

- Atenolol: 5 mg slow IV push over 5 minutes; wait 10 minutes and if tolerated, second dose of 5 mg slow IV over 5 minutes.
- Metoprolol: 5 mg slow IV push at 5 minute intervals to a total of 15 mg.
- Propranolol: 0.1 mg/kg slow IV push divided into three equal doses at 2–3 minute intervals with rate not to exceed 1 mg/min.
- Esmolol: 500 mcg/kg over 1 minute followed by maintenance infusion of 50 mcg/kg/min for 4 minutes; if inadequate, second bolus of 500 mcg/kg over 1 minute with maintenance of 100 mcg/kg/min for 4 minutes, bolus 500 mcg/kg and titration of infusion (addition of 50 mcg/kg/min) can be repeated up to maximum maintenance infusion of 300 mcg/kg/min.

Adverse effects: Bradycardias, AV conduction delays, hypotension; contraindicated in second- or third-degree heart block, hypotension, severe CHF, and lung disease with bronchospasm; caution with preexisting sinus bradycardia and sick sinus syndrome; may be harmful for patients with atrial fibrillation or atrial flutter associated with known WPW.

Atropine

- Action: Reverses cholinergic-mediated decreases in heart rate, systemic vascular resistance, and blood pressure.

Use in ACLS

1. Symptomatic sinus bradycardia, AV block at the nodal level, or organophosphate poisoning

Dose

- 0.5–1 mg IV every 3–5 minutes for bradycardia to a total dose of 0.04 mg/kg or 3 mg.

Adverse effects: Worsening of ischemia; rarely, VF, VT.

ACLS DRUG LIST: CARDIOACTIVE DRUGS

Epinephrine

Action: α-adrenergic receptor-stimulating properties that increase myocardial and cerebral blood flow during CPR.

Use in ACLS

1. Cardiac arrest
2. Symptomatic bradycardia after atropine, dopamine, and pacing, or pacing not available
3. Severe hypotension
4. Anaphylaxis associated with hemodynamic instability or respiratory distress

Dose

- In cardiac arrest: 1:10,000: 1 mg IV push every 3–5 minutes IV/IO.
- Symptomatic bradycardia/anaphylaxis: 2–10 mcg/min infusion.

  Adverse effects: May cause myocardial ischemia, angina, and increased cardiac demand.

Norepinephrine

Action: α- and β-receptor-stimulating actions; vasoconstrictor and inotropic agent.

Use in ACLS

1. Severe hypotension (systolic <70 mmHg) and low total peripheral resistance.

Dose

- Initially, 0.5–1 mcg/min infusion titrated to effect.

  Adverse effects: Ischemic necrosis and sloughing of tissues with extravasation, possibly increased myocardial oxygen requirements.

Dopamine

Action: Dopaminergic, α- and β-receptor-stimulating actions.

Use in ACLS as BP Agent

1. Hypotension with symptomatic bradycardia
2. After return of spontaneous circulation for post-resuscitation hypotension or shock

Dose

- 5–20 mcg/kg/min infusion

  Adverse effect: Tachycardia

Dobutamine

Action: Catecholamine and potent inotropic agent; predominant β-adrenergic receptor-stimulating effects that increase myocardial contractility and decrease left ventricular filling pressures.

Use in ACLS

1. Treatment of severe systolic heart failure

Dose

- 2–20 mcg/kg/min infusion
  Adverse effect: Tachycardia

Nitroglycerin

Action: Relaxes vascular smooth muscle.

Use in ACLS

1. Ischemic-type pain or discomfort, acute coronary syndromes, hypertensive emergencies, CHF

Dose

- For suspected angina: 1 tablet (0.4 mg) sublingually and repeated at 3–5 minute intervals if not relieved.
- Continuous infusion at 10–20 mcg/min and increased by 5–10 mcg/min until desired response occurs.

Adverse effects: Hypotension (also consider RV infarct; check R-sided leads), tachycardia, paradoxical bradycardia, hypoxemia, headache

Sodium Nitroprusside

Action: Potent, rapid-acting direct peripheral vasodilator.

Use in ACLS

1. Severe heart failure and hypertensive emergencies

Dose

- 0.1–5 mcg/kg/min infusion up to 10 mcg/kg/min

Adverse effects: Hypotension, headache, nausea, vomiting, abdominal cramps

Calcium

Action: Replenish calcium; cardioprotective effect

Use in ACLS

1. Hyperkalemia
2. Hypocalcemia
3. Calcium channel blocker toxicity

Dose

- 10% solution of calcium chloride in a dose of 8–16 mg/kg (usually 5–10 mL and repeated as necessary at 10 minute intervals). Recheck ECG after calcium in hyperkalemia; if no decrease in peaked T-waves or QRS width, give second dose.

Sodium Bicarbonate

Use in ACLS

1. Preexisting metabolic acidosis
2. Hyperkalemia
3. Tricyclic antidepressant overdose (suspect of QRS >11 ms)

Dose

- 1 mEq/kg initially; redose guided by blood gas and bicarbonate concentration.

Adverse effects: Possibly extracellular alkalosis, including shift of oxyhemoglobin curve, paradoxical intracellular acidosis, exacerbation of central venous acidosis, and inactivation of simultaneously administered catecholamines.

Diuretics: Furosemide

Action: Inhibits reabsorption of sodium in the loop of Henle; direct venodilating effect in acute pulmonary edema.

Use in ACLS

1. Acute pulmonary edema

Dose

- 0.5–1 mg/kg slow IV

Adverse effects: Fluid and electrolyte abnormalities; hypotension

BIBLIOGRAPHY

Panchal AR, Berg KM, Kudenchuk PJ, et al. (2018). 2018 American Heart Association focused update on advance cardiovascular life support use of antiarrhythmic drugs during and immediately after cardiac arrest. *Circulation*, 138, S70–S749.

Panchal AR, Bartos JA, Cabanas JG, et al. (2020). Adult basic and advanced life support: 2020 American Heart Association guidelines for cardiopulmonary resuscitation and emergency cardiovascular care. *Circulation*, 142(suppl. 2), S366–S468.

Pozner, C, Wall, R, Page, R (2021). Advanced cardiac life support (ACLS) in adults. www.UpToDate.com.

Pediatric Pearls: High-Yield Facts from Fever to Drugs

Julie Tokarski, MD and Christopher Strother, MD

NORMAL VITAL SIGNS BY AGE (PEDIATRIC ADVANCED LIFE SUPPORT GUIDELINES)

Broselow–Luten tape is commonly used as a guide to weight and medication dosing. Using this system, medication doses and equipment sizing are color-coded based on the child's height.

Systolic Hypotension

Numbers given are the 5th percentile, mean BP is higher.

- Newborn: <60 mmHg
- Infant: <70 mmHg
- 1–10 years: <70 mmHg + (age in years × 2)
- >10 years: <90

Heart Rate

- Newborn to 3 months: 80–200
- 3 months to 2 years: 75–190
- 2 to 10 years: 60–140
- >10 years: 50–100

Respiratory Rate

- Infant: 30–60
- Toddler: 24–40
- Preschool: 22 to 34
- School age: 18–30
- Teen: 12–16

PEDIATRIC ADVANCED LIFE SUPPORT

- Shock energy
  - Defibrillation
    First shock 2 J/kg
    Second shock 4 J/kg
    Maximum dose 10 J/kg or adult dose

- Synchronized cardioversion
  Begin with 0.5–1 J/kg
  If not effective, can increase to 2 J/kg

INTUBATION

Endotracheal Tube Size and Cuffs

- (age/4) + 4 *or* (age + 16)/4 (some say add 3.5 if you're using a cuffed tube instead of 4)
- About the size of nares or pinky finger
- Use a cuffed tube down to 1 year of age
  - Infant size 3.5–4.0 at one year
  - Newborn size 3.0–3.5 tube
  - Premature neonate size 2.0–2.5 tube

Laryngoscope

- Miller blade to lift large floppy noncartilaginous epiglottis
- Miller 0–1 at birth, 1–2 for infants and toddlers

Other Equipment Shortcuts

- 2 × ETT: NG/OG/Foley
- 3× ETT: ETT depth
- 4 × ETT: chest tube

Initial Ventilator Settings

- Rate:
  Infant: 20–30/min
  Child: 16–20/min
  Adolescent: 8–12/min
- Tidal volume: 5–8 cc/kg initially, adjust as indicated

NEWBORN RESUSCITATION

- Warm, dry, stimulate, suction
- Bag valve mask if HR <100, chest compressions if HR <60
- Use umbilical line for critical access
- Drugs that may be administered via endotracheal tube: lidocaine, epinephrine, atropine, naloxone (LEAN). *Note*: ET meds are discouraged in recent guidelines, umbilical or intraosseous lines are preferred.

FLUID MANAGEMENT

- Fluid bolus: 20 mL/kg for crystalloid (blood often 10 mL/kg)
- Maintenance fluid rate:
  4 mL/kg/hr for first 10 kg of body weight

2 mL/kg/hr for second 10 kg of body weight

1 mL/kg/hour for each kilogram over 20 kg

Example: 35 kg child maintenance fluid rate:

    10 kg: 40 mL/hr

    + 10 kg: 20 mL/hr

    ± 15 kg: 15 mL/hr

    = 35 kg: 75 mL/hr

- IV glucose bolus: rule of 50 = 0.5 g/kg:

  X% dextrose × X cc/kg = 50

      D50 × 1 cc/kg = 50

      D25 × 2 cc/kg = 50

      D10 × 5 cc/kg = 50

      D5 × 10 cc/kg = 50

BURNS

- Parkland formula: weight (kg) × percentage body surface area (BSA) burn × 4 mL = fluids for 24 hours (in mL)
- Administer half over first 8 hours, half over next 16 hours
- Remember: the infant head is 18% BSA (rule of 9s exception)

Example: 40 kg child with 50% BSA burn: 40 kg × 50 × 4 = 8000 mL; 4000 mL given over first 8 hours, remaining 4000 mL over the next 16 hours.

TOXICOLOGY

What a toddler could have eaten is **always** on your differential. Some ingestions can be deadly in a dose. Drugs followed by severe symptoms (treatment listed if other than supportive):

- Tricyclic acids (TCAs): arrhythmia, hypotension, seizure
  - Treatment of wide QRS is $NaHCO_3$ bolus 1–2 mEq/kg, maintain serum pH 7.45–7.55
- Monoamine oxidase inhibitors (MAOIs): hypotension, bradycardia, seizures, severe hyperthermia, respiratory depression
- Chloroquine: seizures, coma, QRS widening, ventricular dysrhythmias, hypotension, shock, cardiac arrest, respiratory arrest
  - Diazepam may exert an antagonist action against chloroquine cardiotoxicity
- Phenothiazines: ventricular dysrhythmias, hypotension, coma
- Clonidine: hypotension, bradycardia, apnea
- Calcium channel blockers: dysrhythmias, acidosis, hypokalemia, hyperglycemia, CNS depression, acute renal failure, rhabdomyolysis
  - Bradycardia: administer calcium chloride, glucagon, and pacemaker as necessary; atropine is usually not effective in this setting
- Sulfonylureas: protracted hypoglycemia
  - Treat with glucose bolus then infusion, octreotide, bicarbonate for urine alkalization (enhances elimination)
- Theophylline: seizures, hypotension, dysrhythmias, metabolic, acidosis, hypokalemia
  - Treatment: dialysis
- Opioids: respiratory depression, apnea
  - Treatment: naloxone

- Iron: shock, acidosis, GI bleed, coagulopathy, hepatotoxicity, coma
  - Decontamination, deferoxamine
- Salicylates (aspirin, oil of wintergreen, Pepto-Bismol): respiratory alkalosis, metabolic acidosis, coma, seizures, hypotension, pulmonary edema, coagulopathy, cerebral edema, and dysrhythmias
  - Treatment: hydrate, bicarbonate (for urine alkalization), dialysis
- Camphor (mothballs): respiratory depression, seizures

TRAUMA CONSIDERATIONS

- Big head, little body compared to adults – C-spine injury more likely than L spine.
- Large liver and spleen, weak abdominal muscles – tend to get liver or spleen lacerations before other bowel injuries; most can be managed nonoperatively (if the patient is stable).
- Flexible rib cage – can get cardiac and lung contusions without rib fracture.

Head Trauma

- PECARN rule – clinical criteria associated with very low risk of significant traumatic brain injury in children
- Age <2
  - Normal mental status
  - Normal behavior per routine caregiver
  - No LOC
  - No severe mechanism of injury
  - No nonfrontal scalp hematoma
  - No evidence of skull fracture
- Age 2–18
  - Normal mental status
  - No LOC
  - No severe mechanism of injury
  - No vomiting
  - No severe headache
  - No signs of basilar skull fracture

ABUSE (NONACCIDENTAL TRAUMA)

- Mandated reporter (you must report to authorities if there is any suspicion)
- Pattern injuries (not **always** intentional, but suspicious injuries):
  - Retinal hemorrhage, subdural hematomas: shaken baby syndrome
  - Spiral femur fracture (not toddler's fracture)
  - Posterior rib fractures
  - Sock/glove/diaper area submersion burns
  - Belt/hand/cord mark patterns
  - Story inconsistent with injury
  - Story inconsistent with developmental milestones (e.g., two-month-old "rolled off the bed")
- Elbow, knee, and shin bruises are normal and common
- Mongolian spots are often confused with back/buttock bruising

RULE OUT SEPSIS (FEVER WITHOUT CLEAR CAUSE WORK-UP)

- Younger than 28 days or toxic-appearing: antibiotics, CBC and culture, UA and culture, spinal fluid (cell count and culture), admission. Consider LFTs if concern for herpes encephalitis or disseminated herpes.
- 29 days to 2 months: risk stratify with CBC and culture, UA and culture. Add procalcitonin if available. If above studies are abnormal, perform lumbar puncture and admit for antibiotics. Otherwise consider discharge with next-day follow-up if well-appearing, labs negative, and reliable follow-up.
- 2–3 months: Consider CBC and culture, UA and culture. Discharge with next-day follow-up if well-appearing and reliable follow-up. Antibiotics as indicated.
- Remember to consider urine in all boys under 6 months, uncircumcised boys up to 1 year of age, and girls up to 2 years with significant fever and no other clear cause.

PERSISTENT CRYING

Consider corneal abrasion, hair tourniquet (fingers, toes, genitals), urinary tract infection, meningitis, child abuse, intussusception, incarcerated hernia, acute otitis media

LIMP: COMMON CAUSES

- Septic joint versus transient synovitis
  - Kocher criteria for hips
    - Nonweight-bearing
    - Erythrocyte sedimentation rate (ESR) >40
    - Fever
    - WBC >12,000
  - 3 of 4 = 93% chance septic arthritis, 2 of 4 = 40%, 1 of 4 = 3%
- Toddler's fracture: nondisplaced oblique distal tibial fracture from minor trauma, usually a twisting mechanism
- Osgood–Schlatter: inflammation of the growth plate at the tibial tuberosity, teens,
  - Overuse injury
- Slipped capital femoral epiphysis: young teens, classically overweight, treat with urgent surgery
- Avascular necrosis of the femoral head (Legg–Calvé–Perthes): idiopathic avascular osteonecrosis
- Developmental dysplasia of the hip
  - Congenital hip dislocation (diagnose with ultrasound in newborn)
  - Ortolani and Barlow maneuvers (manipulation of the hip creates a clunk sound)

CONGENITAL HEART LESIONS

- Cyanotic heart disease (the Ts): right-to-left shunts
  - Tetralogy of Fallot (ventricular septal defect, overriding aorta, pulmonary stenosis, right ventricular hypertrophy)
  - Transposition of the great arteries (complete separation, needs a shunt to be compatible with life)

- Tricuspid atresia (no right atrium to right ventricle flow, needs a shunt, often associated with atrial septal defect)
  - Total anomalous pulmonary venous return (pulmonary veins flow into systemic/right heart, needs a shunt)
  - Truncus arteriosus (single outflow artery straddling both ventricles)
- Prostaglandin E 1 should be considered for infants less than two weeks old presenting with cyanosis or shock as a shunt-dependent lesion may be the cause
- Noncyanotic heart disease: left-to-right shunts
  - Ventricular septal defects
  - Atrial septal defects
  - Patent ductus arteriosus
  - Atrioventricular defect (also called AV canal or endocardial cushion defect)
- Obstructive disease
  - Valvular stenosis (aortic, pulmonary, mitral)
  - Coarctation of the aorta (remember increased upper extremity pulses and BP, decreased in the lower extremity)
  - Hypoplastic left heart syndrome (severe mitral and aortic stenosis or atresia and aortic arch obstruction, inadequate LV)

Twenty Common Emergency Medicine Procedures: Indications, Contraindications, Technique, and Complications

Reuben J. Strayer, MD

DEFIBRILLATION AND CARDIOVERSION

Indications

- Defibrillation
  - Ventricular fibrillation or pulseless ventricular tachycardia
- Cardioversion
  - Patients with ventricular tachycardia, supraventricular tachycardia, or atrial fibrillation/ flutter who are hemodynamically unstable require immediate synchronized cardioversion. Unstable patients are ill-appearing and may have altered mental status; they may be hypotensive, breathless, experiencing ischemic chest pain, or other evidence of hypoperfusion. Electrical cardioversion may be used as an alternative to chemical cardioversion in **stable** patients with these rhythms. Note that pulseless ventricular tachycardia requires defibrillation, not synchronized cardioversion.

Contraindications

- No absolute contraindications exist for defibrillation or cardioversion except when the procedure poses an undue risk to health care providers (e.g., in a wet submersion victim).
- Defibrillation should not be performed on patients who have incompatible advanced directives for end-of-life care.
- Digoxin toxicity is considered a relative contraindication to cardioversion; however, therapeutic use of digoxin confers no additional risk for cardioversion. The treatment of choice in unstable patients with arrhythmia thought to be due to digoxin toxicity is digoxin antibody fragments (Digibind); if this therapy is unavailable or ineffective, the likelihood of benefit of cardioversion exceeds the likelihood of harm in most instances.
- Unless a thrombus has been excluded by transesophageal echocardiography, cardioversion of atrial fibrillation is relatively contraindicated unless the rhythm is known to be less than 48 hours old. In stable, low-risk patients with recent-onset atrial fibrillation, ED-based cardioversion (and discharge) is an alternative to rate control and admission.
- Pregnancy at any stage is not a contraindication to defibrillation or cardioversion.

Equipment

- Monophasic or biphasic defibrillator with appropriately sized pads – infant paddles for patients less than 10 kg/1 year of age, adult paddles for all others
- Conductive gel, saline-wetted pads, or self-adhesive electrode pads
- Procedural sedation agents, if applicable
- Advanced airway equipment and ACLS medications in the event of complications

Appendix G

Technique

- Defibrillation
  - Verify that the defibrillator is not in synchronous/cardioversion mode.
- Set the dose
  - Adults: dose for monophasic defibrillators is 360 J. Dose for biphasic is unit-specific and should be indicated on face of unit; if unclear, use 200 J.
  - Pediatrics: dose is 2 J/kg for the first shock, 4 J/kg for subsequent shocks in monophasic and biphasic machines.
- Apply conductive gel or alternative.
- Wipe away nitropaste or excessive secretions from the patient's chest.
- Position paddles on chest. The "sternum" paddle is placed to the right of the sternum, below the clavicle; the "apex" paddle is placed to the left of the nipple in the midaxillary line, centered on the fifth intercostal space. Anterior–posterior positioning is preferred in stable patients able to sit up; in this configuration the sternum paddle is placed over the precordium, and the apex paddle to the left of the spine, directly posterior to the heart. If paddles are used, 25 lb. of force is recommended to ensure appropriate contact between the paddle and the chest wall.
- Charge paddles/pads.
- Verify that no personnel are in contact with the patient or stretcher: "I'm clear, you're clear, we're all clear."
- Discharge defibrillatory shock. Immediately resume chest compressions after defibrillation; do not delay to check pulse or rhythm.
- Cardioversion – preferred when possible because shock is administered away from the vulnerable repolarization period in the cardiac cycle.
  - Verify that the defibrillator is in synchronous/cardioversion mode.
  - In stable patients, use analgesia/sedation. 10 mg etomidate in a normal size adult is a reasonable choice in most situations. Do not give propofol or midazolam to a hypotensive patient.
  - Set the dose. Atrial fibrillation often requires a higher dose than ventricular and other supraventricular tachycardias, but the general recommendation is to start with 50 J, then 100 J, followed by 200 J for all rhythms, for both monophasic and biphasic machines. Pediatric dosing is 0.5 J/kg, followed by 1 J/kg, 2 J/kg, and 4 J/kg. Remember to verify that the machine is in synchronized mode before each shock – many units will revert to unsynchronized defibrillation after any discharge.
  - Apply conductive gel or alternative, and position the paddles as described earlier.
  - Charge the paddles and verify that personnel are clear, as described earlier.
  - Discharge the synchronized shock. Note that a delay often occurs while the defibrillator evaluates the rhythm for synchronization.
  - If no shock occurs, the R or S wave may be too small to sense. In that case, change the lead that the monitor is sensing or move the arm leads closer to the chest.

Complications

- Injury to skin and soft tissue – minimized by using conductive gel and wiping away excessive secretions (blood, perspiration, vomitus).
- Myocardial injury – minimized by using lowest effective energy dose and fewest number of shocks.
- Cardiac dysrhythmias – any rhythm, including asystole, may follow defibrillation or cardioversion.
- Injury to health care providers – remember to verify that all providers are clear at time of shock.

Notes

- If unwitnessed arrest, or if delay to defibrillation exceeds 5 minutes, some recommendations suggest 5 cycles of CPR (30 compressions and 2 breaths, 5 cycles = 2 minutes) before defibrillation. The best approach for the boards is to initiate chest compressions as soon as possible, while the defibrillator is being readied, then shock appropriate rhythms when possible.
- Before determining a rhythm to be asystole, increase the gain on the monitor and rotate the paddles 90 degrees or check another lead to rule out fine ventricular fibrillation masquerading as asystole.
- If the patient has a pacemaker in situ, position the paddle at least 1 inch away from the pulse generator.
- "Double sequential defibrillation" or "dual external defibrillation" is using two defibrillators and two sets of pads at the same time to deliver twice the energy, in refractory malignant arrhythmias. This is a new, relatively unproven technique that we do not recommend for the boards.
- Examiners may want to see that you understand that minimizing compression pauses is very important. Charge the defibrillator while compressions are ongoing, utilize a countdown to coordinate holding chest compressions and shock, and immediately resume compressions post-shock.

CRICOTHYROTOMY

Indications

- Endotracheal intubation contraindicated
- Unable to intubate and unable to ventilate patient
- Anticipated inability to perform endotracheal intubation and ventilation of the patient

Contraindications

- Absolute
  - Tracheal transection with retraction into the mediastinum
  - Significant damage to larynx or cricoid cartilage
- Relative – may be overlooked when patient's oxygenation status is jeopardized
  - Age <12 (transtracheal jet ventilation preferred)
  - Bleeding diathesis
  - Acute laryngeal disease
  - Distortion of neck anatomy

Equipment

- Minimum: any scalpel and an appropriately sized tracheostomy tube or an endotracheal tube
- #10 scalpel
- Tracheostomy tube (Shiley #5 in adults) or cuffed ETT (6–7 mm in adults)
- Gum elastic bougie
- Needle and syringe with lidocaine for local anesthesia (if time allows)
- Suture or circumferential tie to secure tracheostomy tube in place

- Several prepacked percutaneous cricothyrotomy sets are available – these contain scalpel, needle, syringe, guidewire, and a specially designed tracheostomy tube fitted over a dilator to use with the Seldinger technique

There are several accepted methods for performing cricothyrotomy; however, the open technique is preferred over the percutaneous Seldinger technique and the scalpel–finger–bougie technique has emerged as a popular option for its simplicity and effectiveness, and is what we recommend unless you have particular comfort with an alternative.

Technique

- Hyperextend the neck if there are no contraindications.
- Identify the cricothyroid membrane below the thyroid cartilage and above the cricoid cartilage – one finger-breadth below the laryngeal prominence.
- Infiltrate the skin and subcutaneous tissue with local anesthetic if time permits.
- Sedate the patient if required (ketamine is a good choice if no contraindications).
  - For a right-handed person, position yourself on the patient's right side, next to the patient's right shoulder.
  - Reidentify the landmarks by grasping/stabilizing the larynx with your left thumb and middle finger, using your index finger to find the membrane.
- Leaving your left hand in position but moving your index finger out of the way, use the scalpel in your right hand to make a 1–1.5 inch vertical incision over the cricothyroid membrane.
- Feel the cricothyroid membrane with your left index finger.
- Use the scalpel to make a stab incision in the membrane, twist the scalpel 180 degrees to slightly extend the incision horizontally.
- Remove the scalpel and place your left index finger into the trachea.
- With the bougie's bent tip pointed down toward the patient's feet, slide the bougie along the palmar aspect of your index finger into the trachea; gently advance bougie until you feel hold-up.
- Insert a lubricated endotracheal tube or tracheostomy tube over the bougie, into the trachea.
- Remove the bougie, inflate the tube cuff, and ventilate.

Complications

- Failure to successfully intubate the trachea
- Subcutaneous emphysema
- Bleeding
- Tube blockage/airway obstruction
- Infection (late complication)
- Subglottic stenosis (late complication)

Notes

- Mobilize airway consultants (anesthesia, ENT, general surgery) as early as possible in difficult airway situations.
- Difficult cricothyrotomy can be predicted using the mnemonic SHORT – neck surgery, hematoma, obesity, radiation, and tumor.
- Failure to perform cricothyrotomy when indicated is an important airway pitfall. Do not hesitate to initiate this procedure in a *can't intubate, can't ventilate/oxygenate* situation. In

general, if laryngoscopy fails, and subsequent bag-mask ventilation fails to oxygenate, place a supraglottic airway device such as an LMA. If the supraglottic device fails to oxygenate, immediately proceed to cricothyrotomy.

TRANSCUTANEOUS PACING

Indications

- Hemodynamically significant bradycardia
- Bradyasystolic arrest (minimal benefit)
- Predicted or high risk for hemodynamically significant bradycardia, including second- and third-degree heart block, ingestion of negatively chronotropic drugs or toxins, and pacemaker malfunction
- Overdrive pacing of certain tachydysrhythmias, most commonly torsades de pointes

Contraindications

- No absolute contraindications.
- Warming the bradycardic and hypothermic patient is advised before pacing, as the cold heart is more susceptible to ventricular fibrillation.

Equipment

- Most EDs have combined defibrillator–transcutaneous pacemakers.
- The only other necessary equipment is a set of pacemaker pads to affix to the patient.

Technique

- Place the pads on the patient. The pads will be labeled front/back or anterior/posterior. The anterior pad is placed over the cardiac apex and the posterior pad is placed just medial to the left scapula.
- Verify that the defibrillator is in *pace mode*.
- For pacing bradycardic rhythms, set the rate to 70.
- For pacing bradyasystolic arrest, set the stimulating current to its maximum output and slowly decrease the output until loss of capture, then increase the output to above the needed current.
- For pacing hemodynamically significant but nonarrest bradycardias, start at the minimum current and slowly increase the current until capture is noted.
- For overdrive pacing of certain ventricular and supraventricular tachycardias, set the rate to 40 bpm faster than the patient's heart rate and slowly increase the current until capture. Once capture is achieved, brief trains of 10 overdrive beats of asynchronous pacing are applied.
- If the patient experiences significant discomfort from muscle contractions, provide analgesia/sedation.
- Prepare to initiate transvenous pacing.

Complications

- Failure to recognize an underlying dangerous rhythm (e.g., ventricular fibrillation) that is buried beneath pacer spikes is the most important potential complication. When in doubt, pause the pacemaker to assess the underlying rhythm.

- Induction of dysrhythmias is rare but possible. A defibrillator should always be available when pacing.
- Patient discomfort is common; skin burns are rare but have been reported.

Notes

- Chest compressions can be administered directly over the pads while pacing. The power delivered during a typical pacing impulse is 1/1000th of defibrillation.

PERICARDIOCENTESIS

Indications

- The indication for emergency physician-performed pericardiocentesis is to relieve diagnosed pericardial tamponade in an unstable patient.
- In certain arrest or near-arrest situations, especially in the case of a pulseless electrical activity rhythm with jugular venous distension, pericardiocentesis is indicated as empiric treatment, before the diagnosis is confirmed, if there is any delay to immediate point of care sonography.

Contraindications

- There are no absolute contraindications to pericardiocentesis.
- Uremic patients with a pericardial effusion should be managed with hemodialysis, if circumstances permit, before pericardiocentesis, but only if hemodynamically stable. Do not defer pericardiocentesis for dialysis in hypotensive patients.
- Hemorrhagic tamponade cannot be definitively managed by pericardiocentesis. In the case of traumatic pericardial effusion, pericardiocentesis may be performed on the arrested or near-arrested patient as preparations are made for thoracotomy, but should not delay thoracotomy.

Equipment

- The minimum equipment necessary is a syringe and a spinal needle (7.5–12.5 cm 18 gauge).
- Alternatives include larger-bore catheters and pigtail catheters, which may be left in the pericardial space for continuous drainage.
- ED pericardiocentesis is preferably performed under ultrasound guidance.
- In the absence of an ultrasound machine, electrocardiographic guidance may be achieved by attaching the clamp of one of the precordial leads on an ECG machine to the needle.

Technique

- Head of bed is elevated to 45 degrees, if possible, to bring the heart closer to the anterior chest wall.
- An NG or OG tube is placed if the abdomen is distended.
- Lower xiphoid and epigastric area are prepped with sterile solution.
- Skin, route, and pericardium are infiltrated with local anesthetic in the awake patient.
- The preferred technique is to identify the largest pocket of pericardial fluid closest to the anterior chest wall using ultrasound, and advance the needle directly into that pocket, which is often at a parasternal location, under active ultrasound guidance.

- The classic technique (without ultrasound) is the subxiphoid approach. The needle is inserted between the xiphoid process and the left costal margin at a 30-degree angle to the skin and directed toward the left shoulder.
- The obturator/stylet is removed after the needle is through the skin.
- The needle is advanced while aspirating until pericardial fluid enters the syringe. If using electrocardiographic guidance, the "current of injury" is seen on the ECG tracing – usually a wide-complex PVC with an elevated ST segment – when the needle is against the epicardium. If encountered, the needle should be withdrawn slightly.
- As much fluid as possible is aspirated from the pericardium.
- The needle is removed and a postprocedure x-ray is ordered to rule out pneumothorax.

Complications

- Dry tap
- Pneumothorax
- Dysrhythmia
- Myocardial or coronary vessel laceration
- Hemopericardium
- Air embolism

NEEDLE THORACOSTOMY

Indications

- Suspected or confirmed tension pneumothorax

Contraindications

- None

Equipment

- 10- to 14-gauge angiocatheter
- Syringe

Technique

- Locate the second intercostal space (between the second and third rib) midclavicular line.
- The second rib is the first rib palpable below the clavicle.
- Prepare the site with antiseptic solution, if time permits.
- Insert the needle just superior to the third rib, perpendicular to the chest wall. A rush of air should be appreciated as the tension is relieved.
- Remove the needle, leaving the catheter in place.
- Immediately prepare to insert a chest tube.

Complications

- Cardiac injury/tamponade
- Chest vessel injury/hemorrhage

- Pneumonia
- Arterial air embolism

Notes

- If possible, finger thoracostomy at the site of chest tube insertion followed by the immediate placement of a chest tube is preferred to needle thoracostomy.
- In obese patients, a needle may not have adequate length at the anterior location, and the usual chest tube insertion site (see below) is preferred over the midclavicular line.

TUBE THORACOSTOMY

Indications

- Drainage of pneumothorax
- Drainage of hemothorax
- Drainage of empyema

Contraindications

- No absolute contraindications, especially in unstable patients
- Relative contraindications include coagulopathy and anatomic abnormalities (e.g., emphysematous blebs or pleural adhesions)

Equipment

- Sterile towels, antiseptic, local anesthetic, syringes, needles
- #10 scalpel
- Kelly clamp
- Thoracostomy tube
  - For pneumothorax, 22–24 Fr
  - For empyema or hemothorax, 36–40 Fr (though evolving literature supports using 28–32 Fr tubes in trauma)
- Scissors
- Petroleum and plain gauze
- Tape
- Suture
- Needle driver
- Chest drainage apparatus
- Clear, sterile plastic tubing
- Plastic serrated connectors

Technique

- A chest tube is placed fully sterile – gown, mask, and glove.
- Give patient supplemental oxygen and place the patient on a monitor.
- Elevate head of bed to 45 degrees, if possible.
- Restrain ipsilateral arm over patient's head.

- Sterilize the site. The conventional site is the fourth or fifth intercostal space, mid to anterior axillary line. This is roughly at the level of the nipple.
- Generously infiltrate local anesthetic into the skin, muscle, periosteum, and parietal pleura. Consider procedural sedation/analgesia if appropriate.
- Make at least a 3–4 cm transverse incision directly over the rib one intercostal space below the level to be entered.
- Using the Kelly clamp, tunnel and dissect a pathway immediately superior to the rib above the incision.
- Advancing through the dissected pathway, puncture the pleura with closed Kelly clamp. A rush of air or fluid is expected.
- Spread and withdraw the Kelly clamp to enlarge the rent in the pleura.
- Insert a gloved finger into the pleural rent to verify the track of entry and the absence of solid organs adjacent to the pleural rent.
- Leaving the finger inside the pleural space, guide the chest tube beside the finger into the pleural cavity.
- Advance the tube posteriorly and far enough that the last drainage hole is within the pleura.
- Attach the tube to the water seal device using plastic tubing and connector.
- Confirm placement with a radiograph.
- Secure the tube by closing the skin and securing the chest tube to the skin with a stay suture.
- Apply petrolatum-impregnated gauze underneath plain gauze to the site where the chest tube enters the skin.

Complications

- Infection (pneumonia, empyema, local incision)
- Bleeding (skin, chest vessel laceration, solid organ injury)
- Malposition (subcutaneous, intraabdominal, inadequately advanced)
- Blocked drainage (tube kinking, clots within tube)
- Air leaks
- Re-expansion pulmonary edema

Notes

- Many patients with simple pneumothorax can be managed with observation or catheter-based drainage (usually a "pigtail" catheter) rather than a chest tube. The decision is based on the cause, size, and degree of symptomatology associated with the pneumothorax.

ED THORACOTOMY

Indications

Accepted Indications
- Penetrating thoracic injury
  - Traumatic arrest with previously witnessed cardiac activity (pre-hospital or in-hospital)
  - Unresponsive hypotension (BP < 70 mmHg)
- Blunt thoracic injury
  - Unresponsive hypotension (BP < 70 mmHg)
  - Rapid exsanguination from chest tube (>1500 mL)

- Relative Indications
- Penetrating thoracic injury
  - Traumatic arrest without previously witnessed cardiac activity

Penetrating nonthoracic injury
  - Traumatic arrest with previously witnessed cardiac activity (pre-hospital or in-hospital)
- Blunt thoracic injuries
  - Traumatic arrest with previously witnessed cardiac activity (pre-hospital or in-hospital)

Contraindications

- Blunt injuries
  - Blunt thoracic injuries with no witnessed cardiac activity
  - Multiple blunt trauma
  - Severe head injury
- Lack of timely availability of surgical expertise to provide definitive repair after ED thoracotomy.

Alternative Ultrasound Indications

- If cardiac activity or pericardial fluid, go forward with ED thoracotomy; if not, don't.

Equipment

- Antiseptic solution
- Scalpel with #20 blade
- Mayo scissors, curved
- Rib spreaders
- Vascular clamps
- Needle holder
- 10-inch tissue forceps
- Suture scissors
- Silk suture
- Foley catheter

Technique

- Patient should be intubated/ventilated.
- Prepare the skin with antiseptic.
- Incise the skin and subcutaneous tissue along the fifth intercostal space from sternum to posterior axillary line – just below the nipple in males or the inframammary crease (with breast elevated) in females.
- Momentarily halt respirations and puncture the intercostal muscles at the anterior axillary line with Mayo scissors, then cut the intercostal muscles along the skin incision while separating the muscles from the pleura by following the path of the scissors with your second and third fingers of the nondominant hand.
- Insert the rib spreader with ratchet pointed down and open the chest.
- Lift the lung to identify the pericardium; perform a pericardiotomy by incising and cutting the pericardial sac as anterior as feasible to avoid the phrenic nerve.

- Evacuate pericardial blood, then tamponade any rents in the myocardium by holding your finger on the wound or, if the wound is too large to staunch with direct pressure, holding your finger in the wound. Maintain finger tamponade until the patient is attended by a trauma or heart surgeon. Inserting a foley catheter into the wound, and certainly attempting to suture the heart, has lost favor.
- Perform open-heart massage by compressing the ventricles in between two hands.
- Find the aorta by sweeping the hand along the posterior thoracic wall just superior to the diaphragm, separate from the esophagus, and cross-clamp using vascular clamp. Aortic cross-clamp is a blind procedure, done by feel.
- If significant pulmonary hemorrhage, cross-clamp the affected pulmonary hilum.

Complications

- Trauma to phrenic nerve, coronary and other thoracic arteries, and solid organs
- Wound infection
- Provider blood exposure/needlestick

CENTRAL VENOUS ACCESS USING SELDINGER TECHNIQUE

Indications

- Inability to achieve adequate peripheral venous access
- Central venous pressure monitoring
- Volume loading, when large-bore peripheral access is not available
- Central venous oxygenation saturation monitoring
- Frequent blood sampling requirement
- Infusion of agents that present an extravasation risk (most vasopressors, including dopamine, calcium chloride), hyperosmolar solutions, and total parenteral nutrition
- Placement of transvenous pacemaker or pulmonary artery catheter
- Hemodialysis

Contraindications (All Relative)

- Distorted local anatomy (including prior radiation therapy to the site, long-term venous cannula at that site)
- Coagulopathy, anticoagulation, or thrombolytic therapy (especially for noncompressible subclavian site)
- Suspected proximal vascular injury or vasculitis
- When pneumothorax presents a particular danger, the subclavian site should be avoided

Equipment

- Sterile gown, gloves, mask, drapes/towels
- Lidocaine and antiseptic solution with corresponding needles and syringes
- Introducing needle
- Guidewire
- Dilator
- Catheter

- #11 scalpel
- Suture
- Scissors

Technique (Seldinger/Guidewire Technique)

- Utilizing fully sterile technique, sterilize the area with antiseptic solution and infiltrate the skin overlying the access site with local anesthetic.
- Cannulate the vein with the introducing needle under ultrasound guidance if available. If unavailable, use anatomic landmarks as follows:
  - The subclavian vein is most often cannulated by the infraclavicular approach, where the needle enters the skin at the costochondral junction (where the clavicle dives posteriorly) and is directed toward the suprasternal notch.
  - The internal jugular vein is most often cannulated by the central approach, where the needle enters the skin at the apex of the triangle formed by the two heads of the sternocleidomastoid muscle and the clavicle and is directed toward the ipsilateral nipple at a 30-degree angle to the skin. The carotid artery is palpated with three fingers on the other hand; the needle is directed lateral to the lateral border of the carotid artery at all times.
  - The femoral vein is cannulated by palpating the femoral artery at the inguinal crease and directing the needle cephalad at a 45-degree angle to the skin, 1–2 cm inferior and 0.5–1 cm medial to the femoral artery.
- Stabilize the needle in the vein and remove the syringe; flow of dark nonpulsatile blood should be appreciated.
- Introduce the flexible (usually J-shaped) end of the guidewire into the needle and advance the guidewire one-quarter to one-half its length. If increased ectopy noted on ECG monitor, withdraw wire.
- Remove the needle and stab the skin next to the wire with the scalpel.
- Place the dilator (or the dilator-in-catheter if using an 8.5 Fr introducer) over the wire and advance the dilator into the vessel using a twisting motion. The tip of the wire must protrude from the dilator before the dilator is advanced into the skin to prevent loss of the wire into the circulation.
- Remove the dilator and place the catheter over the wire into the vein.
- Remove the guidewire.
- Confirm placement by aspirating blood from all catheter lumens.
- Sew the vein in place and confirm placement/rule out pneumothorax with a CXR if IJ or SC location.

Complications

- Vessel or thoracic duct injury
- Pneumothorax, hemothorax, hydrothorax (IJ and SC lines)
- Line infection
- Line thrombosis
- Catheter or wire embolism
- Air embolism
- Arrhythmia
- Myocardial perforation

Notes

- Rapid intravascular volume loading is ineffective in standard triple-lumen central lines. An 8.5 Fr introducer sheath (or short, wide-bore peripheral access) should be placed in situations where aggressive volume expansion is necessary.
- In the event of difficulty threading the guidewire, the guidewire must never be retracted with force back through the needle – in this case, the needle and wire must be removed as a unit to prevent shearing of the wire with subsequent wire embolism.

Intravascular wire confirmation is considered best practice. This should be done before dilation either by confirming intraluminal location of the wire using ultrasound, or by placing the short confirmation catheter over the wire and confirming venous location by manometry/pressure transduction, blood gas sampling, or by flushing saline and seeing the fluid swirling on right heart sonography.

INTRAOSSEOUS INFUSION

Indications

- Immediate vascular access is required and IV access is not available.

Contraindications

- Fractured bone
- Recent IO cannula or multiple IO attempts on the same bone
- Overlying infection or burn

Equipment

- Any needle that has a stylet and is sturdy enough to penetrate bone may be used; a product designed specifically for IO access is preferable.

Technique

- The most commonly used site is the proximal tibia, on the anteromedial flat surface, two finger-breadths below the tibial tuberosity. The distal tibia (medial surface), distal femur (midline), proximal humerus, and sternum are alternative sites. Faster flow rates are possible with the proximal humerus and sternum locations.
- The skin is scrubbed with antiseptic and, if the patient is awake, the site is infiltrated with local anesthetic.
- The needle is directed away from the nearest joint, at a 60- to 90-degree angle to the bone.
- Stabilize the bone with the nondominant hand while using the dominant hand to advance the needle through the cortex using a twisting motion (or drill, if IO drill is available).
- Remove the stylet and aspirate marrow content using a syringe.
- If properly positioned, the needle should stand upright without support and fluids should infuse without extravasation.
- Secure and protect the infusion site.
- All medications and blood products can be administered intraosseously.
- Remove when reliable IV access is achieved.

Complications

- Advancing the needle through the entire bone
- Lumen blockage
- Cellulitis or osteomyelitis at the insertion site (rare)
- Fat embolism (rare)

PARACENTESIS

Indications

- Therapeutic: to relieve symptoms from tense ascites, usually dyspnea
- Diagnostic: to characterize new ascites or rule out spontaneous bacterial peritonitis in patients with known ascites

Contraindications

- Overlying skin infection
- Underlying abdominal hematoma or engorged veins
- If gravid uterus or suspected distension of bowel or bladder, ultrasound-guided paracentesis is recommended
- High INR is not a contraindication to paracentesis.

Equipment

- Sterile gown, gloves, mask, drapes/towels
- Lidocaine and antiseptic solution with corresponding needles and syringes
- 18- to 22-gauge needle; either standard 1.5-inch length or 3.5 inch for obese patients; 20–60 cc syringe
- If performing therapeutic tap, tubing and vacuum bottles for collecting fluid

Technique

- The preferred site is the left lower quadrant of the abdomen, lateral to the rectus abdominis muscle, in the midclavicular line, inferior to the umbilicus.
- Utilizing fully sterile technique, sterilize the area with antiseptic solution and infiltrate the skin overlying the access site with local anesthetic.
- Insert the needle perpendicular to the skin and advance in 5 mm increments, aspirating at the end of each movement, until ascitic fluid is reached.
- For therapeutic taps, the needle may be left in the abdomen in cooperative patients.

Complications

- Perforation of vessels or abdominal solid/hollow organs
- Fluid and electrolyte shifts in large volume paracentesis – some advocate the administration of colloid such as albumin if >5 L of fluid is removed
- Local infection
- Abdominal wall hematoma

- Ascitic fluid leak – can be minimized by retracting the skin caudally before inserting the needle, using the "Z-tract" method

Notes

- Paracentesis may be performed without replacing either factors or platelets in the coagulopathic patient.
- The criteria for diagnosis of spontaneous bacterial peritonitis is 250 WBCs/μL with >50% PMNs.
- A serum-albumin gradient >1.1 g/dL rules in portal hypertension as the cause of ascites.

DIAGNOSTIC PERITONEAL LAVAGE

Indications

- Rapid diagnosis of intraperitoneal hemorrhage in the hemodynamically unstable trauma patient (ultrasound more commonly used for this purpose)
- Diagnosis of abdominal organ injury in the trauma patient, especially with the accuracy of abdominal examination compromised due to alteration of mental status or spinal cord injury (CT more commonly used for this purpose)
- Diagnosis of diaphragmatic injury

Contraindications

- Only absolute contraindication is when an urgent laparotomy is mandated
- Prior abdominal surgery/infections
- Obesity
- Coagulopathy
- Second- or third-trimester pregnancy (may still be performed – see later text)

Equipment

- Gown, gloves, mask, drapes, antiseptic, local anesthetic with appropriate syringes, and needles
- Seldinger introducer needle
- #11 scalpel
- Seldinger-type guidewire
- DPL catheter
- 1 L of warm standard normal saline or lactated Ringer's solution
- IV tubing

Technique

- The more commonly used closed technique is described.
- Insert introducer needle attached to 10 mL syringe 1 cm inferior to umbilicus, at a 60-degree angle to the skin directed inferiorly.
- Advance the needle into the peritoneum past the linea alba and peritoneum (two pops should be felt).
- Advance 0.5 cm into the peritoneal cavity and aspirate for frank blood.

- If negative, place guidewire into the peritoneal cavity, directed toward the left or right pelvic gutter.
- Make a stab wound with the scalpel and advance the catheter over the guidewire, using a twisting motion. Aspirate for frank blood.
- If negative, infuse 1 L of warm, isotonic sterile saline solution into peritoneum.
- Agitate the abdomen to mix the fluid and any blood present.
- When 50 cc of fluid remains in the bag, place the bag on the floor to siphon fluid out of the abdomen.
- Remove the catheter and send fluid for analysis.

Complications

- Hollow viscous or solid organ injury
- Intraperitoneal vessel laceration
- Local skin infection at access site
- Lack of fluid return

Notes

- In penetrating trauma, diagnostic peritoneal lavage should not be conducted through the stab or missile entry site.
- An RBC count of >100,000/cc is considered positive with a blunt mechanism or a stab mechanism to the anterior abdomen, flank, or back.
- An RBC count of >5000/cc is considered positive with a gunshot mechanism or with a stab mechanism to the low chest when the indication is to exclude diaphragmatic injury.
- Elevated amylase and alkaline phosphatase levels in the lavage fluid suggest bowel injury.
- A supraumbilical, fully open technique is preferred in the context of pelvic fracture.
- A suprauterine, fully open technique is preferred in second- or third-trimester pregnancy.

LUMBAR PUNCTURE

Indications

- Suspicion of CNS infection such as meningitis/encephalitis
- Suspicion of subarachnoid hemorrhage
- Suspicion of certain CNS inflammatory conditions such as Guillain–Barré syndrome
- Therapy of idiopathic intracranial hypertension (aka pseudotumor cerebri)

Contraindications

- Infection of overlying skin or soft tissue (absolute)
- Unequal pressures between the supratentorial and infratentorial compartments, as evidenced by characteristic findings on CT scan (absolute)
- Indications for CT scan before performing lumbar puncture are as follows:
  - Age >60
  - Immunocompromise
  - Seizure within 1 week
  - Known CNS lesions

- Decreased level of consciousness
- Focal neurologic deficits
- Papilledema or suspected increased ICP
- Coagulopathy (relative, but risks often outweigh benefits if INR>1.5 or platelets <50,000)
- Brain abscess (relative)

Equipment

- Gown, gloves, mask, drapes, local anesthetic, and corresponding needles and syringes
- Spinal needle
- Four specimen tubes
- Three-way stopcock and manometer

Technique

- Position the patient in either the lateral decubitus position with the knees drawn up to the chest (preferred) or the seated position with the back arched by the patient leaning forward onto a table.
- Identify the L3 to L4 interspace by using the imaginary line connecting the iliac crests.
- Scrub the area with antiseptic, infiltrate the skin overlying the site with local anesthetic, and drape the area.
- Infiltrate the deep tissues along the route the spinal needle will take with local anesthetic.
- Insert the spinal needle into the interspace and advance until in the subarachnoid space, usually one-half to three-quarters the length of the needle. Withdraw the stylet frequently as the needle is advanced to check for CSF return. A pop may be appreciated as the needle dissects the ligamentum flavum, immediately posterior to the subarachnoid space.
- If bone is encountered, adjust the angle of the needle. The adjacent interspaces may also be used.
- When CSF is expressed from the needle, attach the three-way stopcock and manometer to measure the opening pressure. Normal pressure is 10–20 cm H_2O.
- Collect CSF for analysis.
- Replace the stylet and withdraw the needle, then cover the site with a bandage.

Complications

- Postlumbar puncture headache
- Backache and radicular symptoms
- Infection – skin and soft tissue infections as well as iatrogenic meningitis
- Herniation syndromes (see contraindications in the earlier text)

Notes

- Antibiotics must never be delayed for lumbar puncture or prelumbar puncture CT when meningitis is strongly suspected.
- Opening pressure cannot be measured when the patient is in the seated position.
- Prophylactic bed rest following lumbar puncture does not reduce the incidence of post-LP headache and is not recommended.
- Use of a non-cutting, blunt-tipped spinal needle has been demonstrated to decrease the incidence of post-LP headache.

DORSAL SLIT OF PHIMOSIS

Indications

- Inability to urinate or pass a needed urinary catheter secondary to tight phimosis

Contraindications

- Dorsal slit should not be undertaken if the condition can wait for a formal circumcision, which is the definitive repair.

Equipment

- Antiseptic solution and gauze
- Lidocaine without epinephrine
- Syringe and small-bore needle (27 gauge preferred)
- Straight hemostat
- Straight scissors
- Needle holder
- 4–0 absorbable suture

Technique

- The incision runs along the dorsal midline aspect of the penis, from the coronal sulcus to the tip of the foreskin.
- Scrub the site with antiseptic and drape the area.
- Infiltrate the region, including the path of the incision, with local anesthesia.
- Advance closed straight hemostat between the glans and the foreskin, carefully avoiding the meatus and urethra. Gently open the hemostat to break up any adhesions.
- Remove the hemostat and reinsert a single jaw of the hemostat between the glans and the foreskin along the path of the foreskin, then close the hemostat, crushing the foreskin for 5 minutes.
- Remove the hemostat and cut the foreskin with scissors along the length of the crushed tissue.
- If the resulting flaps separate and bleed, they may be reapproximated with running absorbable suture.
- Refer the patient for formal circumcision.

Complications

- Bleeding
- Injury to urethra or glans penis

PARAPHIMOSIS REDUCTION

Indications

- All paraphimoses must be reduced to prevent tissue ischemia.

Contraindications

- None

Equipment

- 1% lidocaine jelly
- Crushed ice and water
- Size 8 latex glove

Technique

- Apply topical anesthetic to the paraphimotic foreskin and glans.
- A penile block and/or light sedation may be helpful. Procedural sedation may be necessary in children.
- Compress the foreskin by encircling it with the hand and squeezing for 5 minutes.
- Applying slow, steady pressure, use both thumbs to push glans proximally while using both index and long fingers to pull foreskin distally over glans. Bring foreskin completely out over glans.
- If unsuccessful, fill glove with ice water and invert the thumb. Place penis into ice- water glove at the thumb slot and hold glove around penis for 10 minutes, then reattempt to pull foreskin over glans as described earlier.
- If still unsuccessful, a phimotic ring incision is generally performed by a urologist in the operating room.

Complications

- Injury to the underlying tissue is rare.

TESTICULAR DETORSION

Indications and Contraindications

- Manual detorsion should be attempted on all cases of suspected testicular torsion; however, manual detorsion attempts should never delay operative intervention. All attempts at manual detorsion should occur simultaneously with preparations for immediate operative repair.

Technique

- Light sedation may facilitate the procedure. Some authors caution against the use of procedural sedation or spermatic cord anesthesia, as they obscure the endpoint of the procedure, namely, relief of pain.
- The procedure is more likely to be successful early in the course of the disease, before the onset of significant scrotal swelling.
- Position the patient in a reclining, supine, or, preferably, lithotomy position.
- The testicle usually torses from lateral to medial, and therefore is rotated from medial to lateral, as if opening a book.
- If difficult to perform or increased pain, attempt to rotate the testicle in the opposite direction.
- Simultaneous caudal-to-cranial rotation may be helpful in releasing the cremasteric muscle.
- If a single rotation improves pain or increases Doppler flow but significant pain remains, a further rotation may be attempted.
- In a successful detorsion, pain should subside and the position of the testicle should return to normal. Swelling and induration may take hours to resolve.
- Clinically successful detorsion does not interrupt the requirement for definitive operative scrotal exploration.

LATERAL CANTHOTOMY

Indications

- Retrobulbar hemorrhage (usually from trauma or recent ophthalmic procedure) resulting in decreased visual acuity, increased intraocular pressure, and proptosis
- In an unconscious patient with consistent findings, an IOP >40 also indicates lateral canthotomy.

Contraindications

- Suspected or confirmed globe rupture

Equipment

- Sterile gloves, gown, mask, and drapes
- Local anesthetic with epinephrine, syringe, and needles
- Normal saline
- Straight hemostat
- Straight scissors
- Forceps

Technique

- The patient should be in a supine position.
- Infiltrate the lateral canthus with local anesthetic.
- Irrigate the eye with saline to clear away debris.
- Crimp the lateral canthus with a straight hemostat for 2 minutes to exsanguinate the area and mark the incision line.
- Using scissors, cut the canthus along the crushed area to the orbital rim, taking care to avoid the globe.
- Expose the inferior crus of the lateral canthal tendon by grasping the lower lid with a hemostat and pulling it inferiorly and laterally.
- Cut the inferior crus and evaluate for relief of pressure and symptoms.
- If no improvement, lyse the superior crus.
- Arrange for immediate ophthalmologic evaluation.

Complications

- Mechanical injury to the globe and surrounding structures
- Bleeding
- Infection

RESUSCITATIVE HYSTEROTOMY (PERIMORTEM C-SECTION)

Indications

- Classically, resuscitative hysterotomy is indicated when the fetus is beyond the point of viability (23–24 weeks' gestation); however, this may not be known at the outset of care and the primary goal of resuscitative hysterotomy is to save the mother, not the baby. Therefore, it should be considered in any arrested or nearly arrested woman clearly in late pregnancy, known to be >23 weeks pregnant, uterine fundus above the umbilicus, or with a large baby visible by ultrasound.

- Classically, resuscitative hysterotomy is indicated within 4 minutes of maternal arrest, as fetal survival is thought to be much less likely after 4 minutes of maternal arrest. However, since resuscitative hysterotomy is for mom, not baby, unless maternal resuscitation is thought to be futile, resuscitative hysterotomy should proceed as quickly as feasible in the arrested or nearly arrested pregnant woman, without regard for the "4 minute rule."

Equipment

- Gown, glove, mask with face shield
- #10 scalpel
- Scissors
- Hemostats
- If available: bladder retractor, general retractors, forceps, gauze sponges, suction
- Standard obstetric pack: bulb syringe, 2 Kelly clamps, cord clamp, basin for placenta, towels, and blanket
- Neonatal resuscitation equipment: warmer, meconium aspirator, IO infusion needles, neonatal airway adjuncts

Technique

- CPR continues until the infant is delivered.
- Have an assistant manually displace the gravid uterus to the left. Sliding a wedge underneath the pelvis hinders resuscitation and is not recommended.
- Incise the abdomen in the midline vertically from the symphysis pubis to the umbilicus.
- Cut through all layers of the abdominal wall to expose the uterus.
- If the bladder obstructs access to the uterus, it may be aspirated and reflected inferiorly.
- Make a 5 cm vertical incision to the lower uterine segment, taking care to avoid fetal injury.
- Insert the index and long fingers into the incision and lift the uterine wall away from the fetus.
- Use scissors to extend the incision to the fundus.
- Deliver the infant, suction the mouth and nose, cut and clamp the umbilical cord.
- Hand over infant to neonatal resuscitation team and continue maternal CPR and resuscitation.

Complications

- Fetal injury, especially by the scalpel

OROTRACHEAL INTUBATION

Indications

- Airway protection (intracranial catastrophe/trauma, compression of the airway by focal mass or angioedema, obstructing foreign body)
- Failure of oxygenation (pneumonia, COPD, asthma, CHF, ARDS)
- Failure of ventilation (sedative overdose, high spinal cord injury, ascending neuropathy, paralytic toxin)

- Reduce myocardial oxygen demand (sepsis)
- The patient must leave the department and clinical course uncertain (e.g., for transfer to another hospital or the radiology department)
- Inability to control patient without profound sedation
- Need to perform procedures that involve the posterior oropharynx (charcoal, gastric lavage, endoscopy)

Contraindications

- Inability to open mouth
- Severe soft tissue swelling or distortion of airway anatomy
- Expected to be unable to visualize vocal cords with laryngoscopy, especially if expected difficult bag-valve-mask ventilation and/or difficult cricothyrotomy

Equipment

- Bag-mask device connected to oxygen
- Laryngoscopy handles
- Laryngoscopy blades
- Suction
- Oral airways
- Nasal airways
- Colorimetric capnometer (if continuous capnography not available)
- Endotracheal tubes
- ETT stylet
- ETT securing device (tape if no device available)
- Gum elastic bougie
- Difficult airway equipment (e.g., supraglottic device [e.g. laryngeal mask airway], cricothyrotomy supplies)
- Magill forceps if suspected foreign body

Technique

- Preoxygenate or bag the patient with high-flow oxygen. Supplemental oxygen by high-flow nasal cannula offers an additional oxygenation benefit and should be left on during intubation attempt.
- Position patient so that external auditory meatus is parallel to suprasternal notch.
- Adjust bed height so that patient's head is at operator's lower sternum.
- Administer pretreatment, induction, and paralytic agents, if applicable.
- Open the mouth as wide as possible, using the finger-scissor technique.
- Insert the laryngoscopy blade into the mouth using the left hand and inch the blade posteriorly down the tongue until the epiglottis comes into view.
- Using the right hand, push the thyroid cartilage posteriorly (toward the bed) as needed to improve glottic visualization.
- Insert the laryngoscopy blade into the vallecula and lift the laryngoscope at a 45-degree angle to the horizontal – upward and toward the patient's feet.
- Identify the posterior notch and continue to lift the epiglottis to expose as much of the vocal cords as possible.

- Advance the endotracheal tube through the vocal cords, which has been molded straight to cuff with a 35-degree angle, from the side of the mouth, until the cuff is beyond the vocal cords.
- Inflate the cuff and confirm placement with end-tidal CO_2, then confirm tube depth by auscultating breath sounds.
- Commence postintubation care.

Complications

- Failure to intubate the trachea with resultant hypoxia
- Unrecognized esophageal intubation
- Direct trauma to mouth, teeth, or larynx
- Vomiting with resultant aspiration
- Manipulation of the airway may cause increased intracranial pressure, bradycardia (especially in children), and laryngospasm

Notes

- If difficulty encountered when performing bag-valve-mask ventilation, insert oropharyngeal and nasopharyngeal airways, ensure proper mask size and reposition to improve seal, use jaw thrust and two-person technique, put in dentures, apply gel to bushy beard.
- If failure of laryngoscopy is anticipated, do not attempt rapid sequence intubation. Call for help (ENT or anesthesia) and utilize alternative technique such as an "awake" technique (laryngoscopy or flexible endoscopy/bronchoscopy) without paralysis or surgical airway (especially if anterior facial edema, as in anaphylaxis).
- If laryngoscopy fails, reestablish oxygenation by bag-mask ventilation. If bag-mask ventilation fails, place a supraglottic device. If supraglottic device fails to oxygenate, perform cricothyrotomy.

DENTAL INJURY

- Ellis I fractures require routine dental follow-up.
- Ellis II and III fractures require a dressing (such as calcium hydroxide) if unable to see a dentist immediately, and prompt dental referral.
- Subluxed teeth require splinting with a cement if unable to see a dentist, and prompt dental referral.
- Avulsed teeth require gentle cleaning and replantation, and if unable to see a dentist immediately, splinting with cement and prompt dental referral.

REDUCTION OF JOINT DISLOCATIONS

General Principles

- Neurovascular status should be documented before and after all reduced dislocations.
- Unless urgent conditions contraindicate, prereduction films should be performed on all reduced dislocations.
- Postreduction films should be performed on all reduced dislocations.
- Sedation and analgesia are often indicated to improve patient comfort and the chance of successful reduction.

Anterior Shoulder Dislocation

There are numerous effective techniques; be familiar with several.
- Stimson maneuver: Place the patient prone on a stretcher and hang 5–10 lb. weight from the patient's wrist. Apply gentle internal and external rotation with traction if needed; reduction should occur within 20 minutes.
- Scapular manipulation: Position the patient as for Stimson maneuver, with weights and slight external rotation of the humerus. Stabilize the superior aspect of the scapula with one hand while displacing the inferior tip of the scapula medially.
- External rotation: In a supine patient, hold the arm in complete adduction with the elbow at 90 degrees of flexion. Placing the other hand on the patient's wrist, slowly and gently guide the arm into external rotation.

Posterior Hip Dislocation (Allis Technique)

- The patient is supine. An assistant applies direct pressure to both sides of the anterior pelvis, pushing it into the bed for countertraction.
- The lower leg is grasped just distal to the knee and traction is applied in the direction of the deformity.
- The hip is then brought to 90 degrees of flexion (perpendicular to the bed) and traction is applied in the anterior direction, toward the ceiling.
- With continuous upward traction, the hip is gently internally and externally rotated until reduction is successful.

MCP/DIP/PIP Dislocations

- Exaggerate the deformity (usually hyperextension of the joint).
- At the angle of maximal exaggeration, apply longitudinal traction.
- While holding traction with one hand, use the other hand to reduce the joint by pressing the proximal aspect of the distal bone back into alignment.

Posterior Elbow Dislocation

- An assistant grasps the proximal humerus in a supine patient to provide countertraction.
- Grasp the wrist with one hand and apply steady traction with the elbow slightly flexed.
- Grasp the distal humerus with the other hand and correct any lateral displacement.
- Gently flex the elbow while maintaining in-line traction.

Knee

- Note the difference between knee dislocation – a high-force emergency – and the comparatively minor patellar dislocation. Traction–countertraction is usually sufficient to reduce femoral–tibial dislocation. If unsuccessful, direct displacement of the femur in the appropriate direction may be attempted while the leg is in full traction–countertraction.
- Most knee dislocations reduce spontaneously; the injury and accompanying popliteal artery disruption must be suspected in cases of knee trauma where the ACL and PCL have been disrupted – that is, a "floppy" knee.

Radial Head Subluxation (Nursemaid's Elbow)

- Place the child on the lap of the parent. Cup the elbow with one hand, placing the thumb over the radial head. With the other hand, grasp the wrist and supinate the forearm, followed by complete elbow flexion.
- Hyperpronation of the forearm followed by elbow flexion is less painful and at least as effective as supination/flexion.

Posterior Ankle Dislocation

- The patient is supine; the knee is flexed.
- An assistant applies cranially directed countertraction at the calf.
- The foot is plantar flexed slightly and then traction applied longitudinally.
- A second assistant pushes the distal tibia posteriorly (toward the bed) while the foot is reduced anteriorly while held in traction.

TMJ

- The classic reduction technique is described below, but there are a variety of alternatives.
- The practitioner must achieve leverage about the jaw; therefore the patient is either seated on the ground against a wall, in a chair against a wall with the practitioner standing on a stool, or upright in bed with the practitioner standing on the bed in front of the patient.
- Wrap both thumbs in gauze and place each thumb on the bottom row of teeth while grasping the mandible with the other fingers.
- Displace the mandible directly downward (toward the ground) with gradually increasing force, then reduce the mandible by pushing the chin posteriorly.
- The mandible may close forcefully as a result of masseter spasm; the thumbs may slide laterally into the space between the teeth and the buccal mucosa.

BIBLIOGRAPHY

Roberts JR (2017). *Clinical Procedures in Emergency Medicine*. 7th ed. Elsevier.
Bailitz J, Bokhari F, Scaletta T, Schaider J (2011). *Emergent Management of Trauma*. 3rd ed. McGraw-Hill.
Brown CA, Sakles JC, Mick NW (2017). *The Walls Manual of Emergency Airway Management*. 5th ed. Lippincott Williams & Wilkins.

Index

ABCs heuristic, 16
abdominal aortic aneurysm (AAA), 153–154
    rupture, 153
abdominal pain, 22–24, 245–251, 256–260, 286–290,
        502–506, 542–546
    acute mesenteric ischemia, 416–417
    appendicitis, 224
    child, 135–138, 456–460
    cholecystitis, 65, 68
    complicated diverticulitis, 505–506
    diabetic ketoacidosis, 249
    diarrhea and, 266–269, 461–464
    ectopic pregnancy, 238–240
    elderly patient, 416–417, 602–606
    epigastric pain, 139–144, 251–255, 406–411
    hemolytic uremic syndrome, 464
    myocardial infarction, 254–255
    ovarian torsion, 259–260
    pancreatitis, 410–411
    sigmoid volvulus, 605–606
    small bowel obstruction, 101–102, 203–204
    splenic rupture, 458–460, 535–536
    spontaneous bacterial peritonitis, 546
    testicular torsion, 138
    tubo-ovarian abscess, 289
    vaginal bleeding and, 236–240
    visceral perforation, 142–144
    vomiting and, 45–49, 66–79, 98–102, 199–204, 221–225,
        406–411
abdominal trauma, 529–536
    child, nonaccidental, 458–460
abscess
    perianal/perirectal, 234–235
    retropharyngeal, 128–130
    tubo-ovarian, 289
acetaminophen, 471–472
    febrile seizure, 212
    overdose, 471–472
    toxicity, 472
activated charcoal
    INH toxicity, 585
    tricyclic antidepressant toxicity, 521

acute angle-closure glaucoma, 96–97
acute chest syndrome, sickle cell disease, 324
acute coronary syndrome, 208
acute emesis, diarrhea and, 695–696
acute kidney injury (AKI), hypertensive emergency and,
        556–557
acute mesenteric ischemia, 416–417
acute mountain sickness, 347
    symptoms, 347
adenosine
    advanced cardiac life support, 719
    supraventricular tachycardia management, 395
adnexal torsion, 260
adrenal gland tumor, Cushing syndrome and, 655–656
advanced cardiac life support (ACLS), 716–725
    airway and ventilation, 717
    bradycardia, 718
    cardiac arrest, post-arrest care, 717
    cardiopulmonary resuscitation (CPR), 716
        defibrillation and, 716
    pulseless arrest, 718
    tachycardia, 718
age heuristic, 16
agitation, 241–244 *see also* mental status, altered
AIDS patient, *Pneumocystis* (PCP), 389–390, 578–579
airway management, 717
    penetrating chest trauma, 282
    status epilepticus, 375
    see also intubation
albuterol, acute chest syndrome, bronchospasm, 324
alcohol intoxication, *see* intoxication
alcohol withdrawal, altered mental status and, 427–428,
        705
Allis technique for hip dislocation, 755
altered mental status, *see* mental status, altered
altitude sickness, 347
amebiasis, 269
amiodarone
    advanced cardiac life support, 720
    ventricular tachycardia management, 515, 625
amitryptyline overdose, 521
    symptoms, 521

anal pain, 232–235
analytic thinking, 16
anaphylaxis, 219–220
anhidrosis, heatstroke, 488
animal bite, 283–285
ankle dislocation, 756
ankle fracture, 441
anthrax, 550–551
antibiotic treatment
 acute chest syndrome, 324
 acute mesenteric ischemia, 416
 anthrax, 551
 cat bite, 284
 cavernous sinus thrombosis, 295
 chronic obstructive pulmonary disease, 422
 diverticulitis, 506
 epidural abscess, 82
 Fournier's gangrene, 380
 HIV pneumonia, 389
 intussusception, 385
 Ludwig's angina, 276
 meningitis, 330
 necrotizing enterocolitis, 540–541
 necrotizing fasciitis, 88
 pancreatitis, 410
 pertussis, 147
 pneumonia, 399, 481
 post-transplant fever, 527
 retropharyngeal abscess, 128
 sepsis, 620
 septic arthritis, 313
 septic shock, infant, 73
 spontaneous bacterial peritonitis, 546
 Stevens–Johnson syndrome, 193
 systemic inflammatory response syndrome, 481
 traveler's diarrhea, 268
 tubo-ovarian abscess, 289
 variceal bleeding, 176
 visceral perforation, 143
anticoagulation
 bleeding complications, 58
 carotid artery dissection, 601
 DVT management, 630
 LVAD thrombosis, 610
 pulmonary embolism, 217
antihypertensive medications
 abrupt cessation, 556
 hypertensive emergency, 556–557
antihypertensives, stroke, 433
antimicrobial therapy, meningitis, 330
aortic coarctation, 363–364, 567–568
aortic dissection, 7–8
 risk factors, 700

 treatment, 700
 work-up, 700
apixaban, DVT management, 630
aplastic crisis
 causes, 660
 with sickle cell disease, 660–661
appendicitis, 224–225
 pregnant women, 224
arm pain, 661, 662
 child, 612–615
 radial head subluxation, 613–615
 rhabdomyolysis, 665–666
arthritis
 monoarticular, 313
 septic, 313
aspiration, of foreign body, 466–467
aspirin
 acute cerebellar stroke management, 676
 toxicity, 106–107
asthma, 75, 90, 97–98, 117, 182, 186–188, 194, 199, 218, 266, 359, 703, 752
atenolol, 454, 722
atropine
 advanced cardiac life support, 722
 bradycardia management, 180, 718
avascular necrosis of the femoral head, 134

back pain, 4–14, 302–306, 443–448
 aortic dissection, 7–8
 epidural abscess, 80
 pedestrian struck by vehicle, 435–442
 pyelonephritis, 446–447
 sickle cell disease, 320–325
bacterial meningitis, 330
balloon tamponade, variceal bleeding management, 174
β-blockers
 advanced cardiac life support, 722
 aortic dissection, 6
 hemodynamically unstable patients, 255
 overdose, 180
 stroke, 433
 supraventricular tachycardia management, 395
Beck's triad, 281–282, 494
beer potomania, 646–647
benzodiazepines
 alcohol withdrawal syndrome, 427
 cocaine-induced chest pain, 208
 seizures, 273
 tricyclic antidepressant toxicity, 521
bite wound, 283–285
blindness, transient monocular, carotid artery dissection and, 601
blood glucose determination

with altered mental status, 341

    status epilepticus, 374

blood transfusion, 714

bloody diarrhea, 569–574

Boerhaave's syndrome, 75–79

Bordetella pertussis, 147

bowel necrosis, 605

bowel obstruction, 48, 102, 111, 143, 203–204, 606

    intussusception, 384–385

    small bowel, 101–102, 203–204

bradycardia, 718

    EKG findings, 180

Brudzinski's sign, 330

Brugada syndrome, 516

bruising

    Cushing syndrome, 655–656

    with fatigue and weight gain, 653–656

burns

    facial trauma, 166–171

    hydrofluoric acid exposure, 637–638

    pediatric patients, 728

calcium, advanced cardiac life support, 724

calcium channel blockers

    advanced cardiac life support, 721

    hemodynamically unstable patients, 255

    stroke, 433

    supraventricular tachycardia management, 395

cardiac arrest, 516, 621

    infant, 307–309

    post-arrest care, 717

    pulseless arrest, 718

    see also advanced cardiac life support (ACLS)

cardiac catheterization, 476

cardiac tamponade, 60, 281–282, 335, 493

    penetrating chest trauma, 281–282 *see also* pericardial
        tamponade

cardiogenic shock, LVAD device failure, 610–611

cardiopulmonary resuscitation (CPR), 716

    defibrillation and, 716

    see also advanced cardiac life support (ACLS)

cardioversion, 516, 732–734

    complications, 733

    contraindications, 732

    equipment, 732

    indications, 732

    supraventricular tachycardia, 395

    technique, 733

    ventricular tachycardia, 515

    see also advanced cardiac life support (ACLS)

carotid artery dissection, 600–601

cat bite, 283–285

cauda equina syndrome (CES), 304–306

cavernous sinus thrombosis (CST), 295

cellulitis, post-transplant fever and, 527

central retinal artery occlusion, 119–120

central venous access, 714, 742–744

    complications, 743

    contraindications, 742

    equipment, 742

    indications, 742

    technique, 743

cerebellar infarction, 676

cervical spine fracture, 404–405

chest pain, 205–209, 213–217, 332–336, 473–476

    aortic dissection, 700

    approach to, 698–701

    Boerhaave's syndrome, 75–79

    cocaine-induced, 208–209

    computations and, 513

    esophageal rupture, 701

    myocardial infarction, 699

        anterolateral, 475–476

    myopericarditis, 335–336

    pulmonary embolism, 216–217, 699–700

    sickle cell disease, 320–325

        acute chest syndrome, 324

    spontaneous pneumothorax, 700

chest trauma, penetrating, 60–65, 278–282, 496–501

chest x-ray (CXR)

    acute chest syndrome, 324

    anthrax findings, 551

    chest pain, 78

    congenital heart disease, 568

    esophageal tear, 79

    pericardial effusion, 282

    pertussis, 147

    pneumonia, 399

    pulmonary embolism, 216

    variceal bleeding, 175

child, *see* pediatric patient

child abuse, 458–460, 730

chiropractic manipulation of the neck, carotid artery
    dissection and, 601

Chlamydia trachomatis, tubo-ovarian abscess, 289

cholecystitis, 68

cholera, 269

chronic obstructive pulmonary disease (COPD),
    exacerbation, 421–422

cirrhosis of the liver, variceal bleeding and, 176

Clostridium difficile, 574

cocaine-induced chest pain, 208–209

colchicine, gout management, 596

community-acquired pneumonia, 399, 579

complicated diverticulitis, 505–506

compression ultrasonography, DVT and, 629

computed tomography (CT)
  acute stroke, 676
  back pain, 6
  bowel obstruction, 203
  cavernous sinus thrombosis, 295
  diverticulitis, 506
  meningitis, indications, 330
  ovarian torsion, 260
  renal colic, 368
  splenic injury, 535
confusion, *see* mental status, altered
congenital heart disease, 364, 567–568, 730–731
  chest x-ray findings, 568
congenital hypertrophic pyloric stenosis, 53
congestive heart failure (CHF), 359
constipation, sigmoid volvulus and, 605–606
corticosteroids
  Pneumocystis pneumonia, 579
  see also steroid therapy
cortisol measurement, 655
cough, 396–399, 547–551, 575–580
  infant, 145–148
  pertussis, 147–148
  pneumonia, 398–399
  pulmonary inhalation anthrax, 550–551
crepitus assessment, Fournier's gangrene, 380
CRH stimulation test, 655
cricothyrotomy, 734–736
  complications, 735
  contraindications, 734
  equipment, 734–735
  facial trauma, 165
  indications, 734
  technique, 735
Crohn's disease, perianal abscess and, 232–235
Cullen's sign, 410
Cushing reflex, 59
Cushing syndrome, complications, 656

Dance's sign, 385
decubitus ulcer, sepsis and, 620
deep-vein thrombosis (DVT)
  after surgery, 628–630
  risk factors, 630
  symptoms, 630
deferoxamine therapy, iron overdose, 48, 49
defibrillation, 516, 716, 732–734
  complications, 733
  contraindications, 732
  equipment, 732
  indications, 732
  technique, 733
  torsades, 125

  see also advanced cardiac life support (ACLS)
dehydration, 665–666
  acute kidney injury, 590–591
  LVAD suction event, 695
dental injury, 754
dexamethasone suppression test, 655
dexamethasone treatment, altitude sickness, 347
dextrose
  alcohol withdrawal syndrome management, 427
  hypoglycemia management, 341
diabetes
  cardiac pathology, 254
  cholecystitis and, 69
  and Fournier's gangrene, 380
  necrotizing fasciitis association, 88
diabetic ketoacidosis (DKA), 249
diagnostic peritoneal lavage, 746–747
diarrhea
  abdominal pain and, 266–269, 461–464
  acute, 269
  bacterial, 572, 573
  bloody diarrhea, 569–574
  child, 461–464, 573–574
  E. coli O157:H7 related, 461
  enteroinvasive, 572–574
  iron overdose, 48
  traveler's diarrhea, 268–269, 572
  viral, 573
digoxin toxicity, 352–354
digoxin-specific FAB, 353
diphenhydramine, anaphylaxis management, 220
dislocation reduction, *see* joint dislocation reduction
disseminated intravascular coagulation (DIC), sepsis and, 620
diverticulitis
  complicated, 505–506
    bowel perforation, 505
  uncomplicated, 506
dizziness, 639–641
  elderly patient, 671–676
  pacemaker malfunction, 641
  weakness and, 194–198
  see also lightheadedness
dobutamine, advanced cardiac life support, 723
drooling, with sore throat, 126–130
drowning, 400–405
  hypothermia, 558–563

eclampsia, 510
  seizure, 510
ectopic pregnancy, 238–240
elbow dislocation, 755
elder abuse, 590–591

elderly patient
   abdominal aortic aneurysm, 153–154
   abdominal pain, 412, 602–606
   acute cerebellar stroke, 675–676
   acute mesenteric ischemia, 416–417
   altered mental status, 226–231, 337–342, 347, 348,
      483–489, 616–620
      headache and, 552–557
      subdural hematoma, 229–230
   dehydration, 590–591
   dizziness, 671–676
   fever, 477–482
   heatstroke, 487–488
   hypoglycemia, 341–342
   lightheadedness, 177–181
   sepsis from decubitus ulcer, 620
   shortness of breath, 355–359, 607–611
   sigmoid volvulus, 605–606
   systemic inflammatory response syndrome, 481–482
   visceral perforation, 142–144
   weakness, 587–591
embolism, superior mesenteric artery, 416
endoscopy, variceal bleeding, 175
endotracheal intubation, *see* intubation
Entamoeba histolytica, 269
enterocolitis, necrotizing, 539–541
enteroinvasive diarrhea, 572, 574
epidural abscess, 80
epidural hematoma, 230
epigastric pain, 139–144, 203, 251–255, 406–411
epinephrine
   anaphylaxis management, 220
   cardiac arrest management, 717
erythema multiforme, 192
escharotomy, 170
Escherichia coli, 546
   O157:H7-related, diarrhea, 461
esmolol, 6, 722
esophageal tear, 75–79, 701
ethylene glycol poisoning, 686–687
eye pain, 95
   headache and, 83, 291

facial trauma, 161–165
   bleeding control, 164–165
   burn, 166–171
   facial hemorrhage, 164
   Le Fort III fracture, 164
FAST examination, *see* focused assessment with
      sonography in trauma (FAST) examination
fatigue
   with bruising and weight gain, 653–656
   Cushing syndrome, 655–656

   see also weakness
febrile seizure, 211–212
femoral head, avascular necrosis of, 134
fever
   elderly patient, 477–482
   headache and, 290, 326
   HIV-infected patient, 386–390
   kidney transplant patient, 523–528
   pediatric patient, 297–301, 314–319, 652, 657, 688–691
      Kawasaki disease, 299–300
   pneumonia, 398–399
   post–kidney transplant fever, 527–528
   rash and, 189–193
   Rocky Mountain spotted fever, 318
   sore throat and, 126–130
   spontaneous bacterial peritonitis and, 546
finger dislocation, 755
finger pain, 635–638
   hydrofluoric acid exposure, 637–638
fingerstick blood glucose
   with altered mental status, 341
   with status epilepticus, 374
Fitz–Hugh–Curtis syndrome, 69
flank pain, 149–154, 365–369
   renal colic, 368
fluid therapy
   acute mesenteric ischemia, 417
   anaphylaxis, 220
   Boerhaave's syndrome, 79
   bowel obstruction, 203
   burn injury, 170
   congenital hypertrophic pyloric stenosis, 53
   dehydration, 665
   diabetic ketoacidosis, 249
   diverticulitis, 505
   food poisoning, 695
   HSP, 111
   hypercalcemia, 652
   myocardial infarction, 254
   necrotizing enterocolitis, 541
   pancreatitis, 410
   post-transplant fever, 527
   spinal cord injury, 405
   spontaneous bacterial peritonitis, 546
   Stevens–Johnson syndrome, 193
   traveler's diarrhea, 268
   variceal bleeding, 176
focused assessment with sonography in trauma (FAST)
      examination, 280
   spinal cord injury, 405
   splenic rupture, 535
food poisoning, 695–696
foot pain, 592–596

Fournier's gangrene, 379–380
   crepitus assessment, 380
fracture
   ankle, 441
   cervical spine, 404–405
   dental injury, 754
   pelvic, 441
      with hemorrhage, 441
furosemide, advanced cardiac life support, 725

gallstones, pancreatitis, 410–411
Giardia lamblia, traveler's diarrhea, 268
glomerular filtration rate (GFR), IV hydration and, 666
glucagon, hypoglycemia management, 342
gout, acute, 595
Grave's disease, 454
Grey–Turner's sign, 154
Guillain–Barre syndrome, 197–198

Haemophilus influenzae, chemoprophylaxis, 330
Hamman's crunch, 79
head trauma, subdural hematoma and, 229–230
   see also facial trauma
headache, 95–97, 667–670
   altered mental status and, 552–557
   bacterial meningitis, 330
   carotid artery dissection, 600–601
   cavernous sinus thrombosis, 294–295
   eye pain and, 83, 291
   fever and, 296, 326
   high-altitude cerebral edema, 347
   hypertensive emergency, 556–557
   intracranial hemorrhage, 57–59
   migraine, 669–670
   nausea and, 331, 343
   with neck pain, 597–601
   pediatric patient, 314–319
   Rocky Mountain spotted fever, 318
   and vision changes, 95–97
heart attack, *see* myocardial infarction
heart rate, pediatric patients, 726
heat exhaustion, 665–666
heatstroke/hyperthermia, 487–488
hematemesis, iron overdose, 48
hematochezia, 537–541
hematoma
   epidural, 230
   retroperitoneal, 154
   subdural, 229–230
hematuria, abdominal aortic aneurysm and, 154
hemodialysis, ethylene glycol poisoning, 687
hemolytic uremic syndrome (HUS)
   child, 464, 573
Henoch–Schönlein purpura (HSP), 111

complications, 111
heparin treatment
   carotid artery dissection, 601
   LVAD thrombosis, 610, 696
   pulmonary embolism, 216–217
hernia, strangulated, 102
heuristics, 15–16
high-altitude cerebral edema (HACE), 347
high-altitude pulmonary edema (HAPE), 347
hip dislocation, 755
HIV-infected patient
   fever, 386–390
   pneumonia, 389–390, 578–579
   see also AIDS patient
Horner syndrome, 601
hydrofluoric acid exposure, 637–638
   dermal exposure, 637
   gastrointestinal exposure, 637
   inhalation exposure, 637
   ophthalmic exposure, 637–638
hyperbaric treatment
   altitude sickness, 347
   carbon monoxide poisoning, 159
   indications, 159
   necrotizing fasciitis, 88
hypercalcemia, from squamous cell lung cancer, 651–652
hypercapnia, 187
hypercortisolism, 655–656
hyperkalemia, 93–94
   causes, 93
   digoxin toxicity and, 353
   EKG findings, 93
hypertension, eclampsia, 510
hypertensive encephalopathy, hypertensive emergency
      and, 556–557
hypertensive urgency, 557
hyperthermia, *see* fever; heatstroke
hypocalcemia, 686–687
hypoglycemia
   alcoholic patients, 428
   sulfonylurea related, 341–342
   symptoms, 341
hypokalemia, aspirin toxicity and, 106, 107
hyponatremia, 646–647
hypothermia
   EKG findings, 563
   following cold water immersion, 558–563
   rewarming, 560, 563
   therapeutic, 626

ibuprofen
   febrile seizure, 212
   kidney injury, 666
ice pack test, for myasthenia gravis, 681

illness scripts, 15
indomethacin, gout management, 596
infant
    aortic coarctation, 363–364, 567–568
    cardiac arrest, 307–309
    congenital heart disease, 364, 730–731
    congenital hypertrophic pyloric stenosis, 53
    cough, 145–148
    hematochezia, 537–541
    intussusception, 384
    necrotizing enterocolitis, 539–541
    newborn resuscitation, 727
    pale appearance, poor feeding and, 564–568
    shortness of breath, 360–364
    vomiting, 50–53, 381–385
    weak, 70–74
    see also pediatric patient
inferior myocardial infarction (MI), 180, 254–255
INH, overdose, pediatric patient, 585–586
insulin therapy, diabetic ketoacidosis, 249
intestinal obstruction, see bowel obstruction
intoxication, 241–244, 642–647, 666, 682
    ethylene glycol poisoning, 686–687
    hypo-osmolar hyponatremia, 646–647
intracranial hemorrhage (ICH), 57–59
intraosseous infusion, 744–745
    complications, 745
    contraindications, 744
    equipment, 744
    indications, 744
    technique, 744
intubation, 714, 752–754
    altered mental status and, 22
    anaphylaxis, 220
    asthma, 186–187
    chronic obstructive pulmonary disease, 422
    complications, 754
    contraindications, 753
    equipment, 753
    ethylene glycol poisoning and, 687
    facial trauma, 161, 164
        burn injury, 170
    Guillain–Barre syndrome, 197
    hypothermia, 563
    indications, 752–753
    Ludwig's angina, 277
    pediatric patients, 727
    penetrating chest trauma, 281
    septic infant, 73
    spinal cord injury and, 405
    status epilepticus, 374
    syncope, 122
    technique, 753–754
intussusception, 111

infant, 384
    symptoms, 385
invasive monitoring, 715
ipratropium bromide, chronic obstructive pulmonary
        disease, 422
iron overdose
    morbidity, 48
    poisoning, 48
        stages, 48
isolation
    anthrax patient, 550
    HIV pneumonia patient, 389
    measles patient, 689–690

joint dislocation reduction, 754–756
    ankle, 756
    elbow, 755
    finger, 755
    hip, 755
    knee, 755
    radial head subluxation, 756
        techniques, 615
    shoulder, 755
    temporomandibular joint, 756

Kawasaki disease (KD), 299–300
    incomplete/atypical, 300
Kernig's sign, 330
ketamine, asthma and, 187
kidney, post, transplant fever, 527–528
kidney injury, acute, 666
    dehydration and, 590–591
kidney stones, 368
knee dislocation, 755
knee pain, 310–313
    child, 131–134
    septic arthritis, 313
Koplik spots, measles and, 690
Korsakoff's syndrome, 428
Kussmaul respirations, 687
Kussmaul's sign, 282, 494

labetalol, 6
laparotomy, splenic rupture and, 535
lateral canthotomy, 751
left ventricular assist device (LVAD), 696
    dehydration-related suction event, 695
    LVAD emergency, 687, 692
    LVAD failure, 610–611
    sepsis, 696
leg pain, 626, 627
    DVT after surgery, 628–630
    pedestrian struck by vehicle, 435–442
leg swelling, 84–89

lethargy, carbon monoxide poisoning, 158–159
lidocaine
    advanced cardiac life support, 720
    ventricular tachycardia management, 625
lightheadedness, 177–181 *see also* dizziness
limp, pediatric patient, 730
Listeria monocytogenes, 330
liver cirrhosis, variceal bleeding and, 176
loperamide, 269
lorazepam treatment, status epilepticus, 374
Ludwig's angina, 276–277
lumbar puncture (LP)
    cavernous sinus thrombosis, 295
    childhood seizure, 212
    complications, 748
    contraindications, 747
    equipment, 748
    hypertensive emergency, 556
    indications, 747
    meningitis, 330
    sepsis, congenital heart disease, 364
    septic infant, 73
    technique, 748
lung cancer, hypercalcemia and, 651–652
LVAD, *see* left ventricular assist device (LVAD)

Mackler's triad, 79
magnesium
    advanced cardiac life support, 721
    asthma management, 187
    torsades management, 125
magnesium sulfate
    chronic obstructive pulmonary disease, 422
    eclampsia, 510
magnetic resonance imaging (MRI)
    cauda equina syndrome, 306
    epidural abscess, 82
maxillofacial trauma, 161–165
measles
    complications, 691
    symptoms, 690
mechanical thrombectomy, stroke, 434
meningitis
    anthrax and, 551
    bacterial, 330
mental status, altered, 634, 648, 702–708
    alcohol withdrawal and, 427–428, 705
    assessment, 703
    cardiac disease, 707
    CNS pathology, 706
    dementia and, 708
    differential diagnosis, 703–708
    drug-/toxin-related, 705
        INH overdose, 585–586

opioid overdose, 264–265
elderly patient, 226–231, 337–342, 347, 348, 477–482,
    483–489, 616–620
    drug-/toxin-related, digoxin toxicity, 352–354
    headache and, 552–557
encephalopathies, 707
endocrinopathies, 706
fluid–electrolyte disturbance, 704
Fournier's gangrene, 379–380
glucose-related, 703–704
history, 702
hypercalcemia and, with squamous cell lung cancer,
    651–652
hyperthermia and, 487–488
hyponatremia and, 646–647
immediate actions, 702
infection/sepsis, 704–705
intracranial hemorrhage, 57–59
LVAD emergency, 687, 692
mnemonic, 708
oxygen/carbon dioxide-related, 703
psychiatric causes, 707
sedation and, 708
temperature-related, 707
thyrotoxicosis and, 453–454
unconsciousness, 261–265
vomiting and, pediatric patient, 581–586
mesenteric ischemia, acute, 416–417
metoprolol, 722
middle cerebral artery stroke, 433–434
    carotid artery dissection and, 601
migraine, 669–670
monitoring, invasive, 715
monoarticular arthritis, 313
myasthenia gravis (MG), 680–681
    ice pack test, 681
    symptoms, 681
myasthenic crisis, 681
myocardial infarction, 516, 699
    anterolateral, 475–476
    bradycardia and, 180
    inferior wall, 254–255
    risk factors, 699
    treatment, 699
    work-up, 699
    see also advanced cardiac life support (ACLS)
myocardial injury, myopericarditis, 335
myopericarditis, 335–336

naloxone, 264
    alcohol withdrawal syndrome, 427
    opioid overdose, 264–265
nasogastric tube, congenital hypertrophic pyloric stenosis, 53
nausea

abdominal pain and, 221–225, 406–411
  epigastric pain and, 251–255
  headache and, 331, 343
  see also vomiting
neck pain
  carotid artery dissection, 600–601
  with headache, 597–601
neck swelling, 630, 631
necrotizing enterocolitis, 540–541
necrotizing fasciitis, 87–88
Neisseria gonorrhoeae, tubo-ovarian abscess, 289
Neisseria meningitidis, chemoprophylaxis, 330
neonate, *see* infant
neurogenic shock, 404–405
newborn resuscitation, 727
nitroglycerin
  advanced cardiac life support, 724
  hemodynamically unstable patients, 254
nonsteroidal anti-inflammatory drugs (NSAIDs)
  myopericarditis, 335–336
  renal injury and, 666
norepinephrine, 723
  advanced cardiac life support, 723
  neurogenic shock, 405
nursemaid's elbow, 613–615, 756

obesity, slipped capital femoral epiphysis (SCFE) and, 133
obstructive series, 203
octreotide
  hypoglycemia management, 341
  variceal bleeding management, 176
Ogilvie's syndrome, 606
opioid overdose, 264–265
opioid withdrawal, 265
orotracheal intubation, *see* intubation
Osborne wave, 563
ovarian torsion, 259–260
overdose, 45–49, 468–472
  acetaminophen, 471–472
  amitriptyline, 521
  β-blockers, 180
  INH, pediatric patient, 585–586
  opioids, 264–265
oxygen therapy
  acute chest syndrome, 324
  altitude sickness, 347
  carbon monoxide poisoning, 159
  chronic obstructive pulmonary disease, 422
  HIV pneumonia, 389
  hyperbaric oxygen indications, 159
  status epilepticus, 374

pacemaker malfunction, 641
pain, cauda equina syndrome, 304–306

pallor, infant, poor feeding and, 564–568
palpitations, 380, 391, 395, 511
  supraventricular tachycardia, 395
  ventricular tachycardia, 515–516
pancreatitis, 410–411
paracentesis, 745–746
  complications, 745
  contraindications, 745
  equipment, 745
  indications, 745
  spontaneous bacterial peritonitis, 546
  technique, 745
paracetamol, *see* acetaminophen
paralysis, 429
paraphimosis reduction, 749–750
Parvovirus B19, 660–657
patent ductus arteriosus, 364, 568
pedestrian struck by vehicle, 435–442
pediatric patient, 726–731
  abdominal pain, 135–138, 456–460
  anaphylaxis, 219–220
  aplastic crisis, 660–661
  arm pain, 612–615
  burns, 728
  cough, 145–148
  diarrhea, 461–464, 573–574
  fever, 297–301, 314–319, 652, 657, 688–691
    Kawasaki disease, 299–300
  fluid management, 727
  foreign body aspiration, 466–467
  headache, 314–319
  hemolytic uremic syndrome, 464
  intubation, 727
  knee pain, 131–134
  limp, 730
  measles, 690–691
  normal vital signs by age, 726
  persistent crying, 730
  pertussis, 147–148
  radial head subluxation, 613–615
  rash, 314–319, 652, 657, 688–691
  respiratory distress, 465–467
  retropharyngeal abscess, 128–130
  Rocky Mountain spotted fever, 318
  seizure, 210–212
  sickle cell disease, 660–661
  sore throat, 126–130
  splenic laceration, 458–460
  syncope, 121–125
  testicular torsion, 138
  trauma, nonaccidental, 458–460
  vomiting, 108–112, 314–319
    with altered mental status, 581–586
  see also infant

pelvic fracture, 441
  with hemorrhage, 441
PERC (pulmonary embolism rule-out criteria), 216, 699
perianal abscess, 234–235
pericardial effusion, 282, 335, 494
  myopericarditis, 335
pericardial tamponade, 494 *see also* cardiac tamponade
pericardiocentesis, 494, 737–738
  complications, 738
  contraindications, 737
  equipment, 737
  hemodynamic collapse, 495
  indications, 737
  technique, 737–738
perimortem C-section, 751–752
perirectal abscess, 234–235
peritonitis
  bowel obstruction and, 203
  intussusception and, 384–385
pertussis, 147–148
phimosis, dorsal slit, 749
pit viper snake bite, 115
Pneumocystis jiroveci, 390
pneumonia
  community-acquired, 398–399, 453–454
  HIV-infected patient, 389–390, 578–579
  Pneumocystis (PCP), 389–390, 578–579
  systemic inflammatory response syndrome, 481–482
  thyroid storm precipitation, 453
pneumothorax
  treatment, 700
    decompression, 496
    see also tension pneumothorax; thoracostomy
poisoning, 709–713
  altered mental status and, 705
  carbon monoxide, 158–159
  ethylene glycol, 686–687
  examination, 709
  history, 709
  iron, 48
    stages of, 48
  pediatric patients, 728
  stabilization, 709
  toxidromes, 710, 712
  toxin-associated abnormalities, 710
post–kidney transplant fever, 527–528
potassium elevation, digoxin toxicity and, 353
preeclampsia, 510
pregnancy
  appendicitis and, 224
  diverticulitis and, 505
  ectopic, 238–240
  ovarian torsion and, 260

perimortem C-section, 751–752
  pyelonephritis, 446–447
pressure ulcer, 620
procainamide, advanced cardiac life support, 721
prolonged QT, 125, 516
  hypocalcemia and, 686–687
propranolol, 722
prostaglandin therapy, congenital heart disease, 364, 568
pseudogout, 596
Pseudomonas aeruginosa, 528
pulmonary edema, 359
pulmonary embolism, 216–217, 699–700
  risk factors, 699
  treatment, 700
  work-up, 700
pulmonary inhalation anthrax, 550–551
pulseless ventricular tachycardia (pVT), 624–626
pyelonephritis, 446–447
pyridoxine, INH overdose management, 585

radial head subluxation
  pediatric patient, 613–615
  reduction, 756
    techniques, 615
Ranson's criteria, 410
rash
  child, 314–319, 652, 657
  fever and, 189–193
    child, 314–319, 652, 657, 688–691
  measles, 690–691
  meningitis, 330
  Rocky Mountain spotted fever, 318
rectal pain, 232–235
rehydration therapy, *see* fluid therapy
renal colic, 368
renal injury, acute, 666
respiratory distress
  acute pulmonary edema, 359
  anaphylaxis, 219–220
  anthrax, 551
  child, 465–467
  chronic obstructive pulmonary disease, 418–422
  congenital heart disease, 363–364
  foreign body aspiration, 466–467
  penetrating chest trauma, 496
  see also shortness of breath
respiratory rate, pediatric patients, 726
resuscitation, newborn, 727
resuscitative endovascular balloon occlusion of the aorta
    (REBOA), pelvic fracture, 441
resuscitative hysterotomy (RH), 751–752
retinal artery occlusion, 119–120
retroperitoneal hematoma, 154

retropharyngeal abscess, 128–130

rewarming, following cold water immersion, 563

rhabdomyolysis, 665–666

ringing in the ears, 103–107

rivaroxaban, DVT management, 630

Rocky Mountain spotted fever, 316–318

salicylate overdose, 107

scapular manipulation, 755

seizure, 270–273, 370–375, 507–510, 517–522
    alcohol withdrawal and, 374–375, 427–428, 705
    eclampsia, 510
    febrile, 211–212
    INH toxicity, 585
    pediatric patient, 210–212
    status epilepticus, 374–375
    tenderness to palpation (TTP), 272–273
    tricyclic antidepressant toxicity, 521

Seldinger/guidewire technique, 743

sepsis
    congenital heart disease, 364
    disseminated intravascular coagulation and, 620
    elderly patient, decubitus ulcer, related, 620
    infant, 73, 730
    LVAD patients, 696
    post-transplant fever and, 527
    systemic inflammatory response syndrome and, 481–482

septic arthritis, 313

septic shock, 73, 482

shortness of breath, 182–188, 490–495, 630, 631
    chronic obstructive pulmonary disease, 418–422
        exacerbation, 421–422
    congestive heart failure, 359
    cough and, 547–551
        pulmonary inhalation anthrax, 550–551
    elderly patient, 355–359, 607–611
    HIV pneumonia, 389–390, 578–579
    infant, 360–364
    LVAD device failure, 610–611
    neck swelling and, 630, 631
    penetrating chest trauma, 496
    pericardial tamponade, 494
    superior vena cava syndrome, 633–634
    see also respiratory distress

shotgunning, 16–17

shoulder dislocation, 755

sickle cell disease
    acute chest syndrome, 324
    chest pain, 320–325
    child, 660–661
    reticulocyte index, 660

sick/not sick paradigm, 15

sigmoid volvulus, 605–606

slipped capital femoral epiphysis (SCFE), 133–134
    obesity and, 133

small bowel obstruction, 101–102, 203–204

snake bite, 113–116
    antivenom, 115
    crotalid venom, 115
    elapid venom, 115

social services notification
    child abuse, 459–460
    elder abuse, 591

sodium bicarbonate
    advanced cardiac life support, 725
    tricyclic antidepressant toxicity, 521

sodium nitroprusside, advanced cardiac life support, 724

sore throat
    fever and, 126–130
    retropharyngeal abscess, 128–130

spinal cord injury, 404–405

spinal epidural abscess, 83

splenic injury, blunt abdominal trauma and, 535–536

spontaneous bacterial peritonitis (SBP)
    symptoms, 546

spontaneous pneumothorax, 700
    work-up, 700

stab wound, penetrating chest trauma, 60–65, 278–282, 496–501

status asthmaticus, 186–187

status epilepticus, 374–375
    childhood seizure, 212

steroid therapy
    altitude sickness, 347
    chronic obstructive pulmonary disease, 422
    HIV pneumonia, 390
    meningitis, 330
    Pneumocystis pneumonia, 579
    spinal cord injury, contraindicated, 405

Stevens–Johnson syndrome, 191–193
    triggers, 192

Stimson maneuver, 755

strangulated hernia, 102

stroke
    acute cerebellar, 675–676
    carotid artery dissection and, 601
    middle cerebral artery, 433–434

subarachnoid hemorrhage, 230

subdural hematoma, 229–230

succinylcholine, Guillain–Barre syndrome and, 197

sulfonylurea-related hypoglycemia, 341–342

superior mesenteric artery embolism, 416

superior vena cava syndrome (SVCS), 633–634

supraventricular tachycardia (SVT), 395, 516

swelling, neck, 630, 631

syncope, 121–125

systemic inflammatory response syndrome (SIRS),
    pneumonia-related, 481–482

tachycardia, 718
  stable, 719
  supraventricular, 395
  unstable, 719
  ventricular, 515–516
tamponade
  balloon, 174
  cardiac, 60, 281–282, 335, 493
  pericardial, 494
temporomandibular joint dislocation, 756
tension pneumothorax, 64
  decompression, 64, 500
  see also thoracostomy
  penetrating chest trauma, 499–500
  symptoms, 64
testicular torsion, 138
  manual detorsion, 138, 750
therapeutic hypothermia, 626
thermal burn, 170
thiamine, alcohol withdrawal syndrome, 427
thoracostomy, 60
  needle, 64
    complications, 738–739
    equipment, 738
    indications, 738
    technique, 738
  penetrating chest trauma, 64, 496, 500
  tube, 714, 739–740
    complications, 740
    contraindications, 739
    equipment, 739
    indications, 739
    technique, 739–740
thoracotomy, 740–742
  complications, 742
  contraindications, 741
  equipment, 741
  indications, 740–741
  penetrating chest trauma, 280, 282
  technique, 741–742
throat swelling, 170, 218–220 *see also* sore throat
thrombotic thrombocytopenic purpura (TTP), 272–273,
    573
thyroid storm, 454
thyrotoxicosis, 453–454
tick-borne illness, 318
toothache, 274–277
  Ludwig's angina, 276–277
torsades de pointes, 125, 736
toxicity
  acetaminophen, 472

altered mental status and, 705
aspirin, 106–107
digoxin, 352–354
ethylene glycol, 686
INH, 585–586
pediatric patients, 728
toxin-associated abnormalities, 710
tricyclic antidepressant toxicity, 521
see also poisoning
toxidromes, 710, 712
  identification of, 712–713
tracheal deviation, tension pneumothorax, 64
transcutaneous pacing, 736–737
  bradycardia, 180
  complications, 736
  contraindications, 736
  equipment, 736
  indications, 736
  pacemaker malfunction, 641
  technique, 736
transfusion, *see* blood transfusion
transvenous pacing, bradycardia management, 718
trauma, 714–715
  abdominal, 529
    child, nonaccidental, 458–460
  central access, 714
  chest, penetrating, 60–65, 278–282, 496–501
  clinical controversies, 715
  facial, 161–165
  head, 229–230
  intubation, 714
  invasive monitoring, 715
  pediatric patients, 729
  pitfalls, 715
  transfusion, 714
  tube thoracostomy, 714
  see also fracture
traveler's diarrhea, 268–269, 572
tricyclic antidepressants, toxicity, 521
triptan medications, migraine treatment, 669–670
tube thoracostomy, *see* thoracostomy
tuberculosis, post-transplant patients, 528
tubo-ovarian abscess, 289
Turner's sign, 410

ultrasound (US)
  abdominal aortic aneurysm, 153
  congenital hypertrophic pyloric stenosis, 53
  focused assessment with sonography in trauma (FAST)
    examination, 280
  intussusception, 385
  pancreatitis, 410
unconsciousness
  opioid overdose, 264–265

syncope, 121–125
  see also mental status, altered
ureterovesicular junction, stones, 368
urinary tract infection (UTI), 249

vaginal bleeding, 236–240
variceal bleeding, liver cirrhosis and, 176
variceal upper GI bleed, 175–176
vasopressor therapy, spinal cord injury, 405
ventilatory support
  chronic obstructive pulmonary disease, 422
  congestive heart failure, 359
  myasthenia gravis, 681
  see also intubation
ventricular tachycardia, 515–516
  pulseless, 624–626
vertigo
  acute cerebellar stroke, 675–676
  HINTs testing, 675
Vibrio cholera, 269
visceral perforation, 142–144
visual impairment, 117–120
vomiting
  abdominal pain and, 45–49, 66–79, 98–102, 199–204,
    221–225, 406–411
    appendicitis, 224

cholecystitis, 65, 68
  small bowel obstruction, 101–102
altered mental status and, pediatric patient, 581–586
blood, 172, 176
child, 108–112, 319
infant, 50–53, 381–385
INH overdose, 585–586
iron overdose, 48
pancreatitis, 410–411
Rocky Mountain spotted fever, 318
small bowel obstruction, 203–204

weakness, 90–94, 155–160, 429–434, 677–681
  dizziness and, 194–198
  elderly patient, 587–591
  Guillain–Barre syndrome, 197–198
  infant, 70–74
    sepsis, 73
  myasthenia gravis, 680–681
  stroke, 433–434
weight gain
  with bruising and fatigue, 653–656
  Cushing syndrome, 655–656
Wernicke–Korsakoff syndrome, 705
Wernicke's encephalopathy, 428
Wolff–Parkinson–White syndrome, 516

For EU product safety concerns, contact us at Calle de José Abascal, 56–1°,
28003 Madrid, Spain or eugpsr@cambridge.org.

www.ingramcontent.com/pod-product-compliance
Ingram Content Group UK Ltd.
Pitfield, Milton Keynes, MK11 3LW, UK
UKHW052016290526
471652UK00013B/748